OXFORD MEDICAL PUBLICATIONS

Oxford Handbook of
Urology

Second edition

Oxford Handbook of
Urology

Second edition

John Reynard

Consultant Urological Surgeon
Department of Urology
Churchill Hospital
Oxford, UK

Simon Brewster

Consultant Urological Surgeon
Department of Urology
Churchill Hospital
Oxford, UK

Suzanne Biers

Specialist Registrar in Urology,
Wessex Deanery, UK

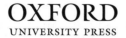

OXFORD
UNIVERSITY PRESS

OXFORD
UNIVERSITY PRESS

Great Clarendon Street, Oxford OX2 6DP

Oxford University Press is a department of the University of Oxford.
It furthers the University's objective of excellence in research, scholarship,
and education by publishing worldwide in

Oxford New York

Auckland Cape Town Dar es Salaam Hong Kong Karachi
Kuala Lumpur Madrid Melbourne Mexico City Nairobi
New Delhi Shanghai Taipei Toronto

With offices in

Argentina Austria Brazil Chile Czech Republic France Greece
Guatemala Hungary Italy Japan Poland Portugal Singapore
South Korea Switzerland Thailand Turkey Ukraine Vietnam

Oxford is a registered trade mark of Oxford University Press
in the UK and in certain other countries

Published in the United States
by Oxford University Press Inc., New York

© Oxford University Press, 2009

The moral rights of the authors have been asserted
Database right Oxford University Press (maker)

First edition published 2006
Second edition published 2009, reprinted 2010

British Library Cataloguing in Publication Data
Data available

Library of Congress Cataloging-in-Publication Data
Data available

Typeset by Cepha Imaging Private Ltd., Bangalore, India
Printed in China
on acid-free paper through
Asia Pacific Offset

ISBN 978–0–19–953494–4

10 9 8 7 6 5 4 3

Acknowledgements

The authors would like to thank Mr Padraig Malone, Dr Andrew Protheroe, Mr Marcus Drake and Mr Rowland Rees, who gave freely of their time and expertise.

Contents

Detailed contents

10 Upper tract obstruction, loin pain, hydronephrosis **457**

**11 Trauma to the urinary tract and other
urological emergencies** **473**

Abbreviations

5AR	5α–reductase
5ARI	5α-reductase inhibitor
AAA	abdominal aortic aneurysm
ACE	angiotensin converting enzyme
ACh	acetylcholine
ACTH	adrenocorticotrophic hormone
ADAM	androgen decline in the aging male
ADH	antidiuretic hormone
ADT	androgen deprivation therapy
ADPKD	autosomal dominant polycystic kidney disease
AFP	alpha fetoprotein
AI	androgen independent
AID	artificial insemination donor
AIDS	acquired immunodeficiency syndrome
AML	angiomyolipoma
ANP	atrial natriuretic peptide
APF	antiproliferative factor
ARC	AIDS-related complex
ARCD	acquired renal cystic disease
ARPKD	autosomal recessive polycystic kidney disease
ART	assisted reproductive techniques
AS	active surveillance
ASAP	atypical small acinar proliferation
ATN	acute tubular necrosis
ATP	adenosine triphosphate
AUA	American Urological Association
AUS	artificial urinary sphincter
BAUS	British Association of Urological Surgeons
BCG	bacillus Calmette–Guérin
BCR	bulbocavernosus reflex
bd	*bis die* (twice daily)
bFGF	basic fibroblastic growth factor
BMSFI	Brief Male Sexual Function Inventory
BNI	bladder neck incision
BOO	bladder outlet obstruction
BP	blood pressure

BPE	benign prostatic enlargement
BPH	benign prostatic hyperplasia
BPO	benign prostatic obstruction
BT	brachytherapy
BTX-A	botulinum toxin-A
BUO	bilateral ureteric obstruction
BXO	balanitis xerotica obliterans
CAH	congenital adrenal hyperplasia
CAPD	chronic ambulatory peritoneal dialysis
CIS	carcinoma *in situ*
CISC	clean intermittent self catheterization
CKD	chronic kidney disease
CNS	central nervous system
CPA	cyproterone acetate
CPB	chronic painful bladder (syndrome)
CPPS	chronic pelvic pain syndrome
CRF	chronic renal failure
CRP	C-reactive protein
CT	computed tomography
CTU	computed tomography urography
CVS	cardiovascular system
CXR	chest x-ray
DCN	dorsal clitoral nerve
DESD	detrusor-external sphincter dyssynergia
DH	detrusor hyperreflexia
DHT	dihyrotestosterone
DIC	disseminated intravascular coagulopathy
DM	diabetes mellitus
DMSA	dimercapto-succinic acid (renogram)
DMSO	dimethyl sulphoxide
DPN	dorsal penile nerve
DTPA	Diethylenetriamine penta-acetic acid
DRE	digital rectal examination
DSD	detrusor sphincter dyssynergia
DSD	disorder of sex development
DVT	deep vein thrombosis
EAU	European Association of Urology
EBRT	external beam radiotherapy
ECF	extracellular fluid
ECG	electrocardiogram

ED	erectile dysfunction
EDTA	ethylene diamine tetra-acetic acid
EGF	epidermal growth factor
EHL	electrohydraulic lithotripsy
EIA	enzyme immunoassay
ELISA	enzyme-linked immunosorbant assay
EMDA	electromotive drug administration
EMG	electromyography
EMU	early morning urine
EORTC	European Organization for Research and Treatment of Cancer
EPS	expressed prostatic secretions
ES	external sphincter
ESR	erythrocyte sedimentation rate
ESRF	end stage renal failure
ESWL	extracorporeal shock wave therapy
FBC	full blood count
FNA	fine needle aspiration
FSH	follicle stimulating hormone
FVC	frequency volume chart
GA	general anaesthetic
GABA	γ-aminobutyric acid
GAG	glycosaminoglycan
GCT	germ cell tumour
GFR	glomerular filtration rate
GI	gastrointestinal
GIFT	gamete intrafallopian transfer
GnRH	gonadotrophin-releasing hormone
GU	gonococcal urethritis (or genitourinary)
HCG	human chorionic gonadotrophin
HIFU	high-intensity focused ultrasound
HIF	hypoxia-inducible factor
HIV	human immunodeficiency virus
HLA	human leucocyte antigen
HPCR	high pressure chronic retention
HPF	high-powered field
HoLAP	holmium laser ablation of the prostate
HoLEP	holmium laser enucleation of the prostate
HPV	human papilloma virus
HR	hormone refractory

HRO	high reliability organization
HRP	horseradish peroxidase
IC	interstitial cystitis
ISC	intermittent catheterization
ICF	intracellular fluid
ICS	International Continence Society
ICSI	intracytoplasmic sperm injection
ICU	intensive care unit
IDC	in-dwelling catheter
IDO	idiopathic detrusor overactivity
IE	inhibited ejaculation
IELT	intravaginal ejaculatory latency time
IGCN	intratubular germ cell neoplasia
IGF	insulin-like glomerular filtration
IIEF	International Index of Erectile Function
ILP	interstitial laser prostatectomy
IPC	intermittent pneumatic calf compression
IPSS	International Prostate Symptom Score
ISC	intermittent self-catheterization
ISD	intrinsic sphincter deficiency
ISF	interstitial fluid
IUI	intra-uterine insemination
IV	intravenous
IVC	inferior vena cava
IVF	*in vitro* fertilization
IVU	intravenous urography
JGA	juxtaglomerular apparatus
K^+	potassium
KGF	keratinocyte growth factor
KTP	potassium titanyl phosphate (laser)
KUB	Kidneys, ureter and bladder (X-ray)
LA	local anaesthetic
LDH	lactate dehydrogenase
LFT	liver function test
LH	luteinizing hormone
LHRH	luteinizing hormone-releasing hormone
LOH	late-onset hypogonadism
LRP	laparoscopic radical prostatectomy
LSD	lysergic acid diethylamide
LUTS	lower urinary tract symptoms

MAB	maximal androgen blockade
MAG3	mercaptoacetyl-triglycyl (renogram)
MAR	mixed antiglobulin reaction (test)
MCDK	multicystic dysplastic kidney
MCUG	micturating cystourethrography
MDCTU	multidetector CT urography
MDP	methylene diphosphonate
MDRD	modification of diet in renal disease
MESA	microsurgical epididymal sperm aspiration
MIS	Müllerian inhibiting substance
MMC	mitomycin C
MNE	monosymptomatic nocturnal enuresis
MPOA	medial pre-optic area
MPR	multiplanar reformatting
MRC	Medical Research Council
MRI	magnetic resonance imaging
MRSA	meticillin-resistant staphylococcus aureus
MRU	magnetic resonance urography
MS	multiple sclerosis
MSA	multisystem atrophy
MSK	medullary sponge kidney
MSU	mid-stream urine
MTOP	Medical Therapy of Prostatic Symptoms
MUCP	maximal urethral closure pressure
MUI	mixed urinary incontinence
NA	noradrenaline
NAAT	nucleic acid amplification test
NaCl	sodium chloride
NGU	non-gonococcal urethritis
NICE	National Institute for Clinical Excellence
NO	nitric oxide
NP	nocturnal polyuria
NSAIDs	non-steroidal anti-inflammatory drugs
NSGCT	non-seminomatous germ cell tumours
NSU	non-specific urethritis
od	*omni die* (once daily)
OAB	overactive bladder
OAT	oligoasthenoteratospermia
OP	open prostatectomy
OSA	obstructive sleep apnoea

P_aCO_2	partial pressure of carbon dioxide (in arterial blood)
P_aO_2	partial pressure of oxygen (in arterial blood)
PAG	peri-aqueductal gray matter
PBS/IC	painful bladder syndrome/interstitial cystitis
PC	prostate cancer
PCNL	percutaneous nephrolithotomy
PD	Parkinson's disease
PDE5	phosphodiesterase type-5
PDGF	platelet-derived growth factor
PE	pulmonary embolism
PESA	percutaneous epididymal sperm aspiration
PFE	pelvic floor exercises
PFS	pressure flow studies
PGE1	prostaglandin E1
PIN	prostatic intraepithelial neoplasia
PLAP	placental alkaline phosphatase
PLESS	Proscar Long-term Efficacy Safety Study
PMC	pontine micturition center
PNE	peripheral nerve evaluation
POP	pelvic organ prolapse
PPV	patent processus vaginalis
PR	per rectum
PREDICT	Prospective European Doxazosin and Combination Therapy
PSA	prostate specific antigen
PTH	parathyroid hormone levels
PTTI	parenchymal transit time index
PTNS	posterior tibial nerve stimulation
PUJ	pelviureteric junction
PUJO	pelviureteric junction obstruction
PUV	posterior urethral valves
PVN	paraventricular nucleus
PVP	photoselective vaporization of the prostate
PVR	post-void residual
PZ	peripheral zone
qds	*quarter die sumendus* (to be taken 4 times per day)
Qmax	maximal flow rate
QoL	quality of life
RBC	red blood count
RBF	Renal blood flow
RCC	renal cell carcinoma

RCT	randomized control trial
RP	radical prostatectomy
RPF	renal plasma flow
RPF	retroperitoneal fibrosis
RPLND	retroperitoneal lymph node dissection
RT	radiotherapy
RTA	renal tubular acidosis
RTK	receptor tyrosine kinase
SARS	sacral anterior root stimulator
SBP	systolic blood pressure
SC	subcutaneous
SCC	squamous cell carcinoma
SCI	spinal cord injury
SHBG	sex hormone binding globulin
SHIM	Sexual Health Inventory for Men
SHO	senior house officer
SIRS	systemic inflammatory response syndrome
SNM	sacral nerve modulation
SNS	sacral nerve stimulation
SOP	standard operating procedures (SOP)
SPC	suprapubic catheter
SPR	specialist registrar
SR	testis-determining gene
SSRI	serotonin re-uptake inhibitor
STI	sexually transmitted infection
SUI	stress urinary incontinence
TB	tuberculosis
TBW	total body water
TC	testicular cancer
TCC	transitional cell carcinoma
tds	*ter die sumendus* (to be taken 3 times per day)
TEDs	thrombo-embolic deterent stockings
TENS	transcutaneous electrical nerve stimulation
TESA	testicular exploration and sperm aspiration
TESE	testicular exploration and sperm extraction
TET	tubal embryo transfer
TGF	transforming growth factor
TIN	testicular intratubular neoplasia (synonymous with IGCN)
TNF	tumour necrosis factor
TNM	tumour, node, metastasis

TOT	transobturator tape
TRUS	trans-rectal ultrasonography
TSC	tuberous sclerosis complex
TULIP	transuretheral ultrasound-guided laser-induced prostatectomy
TUMT	transurethal microwave thermotherapy
TUNA	transurethal radiofrequency needle ablation
TUU	transureteroureterostomy
TURBT	transurethral resection of bladder tumour
TURP	transurethral resection of prostate
TUVP	transurethral electrovaporization of the prostate
TVT	tension-free transvaginal tape
TVTO	Tension-free vaginal tape obturator route
TWOC	trial without catheter
TZ	transition zone
UDT	undescended testis
U&E	urea and electrolytes
UI	urinary incontinence
UPJO	ureteropelvic junction obstruction
US	ultrasound
USS	ultrasound scan
UTI	urinary tract infection
UUI	urge urinary incontinence
UUO	unilateral ureteric obstruction
VCUG	voiding cystourethrography
VEGF	vascular endothelial growth factor
VHL	Von Hippel-Lindau
VLAP	visual laser ablation of the prostate
VTE	venous thromboembolism
VUJ	vesicoureteric junction
VUJO	vesicoureteric junction obstruction
VUR	vesicoureteric reflux
VVF	vesicovaginal fistula
WBC	white blood cell
WW	watchful waiting
YAG	yytrium-aluminium-garnet (laser)
ZIFT	zygote intrafallopian transfer

General principles of management of patients

Communication skills

Communication is the imparting of knowledge and understanding. Good communication is crucial for the surgeon in his or her daily interaction with patients. The nature of any interaction between surgeon and patient will depend very much on the context of the 'interview', whether you know the patient already, and on the quantity and type of information that needs to be imparted. As a general rule the basis of good communication requires the following:

- **Introduction**

Give your name, explain who you are, greet the patient/relative appropriately (e.g. handshake), check you are talking to the correct person.

- **Establish the purpose of the interview**

Explain the purpose of the interview from the patient's perspective and yours, and the desired outcome of the interview.

- **Establish the patient's baseline knowledge and understanding**

Use open questions, let the patient talk and confirm what they know.

- **Listen actively**

Make it clear to the patient that they have your undivided attention—that you are focusing on them. This involves appropriate body language (keep eye contact—don't look out of the window!).

- **Pick up on and respond to cues**

The patient/relative may offer verbal or non-verbal indications about their thoughts or feelings.

- **Elicit the patient's main concern(s)**

What you think should be the patient's main concerns may not be. Try to find out exactly what the patient is worried about.

- **Chunks and checks**

Give information in small quantities and check that this has been understood. A good way of doing this is to ask the patient to explain what they think you have said.

- **Show empathy**

Let the patient know you understand their feelings.

- **Be non-judgemental**

Don't express your personal views or beliefs.

- **Alternate control of the interview between the patient and yourself**

Allow the patient to take the lead where appropriate.

- **Signpost changes in direction**

State clearly when you move onto a new subject.

- **Avoid the use of jargon**

Use language the patient will understand, rather than medical terminology.

- **Body language**

Use body language that shows the patient that you are interested in their problem and that you understand what they are going through. Respect cultural differences; in some cultures eye contact is regarded as a sign of aggression.

- **Summarize and indicate the next steps**

Summarize what you understand to be the patient's problem, and what the next steps are going to be.

Documentation and note keeping

Royal College of Surgeons' guidelines state that each clinical history sheet should include the patient's name, date of birth, and record number. Each entry should be timed, dated, and signed, and your name and position (e.g. SHO for 'senior house officer' or SPR for 'specialist registrar') should be clearly written in capital letters below each entry. You should also document which other medical staff were present with you on ward rounds or when seeing a patient (e.g. 'ward round—SPR (Mr X)/SHO/HO').

Contemporaneous note keeping is an important part of good clinical practice. Medical notes document the patient's problems, the investigations they have undergone, the diagnosis, and the treatment and its outcome. The notes also provide a channel of communication between doctors and nurses on the ward, and between different medical teams. In order for this communication to be effective and safe, medical notes must be clearly written. They will also be scrutinized in cases of complaint and litigation. Failure to keep accurate, meaningful notes, which are timed, dated, and signed, with your name written in capital letters below, exposes you to the potential for criticism in such cases. The standard of note keeping is seen as an indirect measure of the standard of care you have given your patients. Sloppy notes can be construed as evidence of sloppy care, quite apart from the fact that such notes do not allow you to provide evidence of your actions! Unfortunately, the defence of not having sufficient time to write the notes is not an adequate one, and the courts will regard absence of documentation of your actions as indicating that you did not do what you said you did.

Do not write anything that might later be construed as a personal comment about a patient or colleague (e.g. do not comment on an individual's character or manner). Do not make jokes in the patient's notes. Such comments are unlikely to be helpful and may cause you embarrassment in the future when you are asked to interpret them.

Try to make the notes relevant to the situation. So, for example, in a patient with suspected bleeding, a record of blood pressure and pulse rate is important, but a record of a detailed neurological history and examination is less relevant (unless, for example, a neurological basis for the patient's problem is suspected).

The results of investigations should be clearly documented in the notes, preferably in red ink, with a note of the time and date when the investigation was performed.

Avoid the use of abbreviations. In particular, always write LEFT or RIGHT, in capital letters, rather than Lt/Rt or L/R. A handwritten L can sometimes be mistaken for an R and vice versa.

Operation notes

We include the following information on operation notes:
- Patient name, number, and date of birth
- Date of operation
- Surgeon, assistants
- Patient position (e.g. supine, prone, lithotomy, Lloyd–Davies)
- Type of deep vein thrombosis (DVT) prophylaxis (AK–TEDS, Flowtrons, heparin, etc.)
- Type, time of administration, and doses of antibiotic prophylaxis
- Presence of image intensifier, if appropriate
- Type and size of endoscopes used
- Your signature and your name in capitals
- Post-operative instructions and follow-up, if appropriate.

If a consultant is supervising you, but is not scrubbed, you must clearly state that the 'consultant (named) was in attendance'.

Patient safety in surgical practice

The aviation, nuclear, and petrochemical industries are termed 'high reliability organizations' (HROs) because they have adopted a variety of core safety principles that have enabled them to achieve safety success, despite 'operating' in high-risk environments. Surgeons can learn much from HROs and can adopt some of these safety principles in surgical practice, in order to improve safety in the non-technical aspects of care.

Foremost amongst the safety principles of HROs are:

- **Team working**
- **Use of standard operating procedures (SOPs):** day-to-day tasks are carried out according to a set of rules and in a way that is standardized across the organization
- **Cross-checking:** members of the team check that a procedure, drug, or action has been done or administered by 'verbalizing' that action to another team member. This is most familiar when aircraft cabin crew are asked by the pilot to check that the doors of the plane are locked shut ('doors to cross-check') and crew members cross to the opposite door to confirm this has been done. In surgical practice an example of cross-checking could be 'antibiotic given?', confirmed by a specific reply such as '240mg IV gentamicin given'
- **Regular audit and feedback of audit data:** performance data (both good and bad) is collected regularly and *crucially* team members are notified (e.g. in audit meetings) of where they are performing well or badly
- **Establishment of variable hierarchies:** development of a working environment where junior staff are encouraged to 'speak up' if they believe an error is about to occur, without fear of criticism
- **Cyclical training:** frequent and regular training sessions to reinforce safe practice methods.

Chapter 2

Significance and preliminary investigation of urological symptoms and signs

Haematuria I: definition and types

Definition The presence of blood in the urine.

'Macroscopic' (gross) haematuria: the patient has seen blood.

Microscopic or dipstick haematuria: blood identified by urine microscopy or by dipstick testing, either in association with other urological symptoms ('symptomatic microscopic haematuria') or during a routine medical examination (e.g. for insurance purposes; 'asymptomatic microscopic haematuria').

Microscopic haematuria has been variably defined as 3 or more, 5 or more, or 10 or more red blood cells (RBCs) per high-power field.

Urine dipsticks test for haem (i.e. they test for the presence of haemoglobin and myoglobin in urine). Haem catalyses the oxidation of orthotolidine by an organic peroxidase, producing a blue coloured compound. Dipsticks are capable of detecting the presence of haemoglobin from 1 or 2 RBCs.

False +ve urine dipstick: occurs in the presence of myoglobinuria, bacterial peroxidases, povidone, hypochlorite.

False −ve urine dipstick (rare): occurs in the presence of reducing agents (e.g. ascorbic acid —prevents the oxidation of orthotolidine).

Is microscopic or dipstick haematuria abnormal?

A few RBCs can be found in the urine of normal people. The upper limit of normal for RBC excretion is 1 million per 24 h (as seen in healthy medical students). In healthy male soldiers undergoing yearly urine examination over a 12-year period, 40% had microscopic haematuria on at least 1 occasion, and 15% on 2 or more occasions. Transient microscopic haematuria may occur following rigorous exercise, sexual intercourse, or from menstrual contamination.

The fact that the presence of RBCs in the urine is normal explains why a substantial proportion of 'patients' with microscopic and dipstick haematuria, and even macroscopic haematuria will have normal haematuria investigations (i.e. no abnormality is found). No abnormality is found in approximately 50% of subjects with macroscopic haematuria and 70% (or even more) with microscopic haematuria, despite full conventional urological investigation (urine cytology, cystoscopy, renal ultrasonography, and IVU).[1]

1 Khadra MH (2000) A prospective analysis of 1930 patients with hematuria to evaluate current diagnostic practice. *J Urol* **163**:524–7.

Haematuria II: causes and investigation

Urological and other causes of haematuria

Microscopic or dipstick haematuria is common (20% of men >60 years old). Bear in mind that most (70%—and some studies say almost 90%[1,2]) patients with dipstick or microscopic haematuria have no urological pathology. Conversely, a significant proportion of patients with microscopic haematuria have glomerular disease (upwards of 40% or so), despite having normal blood pressure, a normal serum creatinine, and in the absence of proteinuria[3,4] (although it is fair to say that most do not develop progressive renal disease, and those that do usually develop proteinuria and hypertension as 'warning' signs). The management algorithm for patients with negative urological haematuria investigations is shown on p. 14.

- **Cancer:** bladder [transitional cell carcinoma (TCC), squamous cell carcinoma (SCC)], kidney (adenocarcinoma), renal pelvis, and ureter (TCC), prostate
- **Stones:** kidney, ureteric, bladder
- **Infection:** bacterial, mycobacterial (tuberculosis, TB), parasitic (schistosomiasis), infective urethritis
- **Inflammation:** cyclophosphamide cystitis, interstitial cystitis
- **Trauma:** kidney, bladder, urethra (e.g. traumatic catheterization), pelvic fracture causing urethral rupture
- **Renal cystic disease** (e.g. medullary sponge kidney)
- **Other urological causes:** benign prostatic hyperplasia (BPH, the large, vascular prostate), loin pain haematuria syndrome, vascular malformations
- **Nephrological causes of haematuria:** tend to occur in children or young adults and include, commonly, IgA nephropathy, post-infectious glomerulonephritis; less commonly, membrano-proliferative glomerulonephritis, Henoch–Schönlein purpura, vasculitis, Alport's syndrome, thin basement membrane disease, Fabry's disease, etc.
- **Other 'medical' causes of haematuria:** include coagulation disorders—congenital (e.g. haemophilia), anticoagulation therapy (e.g. warfarin), sickle cell trait or disease, renal papillary necrosis, vascular disease (e.g. emboli to the kidney cause infarction and haematuria)
- **Nephrological causes:** more likely in the following situations—children and young adults; proteinuria; red blood cell casts.

What percentage of patients with haematuria have urological cancers?

Microscopic: about 5–10%.
Macroscopic: about 20–25%.[5]

Urological investigation of haematuria

Conventional urological investigation involves urine culture (where, on the basis of associated 'cystitis' symptoms, urinary infection is suspected), urine cytology, cystoscopy, renal ultrasonography, and intravenous urography (IVU).

Diagnostic cystoscopy

Nowadays this is carried out using a flexible, fibre optic cystoscope, unless radiological investigation demonstrates a bladder cancer, in which case one may forego the flexible cystoscopy, and proceed immediately to rigid cystoscopy and biopsy under anaesthetic (transurethral resection of bladder tumour—TURBT).

1   Edwards TJ, Dickinson AJ, Natale S et al. (2006) A prospective analysis of the diagnostic yield resulting from the attendance of 4020 patients at a protocol-driven haematuria clinic. *BJU Int* **97**:301–5.

2   Sultana SR, Goodman CM, Byrne DJ, Baxby K. (1996) Microscopic haematuria: urological investigation using a standard protocol. *Br J Urol* **78**:691–8.

3   Topham PS, Harper SJ, Furness PN et al. (1994) Glomerular disease as a cause of isolated microscopic haematuria. *Q J Med* **87**:329–35.

4   Tomson C, Porter T. (2002) Asymptomatic microscopic or dipstick haematuria on adults: which investigations for which patients? A review of the evidence. *Br J Urol* **90**:185–98.

5   Khadra MH, Pickard RS, Charlton M et al. (2000). A prospective analysis of 1930 patients with hematuria to evaluate current diagnostic practice. *J Urol* **163**:524–7.

What is the role of multidetector CT urography (MDCTU) in the investigation of haematuria?

This is a rapid acquisition CT done following intravenous contrast administration with high spatial resolution. Overlapping thin sections can be 'reconstructed' into images in multiple planes (multiplanar reformatting—MPR) so lesions can be imaged in multiple planes. Has the advantage of a single investigation which potentially could obviate the need for the traditional '4-test' approach to haematuria (IVU, renal ultrasound, flexible cystoscopy, urine cytology), although at the cost of a higher radiation dose (a 7-film IVU = 5–10 mSV, 3 phase MDCTU 20–25 mSV).

There is evidence suggesting that MDCTU has reasonable sensitivity and high specificity for diagnosing bladder tumours[1] (in patients with macroscopic haematuria 93% sensitivity, 99% specificity) and that it has equivalent diagnostic accuracy to retrograde uretero-pyelography (the retrograde administration of contrast via a catheter inserted in the lower ureter, to outline the ureter and renal collecting system).[2] Overall, for patients with haematuria and no prior history of urological malignancy, for the detection of all urological tumours, it has approximately 65% sensitivity and 98% specificity[3]—so it only rarely calls a lesion a tumour when, in fact, the lesion is benign, but it still fails to diagnose a significant proportion of urinary neoplasms (sensitivity for upper tract neoplasms 80%, for bladder tumours 60%).

The role of MDCTU (described by some as the 'ultimate' imaging modality) in the investigation of haematuria remains controversial. MDCTU in all patients with haematuria (microscopic, macroscopic), when most will have no identifiable cause for the haematuria, has a cost (high radiation dose, financial). A targeted approach, aimed at those with risk factors for urothelial malignancy (age >40 years, macroscopic as opposed to microscopic haematuria, smoking history, occupational exposure to benzenes and aromatic amines) might be a better use of this resource, rather than using MDCTU as the first imaging test for both high and low risk patients. Thus, the 'best' imaging probably depends on the context of the patient.

1 Turney BW, Willatt JM, Nixon D, et al. (2006) Computed tomography urography for diagnosing bladder cancer. *BJU Int* **98**:345–8.

2 Cowan NC, Turney BW, Taylor NJ, et al. (2007) Multidetector computed tomography urography for diagnosing upper urinary tract urothelial tumours. *BJU Int 2007*; **99**: 1363-70.

3 Sudakoff GS, Dunn DP, Guralnick ML, et al. (2008). Multidetector computed tomography urography as the primary imaging modality for detecting urinary tract neoplasms in patients with asymptomatic hematuria. *J Urol* **179**:862–7.

Should cystoscopy be performed in patients with asymptomatic microscopic haematuria?

The American Urological Association's (AUA's) *Best Practice Policy on Asymptomatic Microscopic Hematuria*[1] recommends cystoscopy in all high-risk patients (high risk for development of TCC) with microscopic haematuria (see risk factors below).[1] In asymptomatic, low-risk patients <40 it states that 'it may be appropriate to defer cystoscopy', but if this is done, urine should be sent for cytology. However, the AUA also states that 'the decision as to when to proceed with cystoscopy in low-risk patients with persistent microscopic haematuria must be made on an individual basis after a careful discussion between the patient and physician'. It is our policy to inform such patients that the likelihood of finding a bladder cancer is low, but nevertheless we recommend flexible cystoscopy. The patient then makes a decision as to whether or not to proceed with cystoscopy based on their interpretation of 'low risk'.

If no cause for haematuria is found (microscopic or macroscopic) is further investigation necessary?

Some say yes, quoting studies that show serious disease can be identified in a small number of patients where, in addition, retrograde ureterography, endoscopic examination of the ureters and renal pelvis (ureteroscopy), contrast CT, and renal angiography were done. Others say no, citing the absence of development of overt urological cancer during 2–4-year follow-up in patients originally presenting with microscopic or macroscopic haematuria (although without further investigations).[2]

When urine cytology, cystoscopy, renal US, and IVU are all normal, we perform CT scanning of the kidneys and ureters, and retrograde ureterography in:
● Patients at high risk for TCC[3]
● Where microscopic or dipstick haematuria persists at 3 months
● Where macroscopic haematuria persists.

1   Grossfeld GD (2001) Evaluation of asymptomatic microscopic hematuria in adults: the American Urological Association Best Practise Policy-Part II: patient evaluation, cytology, voided markers, imaging, cystoscopy, nephrology evaluation and follow-up. *Urology* **57**:604–10.

2   Khadra MH (2000) A prospective analysis of 1930 patients with hematuria to evaluate current diagnostic practice. *J Urol* **163**:524–7.

3   Risk factors for development of transitional cell cancer of the urothelium (bladder, kidneys, renal pelvis, ureters): +ve smoking history, occupational exposure to chemicals or dyes (benzenes or aromatic amines), analgesic abuse (phenacetin), history of pelvic irradiation, previous cyclophosphamide treatment.

Management algorithm for patients with negative urological haematuria investigations[1]

eGFR forms the foundation for decision making in those patients who have haematuria (macroscopic or dipstick/microscopic) and negative urological investigations. The aim is to identify significant renal disease (CKD—chronic kidney disease), the progression of which might be slowed by careful blood pressure control and other specific treatment.

- Macroscopic haematuria and negative urological investigations or eGFR <60 mL/min/1.73m² —refer to nephrologist
- Dipstick/microscopic haematuria
  - eGFR <60 mL/min/1.73 m² —refer to nephrologist
  - eGFR >60 mL/min/1.73 m²
- Proteinuria
  - Protein:creatinine >45 mg/mmol—refer to nephrologist
  - Protein:creatinine <45 mg/mmol
  - No proteinuria—treat as CKD stage 1 and 2 (treat hypertension, modify cardiovascular risk factors, annual eGFR, and urine analysis for protein).

CKD (Chronic Kidney Disease) classification

1 eGFR >90 mL/min/1.73 m²
2 eGFR 60–89 mL/min/1.73 m²
3 eGFR 30–59 mL/min/1.73 m²
4 eGFR 15–29 mL/min/1.73 m²
5 eGFR <15 mL/min/1.73 m²

1 Joint Specialty Committee on Renal Medicine of the Royal College of Physicians of London and the Renal Association and the Royal College of General Practitioners. *Chronic Kidney Disease in Adults: UK Guidelines for Identification, management and referral.* London: Royal College of Physicians, 2006.

Haemospermia

Definition The presence of blood in the semen.
Usually intermittent, benign, self-limiting, and no cause identified.

Causes

Age <40 years: usually inflammatory (e.g. prostatitis, epididymo-orchitis, urethritis, urethral warts) or idiopathic (though to an extent this reflects the limited investigation that is usually carried out in this age group). Rarely testicular tumour; perineal or testicular trauma.

Age >40 years: as for men aged <40—prostate cancer; bladder cancer; BPH; dilated veins in the prostatic urethra; prostatic or seminal vesicle calculi; hypertension; carcinoma of the seminal vesicles.

Rare causes at any age: bleeding diathesis; utricular cysts; Müllerian cysts; TB; schistosomiasis; amyloid of prostate or seminal vesicles; post-injection of haemorrhoids.

Examination

Examine the testes, epididymis, prostate, and seminal vesicles. Measure blood pressure.

Investigation

Send urine for culture. If the haemospermia resolves, an argument can be made for doing nothing else. If it recurs or persists, arrange a trans-rectal ultrasound (TRUS), flexible cystoscopy, and renal ultrasound. If haematuria co-exists, investigate this as described above.

Treatment

This is directed at the underlying abnormality, if found.

Further reading

Ganabathi K, Chadwick D, Feneley RCL, Gingell JC (1992) Haemospermia. *Br J Urol* **69**:225–30.
Jones DJ (1991) Haemospermia: a prospective study. *Br J Urol* **67**:88–90.

Lower urinary tract symptoms (LUTS)

A plethora of terms have been coined to describe the symptom complex traditionally associated with prostatic obstruction due to BPH. The 'classic' prostatic symptoms of hesitancy, poor flow, frequency, urgency, nocturia, and terminal dribbling have, in the past, been termed 'prostatism' or simply 'BPH symptoms'. One sometimes hears these symptoms being described as due to 'BPO' (benign prostatic obstruction) or benign prostatic enlargement ('BPE'; benign prostatic enlargement) or, more recently, 'LUTS/BPH'. However, these 'classic' symptoms of prostatic disease bear little relationship to prostate size, urinary flow rate, residual urine volume or, indeed, urodynamic evidence of bladder outlet obstruction.[1,2] Furthermore, age-matched men and women have similar 'prostate' symptom scores,[3,4] but women obviously have no prostate. We therefore no longer use the expression prostatism to describe the symptom complex of hesitancy, poor flow, etc. Instead, we call such symptoms 'lower urinary tract symptoms' (LUTS), which is purely a descriptive term avoiding any implication about the possible underlying cause of these symptoms.[5]

The new terminology of 'LUTS' is useful because it reminds the urologist to consider possible alternative causes of symptoms, which may have absolutely nothing to do with prostatic obstruction, and it reminds us to avoid operating on an organ, such as the prostate, when the cause of the symptoms may lie elsewhere.

Baseline symptoms can be 'measured' using a symptom index. The most widely used is the International Prostate Symptom Score (IPSS), a modified version of the AUA Symptom Index[6] (Fig. 2.1).

1 Ganabathi K, Chadwick D, Feneley RCL, Gingell JC (1992) Haemospermia. *Br J Urol* **69**:225–30.

2 Jones DJ (1991) Haemospermia: a prospective study. *Br J Urol* **67**:88–90.

3 Reynard JM, Yang Q, Donovan JL, *et al.* (1998) The ICS-'BPH' study: uroflowmetry, lower urinary tract symptoms and bladder outlet obstruction. *Br J Urol* **82**:619–23.

4 Lepor H, Machi G (1993) Comparison of AUA symptom index in unselected males and females between fifty-five and seventy-nine years of age. *Urology* **42**:36–41.

5 Abrams P (1994) New words for old—lower urinary tracy symptoms for 'prostatism'. *Br Med J* **308**:929–30.

6 Barry MJ, Fowler FJ Jr, O'Leary MP, *et al.* (1992) The American Urological Association symptom index for benign prostatic hyperplasia. *J Urol* **148**:1549–57.

	Not at all	Less than 1 time in 5	Less than half the time	About half the time	More than half the time	Almost always	Score
Incomplete emptying. Over the last month, how often have you had a sensation of not emptying your bladder completely after you finish urinating?	0	1	2	3	4	5	
Frequency. Over the last month, how often have you had to urinate again less than 2 hours after you finished urinating?	0	1	2	3	4	5	
Intermittency. Over the past month, how often have you found you stopped and started again several times when you urinated?	0	1	2	3	4	5	
Urgency. Over the past month, how often have you found it difficult to postpone urination?	0	1	2	3	4	5	
Weak stream. Over the past month, how often have you had a weak urinary stream?	0	1	2	3	4	5	
Straining. Over the past month, how often have you had to push or strain to begin urination?	0	1	2	3	4	5	
Nocturia. Over the past month, how many times did you most typically get up to urinate from the time you went to bed at night until the time you got up in the morning?	0	1	2	3	4	5	
Total IPSS score							

Quality of life due to symptoms	Delighted	Pleased	Mostly satisfied	Mixed— about equally satisfied and dissatisfied	Mostly dissatisfied	Unhappy	Terrible
If you were to spend the rest of your life with your urinary condition just the way it is now, how would you feel about that?	0	1	2	3	4	5	6

Fig. 2.1 The International Prostate Symptom Score (IPSS). (Adapted with permission. Copyright Elsevier 1992).[6]

Other causes of LUTS

In broad terms, LUTS can be due to pathology in the prostate, the bladder, the urethra, other pelvic organs (uterus, rectum), or due to neurological disease affecting the nerves that innervate the bladder. These pathologies can include benign enlargement of the prostate causing bladder outflow obstruction [('BPE' causing bladder outlet obstruction ('BOO')), and infective, inflammatory, and neoplastic conditions of the bladder, prostate, or urethra. While LUTS are, in general, relatively non-specific for particular pathologies, the *context* in which they occur (i.e. associated symptoms) can indicate their cause. For example:

- LUTS in association with macroscopic haematuria, or with dipstick or microscopic haematuria suggests a possibility of bladder cancer. This is more likely if urinary frequency, urgency, and 'bladder' pain (suprapubic pain) are prominent. Carcinoma *in situ* of the bladder—a non-invasive, but potentially very aggressive form of bladder cancer, which very often progresses to muscle invasive or metastatic cancer—classically presents in this way

- Recent onset of bedwetting in an elderly man is often due to high-pressure chronic retention. Visual inspection of the abdomen may show marked distension due to a grossly enlarged bladder. The diagnosis of chronic retention is confirmed by palpating the enlarged, tense bladder, which is dull to percussion, and by drainage of a large volume (often well in excess of 2L) following catheterization

- Rarely, LUTS can be due to neurological disease causing spinal cord or cauda equina compression, or to pelvic or sacral tumours. Associated symptoms include back pain, sciatica, ejaculatory disturbances, and sensory disturbances in the legs, feet, and perineum. In these rare cases, loss of pericoccygeal or perineal sensation (sacral nerve roots 2–4) indicates an interruption to the sensory innervation of the bladder and a magnetic resonance imaging (MRI) scan will confirm the clinical suspicion that there is a neurological problem.

Nocturia and nocturnal polyuria

- Nocturia ≥2 is common and bothersome (sleep disturbance)
- Prevalence of nocturia ≥2:[1,2] men—40% aged 60–70 years, 55% aged >70 years; women—10% aged 20–40 years, 50% aged >80 years
- Nocturia ≥2 is associated with a 2-fold increased risk of falls and injury in the ambulant elderly
- Men who void more than twice at night have a 2-fold increased risk of death (possibly due to the associations of nocturia with endocrine and cardiovascular disease).[3]

The diagnostic approach to the patient with nocturia

Nocturia can be due to urological disease, but more often than not is non-urological in origin. Therefore 'approach the lower urinary tract last' (Neil Resnick, Professor of Gerontology, Pittsburgh[4]).

Causes of nocturia

- **Urological:** benign prostatic obstruction, overactive bladder, incomplete bladder emptying
- **Non-urological:** renal failure, idiopathic nocturnal polyuria, diabetes mellitus, central diabetes insipidus, nephrogenic diabetes insipidus, primary polydipsia, hypercalcaemia, drugs, autonomic failure, obstructive sleep apnoea.

Assessment of the nocturic patient

Ask the patient to complete a frequency volume chart (FVC)—a voiding diary that records time and volume of each void over a 24-h period for 7 days. This establishes:

- If the patient is polyuric or non-polyuric?
- If polyuric, is the polyuria present throughout 24 h or is it confined to night-time (nocturnal polyuria)?

Polyuria is defined empirically as >3 L of urine output per 24 h [Standardization Committee of the International Continence Society (ICS) 2002].

Nocturnal polyuria is empirically defined as the production of more than one-third of 24-h urine output between midnight and 8 a.m. (It is a normal physiological mechanism to reduce urine output at night. Urine output between midnight and 8 a.m.—one-third of the 24-h clock—should certainly be no more than one-third of 24-h total urine output and, in most people, will be considerably less than one-third.)

Polyuria (urine output of >3L per 24h) is due either to a solute diuresis or a water diuresis. Measure urine osmolality: <250 mOsm/kg = water diuresis, >300 mOsm/kg = solute diuresis. Excess levels of various solutes in the urine, such as glucose in the poorly controlled diabetic, lead to a solute diuresis. A water diuresis occurs in patients with primary polydipsia (an appropriate physiological response to high water intake) and diabetes insipidus [antidiuretic hormone (ADH) deficiency or resistance]. Patients on lithium have renal resistance to ADH (nephrogenic DI).

Further reading

Guite HF *et al.* (1988) Hypothesis: posture is one of the determinants of the circadian rhythm of urine flow and electrolyte excretion in elderly female patients. *Age Ageing* **17**:241–48.

Matthiesen TB, Rittig S, Norgaard JP, Pedersen EB, Djurhuus JC (1996) Nocturnal polyuria and natriuresis in male patients with nocturia and lower urinary tract symptoms. *J Urol* **156**:1292–99.

1 Coyne KS, et al. (2003) The prevalence of nocturia and its effect on health-related quality of life and sleep in a community sample in the USA. Br J Urol Int 92:948–54.

2 Jackson S (1999) Lower urinary tract symptoms and nocturia in women: prevalence, aetiology and diagnosis. *Br J Urol Int* **84**:5–8.

3 McKeigue P, Reynard J (2000) Relation of nocturnal polyuria of the elderly to essential hypertension. *Lancet* **355**:486–88.

4 Resnick NM (2002) Geriatric incontinence and voiding dysfunction. In Walsh PC, Retik AB, Vaughan ED, and Wein AJ (eds)*Campbell's Urology* 8th edn. Philadelphia: W.B. Saunders.

Loin (flank) pain

This can present suddenly as severe pain in the flank reaching a peak within minutes or hours (acute loin pain). Alternatively, it may have a slower course of onset (chronic loin pain), developing over weeks or months. Loin pain is frequently presumed to be urological in origin on the simplistic basis that the kidneys are located in the loins. However, other organs are located in this region, pathology within which may be the source of the pain, and pain arising from extra-abdominal organs may radiate to the loins ('referred' pain). So, when faced with a patient with loin pain think laterally—the list of differential diagnoses is long!

The speed of onset of loin pain gives some, although not an absolute, indication of the cause of urological loin pain. Acute loin pain is more likely to be due to something obstructing the ureter, such as a stone. Loin pain of more chronic onset suggests disease within the kidney or renal pelvis.

Acute loin pain

The most common cause of sudden onset of severe pain in the flank is the passage of a stone formed in the kidney, down through the ureter. Ureteric stone pain characteristically starts very suddenly (within minutes), is colicky in nature (waves of increasing severity are followed by a reduction in severity, although seldom going away completely), and it radiates to the groin as the stone passes into the lower ureter. The pain may change in location, from flank to groin, but its location does not provide a good indication of the position of the stone, except where the patient has pain or discomfort in the penis and a strong desire to void, which suggests that the stone has moved into the intramural part of the ureter (the segment within the bladder). The patient cannot get comfortable. They often roll around in agony.

50% of patients with these classic symptoms of ureteric colic do not have a stone confirmed on subsequent imaging studies, nor do they physically ever pass a stone.[1,2] They have some other cause for their pain (see below). A ureteric stone is only very rarely life-threatening, but many of these differential diagnoses may be life-threatening. Acute loin pain is less likely to be due to a ureteric stone in women and in patients at the extremes of age. It tends to be a disease of men (and, to a lesser, extent women) between the ages of ~20 and 60 years, although it can occur in younger and older individuals.

1   Smith RC (1996) Diagnosis of acute flank pain: value of unenhanced helical CT. *Am J Roentgen* **166**:97–100.

2   Thomson JM (2001) Computed tomography versus intravenous urography in diagnosis of acute flank pain from urolithiasis: a randomized study comparing imaging costs and radiation dose. *Australas Radiol* **45**:291–97.

Acute loin pain—non-stone, urological causes

- **Clot or tumour colic:** a clot may form from a bleeding source within the kidney (e.g. renal cell cancer or transitional cell cancer of the renal pelvis). Similarly, a ureteric TCC may cause ureteric obstruction and acute loin pain. Loin pain and haematuria are often assumed to be due to a stone, but it is important to approach investigation of such patients from the perspective of haematuria (i.e. look to exclude cancer)
- **Pelviureteric junction obstruction (PUJO), also known as uretero-pelvic junction obstruction (UPJO):** may present acutely with flank pain severe enough to mimic a ureteric stone. A CT scan will demonstrate hydronephrosis, with a normal calibre ureter below the PUJ and no stone. MAG3 renography confirms the diagnosis
- **Infection:** e.g. acute pyelonephritis, pyonephrosis, emphysematous pyelonephritis, xanthogranulomatous pyelonephritis. These patients have a high fever (>38°C), whereas ureteric stone patients do not (unless there is infection 'behind' the obstructing stone) and are often systemically very unwell. Imaging studies may or may not show a stone, and there will be radiological evidence of infection within the kidney and peri-renal tissues (oedema).

Acute loin pain—non-urological causes

- Vascular
  - Leaking abdominal aortic aneurysm
- 'Medical'
  - Pneumonia
  - Myocardial infarction
  - Malaria presenting as bilateral loin pain and dark haematuria—black water fever
- Gynaecological and obstetric
  - Ovarian pathology (e.g. twisted ovarian cyst)
  - Ectopic pregnancy
- Gastrointestinal
  - Acute appendicitis
  - Inflammatory bowel disease (Crohn's, ulcerative colitis)
  - Diverticulitis
  - Burst peptic ulcer
  - Bowel obstruction
- Testicular torsion
- Spinal cord disease
  - Prolapsed intervertebral disc.

Distinguishing urological from non-urological loin pain

History and examination are clearly important. Patients with ureteric colic often move around the bed in agony. Those with peritonitis lie still. Palpate the abdomen for signs of peritonitis (abdominal tenderness and/or guarding) and examine for abdominal masses [pulsatile and expansile = leaking abdominal aortic aneurysm (AAA)]. Examine the patient's back, chest, and testicles. In women, do a pregnancy test.

Chronic loin pain—urological causes

- Renal or ureteric cancer
  - Renal cell carcinoma
  - Transitional cell carcinoma of the renal pelvis or ureter
- Renal stones
  - Staghorn calculi
  - Non-staghorn calculi
- Renal infection
  - TB
- PUJO
- Testicular pathology (referred pain)
  - Testicular neoplasms
- Ureteric pathology
  - Ureteric reflux
  - Ureteric stone (may drop into the ureter causing severe pain which then subsides to a lower level of chronic pain).

Chronic loin pain—non-urological causes

- Gastrointestinal
  - Bowel neoplasms
  - Liver disease
- Spinal disease
  - Prolapsed intervertebral disc
  - Degenerative disease
  - Spinal metastases.

1   Smith RC (1996) Diagnosis of acute flank pain: value of unenhanced helical CT. *Am J Roentgen* **166**:97–100.

2   Thomson JM (2001) Computed tomography versus intravenous urography in diagnosis of acute flank pain from urolithiasis: a randomized study comparing imaging costs and radiation dose. *Australas Radiol* **45**:291–97.

Urinary incontinence

Definitions

Urinary incontinence (UI): the complaint of any involuntary leakage of urine.

Stress urinary incontinence (SUI): the complaint of involuntary leakage of urine on effort or exertion or sneezing or coughing. SUI can also be a sign, the *observation* of involuntary leakage of urine from the urethra that occurs synchronously with exertion, coughing, etc. A diagnosis of *urodynamic* SUI is made during filling cystometry when there is involuntary leakage of urine during a rise in abdominal pressure (induced by coughing), in the absence of a detrusor contraction.

Urge urinary incontinence (UUI): the complaint of any involuntary leakage of urine accompanied by or immediately preceded by urgency.

Mixed urinary incontinence (MUI): a combination of SUI and UUI.
- Both UUI and MUI cannot be a sign as they both require a perception of urgency by the patient
- 25% of women aged >20 years have UI of whom 50% have SUI, 10–20% pure UUI, and 30–40% MUI
- UI impacts on psychological health, social functioning, and quality of life.

Significance of SUI and UUI

SUI occurs as a result of bladder neck/urethral hypermobility and/or neuromuscular defects causing intrinsic sphincter deficiency (sphincter weakness incontinence). As a consequence, urine leaks whenever urethral resistance is exceeded by an increased abdominal pressure occurring during exercise or coughing, for example.

UUI may be due to bladder overactivity (formerly known as detrusor instability), or less commonly due to pathology that irritates the bladder (infection, tumour, stone). The correlation between urodynamic evidence of bladder overactivity and the sensation of urgency is poor, particularly in patients with MUI. Symptoms resulting from involuntary detrusor contractions may be difficult to distinguish from those due to sphincter weakness. Furthermore, in some patients detrusor contractions can be provoked by coughing, and therefore distinguishing leakage due to SUI from that due to bladder overactivity can be very difficult.

Other types of incontinence

While SUI and especially UUI do not specifically allow identification of the underlying cause, some types of incontinence allow a specific diagnosis to be made.
- **Bedwetting** in an elderly man usually indicates high pressure chronic retention (HPCR)
- A **constant leak** of urine suggests a fistulous communication between the bladder (usually) and vagina (e.g. due to surgical injury at the time of hysterectomy or caesarian section) or, rarely, the presence of an ectopic ureter draining into the vagina (in which case the urine leak is usually low in volume, but lifelong).

Further reading

Hannestad YS, Rortveit G, Sandvik H, Hunskaar S (2000) A community-based epidemiological survey of female urinary incontinence. The Norwegian EPINCONT study. *J Clin Epidemiol* **53**:1150–7.

Genital symptoms

Scrotal pain

- Pathology within the scrotum
  - Torsion of the testicles
  - Torsion of testicular appendages
  - Epididymo-orchitis
  - Testicular tumour
- Referred pain
  - Ureteric colic

Testicular torsion: ischaemic pain is severe (e.g. myocardial infarction, ischaemic leg, ischaemic testis). Torsion presents with sudden onset of pain in the hemiscrotum, sometimes waking the patient from sleep. May radiate to the groin and/or loin. There is sometimes a history of mild trauma to the testis in the hours before the acute onset of pain. Similar episodes may have occurred in the past, with spontaneous resolution of the pain (suggesting torsion/spontaneous detorsion). The testis is very tender. It may be high-riding (lying at a higher than normal position in the testis) and may lie horizontally due to twisting of the cord. There may be scrotal erythema.

Epididymo-orchitis: similar presenting symptoms as testicular torsion. Tenderness is usually localized to the epididymis (absence of testicular tenderness may help to distinguish epididymo-orchitis from testicular torsion, but in many cases it is difficult to distinguish between the two).

see p. 522 for advice on attempting to distinguish torsion from epididymo-orchitis.

Testicular tumour: 20% present with testicular pain.

Acute presentations of testicular tumours

- Testicular swelling may occur rapidly (over days or weeks). An associated (secondary) hydrocele is common. A hydrocele in a young person should always be investigated with an ultrasound to determine whether the underlying testis is normal
- Rapid onset (days) of testicular swelling can occur. Very rarely present with advanced metastatic disease (high volume disease in the retroperitoneum, chest, and neck causing chest, back, or abdominal pain or shortness of breath)
- Approximately 10–15% of testis tumours present with signs suggesting inflammation (i.e. signs suggesting a diagnosis of epididymo-orchitis—a tender, swollen testis, with redness in the overlying scrotal skin and a fever).

Priapism

Painful, persistent, prolonged erection of the penis not related to sexual stimulation (causes summarized in Chapter 13). Two broad categories— low-flow (most common) and high-flow. Low-flow priapism—due to hae-matological disease, malignant infiltration of the corpora cavernosa with malignant disease or drugs. Painful because the corpora are ischaemic. High-flow priapism—due to perineal trauma, which creates an arteriov-enous fistula. Painless.

Diagnosis is usually obvious from the history and examination of the erect, tender penis (in low-flow priapism). Characteristically, the corpora cavernosa are rigid and the glans is flaccid. Examine the abdomen for evidence of malignant disease and perform a digital rectal examination to examine the prostate and check anal tone.

Abdominal examination in urological disease

Because of their retroperitoneal (kidneys, ureters) or pelvic location (bladder and prostate) 'urological' organs are relatively inaccessible to the examining hand when compared with, for example, the spleen, liver, or bowel. For the same reason, for the kidneys and bladder to be palpable implies a fairly advanced disease state.

It is important that the urologist appreciates the characteristics of other intra-abdominal organs when involved with disease, so that they may be distinguished from 'urological' organs.

Characteristics and causes of an enlarged kidney

The mass lies in a paracolic gutter, it moves with respiration, is dull to percussion, and can be felt bimanually. It can also be balloted (i.e. bounced, like a ball (*balla* = ball (*Italian*)) between your hands, one placed on the anterior abdominal wall and one on the posterior abdominal wall.

Causes of an enlarged kidney: renal carcinoma, hydronephrosis, pyonephrosis, perinephric abscess, polycystic disease, nephroblastoma.

Characteristics and causes of an enlarged liver

The mass descends from underneath the right costal margin, you cannot get above it, it moves with respiration, it is dull to percussion, and has a sharp or rounded edge. The surface may be smooth or irregular.

Causes of an enlarged liver: infection, congestion (heart failure, hepatic vein obstruction—Budd–Chiari syndrome), cellular infiltration (amyloid), cellular proliferation, space occupying lesion (polycystic disease, metastatic infiltration, primary hepatic cancer, hydatid cyst, abscess), cirrhosis.

Characteristics and causes of an enlarged spleen

The mass appears from underneath the costal margin, enlarges towards the right iliac fossa, is firm, smooth, and may have a palpable notch. It is not possible to get above the mass, it moves with respiration, is dull to percussion, and it cannot be felt bimanually.

Causes of an enlarged spleen: bacterial infection (typhoid, typhus TB, septicaemia); viral infection (glandular fever); protozoal infection (malaria, kala-azar); spirochaete infection (syphilis, Leptospirosis—Weil's disease); cellular proliferation (myeloid and lymphatic leukaemia, myelosclerosis, spherocystosis, thrombocytopenic purpura, pernicious anaemia); congestion (portal hypertension—cirrhosis, portal vein thrombosis, hepatic vein obstruction, congestive heart failure); cellular infiltration (amyloid, Gaucher's disease); space occupying lesions (solitary cysts, hydatid cysts, lymphoma, polycystic disease).

Characteristics of an enlarged bladder

Arises out of the pelvis, dull to percussion, pressure of examining hand may cause a desire to void.

Abdominal distension: causes and characteristics

- Foetus—smooth, firm mass, dull to percussion, arising out of the pelvis
- Flatus—hyper-resonant (there may be visible peristalsis if the accumulation of flatus is due to bowel obstruction)
- Faeces—palpable in the flanks and across the epigastrium, firm, and may be indentable, there may be multiple separate masses in the line of the colon
- Fat
- Fluid (ascites)—fluid thrill, shifting dullness
- Large abdominal masses (massive hepatomegaly or splenomegaly, fibroids, polycystic kidneys, retroperitoneal sarcoma).

The umbilicus and signs and symptoms of associated pathology

The umbilicus represents the location of 4 foetal structures—the umbilical vein, 2 umbilical arteries, and the urachus, which is a tube extending from the superior aspect of the bladder towards the umbilicus (it represents the obliterated vesicourethral canal).

The urachus may remain open at various points leading to the following abnormalities (Fig. 2.2):[1]

- **Completely patent urachus:** communicates with the bladder and leaks urine through the umbilicus. Usually doesn't present until adulthood (strong contractions of bladder of a child closes the mouth of the fistula)
- **Vesicourachal diverticulum:** a diverticulum in the dome of the bladder. Usually symptomless
- **Umbilical cyst or sinus:** can become infected, forming an abscess or may chronically discharge infected material from the umbilicus. A cyst can present as an immobile, midline swelling between the umbilicus and bladder, deep to the rectus sheath. It may have a small communication with the bladder and, therefore, its size can fluctuate as it can becomes swollen with urine.

Other causes of umbilical masses

Metastatic deposit (from abdominal cancer, metastatic spread occurring via lymphatics in the edge of the falciform ligament, running alongside the obliterated umbilical vein); 'deposit' of endometriosis (becomes painful and discharges blood at the same time as menstruation).

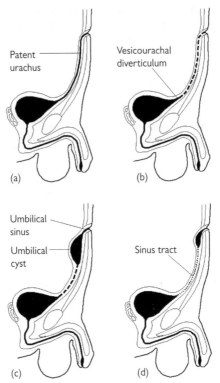

Fig. 2.2 Urachal abnormalities. (Reproduced with permission from Elsevier)[1]

1 Hinman F Jr (1992) *Atlas of Urosurgical Anatomy.* Philadelphia: W.B. Saunders®.

Digital rectal examination (DRE)

The immediate anterior relationship of the rectum in the male is the prostate. The DRE is the mainstay of examination of the prostate.

Explain the need for the examination. Ensure the examination is done in privacy. In the UK, DRE is usually done in the left lateral position—with the patient lying on their left side, and with the hips and knees flexed to 90° or more. Examine the anal region for fistulae and fissures. Apply plenty of lubricating gel to the gloved finger. Lift the tight buttock upwards with your other hand to expose the anus, and gently and slowly insert your index finger into the anal canal, then into the rectum.

Palpate anteriorly with the pulp of your finger and feel the surface of the prostate. Note its consistency (normal or firm), its surface (smooth or irregular), and estimate its size. (It can be helpful to relate its size to common objects (e.g. fruit or nuts!) A normal prostate is the size of a walnut, a moderately enlarged prostate that of a tangerine, and a big prostate the size of an apple or orange.) The normal bilobed prostate has a groove (the median sulcus) between the two lobes and in prostate cancer this groove may be obscured.

Many men find DRE uncomfortable or even painful, and the inexperienced doctor may equate this normal discomfort with prostatic tenderness. Prostatic tenderness is best elicited by gentle pressure on the prostate with the examining finger. If the prostate is really involved by some acute, inflammatory condition such as acute, infective prostatitis, or a prostatic abscess, it will be very tender.

DRE should be avoided in the profoundly neutropenic patient (risk of septicaemia) and in patients with an anal fissure, where DRE would be very painful.

Other features to elicit in the DRE

The integrity of the sacral nerves that innervate the bladder and of the sacral spinal cord can be established by eliciting the bulbocavernosus reflex (the BCR) during a DRE. The sensory side of the reflex is elicited by squeezing the glans of the penis or the clitoris (or in catheterized patients, by gently pulling the balloon of the catheter onto the bladder neck). The motor side of the reflex is tested by feeling for contraction of the anus during this sensory stimulus. Contraction of the anus represents a positive BCR and indicates that the afferent and efferent nerves of the sacral spinal cord (S2–4) and the sacral cord are intact.

Lumps in the groin

Differential diagnosis

Inguinal hernia, femoral hernia, enlarged lymph nodes, saphena varix, hydrocele of the cord (or of the canal of Nück in women), vaginal hydrocele, undescended testis, lipoma of the cord, femoral aneurysm, psoas abscess.

Determining the diagnosis

Hernia

A hernia (usually) has a cough impulse (i.e. it expands on coughing), and (usually) reduces with direct pressure or on lying down unless, uncommonly, it is incarcerated (i.e. the contents of the hernia are fixed in the hernia sac by their size and by adhesions). *Movement* of the lump is not the same as *expansion*. Many groin lumps have a transmitted impulse on coughing (i.e. they move), but do not expand on coughing. Since inguinal and femoral hernias arise from within the abdomen and *descend* into the groin, it is not possible to 'get above' them. For lumps that arise from within the scrotum, the superior edge can be palpated (i.e. it *is* possible to 'get above' them).

Once a hernia has protruded through the abdominal wall, it can expand in any direction in the subcutaneous tissues and therefore the position of the unreduced hernia *cannot* be used to establish whether it is inguinal or femoral. The point of *reduction* of the hernia establishes whether it is an inguinal or femoral hernia.

Inguinal: the hernia reduces through the abdominal wall at a point *above* and *medial* to the pubic tubercle. An indirect inguinal hernia often descends into the scrotum; a direct inguinal hernia rarely does.

Femoral: the hernia reduces through the abdominal wall at a point *below* and *lateral* to the pubic tubercle.

Enlarged inguinal lymph nodes

A firm, non-compressible, nodular lump in the groin. Look for pathology in the skin of the scrotum and penis, the peri-anal area and anus, and the skin and superficial tissues of the thigh and leg.

Saphena varix

A dilatation of the proximal end of the saphenous vein. Can be confused with an inguinal or femoral hernia because it has an expansile cough impulse (i.e. expands on coughing) and disappears on lying down. It is easily compressible and has a fluid thrill when the distal saphenous vein is percussed.

Hydrocele of the cord (or of the canal of Nück in women)

A hydrocele is an abnormal quantity of peritoneal fluid between the parietal and visceral layers of the tunica vaginalis, the double layer of peritoneum surrounding the testis, and which was the processus vaginalis in the foetus. Normally, the processus vaginalis becomes obliterated along its entire length, apart from where it surrounds the testis where a potential space remains between the parietal and visceral layers. If the central part of the processus vaginalis remains patent, fluid secreted by the 'trapped' peritoneum accumulates and forms a hydrocele of the cord (the equivalent in females is known as the canal of Nück). A hydrocele of the cord may therefore be present in the groin.

Undescended testis

May be on the correct anatomical path, but may have failed to reach the scrotum (incompletely descended testis) or may have descended away from the normal anatomical path (ectopic testis). The 'lump' is smooth, oval, tender to palpation, non-compressible, and there is no testis in the scrotum.

Lipoma of the cord

A non-compressible lump in the groin, with no cough impulse.

Femoral aneurysm

Usually in the common femoral artery (rather than superficial or profunda femoris branches) and, therefore, located just below the inguinal ligament. Easily confused with a femoral hernia. Like all aneurysms they are expansile (but unlike hernias they do not expand on coughing).

Psoas abscess

The scenario is one of a patient who is unwell with a fever, with a soft, fluctuant, compressible mass in the femoral triangle.

Lumps in the scrotum

Differential diagnosis

Inguinal hernia, hydrocele, epididymal cyst, testicular tumour, varicocele, sebaceous cyst, tuberculous epididymo-orchitis, gumma of the testis, carcinoma of scrotal skin.

Determining the diagnosis

Inguinal hernia

An indirect inguinal hernia often extends into the scrotum. It usually has a cough impulse (i.e. it expands on coughing) and usually reduces with direct pressure or on lying down. It is not possible to get above the lump.

Hydrocele

A hydrocele is an abnormal quantity of peritoneal fluid between the parietal and visceral layers of the tunica vaginalis, the double layer of peritoneum surrounding the testis and which was the processus vaginalis in the foetus. Normally the processus vaginalis becomes obliterated along its entire length, apart from where it surrounds the testis where a potential space remains between the parietal and visceral layers.

Usually painless, unless the underlying testicular disease is painful. A hydrocele has a smooth surface and it is difficult or impossible to feel the testis which is surrounded by the tense, fluid collection (unless, rarely, the hydrocele is very lax). The superior margin can be palpated (i.e. you can get above the lump). It is possible to trans-illuminate a hydrocele (i.e. the light from a torch applied on one side can be seen on the other side of the hydrocele).

May be primary (idiopathic) or secondary. Primary hydroceles develop slowly (over the course of years, usually), and there is no precipitating event such as epididymo-orchitis or trauma, and the underlying testis appears normal on ultrasound (no testicular tumour). Secondary hydroceles (infection, tumour, trauma) represent an effusion between the layers of the tunica vaginalis (the visceral and parietal layers), analogous to a pleural or peritoneal effusion. In filariasis (infection with the filarial worm *Wuchereria bancrofti*), obstruction of the lymphatics of the spermatic cord give rise to the hydrocele.

Epididymal cyst

(Also known as a spermatocele if there are spermatozoa in the contained fluid.) Derived from the collecting tubules of the epididymis and contain clear fluid. They develop slowly (over years), lie within the scrotum (you can get above them), and usually lie above and behind the testis. They are often multiple (multiloculated).

Orchitis

In the absence of involvement of the epididymitis, due to a viral infection e.g. mumps. Often occurs with enlargement of the salivary glands.

Tuberculous epididymo-orchitis

Infection of the epididymis (principally) by TB, which has spread from the blood or urinary tract. The *absence* of pain and tenderness is noticeable. The epididymis is hard and has an irregular surface. The spermatic cord is thickened and the vas deferens also feels hard and irregular (a 'string of beads').

Testicular tumour (seminoma, teratoma)

A solid mass, arising from within the scrotum that, if very large, may extend up into the spermatic cord. They may present with symptoms which mimic an acute epididymorchitis (i.e. pain and tenderness in the testis and fever). Not infrequently the patient reports a history of minor trauma to the testis in the days or weeks preceding the onset of symptoms. They may have undergone an orcidopexy as a child (fixation of the testis in the scrotum for an undescended testis).

The lump is usually firm or hard, and may have a smooth or irregular surface. Examine for abdominal and supraclavicular lymph nodes.

Gumma of the testis

Rare; syphilis of the testis resulting in a round, hard, insensitive mass involving the testis (a so-called 'billiard ball'); difficult to distinguish from a tumour.

Varicocele

Dilatation of the pampiniform plexus—the collection of veins surrounding the testis and extending up into the spermatic cord (essentially varicose veins of the testis and spermatic cord). Small, symptomless varicoceles occur in approximately 20% of normal men and are more common on the left side. They may cause a dragging sensation or ache in the scrotum. Said to feel like a 'bag of worms'. The varicocele disappears when the patient lies down.

Sebaceous cyst

Common in scrotal skin. They are fixed to the skin and have a smooth surface.

Carcinoma of scrotal skin

Appears as an ulcer on the scrotal skin, often with a purulent or bloody discharge.

Urological investigations

Assessing kidney function

When we talk about measuring kidney function, what we mean is measurement of glomerular filtration rate (GFR). This is regarded as the best measure of kidney function, and we grade the degree of renal impairment and renal failure according to the GFR. Normal GFR in young men is approximately 130 mL/min per 1.73 m^2 of body surface area. In young women it is 120 mL/min per 1.73 m^2 of body surface area. Mean GFR declines with age (Fig. 3.1).

The ideal filtration marker is excreted by filtration alone. Exogenous markers that can be used to measure include inulin, iothalamate, ethylene diamine tetra-acetic acid (EDTA), diethylene triamine penta-acetic acid, and iohexol. Measurement of GFR using exogenously administered markers is complex and expensive, and is difficult to do in routine clinical practice.

Urinary clearance of endogenous markers, such as creatinine, can be used to estimate GFR. Creatinine is a 113D amino acid derivative that is freely filtered at the glomerulus. A timed urine collection and measurement of serum creatinine concentration allows calculation of GFR according to the formula:

Clearance (GFR) = $U \times V/P$

where U is the concentration of urine in urine, P the concentration in plasma and V the urine flow.

As an alternative, estimation of GFR can be made from simple measurement of serum creatinine, since the main mechanism of creatinine excretion is by glomerular filtration and GFR has a reciprocal relationship with serum creatinine. Thus, as GFR falls (indicating worsening renal function), creatinine rises. However, creatinine is not the ideal filtration marker, since it is also excreted by proximal tubular secretion, as well as by glomerular filtration and therefore creatinine clearance exceeds GFR, i.e. creatinine clearance tends to overestimate GFR.

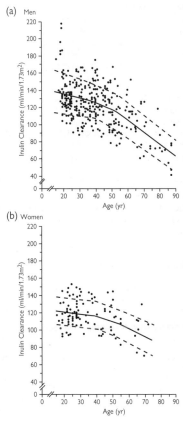

Fig. 3.1 Normal values of GFR in men and women. Adapted from L.G. Wesson (1969) *Physiology of the human kidney*. New York: Greene and Stratton with permission.

Estimated GFR (eGFR)

Since the endogenous production of creatinine is determined by muscle mass, serum levels of creatinine will not only vary according to renal function (glomerular filtration), but also according to age, body size, ethnic group, and sex. Taking account of these factors can overcome some of the limitations of measurement of serum creatinine alone.

Two equations have been widely used for calculating eGFR—the Cockcroft–Gault formula and the Modification of Diet in Renal Disease (MDRD) equation. Both were developed from populations of patients with chronic kidney disease. They are less accurate estimates of renal function in populations *without* chronic kidney disease.

Cockcroft–Gault formula (over-estimates GFR because of tubular secretion of creatinine and the value is not adjusted for body surface area)

$$C_{CR} \text{ in mL/min} = [(140 - \text{age}) \times \text{weight}]/(0.84 \times S_{Cr}) \text{ if male}$$

$$C_{CR} \text{ in mL/min} = [(140 - \text{age}) \times \text{weight}]/ (0.85 \times S_{Cr}) \text{ if female}$$

where S_{Cr} = serum creatinine (mM/L) and C_{Cr} = creatinine clearance.

The Modification of Diet in Renal Disease (MDRD) equation (modified in 2005): adjusts for body surface area:

$$\text{GFR (mL/min/1.73 m}^2) = 30{,}849 \times (S_{Cr})^{-1.154} \times (\text{age})^{-0.203}$$
$$(\times \ 0.742 \text{ if female}; \times 1.212 \text{ if black})$$

The MDRD is reasonably accurate as an estimate of GFR, the mean difference between eGFR and measured GFR ranging from −5 to 1 mL/min/1.73 m^2.

eGFR provides substantial improvements over serum creatinine measurements alone in the clinical assessment of renal function in terms of the detection, evaluation and management of chronic kidney disease.

CKD (Chronic Kidney Disease) Classification

Stage 1 (kidney damage with normal or increased GFR)	eGFR >90 mL/min/1.73m^2
Stage 2 (mild decrease in GFR)	eGFR 60-89 mL/min/1.73m^2
Stage 3 (moderate decrease in GFR)	eGFR 30-59 mL/min/1.73m^2
Stage 4 (severe decrease in GFR)	eGFR 15-29 mL/min/1.73m^2
Stage 5 (kidney failure)	eGFR <15 mL/min/1.73m^2

Urine examination

Dipstick testing

Analysis for pH, blood, protein, glucose, and white cells can be done with dipstick testing.

pH

Urinary pH varies between 4.5 and 8, averaging between 5.5 and 6.5.

Blood

Normal urine contains <3 RBCs per high-powered field (1000 erythrocytes/mL of urine; upper limit of 5000–8000 erythrocytes/mL). +ve dipstick for blood indicates the presence of haemoglobin in the urine. Haemoglobin has a peroxidase-like activity and causes oxidation of a chromogen indicator, which changes colour when oxidized. Sensitivity of urine dipsticks for identifying haematuria (>3 RBCs/HPF is >90%); specificity is lower [i.e. a higher false +ve rate with the dipstick, due to contamination with menstrual blood, dehydration (concentrates what RBCs are normally present in urine)].

Haematuria due to a urological cause does not elevate urinary protein. Haematuria of nephrological origin often occurs in association with casts and there is almost always significant proteinuria.

Protein

Normal, healthy adults excrete about 80–150 mg of protein per day in their urine (normal protein concentration <20 mg/dL). Proteinuria suggests the presence of renal disease (glomerular, tubulo-interstitial, renal vascular) or multiple myeloma, but it can occur following strenuous exercise. Dipstick test is based on a tetrabromophenol blue dye colour change (green colour develops in the presence of protein of >20 mg/dL).

White blood cells

Leukocyte esterase activity detects the presence of white blood cells in the urine. Leukocyte esterase is produced by neutrophils and causes a colour change in a chromogen salt on the dipstick. Not all patients with bacteriuria have significant pyuria. False –ves: concentrated urine, glycosuria, presence of urobilinogen, consumption of large amounts of ascorbic acid. False +ves: contamination.

Nitrite testing

Nitrites in the urine suggest the possibility of bacteriuria. They are not normally found in the urine. Many species of gram –ve bacteria can convert nitrates to nitrites, and these are detected in urine by a reaction with the reagents on the dipstick, which form a red azo dye. The specificity of the nitrite dipstick for detecting bacteriuria is >90% (false +ve nitrite testing is contamination). Sensitivity: 35–85% (i.e. lots of false –ves); less accurate in urine containing fewer than 10^5 organisms/mL.

Cloudy urine that is +ve for white blood cells and is nitrite +ve is very likely to be infected.

Urine microscopy

Red blood cell morphology

Determined by phase-contrast microscopy. RBCs derived from the glomerulus are dysmorphic (they have been distorted by their passage through the glomerulus). RBCs derived from tubular bleeding (tubulointerstitial disease) and those from lower down the urinary tract (i.e. urological bleeding from the renal pelvis, ureters, or bladder) have a normal shape. Glomerular bleeding is suggested by the presence of dysmorphic RBCs, RBC casts, and proteinuria.

Casts

A protein coagulum (principally, Tamm–Horsfall mucoprotein derived from tubular epithelial cells) formed in the renal tubule and 'cast' in the shape of the tubule (i.e. long and thin). The protein matrix traps tubular luminal contents. If the cast contains only mucoproteins it is called a hyaline cast. Seen after exercise, heat exposure, and in pyelonephritis or chronic renal disease. Red blood cell casts contain trapped erythrocytes and are diagnostic of glomerular bleeding, most often due to glomerulonephritis. White blood cell casts are seen in acute glomerulonephritis, acute pyelonephritis, and acute tubulointerstitial nephritis.

Crystals

Specific crystal types may be seen in urine and help diagnose underlying problems (e.g. cystine crystals establish the diagnosis of cystinuria). Calcium oxalate, uric acid, and cystine are precipitated in acidic urine. Crystals precipitated in alkaline urine include calcium phosphate and triple-phosphate (struvite).

Urine cytology

- **Urine collection for cytology:** exfoliated cells lying in urine that has been in the bladder for several hours (e.g. early morning specimens) or in a urine specimen that has been allowed to stand for several hours, are degenerate. Such urine specimens are not suitable for cytological interpretation. Cytological examination can be performed on bladder washings (using normal saline) obtained from the bladder at cystoscopy (or following catheterization) or from the ureter (via a ureteric catheter or ureteroscope). The urine is centrifuged and the specimen obtained is fixed in alcohol and stained by the Papanicolaou technique

- Normal urothelial cells are shed into the urine and under the microscope their nuclei appear regular and monomorphic (diffuse, fine chromatin pattern, single nucleolus)

- Causes of a +ve cytology report (i.e. abnormal urothelial cells seen—high nuclear: cytoplasmic ratio, hyperchromatic nuclei, prominent nucleoli):
  - Urothelial malignancy (TCC, squamous cell carcinoma, adenocarcinoma)
  - Previous radiotherapy (especially if within the last 12 months)
  - Previous cytotoxic drug treatment (especially if within the last 12 months; e.g. cyclophosphamide, busulfan, ciclosporin)
  - Urinary tract stones

- Renal adenocarcinoma (clear cell cancer of the kidney) usually does not exfoliate abnormal cells, although occasionally clusters of clear cells may be seen, suggesting the diagnosis

- High-grade urothelial cancer and carcinoma *in situ* exfoliate cells, which look very abnormal and usually the cytologist is able to indicate that there is a high likelihood of a malignancy. Low-grade bladder TCC exfoliates cells, which look very much like normal urothelial cells. The difficulty arises where the cells look abnormal, but not that abnormal—here, the likelihood that the cause of the abnormal cytology is a benign process is greater

- Sensitivity and specificity of +ve urine cytology for detecting TCC of the bladder depends on the definition of +ve—if only obviously malignant or highly suspicious samples are considered +ve, then the specificity will be high. Urine cytology may be negative in as many as 20% of high-grade cancers. If 'atypical cells' are included in the definition of abnormal, the specificity of urine cytology for diagnosing urothelial cancer will be relatively poor (relatively high number of false +ves) because many cases will have a benign cause (stones, inflammation).

Prostatic specific antigen (PSA)

(📖 see also p. 296–298)

PSA is a 34KD glycoprotein enzyme produced by the columnar acinar and ductal prostatic epithelial cells. It is a member of the human kallikrein family and its function is to liquefy the ejaculate, enabling fertilization. PSA is present in both benign and malignant cells, although the expression of PSA tends to be reduced in malignant cells and may be absent in poorly differentiated tumours. Large amounts are secreted into the semen, and small quantities are found in the urine and blood.

The function of serum PSA is unclear, although it is known to liberate the insulin-like growth factor type 1 from one of its binding proteins. 75% of circulating PSA is bound to plasma proteins (complexed PSA) and metabolized in the liver, while 25% is free and excreted in the urine. Complexed PSA is stable, bound to alpha-1 antichymotrypsin and alpha-2 macroglobulin. Free PSA is unstable, recently found to consist of two iso-forms: pro-PSA is a peripheral zone precursor, apparently elevated in the presence of prostate cancer, and BPSA is the transition zone precursor and associated with benign prostatic hyperplasia. The half-life of serum PSA is 2.2 days. The normal range for the serum PSA assay in men is <4.0 ng/mL, though this varies with age. Table 3.1 shows a published age-specific normal range (95th centile).

In the absence of prostate cancer, serum PSA concentrations also vary physiologically, according to race and prostate volume.

Indications for checking serum PSA

- Patient request, following counselling (📖 see p. 299)
- Lower urinary tract symptoms
- Abnormal digital rectal examination
- Progressive bone pain, especially back pain
- Unexplained anaemia, anorexia, or weight loss
- Spontaneous thrombo-embolism or unilateral leg swelling
- Monitoring of prostate cancer patients.

Table 3.1 The age-adjusted normal range for PSA

Age range	Normal PSA range (ng/mL)
All ages	<4.0
40–49	<2.5
50–59	<3.5
60–69	<4.5
>70	<6.5

Radiological imaging of the urinary tract

Ultrasound

A non-invasive method of urinary tract imaging. While it provides good images of the kidneys and bladder, anatomical detail of the ureter is poor and the mid-ureter cannot be imaged at all by ultrasound because of overlying bowel gas.

Uses of ultrasound

Renal

- Assessment of haematuria
- Determination of nature of renal masses—can differentiate simple cysts (smooth, well-demarcated wall, reflecting no echoes; benign) from solid masses (almost always malignant; cystic masses with solid components or multiple septae or calcification may be malignant), from those casting an 'acoustic shadow' (stones; Fig. 3.2)
- Can determine the presence/absence of hydronephrosis (dilatation of the collecting system) in patients with abnormal renal function (Fig. 3.3)
- Allows ultrasound guided nephrostomy insertion in patients with hydronephrosis and renal impairment or with infected, obstructed kidneys.

Bladder

- Measurement of post-void residual urine volume
- Allows ultrasound guided placement of a suprapubic catheter.

Prostate: TRUS (transrectal ultrasound)

- Measurement of prostate size (where gross prostatic enlargement is suspected on the basis of a DRE, and surgery, in the form of open prostatectomy, is contemplated)
- To assist prostate biopsy (allows biopsy of hypo- or hyper-echoic lesions)
- Investigation of azoospermia (can establish the presence of ejaculatory duct obstruction).

Urethra

Can image the urethra and establish the depth and extent of spongiofibrosis in urethral stricture disease.

Testes

- Assessment of the patient complaining of a 'lump in the testicle (or scrotum)'—can differentiate benign lesions (hydrocele, epididymal cyst) from malignant testicular tumours (solid, echo poor, or with abnormal echo pattern)
- When combined with power Doppler can establish the presence/absence of testicular blood flow in suspected torsion
- Assessment of testicular trauma (rupture is indicated by abnormal echo pattern, due to blood within the body of the testis; surrounding haematoma may be seen—blood within the scrotal soft tissues that has escaped through a tear in the tunica albuginea and the visceral and parietal layers of the tunica vaginalis; haematocele—blood contained by an intact parietal layer of the tunica vaginalis)
- Investigation of infertility—varicoceles and testicular atrophy may be identified.

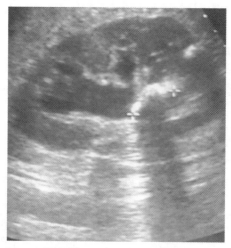

Fig. 3.2 An acoustic shadow cast by a stone within the kidney.

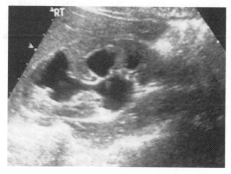

Fig. 3.3 Hydronephrosis. Urine in dilated calyces appears black (hypo-echoic).

Uses of plain abdominal radiography (the 'KUB' X-ray—kidneys, ureters, bladder)

- For detection of stones and determination of their size and (to an extent) their location within the kidneys, ureters, and bladder (Fig. 3.4)
- **Renal calculi:** a calcification overlying the kidneys is intrarenal if it maintains its relationship to the kidney on inspiratory and expiratory films (i.e. if it moves with the kidney). If in doubt as to whether an opacity overlying the outline of the kidney is intrarenal or not, get an ultrasound (look for the characteristic 'acoustic shadow' within the kidney), IVU, or CTU
- **Ureteric calculi:** sensitivity for *detection* of renal calculi is in the order of 50–70% (i.e. the false −ve rate is between 30 and 50%; it misses ureteric stones when these are present in 30–50% of cases). CTU or IVU, which relate the position of the opacity to the anatomical location of the ureters, are required to make a definitive diagnosis of a ureteric stone. However, once the presence of a ureteric stone has been confirmed by another imaging study (CTU or IVU), and as long as it is radio-opaque enough and large enough to be seen, plain radiography is a good way of following the patient to establish whether the stone is progressing distally, down the ureter. It is not useful for 'following' ureteric stones that are radiolucent (e.g. uric acid), small (generally a stone must be 3–4 mm to be visible on plain X-ray), or when the stones pass through the ureter as it lies over the sacrum. Ability of KUB X-ray to 'see' stones is also dependent on amount of overlying bowel gas
- Plain tomography (a plain X-ray taken of a fixed coronal plane through the kidneys) can be useful, but is rarely done nowadays with the availability of ultrasound and CT
- Opacities that may be confused with stones (renal, ureteric) on plain radiography: calcified lymph nodes; pelvic phleboliths (round, lucent centre, usually below the ischial spines)
- Look for the psoas shadow—obscured where there is retroperitoneal fluid (pus or blood; Fig. 3.5).

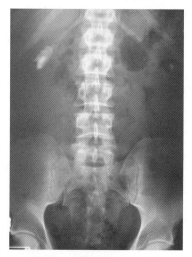

Fig. 3.4 Small staghorn calculus on KUB X-ray.

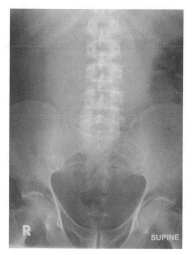

Fig. 3.5 Leaking AAA on plain X-ray; the right psoas shadow cannot be seen due to retroperitoneal haemorrhage.

Intravenous urography (IVU)

Also known as intravenous pyelography (IVP). A control film is obtained before contrast is given. Intravascular contrast is administered followed by a series of X-rays of the kidneys, ureters, and bladder over the following 30 min or so, to image their anatomy and pathology, and to give some indication of renal function.

- Radio-opacity of contrast agents depends on the presence of a tri-iodinated benzene ring in the molecule
- Ionic monomers (sodium and meglumine salts) ionize, thereby producing high osmolality solutions (e.g. iothalamate—Conray®), diatrizoate—Hypaque®, Urografin®)
- Non-ionic monomers—low osmolality (e.g. iopamidol—Niopam, iohexol—Omnipaque®)
- At a concentration of 300 mg of iodine per mL, ionic monomers have an osmolality 5 times higher than plasma, compared with non-ionic monomers, which have an osmolality twice that of plasma
- Excreted from plasma by glomerular filtration.

Films and 'phases' of the IVU

Plain film: looking for calcification overlying the region of the kidneys, ureters, and bladder.

Nephrogram phase: first phase of IVU; film taken immediately following intravenous administration of contrast (peak nephrogram density). The nephrogram is produced by filtered contrast within the lumen of the proximal convoluted tubule (it is a proximal tubular, rather than distal tubular phenomenon).

Pyelogram phase: as the contrast passes along the renal tubule (into the distal tubule) it is concentrated (as water is absorbed, but the contrast agent is not). As a consequence, the contrast medium is concentrated in the pelvicalyceal system, and thus this 'pyelogram' phase (Fig. 3.6) is much denser than the nephrogram phase. The pyelogram phase can be made more dense by dehydrating the patient prior to contrast administration. Pelvic compression can be used to distend the pelvicalyceal system and demonstrate their anatomy more precisely. Compression is released and a film taken (20–30 min; Fig. 3.7).

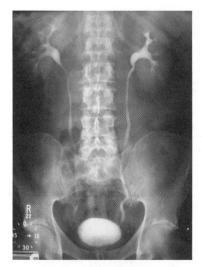

Fig. 3.6 Normal IVU at 15 min.

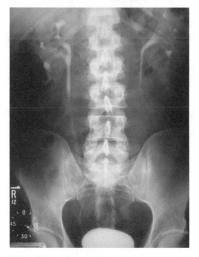

Fig. 3.7 Normal IVU at 20 min. Lower abdominal compression has been released.

Side-effects of administration of intravenous contrast media

- Occur in 1% of patients given non-ionic and 5% given ionic contrast media
- The most serious reactions represent an anaphylactic reaction—hypotension with flushing of the skin (marked peripheral vasodilatation), oedema (face, neck, body, and limbs), bronchospasm, urticaria. Rarely, cardiac arrest can occur. The death rate, as a consequence of these reactions, is 1 in 40,000 to 1 in 70,000 with the ionic media, and 1 in 200,000 with non-ionic contrast agents
- A contrast reaction is more likely to occur in patients with an iodine allergy, previous contrast reaction, asthma, multiple other allergies, and heart disease, and is less likely with non-ionic contrast media. Steroid premedication (at least 12 h before) can reduce the risk of a contrast reaction
- Contrast media are also nephrotoxic. 10% of patients with a raised creatinine will develop an increase in creatinine after an IVU (more likely in diabetics, with dehydration and with large contrast doses). The increase in creatinine usually resolves spontaneously.

Uses of the IVU

- Investigation of haematuria—detection of renal masses, filling defects within the collecting system of the kidney and within the ureters (stones, TCCs)
- Localization of calcification overlying the urinary tract (i.e. is it a stone or not?)
- Investigation of patients with loin pain (e.g. suspected ureteric colic). Increasingly being replaced with CTU, which has superior sensitivity and specificity
- Very good for identification of congenital urinary tract abnormalities (e.g. ureteric anatomy in duplex systems; Fig. 3.8); malrotation; horse-shoe kidneys
- Used for follow-up post-ureteric surgery to identify strictures.

There is a trend towards IVU being replaced by multidetector CT urography (MDCTU—a rapid acquisition CT done following intravenous contrast administration with high spatial resolution), at least in the investigation of haematuria and of loin pain. To a large extent, whether one uses an IVU or MDCTU depends on the availability of the latter in your radiology department.

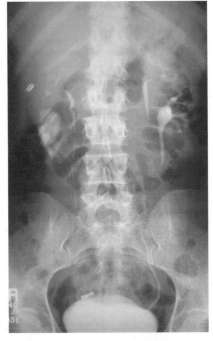

Fig. 3.8 Bilateral duplex as seen on a tomogram from an IVU.

Other urological contrast studies

Videocystourethrography (VCUG) (Fig. 3.9)

To identify the presence of vesicoureteric reflux during filling and emptying of the bladder, and presence and site of obstruction in the outlet of the bladder and within the urethra, particularly in patients with neuropathic bladder problems (e.g. spinal cord injury).

Cystography

Retrograde filling of the bladder, via a catheter, with contrast. Identifies vesicocolic and vesicovaginal fistulae and bladder rupture (extraperitoneal and intraperitoneal).

Urethrography (Fig. 3.10)

Retrograde filling of the urethra with contrast, to identify the site and length of urethral strictures (Fig. 3.11), or presence, extent, and site of urethral injury (in pelvic fracture, for example).

Ileal loopogram

Retrograde filling of an ileal conduit with contrast to establish the presence of free reflux into the ureters (a normal finding; absence of free reflux suggests obstruction at the uretero-ileal junction due to ischaemic stenosis or recurrent TCC in the ureters at the uretero-ileal junction) and the presence of TCCs in the ureters or renal pelvis (an occasional finding in patients who have had a cystectomy for bladder TCC with ileal conduit urinary diversion).

Retrograde ureterography

Retrograde instillation of contrast into the ureters by a ureteric catheter inserted into the ureter via a cystoscope (rigid or flexible). Provides excellent definition of the ureter and renal pelvis for detection of ureteric and renal pelvic TCCs or radiolucent stones in patients with persistent haematuria where other tests have shown no abnormality. Also used to diagnose presence and site of ureteric injury (obstruction, ureteric leak) in cases of ureteric injury (e.g. post hysterectomy or caesarean section).

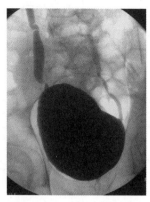

Fig. 3.9 VCUG showing bilateral ureteric reflux.

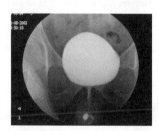

Fig. 3.10 Normal urethrogram.

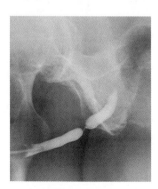

Fig. 3.11 A urethrogram showing a bulbar urethral stricture.

Computed tomography (CT) and magnetic resonance imaging (MRI)

Computed tomography

Widely used for investigation of urological symptoms and disease. It can detect very small differences in X-ray absorption values of tissues, providing a very wide range of densities (and, therefore, differentiation between tissues) when compared with plain radiography. The computer calculates the absorption value (attenuation) of each pixel and reconstructs this into an image. The attenuation values are expressed on a scale from −1000 to +1000 Hounsfield units (water = 0, air = −1000, bone = +1000). More recently, advances in computing power have enabled the data to be reformatted so that images can be produced in sagittal and coronal planes, as well as in the more familiar horizontal plane (Figs 3.12 and 3.13).

'Plain' CT scans (without contrast) can detect calcification and calculi within the urinary tract.

Administration of intravenous contrast is used to investigate haematuria, to evaluate the nature of solid renal lesions and to determine the nature of soft tissue masses (e.g. to differentiate bowel from lymph nodes in cancer staging CTs). 'Spiral' or 'helical' CT (also known as multidetector CT urography—MDCTU—when done following intravenous contrast administration) is very rapid scanning, while the table on which the patient is lying is moved though the scanner. Multiple images ('slices') of the patient are taken. A large volume of the body can be imaged in a single breath hold, thus eliminating movement artefact and increasing spatial resolution—particularly useful for identifying suspected ureteric stones in patients with acute loin pain and (with contrast) for determining the nature of renal masses.

Overlapping thin sections can be 'reconstructed' into images in multiple planes (multiplanar reformatting—MPR) so lesions can be imaged in multiple planes (sagittal, coronal), as opposed to the traditional transverse sections.

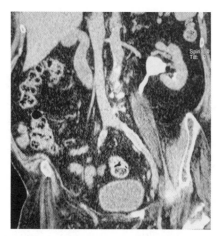

Fig. 3.12 Coronal CT image of abdomen showing the left kidney, aorta, and IVC.

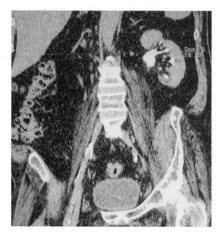

Fig. 3.13 Coronal CT image of abdomen showing the left kidney and paravertebral muscles.

Uses of CT

Haematuria

Investigation of site and cause of urinary tract bleeding. Has the advantage of a single investigation which potentially could obviate the need for the traditional '4-test' approach to haematuria (IVU, renal ultrasound, flexible cystoscopy, urine cytology), although at the cost of a higher radiation dose. There is evidence suggesting that MDCTU has reasonable sensitivity and high specificity for diagnosing bladder tumours[1] (in patients with macroscopic haematuria 93% sensitivity, 99% specificity) and that it has equivalent diagnostic accuracy to retrograde uretero-pyelography (the retrograde administration of contrast via a catheter inserted in the lower ureter, to outline the ureter and renal collecting system).[2] Overall, for patients with haematuria and no prior history of urological malignancy, for the detection of all urological tumours it has approximately 65% sensitivity and 98% specificity[3]—so it only rarely calls a lesion a tumour when, in fact, the lesion is benign, but it still fails to diagnose a significant proportion of urinary neoplasms (sensitivity for upper tract neoplasms 80%, for bladder tumours 60%). The role of MDCTU (described by some as the 'ultimate' imaging modality) in the investigation of haematuria remains controversial. MDCTU in all patients with haematuria (microscopic, macroscopic), when most will have no identifiable cause for the haematuria, has a cost (high radiation dose, financial). A targeted approach, aimed at those with risk factors for urothelial malignancy (age >40 years, macroscopic as opposed to microscopic haematuria, smoking history, occupational exposure to benzenes and aromatic amines) might be a better use of this resource, rather than using MDCTU as the first imaging test for both high *and* low risk patients. Thus, the 'best' imaging probably depends on the context of the patient.

Renal

- Investigation of renal masses—characterizes solid from cystic lesions; differentiates benign (e.g. angiomyolipoma) from malignant solid masses (e.g. renal cell carcinoma)
- Staging of renal cancer (establishes local, nodal, and distant spread)
- Assessment of stone size and location (within the collecting system or within the parenchyma of the kidney)
- Detection and localization of site of intrarenal and perirenal collections of pus (pyonephrosis, perinephric abscess)
- 'Staging' (grading) of renal trauma
- Determination of cause of hydronephrosis.

Ureters

Locates and measures size of ureteric stones.

Bladder

Bladder cancer staging (establishes local, nodal, and distant spread).

Uses of MRI

- Staging of pelvic cancer—bladder and prostate cancer staging (establishes local, nodal, and distant spread). As with CT, oedema and fibrosis cannot be reliably distinguished from tumour within the bladder wall, leading to 'overstaging' of cancer. Again, as with CT, microscopic disease cannot be identified, leading to 'understaging' of cancer
- Localization of undescended testes
- Identification of ureteric stones, where ionizing radiation is best avoided (e.g. pregnant women with loin pain).

1 Turney BW, Willatt JM, Nixon D, et al. (2006) Computed tomography urography for diagnosing bladder cancer. *Br J Urol Int* **98**:345–8.

2 Cowan NC, Turney BW, Taylor NJ, et al. (2007) Multidetector computed tomography urography for diagnosing upper urinary tract urothelial tumours. *Br J Urol Int 2007*; **99**: 1363–70.

3 Sudakoff GS, Dunn DP, Guralnick ML, et al. (2008) Multidetector computed tomography urography as the primary imaging modality for detecting urinary tract neoplasms in patients with asymptomatic hematuria. *J Urol* **179**:862–7.

Radioisotope imaging

A variety of organic compounds can be 'labelled' with a radioactive isotope that emits gamma rays, allowing the radiation to penetrate through tissues and reach a 'gamma' camera placed adjacent to the patient. The most commonly used radioisotope is technetium—^{99m}Tc (half-life 6 h, gamma ray emission energy 0.14 MeV). The excretion characteristics of the organic compound to which the ^{99m}Tc is bound determine the clinical use.

MAG3 renogram

^{99m}Tc is bound to mercapto acetyl triglycine. Over 90% of mercaptoacetyl-triglycyl (MAG3) becomes bound to plasma proteins following intravenous injection. It is excreted from the kidneys principally by tubular secretion (glomerular filtration is minimal). Following intravenous injection MAG3 is very rapidly excreted (appearing in the kidney within 15 s of the injection and starting to appear in the bladder within about 3 min). Approximately two-thirds of the injected dose of MAG3 is taken up by the kidneys with each passage of blood through the kidney. The radioactivity over each kidney thus increases rapidly. The peak of radioactivity represents the point at which delivery of MAG3 to the kidney from the renal artery is equivalent to excretion of MAG3. The radioactivity starts to decline as excretion outstrips supply. Thus, a time-activity curve can be recorded for each kidney. This time-activity curve is known as a renogram.

Images are collected onto a film at 30-s intervals for the first 3 min and then at 5-min intervals for the remainder of the study (usually a total of 30 min).

A normal renogram has 3 phases
- **First phase:** a steeply rising curve lasting 20–30 s
- **Second phase:** a more slowly rising curve, rising to a peak. If the curve does not reach a peak the second phase is said to rise continually. A normal second phase ends with a sharp peak.
- **Third phase:** a curve that descends after the peak. There can be no third phase if there is no peak.

Description of the renogram
No comment is made about the first phase. The second phase is described as being absent, impaired, or normal. The third phase is described as being absent, impaired, or normal.

The time to the peak depends on urine flow and level of hydration, and is a crude measure of the time it takes the tracer to travel through the parenchyma of the kidney and through the renal pelvis. The time to the peak of the renogram normally varies between 2 and 4.5 min.

If the renogram continues beyond the time at which the peak should normally occur, then there may be a distal obstruction (e.g. at the PUJ or lower down the ureter). In this situation, an injection of 40mg of frusemide is given (at about 18 min) and if the curves start to fall rapidly, this is taken as proof that there is no obstruction. If it continues to rise, there is obstruction. If it remains flat (neither rising or falling), this is described as an 'equivocal' result.

Parenchymal transit time can also be measured (PTTI—parenchymal transit time index). The normal range for PTTI is 40–140 s and averages 70 s.

PTTI is prolonged (to >156 s) in obstruction and in renal ischaemia. A normal PTTI excludes obstruction.

Uses
- 'Split' renal function (i.e. the % function contributed by each kidney)
- Determination of presence of renal obstruction—based on shape of renogram curve and PTTI.

DMSA scanning

Dimercapto succinic acid (DMSA) is labelled with ^{99m}Tc. It is taken up by the proximal tubules and retained there, with very little being excreted in the urine. A 'static' image of the kidneys is thus obtained (at about 3–4h post intravenous injection of radioisotope). It demonstrates whether a 'lesion' contains functioning nephrons or not.

Uses
- 'Split' renal function (i.e. the % function contributed by each kidney)
- Detection of scars in the kidney (these appear as defects in the cortical outline, representing areas in which the radioisotope is not taken up).

Radioisotope bone imaging

^{99m}Tc-labelled methylene disphosphonate (MDP) is taken up by areas of bone where there is increased blood supply and increased osteoblastic activity. There are many causes of a focal increase in isotope uptake—bone metastases, site of fractures, osteomyelitis, TB, benign bone lesions (e.g. osteoma). Metastases from urological cancers are characterized by their predilection for the spine and the fact that they are multiple (single foci of metastasis are rare). Prostate cancer classically metastasizes in this way.

Uroflowmetry

Measurement of flow rate (Fig. 3.14). Provides a visual image of the 'strength' of a patient's urinary stream. Urine flow rate is measured in mL/s and is determined using commercially available electronic flowmeters (Fig. 3.15). These flowmeters are able to provide a print-out recording the voided volume, maximum flow rate, and time taken to complete the void, together with a record of the flow pattern. Maximum flow rate, Q_{max}, is influenced by the volume of urine voided, by the contractility of the patient's bladder and by the conductivity (resistance) of their urethra.

A number of nomograms are available which relate voided volume to flow rate (Fig. 3.16).

Interpretation and misinterpretation of urine flow rate

The 'wag' artefact (📖 see Fig. 3.14b) is seen as a sudden, rapid increase in flow rate on the uroflow tracing and is due to the urine flow suddenly being directed at the centre of the flowmeter, producing a sudden artefactual surge in flow rate.

In men with 'prostatic' symptoms, for the same voided volume, flow rate varies substantially on a given day (by as much as 5 mL/s if 4 flows are done[1]). Most guidelines recommend measuring at least 2 flow rates, and using the highest as representing the patient's best effort.

What does a low flow mean?

Uroflowmetry alone cannot tell you why the flow is abnormal. It cannot distinguish between low flow due to bladder outlet obstruction and that due to a poorly contractile bladder.

The principal use of urine flow rate measurement is in the assessment of elderly men with suspected prostatic obstruction ('LUTS/BPH'), but there is debate about its usefulness as a test for predicting outcome of various treatments. Some studies suggest that men with poor outcomes are more likely to have had higher flows pre-operatively compared with those with good outcomes, whereas other studies report equivalent improvements in symptoms whether or not pre-operative flow rate is high or low. A recent Veterans Administration trial comparing TURP with watchful waiting in men with LUTS/BPH found that flow rate could not predict the likelihood of a good symptomatic outcome after TURP.[2]

As a consequence, different guidelines give different guidance with regard to performing uroflowmetry in men with LUTS/BPH. It is regarded as an optional test by the AUA (American Urological Association),[3] recommended by the 4th International Consultation on BPH,[4] and the EAU (European Association of Urology) BPH Guidelines state that it 'is obligatory prior to undertaking surgical treatment'.[5]

1 Reynard JM, Peters TJ, Lim C, Abrams P (1996) The value of multiple free-flow studies in men with lower urinary tract symptoms. *Br J Urol* **77**:813–18.

2 Bruskewitz RC, Reda DJ, Wasson JH, *et al.* (1997) Testing to predict outcome after transurethral resection of the prostate. *J Urol* **157**:1304–8.

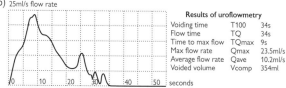

(a) 25ml/s flow rate

Results of uroflowmetry

Voiding time	T100	13s
Flow time	TQ	13s
Time to max flow	TQmax	8s
Max flow rate	Qmax	18.1ml/s
Average flow rate	Qave	11.7ml/s
Voided volume	Vcomp	151ml

(b) 25ml/s flow rate

Results of uroflowmetry

Voiding time	T100	34s
Flow time	TQ	34s
Time to max flow	TQmax	9s
Max flow rate	Qmax	23.5ml/s
Average flow rate	Qave	10.2ml/s
Voided volume	Vcomp	354ml

Fig. 3.14 (a) A uroflow trace; (b) a uroflow trace with a 'wag' artefact. The true Qmax is not 23.5 mL/s as the read-out suggests, but is nearer 18mL/s.

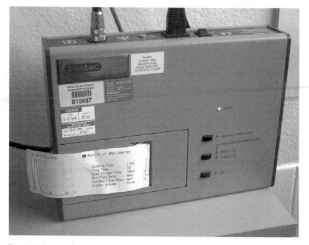

Fig. 3.15 Dantec flowmeter.

3 McConnell JD, Barry MJ, Bruskewitz RC, *et al.* (1994) *Benign prostatic hyperplasia: diagnosis and treatment. Clinical practice guideline.* Rockville: Agency for Health Care Policy and Research.

4 Denis L (ed.) (1997) *Fourth International Consultation on Benign Prostatic Hyperplasia (BPH),* Paris 1997.

5 EAU guidelines for diagnosis of BPH (2001) *Eur Urol* **40**:256–63.

Generally speaking, urine flow rate measurement is regarded as having insufficient diagnostic accuracy for it to be useful in the assessment of female lower urinary tract dysfunction. Although urine flow measurement can be used to assess voiding function in men with urethral strictures, it has limited value in younger men because in this age group the bladder can compensate for a marked degree of obstruction by contracting more forcefully. Thus, a young man may have a normal flow rate despite have a marked urethral stricture.

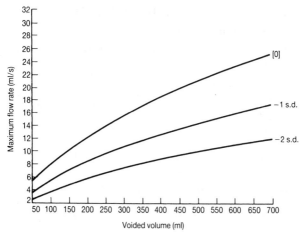

Fig. 3.16 The Bristol flow rate nomogram for men over 50 years. (Reproduced with permission).[1]

1 Fitzpatrick J (ed.) (1992) *Societe Internationale D'Urologie Reports. Non-surgical Treatment of BPH.* Edinburgh: Churchill Livingstone.

Post-void residual urine volume measurement

Post-void residual urine (PVR) volume is the volume of urine remaining in the bladder at the end of micturition. In normal individuals there should be no urine remaining in the bladder at the end of micturition. A PVR may be caused by detrusor under-activity (due to ageing—as the older bladder is less able to sustain a contraction than the younger bladder or neurological disease affecting bladder innervation), bladder outlet obstruction, or a combination of both. In clinical practice, PVR volume is measured by ultrasound after the patient has attempted to empty their bladder. A commonly used formula for calculating bladder volume is:[1,2,3,4,5]

$$\text{Bladder volume (mL)} = \text{bladder height (cm)} \times \text{width (cm)} \times \text{depth (cm)} \times 0.7$$

Interpretation and misinterpretation of PVR volume

PVR volume shows considerable day-to-day variability, with volumes recorded on different days over a 3-month period varying between 150 and 670 mL.[1]

Clinical usefulness of PVR volume measurement

PVR volume measurement cannot predict symptomatic outcome from TURP. For these reasons, residual urine volume measurement is regarded as an optional test in the AUA guidelines, but is recommended by the 4th International Consultation on BPH.[2]

Residual urine volume measurement is useful (along with measurement of serum creatinine) as a safety measure. It indicates the likelihood of back pressure on the kidneys and thus it tells the urologist whether it is safe to offer watchful waiting rather than TURP. In men with moderate LUTS, it is safe not to operate where the post-void residual volume is less than 350 mL, and this probably holds true for those with higher PVR volumes (<700 mL).[3]

Does an elevated residual urine volume predispose to urinary infection?

Though intuition would suggest yes, what evidence there is relating residual volume to urine infection suggests that an elevated residual urine may not, at least in the neurologically normal adult, predispose to urine infection.[4,5]

1 Dunsmuir WD, Feneley M, Corry DA, et al. (1996) The day-to-day variation (test–retest reliability) of residual urine measurement. Br J Urol **77**:192–3.

2 Denis L (ed.) (1997) Fourth International Consultation on Benign Prostatic Hyperplasia (BPH), Paris, 1997.

3 Bates TS, Sugiono M, James ED, et al. (2003) Is the conservative management of chronic retention in men ever justified? Br J Urol Int **92**:581–3.

4 Riehmann M, Goetzmann B, Langer E, et al. (1994) Risk factor for bacteriuria in men. Urology **43**:617–20.

5 Hampson SJ, Noble JG, Rickards D, Milroy EG (1992) Does residual urine predispose to urinary tract infection. Br J Urol **70**:506–8.

Cystometry, pressure flow studies, and videocystometry

- **Cystometry**: the recording of bladder pressure during bladder filling
- **Pressure-flow studies (PFS)**: the simultaneous recording of bladder pressure during voiding
- **Videocystometry**: fluoroscopy (X-ray screening) combined with PFS during voiding (📖 see Fig. 3.9, p. 57).

These techniques provide the most precise measurements of bladder and urethral sphincter behaviour during bladder filling and during voiding. Cystometry precedes the pressure-flow study. Bladder pressure (Pves, measured by a urethral or suprapubic catheter) and abdominal pressure (Pabd, measured by a pressure line inserted into the rectum) are recorded as the bladder fills (cystometric phase) and empties (voiding phase), and flow rate is simultaneously measured during the voiding phase. The pressure developed by the detrusor (the bladder muscle), Pdet, cannot be directly measured, but it can be derived by subtracting abdominal pressure from the pressure measured within the bladder (the intravesical pressure). This allows the effect of rises in intra-abdominal pressure caused by coughing or straining to be subtracted from the total (intravesical) pressure, so that a 'pure' detrusor pressure is obtained.

All pressures are recorded in cmH_2O and flow rate is measured in mL/s. The pressure lines are small-bore, fluid-filled catheters attached to an external pressure transducer or catheter-tip pressure transducers can be used.

A computerized print-out of intravesical pressure (Pves), intra-abdominal pressure (Pabd), and detrusor pressure (Pdet) and flow rate (Qmax) is obtained (Fig. 3.17). During bladder filling, the presence of overactive bladder contractions can be detected. During voiding, the key parameters are Qmax and the detrusor pressure at the point at which Qmax is reached, Pdet Qmax. This pressure, relative to Qmax, can be used to define the presence of bladder outlet obstruction by using a variety of nomograms, of which the ICS nomogram is most widely used.

Fill & void cys to + video (spinal)#1

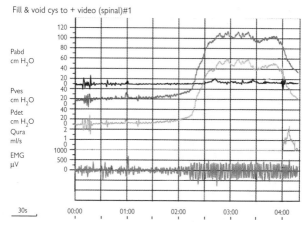

Fig. 3.17 A computerized print-out of intravesical pressure (Pves), intra-abdominal pressure (Pabd), subtracted detrusor pressure (Pdet), and flow rate (Qmax).

Chapter 4

Bladder outlet obstruction

Regulation of prostate growth and development of benign prostatic hyperplasia (BPH)

BPH is characterized by an increase in epithelial and stromal cell numbers (hyperplasia) in the peri-urethral area of the prostate. New epithelial gland formation is normally only seen during foetal development. The development of new glands in the adult prostate has given rise to the concept of 'reawakening' of the inductive effect of the prostatic stroma on the prostatic epithelium.

The increase in prostate cell number could reflect proliferation of epithelial and stromal cells, impairment of programmed cell death, or a combination of both. During the early phases of development of BPH, cell proliferation occurs rapidly. In established BPH, cell proliferation slows down and there is impairment of programmed cell death (androgens and oestrogens actively inhibit cell death).

The role of androgens in BPH (Fig. 4.1)

Testosterone can bind directly to the androgen receptor, or may be converted to a more potent form, dihydrotestosterone (DHT), by the enzyme 5α-reductase (5AR). There are two isoforms of 5AR, type I or 'extra-prostatic' 5AR (which is absent in prostatic tissue and present in, for example, skin and liver) and type II or 'prostatic' 5AR (which is found exclusively on the nuclear membrane of stromal cells, but not within prostatic epithelial cells). Type I 5AR is not inhibited by finasteride, whereas type II 5AR is.

Testosterone diffuses into prostate and stromal epithelial cells. Within *epithelial* cells it binds directly to the androgen receptor. In prostate *stromal* cells a small proportion binds directly to the androgen receptor, but the majority binds to 5AR (type II) on the nuclear membrane, is converted to DHT, and *then* binds (with greater affinity and, therefore, greater potency than testosterone) to the androgen receptor in the stromal cell. Some of the DHT formed in the stromal cells diffuses out of these cells and into nearby epithelial cells (a paracrine action). The androgen receptor/testosterone or androgen receptor/DHT complex then binds to specific binding sites in the nucleus, thereby inducing transcription of androgen-dependent genes and subsequent protein synthesis.

It is thought that stromal/epithelial interactions may be mediated by soluble growth factors—small peptides that stimulate or inhibit cell division and differentiation. Growth stimulating factors include basic fibroblastic growth factor (bFGF), epidermal growth factor (EGF), keratinocyte growth factor (KGF), and insulin-like growth factor (IGF). Transforming growth factors (e.g. TGFb) normally inhibit epithelial cell proliferation and it is possible that, in BPH, TGFb is down-regulated.

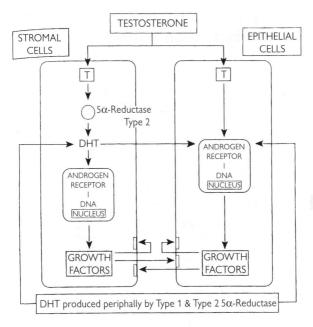

Fig. 4.1 Testosterone (T) diffuses into the prostate epithelial and stromal cell. (see text) (Reproduced with permission.[1])

1 Walsh PC, Retik AB, Vaughan D, *et al.* (eds.) (2002) *Campbell's Urology, 8th Edition,* p. 1299. Philadelphia: WB Saunders/Elsevier.

Pathophysiology and causes of bladder outlet obstruction (BOO) and BPH

The principle cause of BOO in men is BPH. Less common causes are urethral stricture and malignant enlargement of the prostate. BOO in women is altogether less common, the causes including pelvic prolapse (cystocoele, rectocoele, uterine), the prolapsing organ directly compressing the urethra; urethral stricture; urethral diverticulum; post-surgery for 'stress' incontinence; Fowler's syndrome (impaired relaxation of external sphincter occurring in premenopausal women, often in association with polycystic ovaries); and pelvic masses (e.g. ovarian masses). In either sex, neurological disease (spinal cord injury, spina bifida, MS) can cause failure of relaxation of the external sphincter during voiding (detrusor sphincter dysynergia, DSD).

The pathophysiological basis of BOO due to benign prostatic enlargement (BPE) secondary to BPH (benign prostatic obstruction, BPO) has been studied more than any other type of obstruction. BPO has dynamic and static components:

- **Dynamic component of BPO:** 1-adrenoceptor mediated prostatic smooth muscle contraction. Smooth muscle accounts for approximately 40% of the area density of the hyperplastic prostate and human prostate contracts following administration of alpha adrenergic agonists. This effect is the rationale for α-adrenoceptor blocker treatment for symptomatic BPO
- **Static component of BPO:** mediated by the volume effect of BPE.

Pathophysiological consequences of BOO

John Hunter (1786), who founded the Royal College of Surgeons of England, noted that 'The disease of the bladder arising from obstruction alone is increased irritability and its consequences, by which it admits of little distension, becomes quick in its action and thick and strong in its coats'. BOO causes thickening of the wall of the bladder. Microscopically, smooth muscle cells enlarge and there is an increase in connective tissue (collagen and elastin) between the smooth muscle bundles. In some cases, this may lead to poor compliance, with development of high bladder and intra-renal pressures. Progressive hydronephrosis can develop, with impairment of renal function and even renal failure (high pressure chronic urinary retention).

Experimentally created BOO causes development of bladder overactivity (unstable bladder contractions during bladder filling). This may be due to prolonged increased intravesical pressure during voiding causing ischaemia and leading to ischaemic damage to neurons within the bladder (i.e. denervation). Symptomatically, many patients with BOO develop frequency, urgency, and urge incontinence.

Benign prostatic obstruction (BPO): symptoms and signs

Clinical practice guidelines

Developed to standardize the approach to diagnosis (and treatment) of men presenting with symptoms suggestive of BPH (see box).[1] Every guideline agrees that a history should be taken, an examination performed, and that the severity of urinary symptoms should be formally assessed using the IPSS (the International Prostate Symptom Score). This includes a measure of the 'bother' caused by the patient's symptoms (i.e. the degree to which the symptoms are troubling).

Urinary symptoms—what do they mean?

During the 1990s, the classic 'prostatic' symptoms of frequency, urgency, nocturia, hesitancy, poor flow, an intermittent flow, and terminal dribbling—traditionally said to indicate the presence of BOO due to benign prostatic enlargement—were shown to bear little relationship to prostate size, flow rate, residual urine volume, or indeed urodynamic evidence of BOO. Age-matched elderly men and women have similar symptom scores (IPSS), despite the fact that women have no prostate and rarely have BOO.

Prostatism v. lower urinary tract symptoms (LUTS) versus LUTS/BPH

'Prostatism' has therefore been replaced by the expression 'LUTS', which avoids any implication about the cause of these symptoms. More recently, the expression 'LUTS/BPH' has been used to describe the symptoms of BPH. It doesn't really matter whether you use 'prostatism', 'LUTS', or 'LUTS/BPH', as long as you remember that urinary symptoms may have non-prostatic causes. Try to avoid treating the prostate when the problem may lie elsewhere.

Ask specifically about the presence of:

- **Bedwetting:** suggests the presence of high pressure chronic retention (look for distension of the abdomen due to a grossly enlarged bladder that is tense on palpation and dull to percussion)
- **Marked frequency and urgency, particularly when also combined with bladder pain:** look for carcinoma *in situ* of the bladder (urine cytology, flexible cystoscopy, and bladder biopsy)
- **Macroscopic haematuria:** sometimes due to a large vascular prostate, but exclude other causes (bladder and kidney cancer and stones) by flexible cystoscopy and upper tract imaging
- **Back pain and neurological symptoms** (sciatica, lower limb weakness or tingling)**:** rarely, LUTS can be due to neurological disease.

---

1 Irani J, Brown CT, van der Meulen J, Emberton M (2003) A review of guidelines on benign prostatic hyperplasia and lower urinary tract symptoms: are all guidelines the same? *Br J Urol Int* **92**:937–42.

Websites for BPH clinical practice guidelines

AUA guidelines. http://hstat.nlm.NIH.gov/ftrs/arahcpr

EAU guidelines. http://www.uroweb.org/files/uploaded_files/*BPH*.pdf

WHO (International Consensus Committee) guidelines.
   http://www.who.int/ina-ngo/ngo/ngo048.htm

Australian guidelines. http://www.health.gov.au/nhmrc/ publications/pdf/
   cp42.pdf

German guidelines. http://dgu.springer.de/Leit/pdf/3_99.pdf

Singapore guidelines. http://www.urology-singapore.org.html/
   guidelines_*BPH*.htm

Malaysian guidelines. http://www.mohtrg.gov.my/guidelines/bph98.pdf

UK guidelines. http://www.rcseng.ac.uk/publications/

Diagnostic tests in men with LUTS thought to be due to BPH

Clinical practice guidelines

Developed as an attempt to standardize the approach to diagnosis and treatment of men presenting with symptoms suggestive of BPH[1]. All agree that a history should be taken, an examination performed, and all recommend assessment of symptom severity using the IPSS (International Prostate Symptom Score). This includes a measure of the 'bother' caused by the patient's symptoms. There is considerable variation between guidelines in terms of recommended diagnostic tests. High-quality guidelines (e.g. based on results of randomized trials) recommend few diagnostic tests[2]—urine analysis, completion of a voiding diary (frequency–volume chart) to detect the presence of polyuria and nocturnal polyuria (which may be the cause of a patient's increased frequency or nocturia), and measurement of serum creatinine. They regard flow rate measurement and assessment of residual urine volume as optional tests.

Digital rectal examination (DRE) and PSA

Done to detect nodules that may indicate an underlying prostate cancer and to provide a rough indication of prostate size. Size alone is not an indication for treatment, but if surgical treatment is contemplated, marked prostatic enlargement can be confirmed by transrectal ultrasound scan (prostate volume in the order of 100 mL or more increases the likelihood of an open prostatectomy). Discuss the pros and cons of PSA testing with the patient.

Serum creatinine

Baseline measure of renal function and to detect renal failure secondary to high pressure urinary retention.

Post-void residual urine volume (PVR)

Varies considerably (by as much as 600 mL between repeat measurements) on the same or on different days[3]. It cannot predict symptomatic outcome from TURP. Along with serum creatinine it indicates whether watchful waiting is safe. It is safe *not* to operate where the PVR volume is <350 mL,[4,5] since the majority of men show no worsening of creatinine, no increase in PVR, no worsening of symptoms, and do not require TURP.

Flow rate measurement

This is variously regarded as *optional*, *recommended*, and *obligatory* prior to undertaking surgical treatment for BPH. Like PVR, measurement flow rate varies substantially on a given day,[6] cannot distinguish between BOO and a poorly contractile bladder, and is not good at predicting the likelihood of a good symptomatic outcome after TURP.

Pressure flow studies

Reasonably good at predicting symptomatic outcome after TURP. However, most patients without obstruction have a good outcome and the time, cost, and invasiveness of pressure flow studies is perceived by most urologists as not justifying their routine use.

Renal ultrasonography

To detect hydronephrosis if serum creatinine is elevated. The percentage of patients having upper tract dilatation on ultrasound according to serum creatinine is: creatinine <115 mmol/L: 0.8%, creatinine 115–130 mmol/L: 9%, and creatinine >130 mmol/L: 33%.[7]

1 Roehrborn CG, Bartsch G, Kirby R, *et al.* (2001) Guidelines for the diagnosis and treatment of benign prostatic hyperplasia: a comparative international overview. *Urology* **58**:642–50.

2 Irani J, Brown CT, van der Meulen J, Emberton M (2003) A review of guidelines on benign prostatic hyperplasia and lower urinary tract symptoms: are all guidelines the same? *Br J Urol Int* **92**:937–42.

3 Dunsmuir WD, Feneley M, Corry DA, *et al.* (1996) The day-to-day variation (test–retest reliability) of residual urine measurement. *Br J Urol* **77**:192–3.

4 Bates TS, Sugiono M, James ED, *et al.* (2003) Is the conservative management of chronic retention in men ever justified? *Br J Urol Int* **92**:581–3.

5 Wasson JH, Reda DJ, Bruskewitz RC, *et al.* (1995) A comparison of transurethral surgery with watchful waiting for moderate symptom of benign prostatic hyperplasia. The Veterans Administration Cooperative Study Group on Transurethral Resection of the Prostate. *N Engl J Med* **332**:75–9.

6 Reynard JM, Peters TJ, Lim C, Abrams P (1996) The value of multiple free-flow studies in men with lower urinary tract symptoms. *Br J Urol* **77**:813–18.

7 Koch WF, Ezz el Din KE, De Wildt MJ, *et al.* (1996) The outcome of renal ultrasound in the assessment of 556 consecutive patients with benign prostatic hyperplasia. *J Urol* **155**:186–9.

Why do men seek treatment for their symptoms?

Men seek treatment for their LUTS for several reasons:
- The symptoms may be bothersome
- They may fear that the symptoms are a warning that acute urinary retention will develop
- They may be concerned that their symptoms indicate that they have prostate cancer.

Establish what the patient wants from his consultation with you. Once reassured that the likelihood of urinary retention and prostate cancer is low, he may not want treatment for symptoms that, on the surface, may appear quite bad and he may be happy to adopt a policy of watchful waiting.

Goals of treatment
- To improve bothersome symptoms
- To prevent symptom progression
- To reduce long-term complications (urinary retention, renal insufficiency).
- Management options include watchful waiting, life style modification, drug treatments (alpha-adrenergic blockers, 5 alpha reductase inhibitors, anticholinergics, plant extracts), minimally invasive surgery, TURP, open prostatectomy. The choice of treatment is determined by the patient based on his perception of how bad (bothersome) his symptoms are, balanced against the perceived benefit and risks of the various options. Drug treatments have the least impact on symptoms, but are generally safe. Minimally invasive surgery has a somewhat greater impact, with a higher risk of side-effects. TURP and open prostatectomy have the greatest impact on symptoms, but at the risk of potentially serious complications.

Bothersome symptoms

Bothersomeness does not necessarily equate with symptom severity as assessed by symptom scores. Thus, a man with a low symptom score may find his symptoms very bothersome and may want treatment, whereas another man with a high symptom score may not be bothered and may want no treatment. If one symptom is particularly bad, but the other 6 symptoms in the 7-symptom score are minimal, overall symptom score will obviously be relatively low, but the patient may find that one symptom very bothersome (e.g. urgency and nocturia tend to be more bothersome than hesitancy or poor flow).

'Are my symptoms due to prostate cancer?'

No particular LUTS are specific for prostate cancer. Even if it later turns out that he does have prostate cancer, a patient's symptoms might be due to co-existent BPH or some other LUT pathology. If he is concerned about the possibility of prostate cancer, counsel him with regard to PSA testing and prostate biopsy.

'Am I likely to develop retention of urine?'

Many patients are understandably concerned that their urinary symptoms may be a harbinger for the development of acute urinary retention. This may influence their decision to seek help for symptoms which they may perceive as indicating a risk of subsequent retention and it may affect the type of treatment they choose. Table 4.1 can help give the patient some idea of his risk of developing urinary retention.

Table 4.1 Yearly risk of retention according to age and symptom score (i.e. number of men experiencing an episode of retention every year)*

Age (years)	Mild symptoms (AUA symptom score 7 or less)	Moderate or severe symptoms (AUA symptom score >7)
40–49	3 men in every 1000	3 men in every 1000
70–79	9 men in every 1000	34 men in every 1000

Adjusting for age and flow rate, those with an AUA symptom score of 8 or more had a 2.3-fold increased risk of going into urinary retention when compared with those with an AUA score of 7 or less. Those men with a peak flow rate of <12 mL/s had a 4-fold increased risk of urinary retention when compared with those with a flow rate of >12 mL/s. Prostate volume over 30 mL was associated with a 3-fold increased risk of urinary retention compared with those with prostate volumes less than 30 mL.

* This table is taken from Jacobsen's report, a 4-year prospective study of a cohort of >2000 men.[1] The presence of LUTS, a low flow rate, an enlarged prostate, and old age were associated with an increased risk of urinary retention.

1 Jacobsen SJ, Jacobson DJ, Girman CJ, *et al.* (1997) Natural history of prostatism: risk factors for acute urinary retention. *J Urol* **158**:481–7.

Watchful waiting for uncomplicated BPH

A number of studies have shown that in a substantial proportion of men, symptoms do not progress, even for those with severe symptoms:

- **Ball:**[1]107 men followed with watchful waiting over 5 years. In none was there an absolute indication for surgery. Half of the patients were obstructed on urodynamic testing. A third of the patients got better, just under a half stayed the same, a quarter got worse (of whom 8 underwent TURP). 2% went into retention
- **PLESS study** (Proscar long-term efficacy and safety study):[2] 1500 men with moderate to severe symptoms were randomized to placebo (and a similar number to active drug). Those on placebo had an average fall in symptom score of 1 point at 4 years
- **Wasson study of watchful waiting versus TURP:**[3] for men with moderate symptoms, the risk of progression to retention, worsening symptoms, or need for TURP was relatively low in those who chose watchful waiting. 40% noticed an improvement in their symptoms, 30% got worse, and TURP was required in about a quarter
- **Five centres' study:**[4] 500 men referred by their family doctors for consideration for TURP were managed non-operatively after viewing an educational programme. Over the following 4-year period a proportion of the men chose drug treatment or surgery. For men with mild, moderate, or severe symptoms, 10%, 24%, and 39%, respectively, had undergone surgery at the end of 4 years. For the same symptom categories, 63%, 45%, and 33% were still not receiving any treatment at the end of 4 years. Almost a quarter of men who initially presented with severe symptoms noted an improvement in their symptoms, to mild or moderate.

On the basis of these studies we can say that symptoms, even if severe, do not necessarily get worse even over fairly long periods of time. This forms the foundation of watchful waiting as an option for many patients, even if the symptoms at baseline are severe. The IPSS (International Prostate Symptom Score) measures both symptom 'severity', but more importantly the *bother* that the symptoms cause the patient. Thus, if a patient has a high symptom score (severe symptoms), but is not bothered by these symptoms, there is no indication for treatment. Some patients on the other hand have a low symptom score but may find even this degree of symptoms very bothersome. Treatment is indicated in such cases (usually starting with medical therapy such as an alpha blocker or 5 alpha reductase inhibitor).

1   Ball AJ, Feneley RC, Abrams PH (1981) Natural history of untreated 'prostatism'. *Br J Urol* **53**:613–16.

2   McConnell JD, Bruskewitz R, Walsh PC, *et al.* (1998) The effect of finasteride on the risk of acute urinary retention and the need for surgical treatment among men with benign prostatic hyperplasia (PLESS). *N Engl J Med* **338**:557–63.

3   Wasson JH, Reda DJ, Bruskewitz RC, *et al.* (1995) A comparison of transurethral surgery with watchful waiting for moderate symptoms of benign prostatic hyperplasia. The Veterans Affairs Cooperative Study Group on Transurethral Resection of the Prostate. *N Engl J Med* **332**:75–79.

4   Barry MJ, Fowler FJJ, Bin L, *et al.* (1997) The natural history of patients with benign prostatic hyperplasia as diagnosed by North American urologists. *J Urol* **157**:10–14.

Medical management of BPH: alpha blockers

The rationale for blocker therapy in BPH

As described earlier, BPO is caused partly by α1-adrenoceptor mediated prostatic smooth muscle contraction, and this is the rationale for α-adrenoceptor blocker treatment for symptomatic BPO.

There are two broad subtypes of α-adrenoceptor (AR)—α1 and α2. Molecular cloning studies have identified three α1-AR subtypes—α1a (predominant in human stroma and, therefore, mediates prostate smooth muscle contraction), α1b (predominant in human prostate epithelium), and α1L (believed to be a conformational state of the α1a-AR). The AR subtypes mediating efficacy and side-effects of α-adrenoceptor blocking drugs are unknown.

Alpha blocker classification

Alpha blockers are categorized by their selectivity for the AR, and by their elimination half-life.

- Non-selective: phenoxybenzamine—effective symptom control, but high side-effect profile
- α1: prazosin, alfuzosin, indoramin
- Long-acting α1: terazosin, doxazosin, alfuzosin SR
- Subtype selective: tamsulosin—relatively selective for α1a-AR subtype compared to the α1b subtype.

No study has directly compared one alpha blocker with another in terms of efficacy or side-effects. Terazosin and doxazosin require dose titration to minimize dizziness and syncope at the start of treatment.

Indications for treatment

Bothersome lower urinary tract symptoms where watchful waiting has failed or the patient wishes to have treatment.

Efficacy

Percentage of patients who respond to alpha blockers

Patients are able to perceive a 4-point improvement in the International Prostate Symptom Score (IPSS). If 'response' is defined as >25% improvement in symptoms relative to placebo, most studies describe response rates of 30–40%.[1] The mean probability for improvement in symptom score after TURP is in the order of 80% (i.e. 8 out of 10 men will notice an improvement in their symptoms after TURP). For those men who respond, the alpha blockers have a much more rapid onset than do the 5α-reductase inhibitors. Their effect will be maximal within a month of starting treatment.

Improvements in symptom score in men who 'respond' to alpha blockers

The average improvement in symptom score after TURP is about 85%.[2] While some of this may represent a placebo response, this improvement is considerably better than that seen with the alpha blockers, which result in a 10–30% improvement in symptom score relative to placebo.[3] This equates to a 4–5 points' improvement in symptom score over placebo.

Side-effects

A substantial proportion of men stop taking their medication either because of side-effects (15–30% report some constellation of side-effects) or because of a perceived lack of effectiveness (approximately 50% of men stop taking an alpha blocker within 3 years because of a perception that it has not worked[4]). Side-effects include asthenia (weakness, in 5%), dizziness (6%), headache (2%) and postural hypotension (1%), and retrograde ejaculation (8%). There is little data on the safety of concomitant use of the alpha blockers with drugs for erectile dysfunction.

1 Lowe F (1999) Alpha-1-adrenoceptor blockade in the treatment of benign prostatic hyperplasia. *Prostate Cancer and Prostatic Diseases* **2**:110–19.

2 McConnell JD, Barry MD, Bruskewitz RC, *et al.* (1994) *The BPH Guideline Panel. Benign Prostatic Hyperplasia: diagnosis and treatment. Clinical Practice Guideline.* Agency for Health Care Policy and Research, publication No.94–0582, 1994, Rockville, Maryland. Public Health Service, US Department of Health and Human Sciences.

3 Boyle P, Robertson C, Manski R, *et al.* (2001) Meta-analysis of randomized trials of terazosin in the treatment of benign prostatic hyperplasia. *Urology* **58**:717–22.

4 de la Rosette, Kortmann B, Rossi C, *et al.* (2002) Long term risk of retreatment of patients using alpha blockers for lower urinary tract symptoms. *J Urol* **167**:1734-9.

Medical management of BPH: 5α-reductase inhibitors

5α-reductase inhibitors inhibit the conversion of testosterone to dihydrotestosterone, the more potent androgen in the prostate. This causes shrinkage of the prostatic epithelium and therefore a reduction in prostate volume, thereby reducing the 'static' component of benign prostatic enlargement. This takes some months to occur, so urinary symptoms will not improve initially. Finasteride is a competitive inhibitor of the enzyme 5α-reductase (type II isoenzyme), which converts testosterone to DHT. Finasteride therefore lowers serum and intraprostatic DHT levels. Epristeride is a dual inhibitor of 5α-reductase. Whether it has any clinically significant advantages over finasteride remains to be established.

Efficacy

A number of large studies have shown symptom improvement over placebo in the order of 2–3 points on the IPSS and improvements in flow rate in the order of 1–2 mL/s [SCARP[1] (Scandinavian BPH Study Group), PROSPECT[2] (Proscar safety plus efficacy Canadian two-year study), PROWESS Study Group,[3] and more recently, PLESS[4] (Proscar long-term efficacy and safety study)]. The PLESS data also shows a small reduction in the risk of urinary retention.

Side-effects

Generally speaking, fairly mild. Principally centre around sexual problems (e.g. loss of libido, 5%; impotence, 5%; reduced volume of ejaculate in a few percent).

5α-reductase inhibitors and the risk of urinary retention

The PLESS data[5] have been widely publicized as showing a substantial reduction in the risk of urinary retention. In this 4-year follow-up study, 42 of 1471 men on finasteride went into urinary retention (3%), while 99 of 1404 on placebo experienced an episode of retention (7%). This represents an impressive 43% *relative* reduction in risk in those taking finasteride. However, the *absolute* risk reduction over a 4-year period is a less impressive 4%. So, finasteride does reduce the risk of retention, *but it is reducing the risk of an event which is actually quite rare* as suggested by the fact that 93% of men on placebo in this study did not experience retention over a 4-year period. Put another way, to prevent 1 episode of retention, 25 men would have to continue treatment with finasteride for 4 years.

5α-reductase inhibitors for haematuria due to BPH

Shrinking large vascular prostates probably helps reduce the frequency of haematuria in men with BPH.[55]

1 Andersen JT, Ekman P, Wolf H, *et al.* (1995) Can finasteride reverse the progress of benign prostatic hyperplasia? A two-year placebo-controlled study. The Scandinavian BPH Study Group. *Urology* **46**:631–7.

2 Nickel J, Fradet Y, Boake RC, *et al.* (1996) Efficacy and safety of finasteride therapy for benign prostatic hyperplasia: results of a 2-year randomised controlled trial (the PROSPECT study). PROscar Safety Plus Efficacy Canadian Two Year Study. *Can Med Assoc J* **155**:1251–9.

3 Marberger MJ (1998) Long-term effects of finasteride in patients with benign prostatic hyperplasia: a double-blind, placebo-controlled, multicenter study. PROWESS Study Group. *Urology* **51**:677–86.

4 McConnell JD, Bruskewitz R, Walsh PC, *et al.* (1998) The effect of finasteride on the risk of acute urinary retention and the need for surgical treatment among men with benign prostatic hyperplasia (PLESS). *N Engl J Med* **338**:557–63.

5 Foley SJ, Soloman LZ, Wedderburn AW, *et al.* (2000) Finasteride for haematuria due to BPH. A prospective study of the natural history of hematuria associated with BPH and the effect of finasteride. *J Urol* **163**:496–8.

Medical management of BPH: combination therapy

A combination of an alpha blocker and a 5α-reductase inhibitor. The studies:

- **MTOPS study**[1] (Medical Therapy of Prostatic Symptoms): this combination prevented progression of BPH (progression being defined as a worsening of symptom score by 4 or more, or the development of complications such as UTI or acute urinary retention)
- **Veterans Affairs Combination Therapy Study:**[2] 1200 men randomized to placebo, finasteride, terazosin, or both terazosin and finasteride. At 1-year follow-up, relative to placebo, finasteride had reduced the symptom score by an average of 3 points, whereas terazosin alone or in combination with finasteride had reduced the symptom score by an average of 6 points
- **PREDICT study**[3] (Prospective European Doxazosin and Combination Therapy): randomized >1000 men to placebo, finasteride, doxazosin, or both finasteride and doxazosin. Difference in symptom score at baseline and 1-year were: placebo –5.7, finasteride –6.6, doxazosin –8.3, combination therapy –8.5
- **ALFIN study**[4] (Alfuzosin, Finasteride, and combination in the treatment of BPH): 1000 men randomized to alfuzosin, finasteride, or both. At 6 months, the improvement in the IPSS was not significantly different in the alfuzosin versus the combination group.

Thus, most studies, except for MTOPS, suggest that combination therapy is no more useful than an alpha blocker alone. Disadvantages of combination therapy—greater risk of side effects, no additional benefit over alpha blockers alone in most men, need for treatment for >1 year before an improvement in symptoms is seen, sexual side effects.

In the Prostate Cancer Prevention Trial[5] 18,000 men were randomized to finasteride or placebo over a 7-year period. Those in the finasteride group had a lower prevalence of prostate cancer detected on prostate biopsy (26.5% of men receiving finasteride had a positive biopsy v. 29.5% in the placebo group). However, higher-grade tumours (i.e. biologically more aggressive than low-grade cancers) were more common in the finasteride group (there was a 1.3% increase in high grade cancers in the finasteride group). The jury is out on whether finasteride causes higher-grade cancers, or whether these findings are a histological or sampling artefact. Finasteride increases the ability (increased sensitivity) of both PSA, DRE, and prostate biopsy to diagnose high grade prostate cancer[6,7]—so called cytoreduction of the prostate leading to a greater likelihood of finding high grade cancer (the argument is that finasteride has less of an effect on PSA reduction in men with high grade than low grade cancers, so men with high grade cancer are more likely to have an elevated PSA, and therefore to undergo prostate biopsy and thus cancer detection).

1 McConnell JD, Roehrborn CG, Bautista OM, et al. (2003) The long-term effect of doxazosin, finasteride, and combination therapy on the clinical progression of benign prostatic hyperplasia. New Engl J Med **349**:2387–98.

2 Lepor H, Williford WO, Barry MJ, et al. (1996) The efficacy of terazosin, finasteride, or both in benign prostatic hypertrophy. N Engl J Med **335**:533–39.

3 Kirby RS, Roerborn C, Boyle P, et al. (2003) Efficacy and tolerability of doxazosin and finasteride, alone or in combination, in treatment of symptomatic benign prostatic hyperplasia: the Prospective European Doxazosin and Combination Therapy (PREDICT) trial. Urology **61**:119–26.

4 Debruyne FM, Jardin A, Colloi D, et al. (1998) Sustained-release alfuzosin, finasteride and the combination of both in the treatment of benign prostatic hyperplasia. Eur Urol **34**:169–75.

5 Thompson IM, Goodman PJ, Tangen CM, et al. (2003) The influence of finasteride on the development of prostate cancer. N Engl J Med **349**:215–24.

6 Thompson IM, Chi C, Ankerst DP, et al. (2006) Effect of finasteride on the sensitivity of PSA for detecting prostate cancer. J Natl Cancer Inst **98**:1128.

7 Thompson IM, Tangen CM, Goodman PJ, et al. (2007) Finasteride improves the sensitivity of digital rectal examination for prostate cancer detection. J Urol **177**:1749.

Medical management of BPH: alternative drug therapy

Anticholinergics

For a man with frequency, urgency, and urge incontinence—symptoms suggestive of an overactive bladder—consider prescribing an anticholinergic (e.g. oxybutynin, tolterodine, trospium chloride, or flavoxate). There is the concern that these drugs could precipitate urinary retention in men with BOO (because they block parasympathetic/cholinergic mediated contraction of the detrusor), but the risk of this occurring is probably very low, even in men with urodynamically proven BOO.[1]

Phytotherapy

An alternative drug treatment for BPH symptoms, and one which is widely used in Europe and increasingly in North America, is phytotherapy. 50% of all medications consumed for BPH symptoms are phytotherapeutic ones.[2] These agents are derived from plants and include the African plum (*Pygeum africanum*), purple cone flower (*Echinacea purpurea*), South African star grass (*Hipoxis rooperi*), and saw palmetto berry (*Seronoa Repens, Permixon*).

Saw palmetto contains an anti-inflammatory, antiproliferative, oestrogenic drug with 5α-reductase inhibitory activity, derived from the American dwarf palm. It has been compared with finasteride in a large double-blind, randomized trial, and equivalent (40%) reductions in symptom score were found with both agents over a 6-month period. However, a recent randomized trial suggested saw palmetto was no more effective than placebo.[3]

A meta-analysis of 18 randomized controlled trials of almost 3000 men suggests that *Seronoa repens* produces similar improvements in symptoms and flow rates to those produced by finasteride.[4]

South African star grass (*Hipoxis rooperi*, marketed as Harzol®) contains beta-sitosterol, which may induce apoptosis in prostate stromal cells, by causing elevated levels of TGF-α_1. In a double-blind, RCT symptom improvement was 5 points over that with placebo.

For other agents (e.g. *Urtica dioica*—stinging nettle; the African plum) the studies have not been placebo controlled and lack sufficient statistical power to prove conclusively that they work.[2]

1 Reynard J (2004) Does anticholinergic medication have a role for men with lower urinary tract symptoms/benign prostatic hyperplasia either alone or in combination with other agents? *Curr Opin Urol* **14**:13–16.

2 Lowe FC, Fagelman E (1999) Phytotherapy in the treatment of benign prostatic hyperplasia: an update. *Urology* **53**:671–8.

3 Bent S, Kane C, Shinohara K, *et al.* (2006) Saw palmetto for benign prostatic hyperplasia. *N Engl J Med* **354**:557-66.

4 Wilt JW, Ishani A, Stark G, *et al.* (1998) Saw palmetto extracts for treatment of benign prostatic hyperplasia: a systematic review. *JAMA* **280**:1604–8.

Minimally invasive management of BPH: surgical alternatives to TURP

In 1989, Roos reported a seemingly higher mortality and re-operation rate after TURP when compared with open prostatectomy.[1] This, combined with other studies suggesting that symptomatic outcome after TURP was poor in a substantial proportion of patients and that TURP was associated with substantial morbidity, prompted the search for less invasive treatments.

The two broad categories of alternative surgical techniques are minimally invasive and invasive. All are essentially heat treatments, delivered at variable temperature, and power and producing variable degrees of coagulative necrosis (minimally invasive) of the prostate or vaporization of prostatic tissue (invasive).

Transurethral radiofrequency needle ablation (TUNA) of the prostate

Low-level radiofrequency is transmitted to the prostate via a transurethral needle delivery system; the needles which transmit the energy being deployed in the prostatic urethra once the instrument has been advanced into the prostatic urethra. It is done under local anaesthetic, with or without intravenous sedation. The resultant heat causes localized necrosis of the prostate.

Improvements in symptom score and flow rate are modest. Side-effects include bleeding (one third of patients), urinary tract infection (UTI, 10%), and urethral stricture (2%). No adverse effects on sexual function have been reported.[2] The UK National Institute for Clinical Excellence[3] has endorsed TUNA as a minimally invasive treatment option for symptoms associated with prostatic enlargement. Concerns remain with regard to long-term effectiveness.

Transurethral microwave thermotherapy (TUMT)

Microwave energy can be delivered to the prostate via an intraurethral catheter (with a cooling system to prevent damage to the adjacent urethra), producing prostatic heating and coagulative necrosis. Sub-sequent shrinkage of the prostate and thermal damage to adrenergic neurons (i.e. heat-induced adrenergic nerve block) relieves obstruction and symptoms.

Many reports of TUMT treatment are open studies, *all* patients receiving treatment (no 'sham' treatment group where the microwave catheter is inserted, but no microwave energy is given—this results in 10-point symptom improvements in approximately 75% of men). Compared with TURP, TUMT results in symptom improvement in 55% of men and TURP in 75%. Sexual side-effects after TUMT (e.g. impotence, retrograde ejaculation) are less frequent than after TURP, but catheterization period is longer and UTI and irritative urinary symptoms are more common.[4] European Association of Urology Guidelines state that TUMT 'should be reserved for patients who prefer to avoid surgery or who no longer respond favourably to medication'. TUMT is still a popular treatment in the United States.

High-intensity focused ultrasound (HIFU)

A focused ultrasound beam can be used to induce a rise in temperature in the prostate, or indeed in any other tissue to which it is applied. For HIFU treatment of the prostate a transrectal probe is used. A general anaesthetic or heavy intravenous sedation is required during the treatment. It is regarded as an investigational therapy.

1   Roos NP, Wennberg J, Malenka DJ, *et al.* (1989) Mortality and reoperation after open and transurethral resection of the prostate for benign prostatic hyperplasia. *New Engl J Med* **320:**1120–4.

2   Fitzpatrick JM, Mebust WK (2002) Minimally invasive and endoscopic management of benign prostatic hyperplasia. In Walsh PC, Retik AB, Vaughan ED, Wein AJ (eds) *Campbell's Urology*, 8th edn. Philadelphia: Saunders.

3   *Transurethral radiofrequency needle ablation of the prostate. National Institute for Clinical Excellence Interventional Procedure Guidance,* October 2003.

4   D'Ancona FCH, Francisca EAE, Witjes WPJ, *et al.* (1998) Transurethral resection of the prostate vs high-energy thermotherapy of the prostate in patients with benign prostatic hyperplasia: long-term results. *Br J Urol* **81:**259–64.

Invasive surgical alternatives to TURP

Transurethral electrovaporization of the prostate (TUVP)

Vaporizes and dessicates the prostate. TUVP seems to be as effective as TURP for symptom control and relief of BOO, with durable (5-year) results. Operating time and in-patient hospital stay are equivalent. Requirement for blood transfusion may be slightly less after TUVP.[1,2] TUVP does not provide tissue for histological examination so prostate cancers cannot be detected. The National Institute for Clinical Excellence in the UK has endorsed TUVP as a surgical treatment option for prostatic symptoms.[3]

Laser prostatectomy

Several different techniques of 'laser prostatectomy' evolved during the 1990s. Essentially, in the year 2008 we are left with just two—holmium laser prostatectomy and the green light laser.

Transurethral ultrasound-guided laser-induced prostatectomy (TULIP)

Performed using a probe consisting of a Nd:YAG laser adjacent to an ultrasound transducer.

Visual laser ablation of the prostate (VLAP)

This side-firing system used a mirror to reflect or a prism to refract the laser energy at various angles (usually 90°) from a laser fibre located in the prostatic urethra onto the surface of the prostate. The principle tissue effect was one of coagulation with subsequent necrosis.

Contact laser prostatectomy

Produces a greater degree of vaporization than VLAP, allowing the immediate removal of tissue.

Interstitial laser prostatectomy (ILP)

Performed by transurethral placement of a laser fibre directly into the prostate that produces a zone of coagulative necrosis some distance from the prostatic urethra.

TULIP, VLAP, contact laser prostatectomy, and ILP have been succeeded by holmium laser prostatectomy.

1 Hammadeh MY, Madaan S, Hines J, Philp T (2000) Transurethral electrovaporization of the prostate after 5 years; is it effective and durable? *BJU Int* **86**: 648–51.

2 McAllister WJ, Karim O, Plail RO, *et al.* (2003) Transurethral electrovaporization of the prostate: is it any better than conventional transurethral resection of the prostate? *BJU Int* **91**: 211–14.

3 National Institute for Clinical Excellence Interventional Procedure Guidance 14, London, October 2003.

KTP laser vaporization of the prostate

Also known as 'Greenlight' photoselective vaporisation of the prostate (PVP). A ytrium-aluminium-garnet (YAG) laser light is shone through a potassium titanyl phosphate (KTP) crystal, doubling the frequency and halving the emitted light wavelength to 532 nm. This is in the green part of the visible spectrum, and is strongly absorbed by haemoglobin producing efficient prostate tissue vaporisation (☐ see Fig. 4.2). KTP energy is poorly absorbed by water/saline (the irrigant), and, therefore, a non-contact vaporization is possible. The benefits include less heating of the delivery fibre, which can last for a longer period of time. 80 and 120 W laser systems are available. In the 80 W system, approximately 100 KJ will be delivered to the average prostate in 30 min by rapid pulses of 'quasi-continuous' energy. Laser heat is concentrated over a small area, which allows rapid vaporization of tissue with minimal coagulation of underlying structures (2 mm rim of coagulated tissue is left), but creating effective haemostasis.

Indications

NICE has endorsed KTP laser prostatectomy for symptomatic benign prostatic enlargement.[1] It can be used for larger prostates (>100 mL),[2] and higher risk patients on anticoagulants.[3]

Technique

Using a KTP/532 80 W laser (Laserscope®), a 6F side-firing fibre is placed through a 24F continuous irrigation cystoscope, with normal saline irrigation. Generally, the median lobe is treated first, then the lateral lobes, using a sweeping movement of the laser fibre across the prostate, starting at the bladder neck and working distally to the level of the verumontanum. No tissue is available for histology.

1 *National Institute for Health and Clinical Excellence Interventional Procedure Guidance* 120, May 2005.

2 Sandhu JS, Ng C, Vanderbrink BA, *et al.* (2004). High-power potassium-titanyl-phosphate photoselective laser vaporisation of prostate for treatment of benign prostatic hyperplasia in men with large prostates. *J Urol* **64**:1155–9.

3 Sandhu JS, Ng CK, Gonzalez RR, *et al.* (2005). Photoselective laser vaporization prostatectomy in men receiving anti-coagulants. *J Endourol* **19**:1196–8.

Advantages over TURP

KTP laser prostatectomy can be performed safely as a day surgery operation, and in selected cases, a catheter may not be needed post-operatively, or can be removed within 24 h. It provides a virtually bloodless operation with no reported need for blood transfusion, even in anticoagulated patients. Irrigation with saline or water avoids the risk of TUR syndrome. The incidence of retrograde ejaculation is lower than TURP (8.3–52%),[1,2] with no reported cases of new erectile dysfunction. When directly compared to TURP, equivalent short-term efficacies are seen, but with significantly shorter catheterization times and in-patient stays in the laser group.[3,4]

Outcomes

Short and medium-term outcomes (up to 5 years follow-up) demonstrate sustained and statistically significant improvements in symptom scores (IPSS/AUA), flow rate and post void residual volumes.[1–6]

Post operative complications

Haematuria (1–11%); dysuria (2–21%); acute urinary retention (1–11%); re-operation rate (0–5% at 1 year).

1 Sandhu JS, Ng CK, Gonzalez RR, *et al.* (2005). Photoselective laser vaporization prostatectomy in men receiving anti-coagulants. *J Endourol* **19**:1196–8.

2 Sarica K, Alkan E, Lüleci H, *et al.* (2005). Photoselective vaporization of the enlarged prostate with KTP laser: long-term results in 240 patients. *J Endourol* **19**:1199–202.

3 Bachmann A, Schürch L, Ruszat R, *et al.* (2005). Photoselective vaporisation (PVP) versus transurethral resection of the prostate (TURP): a prospective bi-centre study of perioperative morbidity and early functional outcome. *Eur Urol* **48**:965–72.

4 Bouchier-Hayes DM, Anderson P, Van Appledorn S, *et al.* (2006). KTP laser versus transurethral resection: early results of a randomised trial. *J Endourol* **20**:580–5.

5 Sandhu JS, Ng C, Vanderbrink BA, *et al.* (2004). High-power potassium-titanyl-phosphate photoselective laser vaporisation of prostate for treatment of benign prostatic hyperplasia in men with large prostates. *J Urol* **64**:1155–9.

6 Malek RS, Kuntzman RS, Barrett DM (2005). Photoselective potassium-titanyl-phosphate laser vaporisation of the benign obstructive prostate: observations on long-term outcomes. *J Urol* **174**:1344–8.

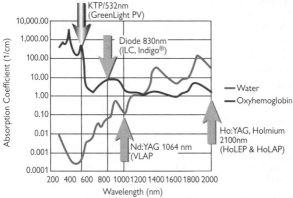

Fig. 4.2 Absorption curve of water and oxyhaemoglobin. From Laserscope ®
Physician training manual 2006. \(Reproduced with permission from the American
Medical Systems Inc, Minnesota).

Holmium (Ho): YAG laser

The holmium laser is a pulsed solid state laser with a wavelength of 2100 nm, which is strongly absorbed by water. It is absorbed into prostate tissue to a depth of 0.4 mm, and the heat created (>100°C) causes good tissue vaporization, whilst causing coagulation of small-medium sized blood vessels. The coagulative depth is about 2–3 mm beyond the tissue that has been vaporized. The irrigant is normal saline, so the risk of TUR syndrome is avoided.

Holmium laser ablation of the prostate (HoLAP)

A side-firing dual-wavelength fibre is used in a near-contact mode to vaporize prostatic tissue circumferentially to produce a satisfactory channel. Original techniques used 60 W lasers, however lasers up to 100W are now available. Symptom improvements are sustained in the long-term,[1] and when directly compared with TURP, similar efficacy was seen in the short-term, but with shorter hospital stay and catheters times in the HoLAP group, and less bleeding than for TURP.[2] Studies suggest overall it is most effective for smaller prostate glands.

Holmium laser enucleation of the prostate (HoLEP)*

HoLEP is particularly useful for treating larger prostates. An end-firing laser fibre is used to cut groves into the prostate down to the level of the capsule. The prostate lobes are then dissected off and pushed into the bladder where a mechanical morcellator is used to fragment and aspirate the tissue. HoLEP is technically more difficult to master than laser vaporization and has a longer learning curve, but the overall results are at least equivalent to TURP with fewer associated risks.

At short-term follow-up, HoLEP has proven equivocal results to TURP, however the HoLEP group had shorter catheterisation times and hospital stays, and a larger volume of prostatic tissue was removed.[3] Long-term follow-up (7 years) demonstrates sustained significant improvements in symptom scores and flow rates.[4] In a direct comparison with open prostatectomy, HoLEP has also demonstrated equivalent improvement in symptom scores and flow rates at 3 years follow-up.[5]

Holmium laser resection of the prostate (HoLRP)*

This technique copies that of TURP, whereby the precise cutting ability of the holmium laser is used to remove pieces of prostate down to the capsule, to create a large and relatively bloodless channel. It can be used on prostate glands of all sizes. Again, it has short catheterization times and hospital stays, and is associated with minimal post-operative dysuria.[6]

1 Tan AHH, Gilling PJ, Kennett KM, *et al.* (2003). Long-term results of high-power holmium laser vaporization (ablation) of the prostate. *BJU Int* **92:**707–9.

2 Mottet N, Anidjar M, Bourdon O, *et al.* (1999). Randomised comparison of transurethral electroresection and holmium:YAG laser vaporization for symptomatic benign prostatic hyperplasia. *J Endourol* **13:**127–30.

3 Wilson LC, Gilling PJ, Williams A, *et al.* (2006). A randomised trial comparing holmium laser enucleation versus transurethral resection in the treatment of prostates larger than 40 grams: results at 2 years. *Eur Urol* **50:**569–73.

4 Elzayat EA, Habib EI, Elhilali MM (2005). Holmium laser enucleation of the prostate: a size-independent new 'gold standard'. *Urology* **66:**108–13.

5 Kuntz RM, Ahyai S, Lehrich K (2006). Transurethral holmium laser enucleation of the prostate compared with transvesical open prostatectomy: 3 years follow-up of a randomised trial. *Proc SPIE* 6078:11.

6 Gilling PJ, Cass CB, Cresswell MD, *et al.* (1996). The use of holmium laser in the treatment of benign prostatic hyperplasia. *J Endourol* **5**: 459-61.

*Endorsed by NICE for the treatment of benign prostatic obstruction (National Institute for Health and Clinical Excellence Interventional Procedure Guidance 17, November 2003).

TURP and open prostatectomy

TURP

Removal of the obstructing tissue of BPH or obstructing prostate cancer from within the prostatic urethra, leaving the compressed outer zone intact (the 'surgical capsule'). An electrically-heated wire loop is used, through a resectoscope, to cut the tissue and diathermy bleeding vessels. The cut 'chips' of prostate are pushed back into the bladder by the flow of irrigating fluid and at the end of resection are evacuated using specially designed 'evacuators'—a plastic or glass chamber attached to a rubber bulb, which allows fluid to be flushed in and out of the bladder.

Indications for TURP

- Bothersome lower urinary tract symptoms that fail to respond to changes in life style or medical therapy
- Recurrent acute urinary retention
- Renal impairment due to BOO (high pressure *chronic* urinary retention)
- Recurrent haematuria due to benign prostatic enlargement
- Bladder stones due to prostatic obstruction.

Open prostatectomy

Indications

- Large prostate (>100 g)
- TURP not technically possible (e.g. limited hip abduction)
- Failed TURP (e.g. because of bleeding)
- Urethra too long for the resectoscope to gain access to the prostate
- Presence of bladder stones which are too large for endoscopic cysto-litholapaxy, combined with marked enlargement of the prostate.

Contraindications

- Small fibrous prostate
- Prior prostatectomy in which most of the gland has been resected or removed; this obliterates the tissue planes
- Carcinoma of the prostate.

Techniques

Suprapubic (transvesical)

The preferred operation if enlargement of the prostate involves mainly the middle lobe. The bladder is opened, the mucosa around the protruding adenoma is incised and the plane between the adenoma and capsule is developed to enucleate the adenoma. A 22Ch urethral and a suprapubic catheter are left, together with a retropubic drain. Remove the urethral catheter in 3 days and clamp the suprapubic at 6 days, removing it 24 h later. The drain can be removed 24 h after this (day 8).

Simple retropubic

Popularized by Terence Millin (Ireland 1947). Compared with the suprapubic (transvesical) approach it allows more precise anatomic exposure of the prostate, thus giving better visualization of the prostatic cavity, which allows more accurate removal of the adenoma, better control of bleeding points, and more accurate division of the urethra, so reducing the risk of incontinence.

As well as the contraindications noted above, the retropubic approach should not be employed when the middle lobe is very large because it is difficult to get behind the middle lobe and so to incise the mucosa (safely) distal to the ureters.

The prostate is exposed by a Pfannenstiel or lower midline incision. Haemostasis is achieved before enucleating the prostate, by ligating the dorsal vein complex with sutures placed deeply through the prostate. The prostatic capsule and adenoma are incised transversely with the diathermy just distal to the bladder neck. The plane between the capsule and adenoma is found with scissors and developed with a finger. Sutures are used for haemostasis. A wedge of bladder neck is resected. A catheter is inserted and left for 5 days, and the transverse capsular incision is closed. A large tube drain (30Ch Robinson's) is left for 1–2 days.

Complications
- Haemorrhage
- Urinary infection
- Rectal perforation (close and cover with a colostomy).

Acute urinary retention: definition, pathophysiology, and causes

Definition

Painful inability to void, with relief of pain following drainage of the bladder by catheterization.

The combination of reduced or absent urine output with lower abdominal pain is not, in itself, enough to make a diagnosis of acute retention. Many acute surgical conditions cause abdominal pain and fluid depletion, the latter leading to reduced urine output, and this reduced urine output can give the erroneous impression that the patient is in retention, when in fact they are not. Thus, central to the diagnosis is the presence of a *large* volume of urine, which when drained by catheterization, leads to resolution of the pain. What represents 'large' has not been strictly defined, but volumes of 500–800 mL are typical. Volumes <500 mL should lead one to question the diagnosis. Volumes >800 mL may be defined as acute-on-chronic retention.

Pathophysiology

Normal micturition requires:
- Afferent input to the brainstem and cerebral cortex
- Co-ordinated relaxation of the external sphincter
- Sustained detrusor contraction
- The absence of an anatomic obstruction in the outlet of the bladder.

Four broad mechanisms can lead to urinary retention:
- Increased urethral *resistance* [i.e. bladder outlet obstruction (BOO)]
- Low bladder *pressure* (i.e. impaired bladder contractility)
- Interruption of sensory or motor innervation of bladder
- Central failure of co-ordination of bladder contraction with external sphincter relaxation.

Causes in men

- Benign prostatic enlargement
- Malignant enlargement of prostate
- Urethral stricture; prostatic abscess.

Urinary retention in men is either *spontaneous* or *precipitated* by an event. Precipitated retention is less likely to recur once the event, which caused it has been removed. Spontaneous retention is more likely to recur after trial of catheter removal, and therefore to require definitive treatment (e.g. TURP). Precipitating events include anaesthetic and other drugs (anticholinergics, sympathomimetic agents, such as ephedrine in nasal decongestants); non-prostatic abdominal or perineal surgery; immobility following surgical procedures.

Causes of acute urinary retention in either sex

- Haematuria leading to clot retention
- Drugs (as above)
- Pain (adrenergic stimulation of the bladder neck)
- Post-operative retention (see below)
- Sacral cord (S2–4) injury
- Sacral (S2–4) nerve or compression or damage, resulting in detrusor areflexia—cauda equina compression (due to prolapsed L2–L3 disc or L3–L4 intervertebral disc pressing on sacral nerve roots of the cauda equina, trauma to vertebrae, benign or metastatic tumours)
- Suprasacral spinal cord injury (results in loss of coordination of external sphincter relaxation with detrusor contraction—so-called detrusor-sphincter dyssynergia (DSD)—so external sphincter contracts when bladder contracts)
- Radical pelvic surgery damaging pelvic parasympathetic plexus (radical hysterectomy, abdomino-perineal resection): unilateral injury to pelvic plexus (preganglionic parasympathetic and postganglionic sympathetic neurons) denervates motor innervation of detrusor muscle
- Pelvic fracture rupturing urethra (more likely in men than women)
- Neurotropic viruses involving sensory dorsal root ganglia of S2–4 (herpes simplex or zoster)
- Multiple sclerosis (can affect any part of CNS—Fig. 4.3); retention caused by detrusor areflexia or DSD
- Transverse myelitis
- Diabetic cystopathy (causes sensory and motor dysfunction)
- Damage to dorsal columns of spinal cord causing loss of bladder sensation (tabes dorsalis, pernicious anaemia).

Causes in women

- Pelvic prolapse (cystocoele, rectocoele, uterine); urethral stricture; urethral diverticulum
- Post-surgery for 'stress' incontinence
- Pelvic masses (e.g. ovarian masses)
- Fowler's syndrome
- *Fowler's syndrome:* increased electromyographic activity can be recorded in the external urethral sphincters of these women (which on ultrasound are of increased volume) and is hypothesized to cause impaired relaxation of external sphincter. Occurs in premenopausal women, often in association with polycystic ovaries.

Risk factors for post-operative retention

Instrumentation of lower urinary tract; surgery to perineum or anorectum; gynaecological surgery; bladder over-distension; reduced sensation of bladder fullness; pre-existing prostatic obstruction; epidural anaesthesia. Post-partum retention is not uncommon, particularly with epidural anaesthesia and instrumental delivery.

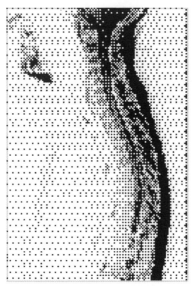

Fig. 4.3 MRI of cervical and sacral cord in a young patient presenting with urinary retention. The patient had undiagnosed MS. Signal changes are seen in the cervical, thoracic, and lumbosacral cord.

Acute urinary retention: initial and definitive management

Initial management

Urethral catheterization to relieve pain (suprapubic catheterization if urethral route not possible). Record the volume drained—this confirms the diagnosis, determines subsequent management, and provides prognostic information with regard to outcome from this treatment.

Definitive management in men

Discuss trial without catheter (TWOC) with the patient. Precipitated retention often does not recur; spontaneous retention often does. 50% with *spontaneous* retention will experience a second episode of retention within the next week or so, and 70% within the next year. A maximum flow rate (Qmax) <5 mL/s and low voiding detrusor pressure predict subsequent retention. Thus, while most will require definitive treatment (e.g. TURP), a substantial minority will get away without needing surgery.

In men, mortality in the first year after acute urinary retention is 2–3 times higher than the general male population. Not surprisingly it increases with age. A substantial proportion of this increased mortality seems to be linked to co-morbidity in these men.[11] Thus, when deciding whether to 'subject' a man to TURP for retention, remember that acute retention represents a harbinger of severe systemic disease. A careful assessment for co-morbidity (cardiovascular disease, diabetes, chronic pulmonary disease) should be made and referral for appropriate specialist advice on management of this co-morbidity should be considered.

Table 4.1 1 year mortality rates in men with acute retention

Age	Spontaneous acute retention	Precipitated acute retention
45-54	4%	10%
85 or over	33%	45%
All ages	15%	25%

Options to avoid TURP

- Prostate shrinking drugs followed by a TWOC several months later (5α-reductase inhibitors in those with benign feeling prostates, LHRH agonists in those with malignant feeling prostates on DRE, confirmed by TURS-guided prostate biopsy)
- Prostatic stents
- Long-term urethral or suprapubic catheter
- Clean, intermittent self-catheterization (CISC)—not a realistic option for most men, but some will be able and happy to do this.

Definitive management in women

CISC either until normal voiding function recovers, or permanently if it does not. Fowler's syndrome—sacral neuromodulation (e.g. Medtronic Interstim).

Risks and outcomes of TURP for retention

Relative risks of TURP for retention v. TURP for lower urinary tract symptoms (LUTS): post-operative complications 26:1; blood transfusion 2.5:1; in-hospital death 3:1. [1,2]

Failure to void after initial catheter removal: high retention volume, greater age, and low maximum detrusor pressure are predictive for failure to void after TURP. 10% in those with acute retention of urine and 40% in those with acute-on-chronic retention fail to void after initial post-TURP TWOC. Overall, 1% of men will fail to void after subsequent TWOCs and will require long-term catheterization. [3]

1 Armitage JN, Sibanda N, Cathcart P, et al. (2008) Mortality in men admitted to hospital with acute urinary retention: database analysis. *BMJ* **335**:1199–202.

2 Pickard R, Emberton M, Neal D (1998) The management of men with acute urinary retention. *Br J Urol* **81**:712–20.

3 Reynard JM (1999) Failure to void after transuretural resection of the prostate and mode of presentation. *Urology* **53**:336–9.

Indications for and technique of urethral catheterization

Indications

- Relief of urinary retention
- Prevention of urinary retention—a period of post-operative catheterization is commonly employed after many operations where limited mobility makes normal voiding difficult
- Monitoring of urine output (e.g. post-operatively); prevention of damage to the bladder during caesarean section
- Bladder drainage following surgery to the bladder, prostate, or urethra (e.g. TURP, TURBT, open bladder stone removal, radical prostatectomy)
- Bladder drainage following injuries to the bladder.

Technique

Explain the need for and method of catheterization to the patient. Use the smallest catheter—in practical terms usually a 12Ch, with a 10 mL balloon. For longer catheterization periods (weeks) use a silastic catheter to limit tissue 'reaction', thereby reducing risk of a catheter-induced urethral stricture. If clot retention, use a 3-way catheter (20Ch or greater) to allow evacuation of clots and bladder irrigation to prevent subsequent catheter blockage.

Technique is aseptic. One gloved hand is sterile, the other is 'dirty'. Dirty hand holds penis or separates labia to allow cleansing of urethral meatus; this hand should not touch catheter. Use sterile water or sterile cleaning solution to 'prep' skin around meatus.

Apply lubricant jelly to urethra. Traditionally this contains local anaesthetic (e.g. 2% lidocaine), which takes between 3 and 5 min to work. However, a randomized, placebo controlled trial showed that 2% lignocaine was no more effective for pain relief than anaesthetic-free lubricant,[1] suggesting that it is lubricant action that prevents urethral pain. If using local anaesthetic lubricant, warn patient that it may 'sting'. Local anaesthetic lubricant is contraindicated in patients with allergies to local anaesthetics and in those with urethral trauma, where there is a (theoretical) risk of complications arising from systemic absorption of lignocaine. When instilling jelly, do so gently—a sudden, forceful depression of the plunger of the syringe can rupture the urethra! In male, 'milk' gel towards posterior urethra, while squeezing meatus to prevent it from coming back out of meatus.

Insert the catheter using sterile hand, until flow of urine confirms it is in the bladder. Failure of urine flow may indicate that the catheter balloon is in the urethra. Intra-urethral inflation of balloon can rupture urethra. If no urine flows attempt aspiration of urine using a 50-mL bladder syringe (lubricant gel can occlude eye-holes of catheter). Absence of urine flow indicates either catheter is not in the bladder or, if indication for catheterization is retention, that the diagnosis is wrong (there will usually be a few mL of urine in the bladder even in cases where the absence of micturition is due to oliguria or anuria, so complete absence of urine flow usually indicates the catheter is not in the bladder). If the catheter will not pass into the bladder, and you are sure that the patient is in retention, proceed with suprapubic catheterization.

1 Birch BR (1994) Flexible cystoscopy in men: is topical anaesthesia with lignocaine gel worthwhile? *Brit J Urol* **73**:155.

Indications for and technique of suprapubic catheterization

Indications

- Failed urethral catheterization in urinary retention
- Preferred site for long-term catheters
- Long-term *urethral* catheters commonly lead to acquired hypospadias in males (ventral splitting of glans penis) and patulous urethra in females (leading to frequent balloon expulsion and bypassing of urine around the catheter); hence, suprapubic site is preferred for long-term catheters.

Contraindications

Suprapubic catheterization is best avoided in:

- Patients with clot retention, the cause of which may be an underlying bladder cancer (the cancer could be 'spread' along the catheter track to involve the skin)
- Patients with lower midline incisions (bowel may be 'stuck' to the deep aspect of the scar, leading to the potential for bowel perforation)
- Pelvic fractures, where the catheter may inadvertently enter the large pelvic haematoma which always accompanies severe pelvic fracture. This can lead to infection of the haematoma, and the resulting sepsis can be fatal. Failure to pass a urethral catheter in a patient with a pelvic fracture usually indicates a urethral rupture (confirmed by urethrography) and is an indication for formal open, suprapubic cystotomy.

Technique

Prior to insertion of trocar, be sure to confirm the diagnosis by:

- Abdominal examination (palpate and percuss lower abdomen to confirm bladder is distended)
- Ultrasound (in practice, usually not available)
- Aspiration of urine (using a green needle).

Patients with lower abdominal scars may have bowel interposed between the abdominal wall and bladder, and this can be perforated if the trocar is inserted near the scar and without prior aspiration of urine. In such cases, ultrasound guided catheterization may be sensible.

Use a wide-bore trocar if you anticipate that the catheter will be in place for more than 24 h (small-bore catheters will block within a few days). Aim to place the catheter about 2–3 finger-breadths above the pubis symphysis. Placement too close to the symphysis will result in difficult trocar insertion (the trocar will hit the symphysis). Instil a few mL of local anaesthetic into skin of intended puncture site and down to rectus sheath. Confirm location of bladder by drawing back on needle to aspirate urine from bladder. This helps guide the angle of trocar insertion. Make a 1-cm incision with a sharp blade through the skin. Hold trocar handle in your right hand and steady needle end with your left hand (this hand helps prevent insertion too deeply). Push the trocar in the same direction in which you previously aspirated urine. As soon as urine issues from the trocar, withdraw the latter, holding the attached sheath in place. Push the catheter in as far as it will go. Inflate the balloon. Peel away the side of the sheath and remove it.

Complications of urethral and suprapubic catheters

At the time of insertion

- Bowel perforation that accounts for the reported mortality of suprapubic catheter insertion of 1–2%.[1,2] Try to avoid the temptation to describe SPC insertion as a 'minor' procedure!
- Persistent haematuria (may require bladder washouts and even very occasionally return to theatres for cystoscopic diathermy of the bleeding point, if it can be found).

Long term problems and complications

- **Recurrent UTIs.** The definition of what represents a 'UTI' is a source of much confusion and the cause of much inappropriate prescribing of antibiotics, which inevitably leads to the development of resistant bacteria in the urine. Inevitably, any foreign body in the bladder will become colonized with bacteria very rapidly. We do not regard the mere presence of bacteria or pus cells (of whatever number) as indicative of a UTI (the presence of bacteria in the absence of constitutional symptoms of feeling unwell, a fever, and cloudy, smelly urine is not regarded as 'active' infection, but rather is better termed 'colonization'). Avoid the temptation to prescribe antibiotics for mere colonization. Symptomatic UTIs (fever, feeling generally unwell, smelly, cloudy urine) can be a very difficult problem to manage. Not infrequently patients (particularly those with spinal cord injuries managed with long-term catheter drainage) report such symptoms in the absence of *any* bacterial growth in the urine. Others report feeling perfectly well, for months on end, in the face of urine that is full of bacteria! Remember, although short courses of antibiotics (7–10 days) may resolve what we think may be the symptoms of UTI, no amount of antibiotics will, over the long term, be able to sterilize the urine of a patient with a foreign body such as a catheter in it. Low dose antibiotics (a quarter of the normal daily treatment dose) may keep the symptoms at bay or reduce the frequency of 'infective' episodes (but long-term use of nitrofurantoin or trimethoprim—two popular low dose antibiotics—is associated, albeit rarely, with severe side-effects such as blood dyscrasias or pulmonary fibrosis). In some patients, the only solution is to change bladder management. There is a greater risk of pyelonephritis in the chronically catheterized patient.

1   Ahluwalia RS, Johal N, Kouriefs C et al. (2006) The surgical risk of suprapubic catheter insertion and long-term sequelae. *Ann R Coll Surg Engl* **88**: 171–6.

2   Sheriff MK, Foley S, McFarlene J, et al. (1998) Long-term suprapubic catheterization: clinical outcome and satisfaction survey. *Spinal Cord* **36**: 171–6.

- **Catheter blockages** due to encrustation of the lumen of the catheter with bacterial biofilms. Proteus mirabilis, Morganella and Providencia species secrete a polysaccharide matrix. Within this urease producing bacteria generate ammonia from nitrogen in urine, raising urine pH and precipitating magnesium and calcium phosphate crystals. The matrix-crystal complex blocks the catheter. Catheter blockage causes bypassing, which soils the patient's clothes. Bladder distension can cause autonomic dysreflexia in patients with thoracic or cervical spinal cord injuries, leading to extreme rises in blood pressure that, believe it or not, can cause stroke and death! Regular bladder washouts and increased catheter size sometimes help. There is a suggestion, based on *in vitro* experiments on catheters in the laboratory that intermittent catheter drainage (by the use of a valve inserted between the catheter and the drainage bag) can reduce the likelihood of catheter blockages. Whether this holds true in patients remains to be documented
- **Bladder stone formation**, necessitating surgical removal (endoscopic or open cystolithotomy) occurs in 1 in 4 patients followed over a 5-year period[1]
- **'Track' problems at the time of catheter changes:** difficultly removing the catheter (some catheter balloons have a 'memory', retaining a an awkward shape such that they resist removal); difficulty reinserting the catheter (may require re-positioning of the SPC site
- In female patients managed by a long-term urethral catheter, the pressure of the catheter can cause urethral and bladder neck erosion, leading to a so-called patulous urethra. In the male, a long-term urethral catheter can lead to pressure atrophy of the meatus of the penis, leading to an acquired hypospadias ('kippering' of the glans penis and even the shaft of the penis). While a mild acquired hypospadias has no great functional effect, cosmetically it does
- **Catheter bypassing**, either around the suprapubic site or per-urethra. Management is empirical. Try as small a balloon size as possible. If the leakage is due to bladder spasms then a smaller balloon may, possibly, reduce their intensity and frequency. Anticholinergics may help as may intravesical botox injections. Other options include condom sheath drainage (in men) or bladder neck closure. This is not the minor operation ('just a few stitches') that patients are sometimes led to believe and often—30% of cases—the closure breaks down so the leak persists). Bladder neck closure is irreversible and access to the bladder via the suprapubic track is not always easy, particularly if access to the ureteric orifices is required for upper tract endoscopy
- **Bladder cancer** (squamous cell carcinoma of the bladder): there is conflicting evidence regarding the incidence of bladder cancer in spinal cord injured patients some studies suggesting an increased risk and others suggesting the risk is the same as in the non-spinal injured population.[2] The author feels that the risk of squamous cell cancer is greater than in the ambulant, non-catheterized population, but that the risk is still low. The pathogenesis is likely to involve chronic bacterial colonization of the bladders of spinal patients, whether managed with indwelling catheters, ISC, or sheath drainage, and so the presence of the catheter *per se* is not enough to induce development of a cancer. Screening cystoscopy studies have either failed to result in

a down-staging of bladder cancer when compared with non-screened patients or have simply not detected any cases of bladder cancer was detected. Screening cystoscopy remains a subject of debate.[3]

Further reading

Hamid R, Bycroft J, Arya M, Shah PJ. (2003) Screening cystoscopy and biopsy in patients with neuropathic bladder and chronic suprapubic indwelling catheters: is it valid? *J Urol* **170**(2 Pt 1):425–7.

Ord J, Lunn D, Reynard J. (2003) Bladder management and risk of bladder stone formation in spinal cord injured patients. *J Urol* **170**:1734–7.

Sabbuba NA, Stickler DJ, Long M, *et al.* (2005) Does the valve-regulated release of urine from the bladder reduce the encrustation and blockage of indwelling catheters by crystalline Proteus mirabilis biofilms? *J Urol* **173**:262–6.

Stickler DJ, Zimakoff J. (1994) Complications of urinary tract infections associated with devices for long-term bladder management. *J Hosp Infect* **28**:177–94.

Warren JW, Muncie HL, Hebel JR, Hall-Craggs M. (1994) Long-term urethral catheterisation increases risk of chronic pyelonephritis and renal inflammation. *J Am Geriatr Soc* **42**:1286–90.

1   Ord J, Lunn D, Reynard J. (2003) Bladder management and risk of bladder stone formation in spinal cord injured patients. J Urol 170:1734–7.

2   Subramonian K, Cartwright RA, Harnden P, Harrison SCW. (2004) Bladder cancer in patients with spinal cord injuries. *Br J Urol Int* **93**:739–43.

3   Hamid R, Bycroft J, Arya M, Shah PJ. (2003) Screening cystoscopy and biopsy in patients with neuropathic bladder and chronic suprapubic indwelling catheters: is it valid? *J Urol* **170**(2 Pt 1):425–7.)

Management of nocturia and nocturnal polyuria

Nocturia can be particularly resistant to treatment.

First, establish whether the patient is polyuric (>3 L or urine/24 h) by getting them to complete a frequency volume chart. If they are polyuric, this may account for their daytime and night-time voiding frequency. Establish whether they have a solute or water diuresis, and the causes thereof (see box).

If non-polyuric (<3 L urine output/24 h), determine the *distribution* of urine output over the 24-h period. If >1/3 of urine output is between the hours of midnight and 8 a.m. then the patient has nocturnal polyuria (NP).

Non-polyuric nocturia

BPH medical therapy

The impact of alpha blockers, 5α-reductase inhibitors, and anticholinergics on nocturia is modest.

TURP

Nocturia persists in 20–40% of men after TURP.

Medtronic Interstim therapy for nocturia

Patients pre-selected on the basis of a favourable symptomatic response to a test stimulation can experience a reduction in nocturia,[1] but not all patients respond to the test stimulation and the treatment is expensive and not yet widely available in all countries.

Treatment for nocturnal polyuria (NP)

The evidence base for NP treatments is limited (very few randomized, placebo controlled trials).

Fluid restriction

Many patients have reduced their afternoon and evening fluid intake in an attempt to reduce their night-time diuresis.

Diuretics

Diuretics, taken several hours before bedtime, reduce nocturnal voiding frequency in some patients.[2]

DDAVP

A synthetic analogue of arginine vasopressin (endogenous ADH), which if taken at night can reduce urine flow by its antidiuretic action. It has been suggested that NP may be caused by a lack of endogenous production of ADH in elderly people. However, adults both with and without NP have no rise in ADH at night (i.e. ADH secretion remains remarkably *constant* throughout the day in adults with and without NP). Furthermore, the diuresis in adults with NP is a *solute* diuresis due to a nocturnal natriuresis.[3] Thus, lack of ADH secretion at night is *not* the cause of the diuresis in nocturnal polyuric adults and, therefore, from a theoretical perspective there is no logical basis for using desmopression in NP.[4] There is limited evidence that it reduces night-time voiding frequency (at least in responder enrichment studies) and increases sleep duration in a proportion of patients with NP.[5]

Side effects: hyponatraemia (Na < 130 mmol/L) in 5% of patients. Measure serum Na 3 days after starting DDAVP and stop if hyponatraemia develops.

Nocturia and sleep apnoea

Obstructive sleep apnoea (OSA) is highly prevalent in those over 65 years of age. It is often manifested by snoring. There is a strong association between OSA symptoms and nocturia.[6] Large negative intrathoracic pressure swings may trigger a cardiac-mediated natriuresis and, hence, cause NP.

Investigation of the polyuric patient (= urine output of >3 L per 24h)

Urine osmolarity?
>250 mosm/kg = solute diuresis
<250 mosm/kg = water diuresis
Solute diuresis—poorly controlled diabetes mellitus; saline loading (e.g. post-operative diuresis); the diuresis following relief of high pressure chronic retention
Water diuresis—primary polydipsia; diabetes insipidus (nephrogenic— e.g. lithium therapy, central—ADH deficiency)

1   Spinelli M (2003) New sacral neuromodulation lead for percutaneous implantation using local anesthesia: description and first experience. *J Urol* **170**:1905–7.

2   Reynard JM, Cannon A, Yang Q, Abrams P (1998) A novel therapy for nocturnal polyuria: a double-blind randomized trial of frusemide against placebo. *Br J Urol* **81**:215–18.

3   Matthiesen TB, Rittig S, Norgaard JP, Pedersen EB, Djurhuus JC (1996) Nocturnal polyuria and natriuresis in male patients with nocturia and lower urinary tract symptoms. *J Urol* **156**:1292–9.

4   McKeigue P, Reynard J (2000) Relation of nocturnal polyuria of the elderly to essential hypertension. *Lancet* **355**:486–8.

5   Mattiasson A (2002) Efficacy of desmopressin in the treatment of nocturia: a double-blind placebo-controlled study in men. *Br J Urol* **89**:855–62.

6   Umlauf M (1999) Nocturia and sleep apnea symptoms in older patients: clinical interview. *Sleep* **22**:S127.

High pressure chronic retention (HPCR)

This is maintenance of voiding, with a bladder volume of >800 mL and an intravesical pressure above 30 cmH$_2$O, accompanied by hydronephrosis.[1,2] Over time this leads to renal failure. When the patient is suddenly unable to pass urine, acute-on-chronic high pressure retention of urine has occurred.

A man with high pressure retention who continues to void spontaneously may be unaware that there is anything wrong. He will often have no sensation of incomplete emptying and his bladder seems to be insensitive to the gross distension. Often the first presenting symptom is that of bedwetting. This is such an unpleasant and disruptive symptom that it will cause most people to visit their doctor. Visual inspection of the patient's abdomen may show marked distension due to a grossly enlarged bladder. The diagnosis of chronic retention can be confirmed by palpation of the enlarged, tense bladder, which is dull to percussion.

Acute treatment

Catheterization relieves the pressure on the kidneys and allows normalization of renal function. A large volume of urine is drained from the bladder (often in the order of 1–2 L, and sometimes much greater). The serum creatinine is elevated and an ultrasound will show hydronephrosis with a grossly distended bladder if the scan is done before relief of retention.

Anticipate a profound diuresis following drainage of the bladder. This is due to:

- Excretion of salt and water that has accumulated during the period of renal failure
- Loss of the corticomedullary concentration gradient, due to continued perfusion of the kidneys with diminished flow of urine through the nephron (this washes out the concentration gradient between the cortex and medulla)
- An osmotic diuresis caused by elevated serum urea concentration.

A small percentage of patients have a postural drop in blood pressure. It is wise to admit patients with HPCR for a short period of observation, until the diuresis has settled. A few will require intravenous fluid replacement if they experience a symptomatic fall in blood pressure when standing.

Definitive treatment

TURP or a long-term catheter. In those unable to void who have been catheterized, a trial without catheter is clearly not appropriate in cases where there is back pressure on the kidneys. Very rarely a patient who wants to avoid a TURP and does not want an in-dwelling catheter will be able to empty their bladder by intermittent self-catheterization, but such cases are exceptional.

1   Mitchell JP (1984) Management of chronic urinary retention. *BMJ* **289**:515–16.

2   Abrams P, Dunn M, George N (1978) Urodynamic findings in chronic retention of urine and their relevance to results of surgery. *BMJ* **2**:1258–60.

Bladder outlet obstruction and retention in women

Relatively rare (~5% of women undergoing pressure flow studies have BOO, compared with 60% of unselected men with LUTS).[1,2]

It may be symptom-free, and present with LUTS or as acute urinary retention. In broad terms, the causes are related to obstruction of the urethra (e.g. urethral stricture, compression by a prolapsing pelvic organ, such as the uterus, post-surgery for stress incontinence) or have a neurological basis (e.g. injury to sacral cord or parasympathetic plexus, degenerative neurological disease, e.g. MS, diabetic cystopathy).

Voiding studies in women

Women have a higher Qmax, for a given voided volume, than do men. Women with BOO have lower Qmax than those without BOO. There are no universally accepted urodynamic criteria for diagnosing BOO in women.

Treatment of BOO in women

Treat the cause (e.g. dilatation of a urethral stricture; repair of a pelvic prolapse). Where this it is not possible (because of a neurological cause such as MS or spinal cord injury), the options are:
- Intermittent self-catheterization (ISC) or intermittent catheterization by a carer
- In-dwelling catheter (preferably suprapubic, rather than urethral)
- Mitrofanoff catheterizable stoma.

Where urethral intermittent self-catheterization is technically difficult, a catheterizable stoma can be constructed between the anterior abdominal wall and the bladder, using the appendix, Fallopian tube, or a narrowed section of small intestine. This is the Mitrofanoff procedure. It is simply a new urethra, which has an abdominal location, rather than a perineal one, and is therefore easier to access for ISC.

For women with a suprasacral spinal cord injury with preserved detrusor contraction and urinary retention due to detrusor-sphincter dyssynergia (DSD), sacral deafferentation combined with a Brindley stimulator can be used to manage the resulting urinary retention.

Fowler's syndrome

A primary disorder of sphincter relaxation (as opposed to secondary to, for example, SCI). Increased electromyographic activity (repetitive discharges on external sphincter EMG) can be recorded in the external urethral sphincters of these women (which on ultrasound are of increased volume) and is hypothesized to cause impaired relaxation of external sphincter. Occurs in premenopausal women, typically aged 15–30, often in association with polycystic ovaries (50% of patients), acne, hirsutism, and menstrual irregularities. May also be precipitated by childbirth or gynaecological or other surgical procedures. They report no urgency with bladder volumes >1000 mL, but when attempts are made to manage their retention by ISC, they experience pain, especially on withdrawing the catheter.
Pathophysiology: may be due to a channelopathy of the striated urethral sphincter muscle leading to involuntary ES contraction.

Treatment: ISC, sacral neuromodulation with Medtronic Interstim (90% void post implantation and 75% are still voiding at 3 years' follow-up). The mechanism of action of sacral neuromodulation in urinary retention is unknown.

1   Madersbascher S, Pycha A, Klingler CH, *et al.* (1998) The aging lower urinary tract: a comparative urodynamic study of men and women. *Urology* **51**:206–12.

2   Swinn MJ, Fowler C, *et al.* (2002) The cause and treatment of urinary retention in young women. *J Urol* **167**:151–6.

Urethral stricture disease

A urethral stricture is an area of narrowing in the calibre of the urethra due to formation of scar tissue in the tissues surrounding the urethra. The disease process of anterior urethral stricture disease is different to that in the posterior urethra.

Anterior urethra

The process of scar formation occurs in the spongy erectile tissue (corpus spongiosum) of the penis that surrounds the urethra—spongiofibrosis:

- Inflammation (e.g. balanitis xerotica obliterans—BXO), gonococcal infection leading to gonococcal urethritis (less common nowadays because of prompt treatment of gonorrhea)
- Trauma
  - Straddle injuries—blow to bulbar urethra (e.g. cross-bar injury)
  - Iatrogenic—instrumentation (e.g. traumatic catheterization, traumatic cystoscopy, TURP, bladder neck incision).

The role of non-specific urethritis (e.g. *Chlamydia*) in the development of anterior urethral strictures has not been established.

Posterior urethra

Fibrosis of the tissues around the urethra results from trauma—pelvic fracture or surgical (radical prostatectomy, TURP, urethral instrumentation). These are essentially *distraction* injuries, where the posterior urethra has been pulled apart and the subsequent healing process results in the formation of a scar, which contracts and thereby narrows the urethral lumen.

Symptoms and signs of urethral stricture

- Voiding symptoms—hesitancy, poor flow, post-micturition dribbling
- Urinary retention—acute, or high pressure acute-on-chronic
- Urinary tract infection—prostatitis, epididymitis.

Management of urethral strictures

Where the patient presents with urinary retention, the diagnosis is usually made following a failed attempt at urethral catheterization. In such cases, avoid the temptation to 'blindly' dilate the urethra. Dilatation may be the wrong treatment option for this type of stricture—it may convert a short stricture, which could have been cured by urethrotomy or urethroplasty, into a longer and more dense stricture, thus committing the patient to more complex surgery and a higher risk of recurrent stricturing. Place a suprapubic catheter instead, and image the urethra with retrograde and antegrade urethrography to establish the precise position and the length of the stricture.

Similarly, avoid the temptation to inappropriately dilate a urethral stricture diagnosed at flexible cystoscopy (urethroscopy). Arrange retrograde urethrography so appropriate treatment can be planned.

Treatment options

Urethral dilatation: designed to stretch the stricture without causing more scarring; bleeding post-dilatation indicates tearing of the stricture (i.e. further injury has been caused) and restricturing is likely.

Internal (optical) urethrotomy: stricture incision, with an endoscopic knife or laser. Divides the stricture, followed by epithelialization of the incision. If deep spongiofibrosis is present, the stricture will recur. Best suited for short (<1.5 cm) bulbar urethral strictures with minimal spongiofibrosis.[1] Leave a catheter for 3–5 days (longer catheterization does not reduce long-term restricturing). Consider ISC for 3–6 months, starting several times daily, reducing to once or twice a week towards the end of this period.

Excision and reanastomosis or tissue transfer: excises the area of spongiofibrosis with primary reanastomosis or closure of defect with buccal mucosa or pedicled skin flap; best chance of cure.

A stepwise progression up this 'reconstructive ladder' (the process of starting with a simple procedure and moving onto the next level of complexity when this fails) is not appropriate for every patient. For the patient who wants the best chance of long-term cure, offer excision, and reanastomosis or tissue transfer up front. For the patient who is happy with lifelong 'management' of his stricture (with repeat dilatation or optical urethrotomy), offer dilatation or optical urethrotomy.

Balanitis xerotica obliterans (BXO)

Genital lichen sclerosis and atrophicus in the male. Hyperkeratosis is seen histologically. Appears as a white plaque on the foreskin, glans of the penis, or within the urethral meatus. Most common cause of stenosis of the meatus. Foreskin becomes thickened and adheres to the glans, leading to phimosis (a thickened, non-retractile foreskin). Patients with long-standing BXO and meatal stenosis often have more proximal urethral strictures.

1   Pansadoro V, Emiliozzi P (1996) Internal urethrotomy in the management of anterior urethral strictures: long term follow-up. *J Urol* **156**:73–75.

Incontinence

Classification

Definition

Urinary incontinence (UI) is the complaint of any involuntary leakage of urine.[1] It results from a failure to store urine during the filling phase of the bladder due to abnormality of bladder smooth muscle (detrusor) or the urethral sphincter. Urine loss is either urethral or extra-urethral (secondary to anatomical abnormalities including ectopic ureters, rectovesical or vesicovaginal fistulae).

Prevalence

There is wide variation in the reported prevalence of UI worldwide. It affects about 3.5 million people in the UK, females > males, and increases with age (Table 5.1).[2] Several other studies demonstrate a trend for a general increase in UI during adulthood, stabilizing between the ages of 50 and 70 years old, before increasing in prevalence again.

Classification

Stress urinary incontinence (SUI): involuntary urinary leakage on effort, exertion, sneezing or coughing.[1] It is due to hypermobility of the bladder base, pelvic floor, and/or intrinsic urethral sphincter deficiency. When confirmed on urodynamic testing, it is referred to as urodynamic stress incontinence. It can be further categorized (using video-urodynamics) into:
- **Type 0**: report of urinary incontinence, but without clinical signs
- **Type I**: leakage that occurs during stress with <2 cm descent of the bladder base below the upper border of the symphysis pubis
- **Type II**: leakage on stress accompanied by marked bladder base descent (>2 cm) that occurs only during stress (II_a) or is permanently present (II_b)
- **Type III**: bladder neck and proximal urethra are already open at rest (with or without descent), which is also known as intrinsic sphincter deficiency (ISD).

Urge urinary incontinence (UUI): involuntary urine leakage accompanied by, or immediately preceded by urgency[1] (a sudden, strong desire to void). It is due to an overactive detrusor muscle. The urodynamic diagnosis is termed detrusor overactivity incontinence. It is a component of the overactive bladder syndrome (📖 see OAB, p. 148).

Mixed urinary incontinence (MUI): involuntary leakage associated with urgency, and also with exertion, effort, sneezing or coughing.[1] It contains symptoms of both SUI and UUI.

Overflow incontinence: is leakage of urine when the bladder is abnormally distended with large residual volumes. Typically, men present with chronic urinary retention (with a degree of detrusor failure) and dribbling incontinence. This can lead to back pressure on the kidneys and renal failure in 30% of patients. Bladder outlet obstruction must be corrected; detrusor failure can be managed with clean intermittent self-catheterization (CISC) or in-dwelling catheter.

Nocturnal enuresis: the complaint of loss of urine occurring during sleep.[1] The prevalence in adults is about 0.5%,[3] and 7–10% in children aged

7 years old.[4] Nocturnal enuresis can be further classified into primary types (never been dry for longer than a 6-month period) or secondary (the re-emergence of bed wetting after a period of being dry for at least 6–12 months; see p. 658).

Post-micturition dribble: the complaint of a dribbling loss of urine that occurs after voiding. It predominantly affects males and is due to pooling of urine in the bulbous urethra after voiding. It affects 17% of healthy adults,[5] and 67% of those with existing LUTS.[6]

Table 5.1 Prevalence of urinary incontinence in UK

Age (years)	Females	Males
15–44	5–7%	3%
45–64	8–15%	3%
65 +	10–20%	7–10%

1 Abrams P, Cardozo L, Fall M, et al. (2002). The standardization of terminology of lower urinary tract function: report from the standardization sub-committee of the International Continence Society. Neurourol Urodyn **21**:167–78.

2 Royal College of Physicians (1995) Incontinence: Causes, Management and Provision of Services. Report of a working party. London: RCP. Available at: www.rcplondon.ac.uk

3 Hirasing RA, van Leerdam FJM, Bolk-Bennink L, et al. (1997) Enuresis nocturna in adults. Scan J Urol Nephrol **31**:533–6.

4 Abrams P, Cardozo L, Khoury S, Wein A. (2005) Epidemiology of Urinary and Faecal Incontinence and Pelvic Organ Prolapse, 3rd International Consultation on Incontinence, 2005. London: Health Publications Ltd.

5 Furuya S, Ogura H, Tanaka M et al. (1997) Incidence of postmicturition dribble in adult males in their twenties through fifties. Hinyokika Kiyo **43(6)**:407–10.

6 Paterson J, Pinnock CB, Marshall VR (1997) Pelvic floor exercises as a treatment for post-micturition dribble. Br J Urol **79**:892–7.

Causes and pathophysiology

General risk factors for urinary incontinence (UI)

Predisposing factors

- Gender (female>males)
- Race (Caucasian>Afro-Caribbean)
- Genetic predisposition
- Neurological disorders (spinal cord injury, stroke, multiple sclerosis, Parkinson's disease)
- Anatomical disorders (vesicovaginal fistula, ectopic ureter, urethral diverticulum)
- Childbirth (vaginal delivery, increasing parity) and pregnancy
- Anomalies in collagen subtype
- Pelvic, perineal and prostate surgery (radical hysterectomy, prostatectomy, TURP) leading to pelvic muscle and nerve injury
- Radical pelvic radiotherapy.

Promoting factors

- Smoking (associated with chronic cough and raised intra-abdominal pressure)
- Obesity
- Infection (UTI)
- Increased fluid intake
- Medications
- Poor nutrition
- Ageing
- Cognitive deficits
- Poor mobility
- Oestrogen deficiency (menopause).

Pathophysiology

The underlying aetiology for UI can only be absolutely determined by urodynamic studies. Causes include:

Bladder abnormalities

Detrusor overactivity: a urodynamic observation characterized by involuntary bladder muscle (detrusor) contractions during the filling phase of the bladder, which may be spontaneous or provoked, and can consequently cause urinary incontinence. The underlying cause may be neurogenic, where there is a relevant neurological condition, or idiopathic, where there is no defined cause. It leads to the symptoms of urge incontinence and overactive bladder (OAB).

Low bladder compliance: characterized by a decreased volume to pressure relationship, where there is a high increase in bladder pressure during filling due to alterations in elastic properties of the bladder wall, or changes in muscle tone (secondary to myelodysplasia, spinal cord injury, radical hysterectomy, interstitial or radiation cystitis).

Sphincter abnormalities

In females there may be functional abnormalities of urethral hypermobility and/or intrinsic sphincter deficiency (ISD). These are the main causes of SUI.

Urethral hypermobility: due to a weakness of pelvic floor support causing a rotational descent of the bladder neck and proximal urethra during increases in intra-abdominal pressure. If the urethra opens concomitantly, there will be urinary leaking.

Intrinsic sphincter deficiency (ISD): describes an intrinsic malfunction of the sphincter, regardless of its anatomical position, which is responsible for type III SUI. Causes include inadequate urethral compression (previous urethral surgery, ageing, menopause, radical pelvic surgery, anterior spinal artery syndrome) or deficient urethral support (pelvic floor weakness, childbirth, pelvic surgery, menopause). In males, the urethral sphincter may be damaged after prostatic or pelvic surgery (TURP, radical prostatectomy).

Evaluation

History

Aim: to establish the type of incontinence (stress, urge or mixed). Enquire about LUTS (storage or voiding symptoms); triggers for incontinence (cough, sneezing, exercise, position, urgency); frequency and severity of symptoms. Establish risk factors (abdominal/pelvic surgery or radiotherapy, neurological diseases, obstetric and gynaecology history, medications). A validated patient completed questionnaire is helpful (ICIQ-SF,[1,6] ICIQ-FLUTS,[2] ICIQ-MLUTS,[3] SF36 QOL,[4] IPSS[5]).

Physical examination

Women

Perform a chaperoned pelvic examination in the supine, standing, and left lateral position with a Sim's speculum. Ask the patient to cough or strain, and inspect for vaginal wall prolapse (cystocele, rectocele, enterocele), uterine or perineal descent, and urinary leakage (stress test). Internal pelvic examination can be performed to assess the strength of voluntary pelvic floor muscle strength and inspect the vulva for oestrogen deficiency (causing atrophy), which may require topical oestrogen treatment.

Both sexes

Examine the abdomen for a palpable bladder (indicating urinary retention if the patient has recently passed urine). A neurological examination should include assessment of anal tone and reflex, perineal sensation, and lower limb function.

---

1 **ICIQ-SF:** International Consultation on Incontinence Questionnaire (short form) for men and women, to assess symptom score and quality of life (☐ see Fig. 5.1).

2 **ICIQ-FLUTS:** ICIQ on Female Lower Urinary Tract Symptoms. Assesses occurrence and bother of symptoms relating to incontinence and other urinary symptoms in females.

3 **ICIQ-MLUTS:** ICIQ Male Lower Urinary Tract Symptoms.

4 **SF36 QOL:** Short Form 36 health survey questionnaire. Assesses health status in persons with incontinence.

5 **IPSS:** International Prostate Symptom Score (☐ see Fig. 2.1 p. 17).

6 Avery K, Donovan J, Peters TJ, *et al.* (2004) ICIQ: a brief and robust measure for evaluating the symptoms and impact of urinary incontinence. *Neurourol Urodyn* **23**:322–30.

Many people leak urine some of the time. We are trying to find out how many people leak urine, and how much this bothers them. We would be grateful if you could answer the following questions, thinking about how you have been, on average, over the PAST FOUR WEEKS.

1 Please write in your date of birth:

☐☐   ☐☐   ☐☐
DAY   MONTH   YEAR

2 Are you *(tick one)*:   Female ☐   Male ☐

---

3 How often do you leak urine? *(Tick one box)*

never	☐	0
about once a week or less often	☐	1
two or three times a week	☐	2
about once a day	☐	3
several times a day	☐	4
all the time	☐	5

---

4 We would like to know how much urine you think leaks.
How much urine do you usually leak (whether you wear protection or not)? *(Tick one box)*

none	☐	0
a small amount	☐	2
a moderate amount	☐	4
a large amount	☐	6

---

5 Overall, how much does leaking urine interfere with your everyday life?
Please ring a number between 0 (not at all) and 10 (a great deal)

0   1   2   3   4   5   6   7   8   9   10

not at all   a great deal

ICIQ score: sum scores 3+4+5 ☐☐

---

6 When does urine leak? *(Please tick all that apply to you)*

never – urine does not leak	☐
leaks before you can get to the toilet	☐
leaks when you cough or sneeze	☐
leaks when you are asleep	☐
leaks when you are physically active/exercising	☐
leaks when you have finished urinating and are dressed	☐
leaks for no obvious reason	☐
leaks all the time	☐

Thank you very much for answering these questions.

Fig. 5.1 International Consultation on Incontinence Modular Questionnnaire, ICIQ UI SF (short form).[1]

---

1   Reproduced with permission from: Abrams P, Cardozo L, Khoury S, Wein A. (eds) (2005) *3rd International Consultation on Incontinence. Annex 2: International Consultation on Incontinence Modular Questionnaire (ICIQ) UI SF (short form)*. London: Health Publications Ltd, p. 1630.

Basic investigation

Bladder diaries: record the frequency and volume of urine voided, incontinent episodes, pad usage, fluid intake, and degree of urgency (over a 3-day period). Alternatively, pads can be weighed to estimate urine loss (pad testing).

Urinalysis ± culture: treat any infection and reassess symptoms.

Flow rate and post-void residual (PVR) volume: patients need to void >100 mL of urine for an accurate result. A reduced flow rate suggests bladder outflow obstruction or reduced bladder contractility. The volume of urine remaining in the bladder after voiding (PVR) is also informative (<50 mL is normal; >200 mL is abnormal; 50–200 mL requires clinical correlation).

Further investigation

Blood tests, imaging (USS) and cystoscopy: indicated for complicated cases with persistent or severe symptoms, haematuria, bladder pain, voiding difficulties, recurrent UTI, abnormal neurology, previous pelvic surgery or radiation therapy, or suspected extra-urethral incontinence.

Urodynamic investigation (see p. 70): cystometry can measure the minimal pressure at which leakage occurs on straining (abdominal leak point pressure). Pressures >90–100 cmH_2O suggest SUI and hypermobility, <60 cmH_2O suggests ISD. Video-urodynamics can visualize movement of the proximal urethra and bladder neck, and establish the precise aetiology of UI. It can also identify relevant anatomical or neurological abnormalities and risk factors for the development of upper tract deterioration.

Sphincter electromyography (EMG): measures electrical activity from striated muscles of the urethra or perineal floor, and provides information on synchronization between bladder muscle (detrusor) and external sphincter.

Stress and mixed urinary incontinence

Stress urinary incontinence (SUI)

This accounts for up to 50% of reported urinary incontinence (UI) in women, and causes the symptoms of involuntary urinary leakage on effort (e.g. lifting), exertion (e.g. running), sneezing, and coughing. It is associated with an intrinsic loss of urethral strength and/or urethral hypermobility.

Specific risk factors for female SUI

- Childbirth (increased risk with vaginal delivery, forceps delivery)
- Ageing
- Oestrogen withdrawal
- Previous pelvic surgery
- Obesity.

Specific risk factors for male SUI

External urethral sphincter damage (from pelvic fracture, prostatectomy, other pelvic surgery or radiotherapy).

Other risk factors

Neurological disorders causing sphincter weakness (spinal cord injury, multiple sclerosis, spina bifida).

Investigation of SUI (📖 also see p. 130)

Women

- **Stress test:** a leakage of urine from the urethra on cough denotes a positive test
- **Pad test:** number and weight of pads used to estimate urine loss
- **Pelvic exam:** check for pelvic organ prolapse (POP). Elevation of an existing cystocele will unmask any occult sphincter incompetence in those who are continent as a result of obstruction caused by the prolapse. Assess oestrogen status and requirement for topical treatments
- **Q-tip test:** although not performed routinely, the Q-tip angle is a measure of urethral mobility in women. With the patient in lithotomy position and the bladder comfortably full, a well-lubricated sterile cotton-tipped applicator is gently inserted through the urethra into the bladder. Once in the bladder, the applicator is withdrawn to the point of resistance, which is at the level of the bladder neck. The resting angle from the horizontal is recorded. The patient is then asked to strain and the degree of rotation is assessed. Hypermobility is defined as a resting or straining angle of greater than 30° from the horizontal
- **Urethral pressure profile (selected cases only):** microtransducers are mounted in a catheter that is placed into the bladder, then slowly withdrawn, measuring both intravesical and urethral pressures. A measure of urethral closure pressure can be obtained.

Men
- Abdominal exam to detect a palpable bladder
- External genitalia exam to assess for penile abnormalities
- DRE
- Flow rate and post-void residual volume
- Consider imaging of upper tracts if evidence of bladder outlet obstruction.

Conservative treatment
- **Pelvic floor exercises:** ± vaginal weights (Kegel's exercises) are important and can improve symptoms in 30% of women with mild SUI
- **Life-style modification:** includes weight loss, stop smoking, avoid constipation
- **Biofeedback:** the technique by which information on ability and strength of pelvic floor muscle contraction is presented back to the patient as a visual, auditory or tactile signal. Patients may also be helped by the perineometer, which measures pelvic floor contraction
- **Medication:** duloxetine inhibits the re-uptake of both serotonin and noradrenaline. It is given orally 20—40 mg twice daily and acts to increase sphincteric muscle activity during bladder filling
- **Extracorporal magnetic innervation:** involves sitting the patient in a chair, and using a pulsed magnetic field to stimulate the nerves of the sphincter and pelvic floor. Possible benefit in mixed incontinence
- **High frequency electrical stimulation:** produces contraction of the pelvic floor (35–50 Hz). No proven therapeutic benefit in SUI.

Surgical treatment
- Urethral bulking agents (p. 136)
- Retropubic suspension (colposuspension, paravaginal repair in women) (p. 140)
- Suburethral slings (p. 142)
- Artificial urinary sphincters (p. 146).

Mixed urinary incontinence
Approximately 30% of women will report symptoms of mixed urinary incontinence (MUI), with involuntary urinary leakage associated with urgency, and also with exertion, effort, sneezing, or coughing. The underlying aetiologies and evaluation remain the same as for SUI and UUI, but also consider further investigation to rule out pathologies, such as bladder cancer, stones, and interstitial cystitis. The aim of management is to treat the predominant symptoms first.

Surgery for stress incontinence: injection therapy

Indications

The injection of bulking materials into bladder neck and peri-urethral muscles (see Table 5.2) is a minimally invasive surgical technique used to increase outlet resistance. The main indication is for stress incontinence secondary to demonstrable intrinsic sphincter deficiency (ISD), in the presence of normal bladder muscle function. It is used for both adults (male and female) and children.

Table 5.2 Peri-urethral bulking agents

Non-absorbable agents		Absorbable agents	
Product	Material	Product	Material
Macroplastique (Uroplasty)	Silicone	Contigen (Bard)	Bovine cross-linked collagen*
Durasphere-EXP (CMT)	Carbon-coated zirconium beads	Zuidex (Q-Medical)	Hyaluronic acid and dextranomer microspheres
Urethrin (Mentor)	Polytetrafluoroethylene paste (PTFE)	Tegress (Bard)	Ethylene vinyl alcohol copolymer in DMSO
Coaptite (Bioform)	Calcium hydroxylapatite		Autologous fat

*Skin test with non-cross-linked collagen to elicit any possible allergic reaction prior to definitive treatment.

Contraindications
- Active infection (UTI)
- Untreated bladder overactivity
- Bladder neck stenosis.

Injection techniques
- Under local anaesthetic (LA) block or general anaesthesia, agents are injected submucosally under endoscopic guidance (📖 see Figs. 5.2 and 5.3).
- In women, a periurethral (percutaneous) technique can be used with endoscopic or ultrasound guidance
- A 'blind' mid-urethral technique using LA and an instillation device is being utilized to administer Zuidex, and Macroplastique.

The aim is to achieve urethral muscosal apposition and closure of the lumen. In women, 2–4 injections are recommended (depending on agent), while in men, 3–4 circumferential injections are administered. Overall success rates are variable, depending on both the agent and patient selection (reported in ranges of 50–80%[1–4]). Results tend to deteriorate with time, and repeat treatments are often needed.

Complications

- Urinary urgency
- Urinary retention (which may need CISC or SPC insertion)
- Haematuria
- UTI/cystitis
- Distant migration of the injected particles (PTFE, Macroplastique) and risk of granuloma formation (PTFE), although no adverse consequences are reported.

1 Koelbl H, Saz V, Doerfler D, *et al.* (1998) Transurethral injection of silicone microimplants for intrinsic urethral sphincter deficiency. *Obstet Gynaecol* **92**:332–6.

2 Appell RA (1994) Collagen injection therapy for urinary incontinence. *Urol Clin N Am* **21**:177–82.

3 Dmochowski R, Apell RA, Klimberg I, *et al.* (2002) *Initial clinical results from coaptite injections for stress urinary incontinence, comparative clinical study.* Program of the International Continence Society. Heidelberg, Germany, August 2002.

4 Lighter D, Calvosa C, Andersen R, *et al.* (2001) A new injectable bulking agent for treatment of stress urinary incontinence: results of a multicentre, randomized, controlled, double-blind study of Durasphere ™. *Urology* **58**:12–15.

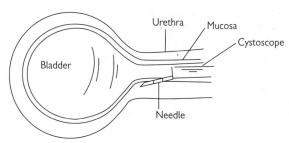

Fig. 5.2 Using cystoscopic guidance, the needle is positioned in the submucosa of the proximal urethra.

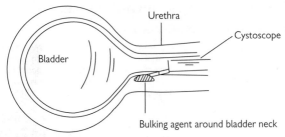

Fig. 5.3 Injections of the bulking agent (Macroplastique) are performed to achieve urethral mucosal apposition.

Surgery for stress incontinence: retropubic suspension

Retropubic suspension procedures are used to treat female stress incontinence caused by urethral hypermobility. The aim of surgery is to elevate, and fix the bladder neck and proximal urethra in a retropubic position, in order to support the bladder neck and regain continence. There is a lower chance of clinical benefit in the presence of significant intrinsic sphincter deficiency (ISD).

Types of surgery

Surgery is considered after conservative methods have failed. There are 3 main operations, all of which can be performed open via a Pfannenstiel or lower midline abdominal incision to approach the bladder neck and develop the retropubic space. Burch colposuspension can also be done laparoscopically. Better results are seen in patients with pure stress incontinence and primary repair (as opposed to 'redo' surgery).

Burch colposuspension

This is the most widely used technique with the best durability. Patients that are selected require good vaginal mobility, as the vaginal wall is elevated and attached to the lateral pelvic wall where the formation of adhesions over time will secure its position. This operation involves exposing the paravaginal fascia and approximating it to the iliopectineal (Cooper's) ligament of the superior pubic rami. Initial success rates for open repair are about 85–90% at 1 year, and 70% at 5 years.[1] Overall success rates are slightly higher for open repair over the laparoscopic approach.[2,3]

Marshall–Marchetti–Krantz (MMK) procedure

Sutures are placed either side of the urethra around the level of the bladder neck and then tied to the hyaline cartilage of the pubic symphysis. Short-term success is about 90%;[1] however, this declines over time and is now considered less effective than the Burch procedure. Complications include a 3% risk of osteitis pubis, which typically presents up to 8 weeks post-operatively with pubic pain radiating to the thigh. Treatment is with simple analgesia, bed rest, and steroids.

Vagino-obturator shelf / paravaginal repair

A variant of the Burch procedure. Sutures are placed by the vaginal wall and paravaginal fascia, and then passed through the obturator fascia to attach to part of the parietal pelvic fascia below the tendinous arch (arcus tendoneus fascia). Cure rates are up to 85%.

Complications

- Urinary retention (5%)
- Dysuria
- Bladder overactivity
- Vaginal prolapse.

1 Lapitan MC, Cody DJ, Grant AM (2005) Open retropubic colposuspension for urinary incontinence in women. *Cochrane Database Syst Rev* **20(3)**: CD002912.

2 Moehrer B, Carey M, Wilson D (2003) Laparoscopic colposuspenion: a systematic review. *BJOG* **110**:230–5.

3 Ankardal M, Ekerydh A, Crafoord K, et al. (2004) A randomized trial comparing open Burch colposuspension using sutures with laparoscopic colposuspension using mesh and staples in women with stress urinary incontinence. *BJOG* **111**:974–81.

Surgery for stress incontinence: suburethral slings

Indications

Sling procedures are mainly used for female stress incontinence associated with poor urethral function (type III or intrinsic sphincter deficiency) or when previous surgical procedures have failed. Also used for incontinence due to urethral damage (following radical pelvic surgery or radiotherapy) and for neurological urethral dysfunction (e.g. due to myelodysplasia) in both sexes. It is important that urethral and bladder function is evaluated prior to surgical repair.

Types of sling

- **Synthetic:** type I (>75 μm pores), soft, monofilamentous polypropylene mesh, i.e. tension-free transvaginal tape (TVT), transobturator tape (TOT) and tension-free vaginal tape obturator route (TVTO)
- **Autologous:** rectus fascia, fascia lata (from the thigh), vaginal wall slings
- **Non-autologous:** allograft fascia lata from donated cadaveric tissue.

Synthetic slings (low-tension suburethral tapes)

Widely practiced procedures as tapes can be inserted under general or local anaesthetic as day-cases, and they are less invasive, with few complications. All techniques use cystoscopy to assist prevention of bladder perforation during sling placement. Post-operatively, patients may temporarily require clean intermittent self catheterization (CISC) until post void residuals are less than 100 mL.

TVT

The tape has long trocars on each end, which are inserted either side of the urethra through an anterior vaginal approach. The tape has long trocars on each end, which are inserted either side of the urethra through an anterior vaginal approach. They perforate through the endopelvic fascia, and are pushed up behind the symphysis pubis and out onto the lower abdominal wall, just above the pubic bone. Once the tape is positioned loosely (tension-free) behind the mid-urethra, its covering is removed, and the ends cut flush to the abdomen.

Outcomes: success rates at 1 year are up to ~90%, and at 5 years are up to 80%.[1] TVT has proven equivalent efficacy to colposuspension.[2]

TOT

A midline anterior vaginal incision is made for dissection around the urethra and 2 small incisions are made lateral to the labia majora at the level of the clitoris. The curved handle device is placed through the skin incision and turned downwards, passing through the anterior part of the obturator foramen, and exiting alongside the urethra on each side, respectively. The tape is attached to the end of each handle and brought back out to the skin surface. It is positioned loosely around the mid-urethra and the ends cut flush with the skin. In TVTO, the tape is passed in a reverse route (from vagina to skin).

Outcomes: TOT has equivalent short-term outcome to TVT.[3]

Autologous and allograft slings

The tissue strip is inserted via an abdominal incision, and tunnelled through the endopelvic fascia on one side, behind the proximal urethra guided via an anterior vaginal incision, and then guided out contralaterally. The two ends are sutured to rectus fascia, using the minimal amount of tension needed to prevent urethral movement. Alternative methods of fixation include bone anchoring, but this is associated with increased risk of osteitis pubis and is now not recommended.

Complications

- Voiding dysfunction (urinary retention, *de novo* bladder overactivity)
- Vaginal, urethral, and bladder erosions
- Bladder perforation
- Damage to bowel or blood vessels.

TOT has a lower risk of bladder perforation than TVT, but carries a slightly higher risk of vaginal injury/erosion and groin pain. TOT and TVT have similar rates of *de novo* urgency.

1 Chene G, Amblard J, Tardieu AS, et al. (2006) Long-term results of tension-free vaginal tape (TVT) for the treatment of female urinary stress incontinence. *Eur J Obstet Gynaecol Reprod Biol.* [Epub]

2 Ward K, Hilton P (2006) Multicentre randomized trial of tension-free vaginal tape and colposuspension for primary urodynamic stress incontinence: five year follow up. *Neurourol Urodynam* **25**:568–9.

3 Latthe PM, Foon R, Toozs-Hobson P (2007) Transobturator and retropubic tape procedures in stress urinary incontinence: a systematic review and meta-analysis of effectiveness and complications. *BJOG* **114**:522–31.

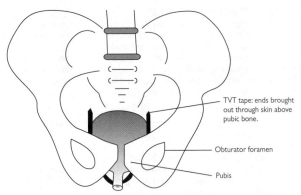

TVT tape: ends brought
out through skin above
pubic bone.

Obturator foramen

Pubis

Fig. 5.4 Tension-free transvaginal tape (TVT) placement.

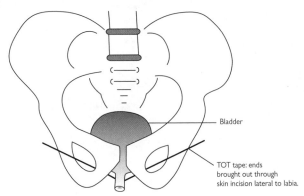

Bladder

TOT tape: ends
brought out through
skin incision lateral to labia.

Fig. 5.5 Transobturator tape (TOT) placement.

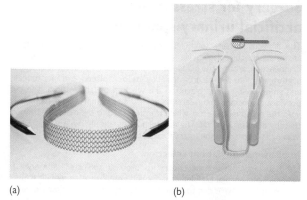

(a) (b)

Fig. 5.6 (a) TVT (Gynaecare TVT Tension-free support for incontinence).
(b) TVTO (Gynaecare TVT obturator system tension-free support for incontinence).
(©ETHICON, INC. Reproduced with permission).

Surgery for stress incontinence: artificial urinary sphincter

The artificial urinary sphincter (AUS; AMS800™; Fig. 5.7) consists of an inflatable cuff placed, via a lower abdominal incision (midline or Pfannenstiel), around the bladder neck in both men and women or bulbar urethra in men, a pressure-regulating balloon placed extraperitoneally, and an activating pump placed in the scrotum or labia majora. The cuff provides a constant circumferential pressure to compress the urethra. To void, the pump is squeezed, which transfers fluid to the reservoir balloon, thereby deflating the cuff. The cuff then automatically refills within 3 min. Voiding takes place in the interval taken for the cuff to refill.

Indications and patient selection

Used for incontinence secondary to urethral sphincter deficiency in patients with normal bladder capacity and compliance. In men, it is used for sphincter damage due to radical prostatectomy or TURP, pelvic radiotherapy, pelvic fracture, and following urethral reconstruction. In women it is used after other treatments for incontinence have failed. It can be used for neuropathic sphincter weakness (e.g. spinal cord injury, spina bifida) if the incontinence is not due to bladder overactivity. If there is combined bladder overactivity and sphincter weakness, treat the bladder first (i.e. lower bladder pressures with anticholinergics, intravesical botulinum injections, augmentation), which in some cases will be enough to achieve continence. If incontinence persists, proceed with AUS at a later date.

Patient evaluation

Patients should undergo urodynamics, cystoscopy and upper tract imaging to evaluate voiding function and identify anatomical abnormalities that might affect the efficacy of the sphincter. Good manual dexterity is required to manipulate the pump and perform CISC if needed. The patient must also have sufficient cognitive function to operate the sphincter themselves, several times daily.

Results

AUS can function well for many years (≥10). Overall long-term success (continued continence, no device malfunction) is 70–90%; revision rates are 20–30%.[1]

Complications and long-term outcomes

Recurrent incontinence due to:
- Urethral atrophy underneath the cuff (10% over the first 5 years post-implantation)
- Mechanical failure (of the pump or slow leak of fluid from the system)
- Urethral erosion (essentially a pressure sore in the urethra due to chronic pressure from the cuff)
- Bladder overactivity or reduced compliance also causing reflux, hydronephrosis and renal impairment.

Investigate recurrent incontinence by cystoscopy (to exclude erosion), X-ray to determine leaks from the system (the balloon loses its round shape), and urodynamics (to detect high bladder pressures).

Erosion: occurs in 5% and most common at 3–4 months, with 75% occurring in the first year. Presents with pain and swelling of scrotum, labia, or perineum, incontinence, and bloody discharge.

Infection: primary implant infection rates are 1–5%. With infection or erosion, remove entire device and wait 3–6 months before reinsertion.

Other: haematoma (scrotum or labia); late urinary retention which may signify obstruction from urethral stricture or bladder neck contracture (higher risk with previous pelvic irradiation).

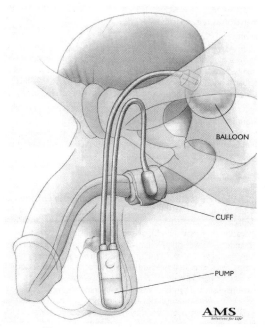

Fig. 5.7 AMS 800™ Urinary Control System Artificial Urinary Sphincter. (Reproduced with permission. Courtesy of American Medical Systems Inc., Minnesota.)

1 Lai HH, Hsu El, Teh BS, *et al.* (2007) 13 years of experience with artificial urinary sphincter implantation at Baylor College of Medicine. *J Urol* **177**:1021–5.

Overactive bladder: conventional treatment

Definition

Overactive bladder (OAB) is a symptom syndrome that includes urgency, with or without urge incontinence, usually with frequency and nocturia. The symptoms are usually caused by bladder (detrusor) overactivity, but can be due to other forms of voiding dysfunction (Fig. 5.8). 17% of the population >40 years old in Europe have symptoms of OAB.[1]

Conventional treatment

Conservative

Patient management involves a multidisciplinary team approach (urologists, gynaecologists, continence nurse specialists, physiotherapists, and community-based health care workers). Pelvic floor exercises (PFE), biofeedback, and daily electrical stimulation therapy at 5–10Hz (which strengthens the pelvic floor and sphincter by increasing tone through sacral neural feedback systems) may provide some benefit.

Behavioural modification

This involves modifying fluid intake, avoiding stimulants (caffeine, alcohol), and bladder training for urgency (delay micturition for increasing periods of time by inhibiting the desire to void).

Medication

50% of patients will benefit from medication.
- **Anticholinergic (antimuscarinic) drugs** act to inhibit bladder contractions and increase bladder capacity (oxybutynin, tolterodine, solifenacin, trospium). Oxybutynin is also available in a transdermal preparation (Kentera® patch), or can be administered directly into the bladder (intravesically) in patients performing intermittent catheterization (5 mg in 30 mL normal saline 8-h after emptying the bladder). *Contraindication*: closed angle glaucoma. *Side effects*: dry mouth, constipation, blurred vision, urinary retention
- **Desmopressin** is a synthetic vasopressin analogue, which acts as an antidiuretic. Intranasal desmopressin can improve nocturia and enuresis associated with detrusor overactivity. Oral desmopressin is effective for nocturia. Check serum sodium level in the first week of treatment as there is increased risk of hyponatraemia in the elderly
- **Baclofen** is a GABA receptor agonist, which is used orally or via intrathecal pump in neuropathic patients with bladder dysfunction and limb spasticity.

1 Milsom I, Abrams P, Cardozo L et al. (2001) How widespread are the symptoms of an overactive bladder and how are they managed? A population-based prevalence study. *BJU Int* **87**:760–6.

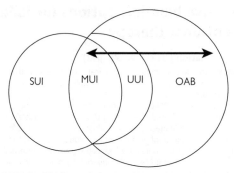

Fig. 5.8 Spectrum of OAB.
SUI = stress urinary incontinence; MUI = mixed urinary incontinence; UUI = urge urinary incontinence; OAB= overactive bladder.

Overactive bladder: options for failed conventional therapy

Neuromodulation (📖 see also p. 602)

Sacral nerve stimulation involves electrical stimulation of the bladder's nerve supply to suppress reflexes responsible for involuntary bladder muscle (detrusor) contraction.*

- The Interstim device (Medtronic) stimulates the S3 afferent nerve, which then inhibits detrusor activity at the level of the sacral spinal cord. An initial percutaneous nerve evaluation is performed, followed by surgical implantation of permanent electrode leads into the sacral foramen, with a pulse generator which is programmed externally.
- SANS™ (Stoller Afferent Nerve Stimulator) is a minimally invasive technique, which is applied near the posterior tibial nerve near the ankle.

Surgery

The aim is to increase functional bladder capacity, decrease maximal detrusor pressure, and protect the upper urinary tract (also 📖 see p. 588–9).

Autoaugmentation enterocystoplasty ('Clam' ileocystoplasty): relieves intractable frequency, urge, and UUI in 90% of patients. The bladder dome is cut open (bivalved) and a detubularized segment of ileum is anastomosed, creating a larger bladder volume.

Autoaugmentation (detrusor myectomy): detrusor muscle is excised from the entire dome of bladder, leaving the underlying bladder endothelium intact. A large epithelial bulge is created which augments bladder capacity. Less commonly performed now as limited long-term efficacy.

Urinary diversion: a non-continent urinary outlet. Typically, both ureters are anastomosed and connected to a short ileal pouch, which is brought out cutaneously as a stoma.

Intravesical pharmacotherapy

Botulinum toxin-A (BTX-A): injected at multiple sites as a bleb under the bladder mucosa or into detrusor, sparing the trigone (📖 see p. 152–3; 590–1). Although widely used in clinical urological practice, it is still pending licence for urological indications.

---

* Sacral nerve stimulation has National Institute of Excellence (NICE) approval for women with detrusor overactivity who have failed conservative treatments.

Overactive bladder: intravesical botulinum toxin-A therapy

Botulinum toxin-A (BTX-A)

Botulinum toxin (BTX) is a neurotoxin produced by a gram positive, rod-shaped anaerobic bacterium *Clostridium botulinum*. There are seven subtypes. Subtypes A and B are used in urology; however, BTX-A is the more potent with longer duration of action.

Main applications for treatment in the urinary tract

- Neurogenic detrusor overactivity (NDO)[1]
- Idiopathic detrusor overactivity (IDO)[2]
- Detrusor-sphincter-dyssynergia (DSD).[3]

Children with NDO associated with myelomeningocele[4] and with IDO[5] have been safely and successfully treated with BTX-A. There is also emerging, but limited evidence for a role in symptomatic benign prostatic enlargement and chronic pelvic pain syndromes (including interstitial cystitis).

Mechanism of action

BTX-A acts by inhibiting the release of acetylcholine (ACh) and other neurotransmitters from presynaptic cholinergic nerve terminals, resulting in regionally decreased muscle contractility and muscle atrophy at the site of BTX-A injection. The chemical dennervation that results is a reversible process.

Adult dosing regimen for detrusor overactivity

- American botulinum toxin A (Botox®, Allergan) 100–300 units
- English botulinum toxin A (Dysport®, Ipsen) up to 1000 units
- Botox® 300 is roughly equivalent to 900 units of Dysport®.

Method of intravesical administration

- Techniques include rigid cystoscopy under GA using a collagen-flexible needle, or LA flexible cystoscopy using an ultra-fine 4-mm needle
- BTX-A is diluted in normal saline (i.e. 300 IU Botox® diluted in 30 mL saline)
- 20–30 random sites on the bladder wall are injected (i.e. ~1 mL (10 IU Botox®) per injection site)
- BTX-A can be injected directly into detrusor muscle or sub-mucosally
- General practice is usually to avoid injecting the trigone (trigone sparing*).

Outcome

- A response is seen within 7 days (maximal response may take 30 days)
- Effects last approximately 6–9 months, and repeat injections are required
- Tolerance to the drug appears unchanged with repeated applications.

Contraindications to treatment

- Myasthenia gravis
- Aminoglucosides/drugs interfering with neuromuscular transmission
- Eaton–Lambert syndrome**

- Breast feeding and pregnancy
- Bleeding disorders (haemophilia; hereditary clotting factor deficiency).

Side effects

- Urinary retention (requiring intermittent self catheterization post-operatively). Higher risk in neuropaths
- Haematuria
- UTI
- General weakness
- Dysphagia
- Diplopia, blurred vision.

---

* A trigone sparing technique should prevent the theoretical risk of iatrogenic vesicoureteric reflux.

** Eaton–Lambert syndrome: small cell bronchial carcinoma associated with defective ACh release at the neuromuscular junction causing proximal muscle weakness.

1 Schurch B, De Seze M, Denys P, et al. (2005). Botulinum toxin type is a safe and effective treatment for neurogenic incontinence: results of a single treatment, randomised, placebo controlled 6-month study. *J Urol* **174**:196–200.

2 Schmid DM, Suermann P, Werner M, et al. (2006). Experience with 100 cases treated with botulinum-A toxin injections in the detrusor for idiopathic overactive bladder syndrome refractory to anticholinergics. *J Urol* **176**:177–85.

3 Dykstra DD, Sidi AA, Scott AB, et al. (1988). Effects of botulinum A toxin on detrusor-sphincter dyssynergia in spinal cord injury patients. *J Urol* **139**:919–22.

4 Riccabona M, Koen M, Schinder M, et al. (2004). Botulinum-A toxin injection into the detrusor: a safe alternative in the treatment of children with myelomeningocele with detrusor hyperreflexia. *J Urol* **171**:845–8.

5 Verleyen P, Hoebeke P, Raes A, et al. (2004). The use of botulinum toxin A in children with a non-neurogenic overactive bladder: a pilot study. *BJU Int* **93**:69, Abstract.

Post-prostatectomy incontinence

Incidence

Urinary incontinence (UI) occurs in <1% after TURP and 0.5% after open prostatectomy (OP) performed for benign prostate disease.[1] Following radical prostatectomy (RP) for malignant disease, UI tends to improve over 12–18 months post-surgery.[2] The overall incidence in open RP is ~10–15%,[2,3] with similar risks reported for laparoscopic RP.[4] Early results from robotic-assisted laparoscopic RP suggest slightly earlier recovery of continence and improved overall continence rates.[5]

Risk factors for UI after RP

- Increasing age
- Pre-existing bladder dysfunction
- Previous radiotherapy (TURP following brachytherapy has a 40% risk of UI)
- Prior TURP
- Advanced stage of disease and surgical technique.

Earlier recovery of continence after open RP is achieved using a perineal approach, nerve-sparing techniques, and sphincter and bladder neck preserving procedures.

Pathophysiology

The main cause of post-radical prostatectomy incontinence is sphincter dysfunction. The proximal sphincter mechanism is removed at prostatectomy (TURP, OP, RP). Post-prostatectomy continence therefore requires a functioning distal (external) urethral sphincter mechanism and low bladder pressure during bladder filling. Direct damage to the external sphincter can occur during prostatectomy (at TURP it occurs particularly during resection between 11 and 2 o'clock positions, when the reference point for the position of the distal sphincter, the verumontanum, cannot be seen). Damage to the innervation of the sphincter can also occur during prostatectomy. Urodynamic studies before and after RP show that maximal urethral closure pressure (MUCP) and functional urethral length (the length of urethra over which the sphincter functions to maintain high pressures) are lower. Nerve-sparing RP (where the neurovascular bundles are specifically identified and preserved) produces better continence rates and longer functional urethral lengths and MUCPs.

A substantial proportion of men also have overactive bladders before prostatectomy and this may remain so after surgery contributing to UI.

Evaluation

Wait for up to 12 months for spontaneous improvement (patients can practice pelvic floor exercises during this time). Act sooner if symptoms are severe:

- **History:** stress-induced leakage (cough, standing from a sitting position) suggests sphincter dysfunction
- **Examination:** observe for leakage on coughing
- **Tests:** post-void residual volume measurement on ultrasound (to exclude retention with overflow); urodynamic studies allow determination of bladder and sphincter function; cystoscopy allows identification of strictures (particularly important if artificial sphincter implantation is contemplated).

Treatment

Sphincter dysfunction

- Pelvic floor exercises
- Insertion of urethral bulking agents
- Bulbourethral sling or tapes to compress or elevate the urethra (InVance™ and AdVance™ male tapes). Clinical evidence is still limited, and they are not yet widely practised
- Artificial urinary sphincter. Insertion is usually deferred until 1 year post-prostatectomy, and it is the most effective long-term treatment (80% success rates).

Bladder dysfunction

- Conservative treatment for bladder overactivity includes behavioural therapy, pelvic floor exercises and anticholinergic medication
- Surgery for intractable cases includes augmentation cystoplasty, or urinary diversion
- Catheterization may be considered in the older patient.

1 Agency for Health Care Policy and Research (AHCPR) (1994). *Benign Prostatic Hyperplasia: diagnosis and treatment*, Clinical Practice Guidelines No.8. Feb. (www.ncbi.nlm.nih.gov).

2 Benoit RM, Naslund MJ, Cohen JK (2000). Complications after radical prostatectomy in the medicare population. *Urology* **56**:116–20.

3 Catalona WJ, Carvalhal GF, Mager DE, *et al.* (1999). Potency, continence and complication rates in 1,870 consecutive radical retropubic prostatectomies. *J Urol* **162**:433–8.

4 Eden CG, Moon DA (2006). Laparoscopic radical prostatectomy: minimum 3-year follow-up of the first 100 patients in the UK. *BJU Int* **97**:981–4.

5 Patel VR, Thaly R, Shah K (2007). Robotic radical prostatectomy: outcomes of 500 cases. *BJU Int* **99**:1109–12.

Vesicovaginal fistula (VVF)

VVF is an abnormal communication between the bladder and vagina. In 10% there is a co-existing ureterovaginal fistula.

Aetiology

In developing countries, the majority are due to obstructed or prolonged childbirth, causing tissue pressure necrosis between vagina and bladder. In developed countries, 75% follow hysterectomy (0.1–0.2% risk; Fig. 5.9).[1,2] Other causes include pelvic surgery or radiotherapy; pessary erosion; advanced pelvic malignancy (cervical carcinoma); pelvic endometriosis; inflammatory bowel disease; trauma; childbirth (5%); low oestrogen states; infection (urinary TB); congenital abnormalities.

Symptoms

Immediate or delayed onset of urinary leakage from the vagina post-operatively; abdominal pain or distension; prolonged bowel ileus (due to some leak of urine into peritoneal cavity as well as through vagina); suprapubic pain; haematuria.

Examination

- Pelvic examination may demonstrate the VVF
- '3-swab test': give oral phenazopyridine which turns the urine orange. After 1 h, place 3 swabs into the vagina, and instil methylene blue into the bladder. If the proximal swab turns blue it indicates VVF; if it is orange, it suggests ureterovaginal fistula
- Cystoscopy may directly identify the fistula tract, and help determine its proximity to the ureteric orifices. Biopsy the tract if history of malignancy
- IVU and/or bilateral retrograde pyelograms to assess ureteric involvement
- **Cystogram (or voiding cystourethrogram, VCUG):** best test for identifying fistula.

Management

Small, uncomplicated VVF may resolve with urethral catheterization (± anticholinergics and antibiotics) or electrocoagulation of the tract (± fibrin sealant). A co-existing ureterovaginal fistula will require ureteric stent or catheter. Most cases proceed to surgery.

Surgery

Overall surgical success for simple VVF repair is 90%. Early repair (within 2–3 weeks) is advocated in selected cases, but traditionally, surgery is delayed 3–6 months (or 6–12 months following radiation therapy).

Transvaginal approach: commonly used. The Vaginal Flap Technique involves incision of the fistula tract and closure with 2 layers of sutures. Interpositional tissue grafts may be mobilized between the bladder and vagina (Martius fat pad graft from labia majora; peritoneal flap; gracilis flap) prior to advancement of a vaginal flap and closure of vaginal wall.

Abdominal approach: more often used for complex cases. The bladder is bisected to the level of the fistula tract, which is then completely excised.

The bladder is closed and an interpositional (omental) graft created. In complex cases, urinary diversion procedures may be needed.

Suprapubic and urethral catheters are placed for 2 weeks, and VCUG performed prior to catheter removal. Offer oestrogen replacement to post-menopausal women. Avoid tampons or sexual intercourse for 3 months.

Post-operative complications: vaginal bleeding; infection; bladder pain; dyspareunia due to vaginal stenosis; graft ischaemia; ureteric injury; fistula recurrence.

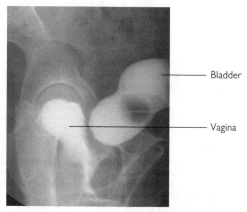

Bladder

Vagina

Fig. 5.9 Cystogram (lateral view) showing leak of contrast from the bladder and into the vagina due to a VVF. This followed a hysterectomy.

1 Tancer ML (1992). Observations on prevention and management of vesicovaginal fistula after total hysterectomy. *Surg Gynaecol Obstet* **175**:501–6.

2 Harris WJ (1995). Early complications of abdominal and vaginal hysterectomy. *Obstet Gynaecol Survey* **50(11)**:795–805.

Incontinence in elderly patients

Prevalence

Urinary incontinence (UI) steadily increases with advancing age (particularly $\geq$ 70 years). It affects about 10–20% of women and 7–10% of men >65 years old and living at home. These figures escalate if older people are institutionalized.

Prevalence for both sexes: residential home 25%; nursing home 40%; long-stay hospital ward 50–70%.[1]

Transient causes of UI ('DIAPPERS')

Delirium

Infection

Atrophic vaginitis or urethritis

Pharmaceuticals (opiates and calcium antagonists cause urinary retention and constipation; anticholinergics cause increased PVR and retention; α-adrenergic antagonist cause reduced urethral resistance in women)

Psychological problems – depression; neurosis; anxiety

Excess fluid input or output (diuretics; CCF; nocturnal polyuria)

Restricted mobility

Stool impaction (constipation)

Established UI

This is unrelated to co-morbid illness and persists over time. There are several types including UUI, SUI, and incontinence associated with impaired bladder emptying (due to under-active bladder, urethral or bladder outlet obstruction). In addition, functional incontinence is associated with factors outside of the urinary tract, such as permanent immobility, cognitive impairment, and environmental changes.

History

Seek out any transient causes and correct before arranging complex assessment and investigation. This can immediately improve function and quality of life, and may be sufficient to restore continence, even if there is co-existing urinary tract dysfunction. Elicit full drug history; co-morbid conditions; psychological, cognitive, functional, social, and environmental status.

Examination

Include mini-mental state evaluation and direct observation of patient dexterity and mobility (Barthel Index). Include abdominal assessment (distended bladder), DRE (impacted faeces), vulval inspection (pelvic organ prolapse, POP; atrophic vaginitis), and neurological testing.

Investigations
- Measure serum creatinine
- Frequency volume chart
- Bladder ultrasound for post-void residual volume
- Urinalysis (screen for infection, haematuria, glycosuria)
- Stress test
- Evaluation of the home environment, and assess need for modifications (occupational therapist and district nurse visits).

Urodynamics should be reserved for patients considered fit for surgery, and where the results will alter clinical treatment.

Management

Conservative

Biofeedback, electrical stimulation of pelvic floor, and behavioural methods are appropriate only if cognition is intact. Pelvic floor exercises (good results if used in conjunction with anticholinergics). Treat any atrophic vaginitis (0.01% estriol cream topically). Optimize mobility and bring the toilet closer to the bed. Try timed and prompted voiding. Absorbent appliances include bed pads and body worn pad products (disposable or re-useable); body worn external urine collection devices (close fitting penile sheath); pessary for POP; in-dwelling catheters where UI is due to obstruction and/or no alternative intervention suitable.

Surgery
- In women, consider colposuspension, suburethral slings/tapes or periurethral bulking agents for SUI, and surgery for POP
- In men, sphincter incompetence can be treated with injection of periurethral bulking agents, bulbourethral slings/tapes, and artificial urinary sphincter.

---

1 Royal College of Physicians (1995) *Incontinence: causes, management and provision of services*, Report of a working party. London: RCP (www.rcplondon.ac.uk).

Management pathways for urinary incontinence

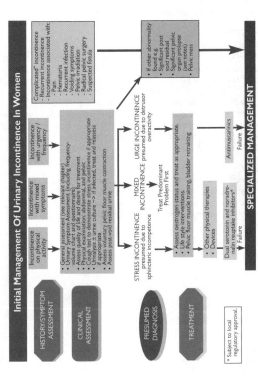

Fig. 5.10 International Continence Society (ICS) recommendations. Reproduced with permission from 3rd International Consultation on Incontinence. Incontinence, edition 2005. Ed. Abrams P, Cardozo L, Khoudry S, Wein A. Health Publications Ltd 2005, p. 1607.

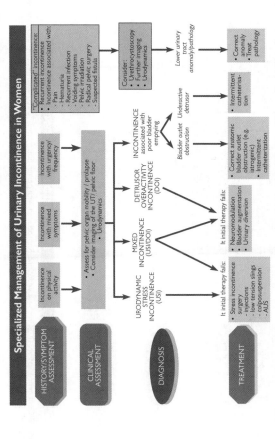

Fig. 5.11 International Continence Society (ICS) recommendations. Reproduced with permission from 3rd International Consultation on Incontinence. Incontinence, edition 2005. Ed. Abrams P, Cardozo L, Khoudry S, Wein A. Health Publications Ltd 2005, p. 1609.

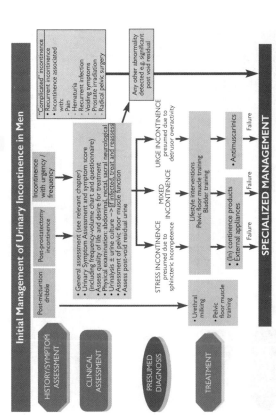

Fig. 5.12 International Continence Society (ICS) recommendations. Reproduced with permission from 3rd International Consultation on Incontinence. Incontinence, edition 2005. Ed. Abrams P, Cardozo L, Khoudry S, Wein A. Health Publications Ltd 2005, p. 1603.

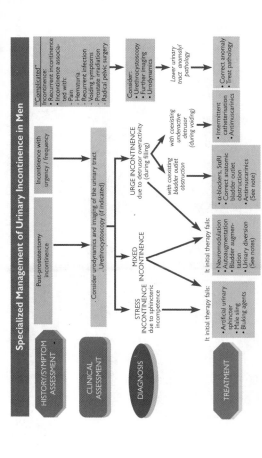

Fig. 5.13 International Continence Society (ICS) recommendations. Reproduced with permission from 3rd International Consultation on Incontinence. Incontinence, edition 2005. Ed. Abrams P, Cardozo L, Khoudry S, Wein A. Health Publications Ltd 2005, p. 1605.

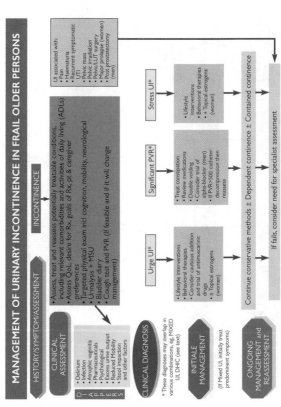

MANAGEMENT OF URINARY INCONTINENCE IN FRAIL OLDER PERSONS

HISTORY/SYMPTOM/ASSESSMENT

INCONTINENCE

CLINICAL ASSESSMENT

- Delirium
- Infection
- Atrophic vaginitis
- Pharmaceuticals
- Psychological
- Excess urine output
- Reduced Mobility
- Stool impaction and other factors

D·I·A·P·P·E·R·S

- Assess, treat and reassess potentially treatable conditions, including relevant comorbidities and activities of daily living (ADLs)
- Assess QoL, desire for Rx, goals of Rx, pt & caregiver preferences
- Targeted physical exam incl cognition, mobility, neurological
- Urinalysis + MSU
- Bladder diary
- Cough test and PVR (if feasible and if it will change management)

UI associated with:
- Pain
- Haematuria
- Recurrent symptomatic UTI
- Pelvic mass
- Pelvic irradiation
- Pelvic/LUT surgery (women)
- Major prolapse (women)
- Post prostatectomy (men)

CLINICAL DIAGNOSIS

* These diagnoses may overlap in various combinations, eg, MIXED UI, DHIC (see text)

Urge UI*   Significant PVR*   Stress UI*

INITIALE MANAGEMENT

(If Mixed UI, initially treat predominant symptoms)

Urge UI*
- Lifestyle interventions
- Behavioral therapies
- Consider cautious addition and trial of antimuscarinic drugs
- ± Topical estrogens (women)

Significant PVR*
- Treat constipation
- Review medications
- Double voiding
- Consider trial of alpha-blocker (men)
- If PVR>500: catheter decompression then reasses

Stress UI*
- Lifestyle interventions
- Behavioral therapies
- ± Topical estrogens (women)

ONGOING MANAGEMENT and REASSESSMENT

Continue conservative methods ± Dependent continence ± Contained continence

If it fails, consider need for specialist assessment

Fig. 5.14 International Continence Society (ICS) recommendations. Reproduced with permission from 3rd International Consultation on Incontinence. Incontinence, edition 2005. Ed. Abrams P, Cardozo L, Khoudry S, Wein A. Health Publications Ltd 2005, p. 1611.

Infections and inflammatory conditions

Urinary tract infection: definitions and epidemiology

Definitions

Urinary tract infection (UTI)

UTI is currently defined as the inflammatory response of the urothelium to bacterial invasion. This inflammatory response causes a constellation of symptoms. Bladder infection (cystitis) causes frequent small volume voids, urgency, suprapubic pain, or discomfort, and urethral 'burning' on voiding (dysuria). Acute kidney infection (acute pyelonephritis) causes symptoms of fever, chills, malaise, and loin pain, often with associated lower urinary tract symptoms (LUTS) of frequency, urgency, and urethral pain on voiding. The strict requirement for >10^5 bacteria/mL of midstream urine (MSU) specimen is no longer required to make a diagnosis of UTI. In symptomatic patients, many clinicians will now make a diagnosis of UTI with bacterial counts of >10^2/mL. Current recommendations for diagnosing UTI from MSU culture is shown in Table 6.1.

Bacteriuria is the presence of bacteria in the urine. Bacteriuria may be asymptomatic or symptomatic. Bacteriuria without pyuria indicates the presence of bacterial *colonization* of the urine, rather than the presence of active infection.

Pyuria is the presence of white blood cells in the urine (implying an inflammatory response of the urothelium to bacterial infection or, in the absence of bacteriuria, some other pathology, such as carcinoma *in situ*, TB infection, bladder stones, or other inflammatory conditions).

An uncomplicated UTI is one occurring in a patient with a structurally and functionally normal urinary tract. The majority of such patients are women who respond quickly to a short course of antibiotics.

A complicated UTI is one occurring in the presence of an underlying anatomical or functional abnormality (e.g. incomplete bladder emptying secondary to bladder outlet obstruction or detrusor-sphincter-dyssynergia in spinal cord injury), renal or bladder stones, colovesical fistula, etc. Other factors suggesting a potential complicated UTI are diabetes mellitus, immunosuppression, hospital-acquired infection, in-dwelling catheter and recent urinary tract intervention. Most UTIs in men occur in association with a structural or functional abnormality, and are therefore defined as complicated UTIs. Complicated UTIs take longer to respond to antibiotic treatment than uncomplicated UTIs, and if there is an underlying anatomical or structural abnormality they will usually recur within days, weeks, or months.

Urinary tract infection may be isolated, recurrent or unresolved.

- **Isolated UTI:** an interval of at least 6 months between infections
- **Recurrent UTI:** >2 infections in 6 months, or 3 within 12 months. Recurrent UTI may be due to re-infection (i.e. infection by a different bacteria) or bacterial persistence (infection by the same organism originating from a focus within the urinary tract). Bacterial persistence is caused by the presence of bacteria within calculi (e.g. struvite calculi); within a chronically infected prostate (chronic bacterial prostatitis);

within an obstructed or atrophic infected kidney; or occurs as a result of a bladder fistula (with bowel or vagina) or urethral diverticulum
- **Unresolved infection:** implies inadequate therapy, and is caused by natural or acquired bacterial resistance to treatment, infection by different organisms, or rapid re-infection.

Prevalence of bacteriuria

Age	Female	Male
Infants (<1 year)	1%	3%
School (<15 years old)	1–3%	<1%
Reproductive	4%	<1%
Elderly	20–30%	10%

General risk factors for bacteriuria
- Female sex
- Increasing age
- Low oestrogen states (menopause)
- Pregnancy
- Diabetes mellitus
- Previous UTI
- The institutionalized elderly
- In-dwelling catheters
- Stone disease (kidney, bladder)
- Genitourinary malformation and voiding dysfunction (including obstruction).

Table 6.1 Recommended criteria for diagnosing urinary tract infection (UTI)[1]

Type of UTI	Urine culture
Acute uncomplicated UTI/cystitis in women	≥10³ cfu/mL
Acute uncomplicated pyelonephritis	≥10⁴ cfu/mL
Complicated UTI	≥10⁵ cfu/mL in women; ≥10⁴ cfu/mL in men
Asymptomatic bacteriuria	≥10⁵ cfu/mL in 2 consecutive MSU cultures ≥24 h apart
Recurrent UTI	<10³ cfu/mL

Cfu/mL = colony forming units/mL; MSU = midstream urine.

1 Naber KG, Bishop MC, Bjerklund-Johansen TE, *et al.* (2007). *Guidelines on the Management of Urinary and Male Genital Tract Infections.* European Association of Urology, http://www.eau.org.

Urinary tract infection: microbiology

Most UTIs are caused by faecal-derived bacteria that are facultative anaerobes (i.e. they can grow under both anaerobic and non-anaerobic conditions; see Table 6.2).

Uncomplicated UTI

Most UTIs are bacterial in origin. The most common cause is *Escherichia coli (E. coli)*, a gram −ve bacillus, which accounts for 85% of community acquired and 50% of hospital-acquired infection. Other common causative organisms include *Staphylococcus saprophyticus*, *Enterococcus faecalis* (also known as *Streptococcus faecalis*—gram +ve), *Proteus mirabilis*, and *Klebsiella* (gram −ve enterobacteriacae).

Complicated UTI

E. coli is responsible for up to 50% of cases. Other causes include *Enterococci* (e.g. *Streptococcus faecalis*), *Staph. aureus*, *Staph. epidermidis* (gram +ve), *Pseudomonas aeruginosa* (gram −ve).

Route of infection

Ascending

The vast majority of UTIs result from infection ascending retrogradely up the urethra. Bacteria, derived from the large bowel, colonize the perineum, vagina, and distal urethra. They ascend along the urethra to the bladder (increased risk in females as urethra shorter) causing cystitis. From the bladder they may ascend, via the ureters, to involve the kidneys (pyelonephritis). Reflux is not necessary for infection to ascend to the kidneys, but it will encourage ascending infection, as will any process that impairs ureteric peristalsis (e.g. ureteric obstruction, gram −ve organisms and endotoxins, pregnancy). Infection that ascends to involve the kidneys is also more likely where the infecting organism has P pili (filamentous protein appendages—also known as fimbriae—which allow binding of bacteria to the surface of epithelial cells).

Haematogenous Uncommon, but is seen with *Staph. aureus*, candida fungaemia, and *Mycobacterium tuberculosis* (causing tuberculosis).

Infection via lymphatics Seen rarely in inflammatory bowel disease and from retroperitoneal abscess.

Table 6.2 Bacterial classification: uropathogens

Cocci	Gram +ve
	Aerobes: Streptococcus (*Enterococcus*/ *Streptococcus faecalis*); Staphylococcus (*S. aureus*; *S. saprophyticus*-causes approximately 10% of symptomatic lower UTIs in young, sexually active women)
	Gram −ve
	Aerobes: Neisseria (*N. gonorrhoeae*)
Bacilli (rods)	Gram +ve
	Anaerobes*: Clostridium, Lactobacillus (usually a vaginal commensal)
	Aerobes: Corynebacteria (*C. urealyticum*)
	Gram −ve
	Aerobes: Enterobacteriaceae (Escherichia, Klebsiella, Proteus), Pseudomonas
	Anaerobes*: Bacteroides
Others	Filamentous bacteria: Mycobacterium (*M. tuberculosis*—acid-fast, aerobic, gram +ve)
	Chlamydiae: *Chlamydia trachomatis* (Fungi: *Candida albicans*)
	Mycoplasma: *Mycoplasma* species Ureaplasma urealyticum (cause UTI in patients with in-dwelling catheters)

*Anaerobic infections of the bladder and kidney are uncommon—anaerobes are normal commensals of the perineum, vagina, and distal urethra. However, infections of the urinary system that produce pus (e.g. scrotal, prostatic, or perinephric abscesses) are often caused by anaerobic organisms (e.g. *Bacteroides* sp., such as *Bacteroides fragilis*, *Fusobacterium* species, anaerobic cocci, and *Clostridium perfringens*).

Factors increasing bacterial virulence

Adhesion factors

Many gram −ve bacteria contain pili on their surface, which aid attachment to urothelial cells of the host. A typical piliated cell may contain 100–400 pili. Pili are 5–10 nm in diameter and up to 2 μm long. *E. coli* produces a number of antigenically and functionally different types of pili on the same cell; other strains may produce only a single type, and, in some isolates, no pili are seen. Pili are defined functionally by their ability to mediate haemagglutination (clumping of red blood cells) of specific types of erythrocytes. Mannose-sensitive (type 1) pili are produced by all strains of *E. coli*. Certain pathogenic types of *E. coli* also produce mannose-resistant (P) pili (associated with pyelonephritis).

Avoidance of host defence mechanisms

- **General:** an extracellular capsule reduces immunogenicity and resists phagocytosis (*E. coli*). *M. tuberculosis* resists phagocystosis by preventing phagolysosome fusion
- **Toxins:** *E. coli* species release cytokines which have a direct pathogenic effect on host tissues
- **Enzyme production:** *Proteus* species produce ureases, which causes breakdown of urea in the urine to ammonia, which then contributes to disease processes (struvite stone formation).

Antimicrobial resistance

- **Enzyme inactivation:** *Staph. aureus, N. gonorrhoeae,* and *enterobacteria* can produce β-lactamase, which hydrolyses the β-lactam bond within the structure of some antibiotics, so inactivating them. The β-lactam antibiotics are penicillins, cephalosporins, and carbapenems
- **Altered permeability:** access of the antibiotic to the bacteria is prevented by alterations in receptor activity or transport mechanisms
- **Alteration of binding site:** genetic variations may alter the antibiotic target, leading to drug resistance.

Host defences Factors that protect against UTI include:

General

- Commensal flora: protect by competing for nutrients, bacteriocin production, and stimulation of immune system
- Mechanical integrity of mucous membranes
- Mucosal secretions: lysozymes split muramic acid links in cell walls of gram +ve organisms; lactoferrin disrupts normal metabolism of bacteria
- Urinary immunoglobulin (IgA) inhibits bacterial adherence.

Specific

- Mechanical flushing effect of urine through the urinary tract (i.e. antegrade flow of urine)
- A mucopolysaccharide coating of bladder (Tamm–Horsfall protein) helps prevent bacterial attachment
- Bladder surface mucin: glycosaminoglycan (GAG) layer is an anti-adherent factor, preventing bacterial attachment to mucosa
- Low urine pH and high osmolarity reduces bacterial growth
- Female commensal flora: *Lactobacillus acidophilus* metabolize glycogen into lactic acid, causing a drop in pH.

Lower urinary tract infection: cystitis

Cystitis: infection and/or inflammation of the bladder.
Presentation: frequent voiding of small volumes, dysuria, urgency, offensive urine, suprapubic pain, haematuria, fever, and incontinence.

Investigation

Dipstick of midstream specimen of urine (MSU)

White blood cells (indirect testing for pyuria)

Leukocyte esterase activity detects the presence of white blood cells in the urine. Leukocyte esterase is produced by neutrophils and causes a colour change in a chromogen salt on the dipstick. Not all patients with bacteriuria have significant pyuria (sensitivity of 75–95% for detection of infection—i.e. 5–25% of patients with infection will have a –ve leukocyte esterase test suggesting, erroneously, that they have no infection).

- False –ves (pyuria present, negative dipstick test)—concentrated urine, glycosuria, presence of urobilinogen, consumption of large amounts of ascorbic acid
- False +ves (pyuria absent, positive dipstick test)—contamination.

Remember, there are many causes for pyuria (and, therefore, a +ve leukocyte esterase test occurring in the absence of bacteria on urine microscopy). This is so-called sterile pyuria and it occurs with TB infection, renal calculi, bladder calculi, glomerulonephritis, interstitial cystitis, and carcinoma *in situ*. Thus, the leukocyte esterase dipstick test may be truly positive, in the absence of infection.

Nitrite testing (indirect testing for bacteriuria)

Nitrites are not normally found in urine and their presence suggests the possibility of bacteriuria. Many species of gram –ve bacteria can convert nitrates to nitrites, and these are detected in urine by a reaction with the reagents on the dipstick which form a red azo dye. The specificity of the nitrite dipstick for detecting bacteriuria is >90% (false +ve nitrite testing can occur with contamination). Sensitivity: 35–85% (i.e. false –ves are common—a negative dipstick in the presence of active infection); less accurate in urine containing <10^5 organisms/mL. So, if the nitrite dipstick test is +ve, the patient probably has a UTI, but a –ve test often occurs in the presence of infection.

Cloudy urine which is +ve for wbcs on dipstick and is nitrite +ve is very likely to be infected.

Microscopy of midstream specimen of urine (MSU)

- False –ves—low bacterial counts may make it very difficult to identify bacteria, and the specimen of urine may therefore be deemed to be negative for bacteriuria, when in fact there is active infection
- False +ves—bacteria may be seen in the MSU in the absence of infection. This is most often due to contamination with commensals from the distal urethra and perineum (urine from a woman may contain thousands of lactobacilli and corynebacteria derived from the vagina). These bacteria are readily seen under the microscope, and although they are gram +ve, they often appear gram –ve (gram-variable) if stained.

If the urine specimen contains large numbers of squamous epithelial cells (cells which are derived from the foreskin, vaginal, or distal urethral epithelium), this suggests contamination of the specimen, and the presence of bacteria in this situation may indicate a false +ve result. The finding of pyuria and red blood cells suggests the presence of active infection.

Further investigation

Determined by the clinical scenario. If this is a one-off infection in an otherwise healthy individual, no further investigations are required. However, further investigations are required if:

- The patient develops symptoms and signs of upper tract infection (loin pain, malaise, fever), and therefore acute pyelonephritis, a pyonephrosis, or perinephric abscess is suspected
- Recurrent UTIs develop (see p. 174)
- The patient is pregnant
- Unusual infecting organism (e.g. Proteus), suggesting the possibility of an infection stone.

These further investigations will include a KUB X-ray ± IVU (looking for infection stones in the kidney; avoid in pregnant women) and a renal ultrasound.

Non-infective cystitis

Symptoms of cystitis can also be caused by:

- Pelvic radiotherapy (radiation cystitis—bladder capacity is reduced and multiple areas of mucosal telangectasia are seen cystoscopically)
- Drug-induced cystitis (e.g. cyclophosphamide treatment, ketamine abuse).

Recurrent urinary tract infection

Recurrent urinary tract infection (UTI) is defined as >2 infections in 6 months, or 3 within 12 months. It may be due to re-infection (i.e. infection by a different bacteria) or bacterial persistence (infection by the same organism originating from a focus within the urinary tract).

Bacterial persistence

Bacterial persistence usually leads to frequent recurrence of infection (within days or weeks) and the infecting organism is usually the same organism as that causing the previous infection(s). There is often an underlying functional or anatomical problem, and infection will often not resolve until this has been corrected. Causes include kidney stones; the chronically-infected prostate (chronic bacterial prostatitis); bacteria within an obstructed or atrophic infected kidney; vesicovaginal or colovesical fistula, and bacteria within a urethral diverticulum.

Re-infection

This usually occurs after a prolonged interval (months) from the previous infection, and is often caused by a different organism than the previous infecting bacterium.

Women with re-infection do not usually have an underlying functional or anatomical abnormality. Re-infections are associated with increased vaginal mucosal receptivity for uropathogens and ascending colonization from faecal flora. These women cannot be cured of their predisposition to recurrent UTIs, but they can be managed by a variety of techniques (see p. 176).

Men with re-infection may have underlying bladder outlet obstruction (due to benign prostatic enlargement or a urethral stricture), which makes them more likely to develop a repeat infection, but between infections their urine is sterile (i.e. they do not have bacterial persistence between symptomatic UTIs). A flexible cystoscopy, post-void bladder ultrasound for residual urine volume and, in some cases, urodynamics or urethrography may be helpful in establishing the potential causes.

As stated above, both men and women with bacterial persistence usually have an underlying functional or anatomical abnormality and they can potentially be cured of their recurrent UTIs, if this abnormality can be identified and corrected.

Management of recurrent urinary tract infection

Management of women with recurrent UTIs due to re-infection

Imaging tests including KUB X-ray, renal ultrasound, and flexible cystoscopy can be performed to check for potential sources of bacterial persistence (i.e. to confirm this is a 'simple' case of re-infection rather than one of bacterial persistence). In the absence of finding an underlying functional or anatomic abnormality, these patients cannot be cured of their tendency to recurrent urinary infection, but they can be managed in several ways:

Avoidance of spermicides used with the diaphragm or on condoms

Spermicides containing nonoxynol-9 reduce vaginal colonization with lactobacilli and may enhance *E. coli* adherence to urothelial cells. Recommend an alternative form of contraception.

Oestrogen replacement therapy

Lack of oestrogen in post-menopausal women causes loss of vaginal lactobacilli and increased colonization by *E. coli*. Oestrogen replacement (topical or systemic) can result in recolonization of the vagina with lactobacilli, and help eliminate colonization with bacterial uropathogens.[1]

Low-dose antibiotic prophylaxis

Oral antimicrobial therapy with full-dose oral tetracyclines, ampicillin, sulphonamides, amoxicillin, and cefalexin causes resistant strains in the faecal flora and subsequent resistant UTIs. However, trimethoprim, nitrofurantoin, low-dose cefalexin, and the fluoroquinolones have minimal adverse effects on the faecal and vaginal flora.

- **Efficacy of prophylaxis:** recurrences of UTI may be reduced up to 90% when compared with placebo.[2] Only small doses of antimicrobial agent are required, generally given at bedtime for 6–12 months. Symptomatic re-infection during prophylactic therapy is managed with a full therapeutic dose with the same prophylactic antibiotic or another antibiotic. Prophylaxis can then be restarted. Symptomatic re-infection immediately after cessation of prophylactic therapy is managed by restarting nightly prophylaxis

- **Trimethoprim:** the gut is a reservoir for organisms that colonize the periurethral area, which may cause episodes of acute cystitis in young women. Trimethoprim eradicates gram –ve aerobic flora from the gut and vaginal fluid (i.e. it eliminates the pathogens from the infective source). Trimethoprim is also concentrated in bactericidal concentrations in the urine following an oral dose. *Adverse reactions:* include gastro-intestinal (GI) disturbance; rash; puritis; depression of haematopoiesis; allergic reactions; rarely: erythema multiforme, toxic epidermal necrolysis, photosensitivity. Use with caution in renal impairment as it can increase creatinine by competitively inhibiting tubular secretion

- **Nitrofurantoin** is completely absorbed and/or inactivated in the upper intestinal tract and, therefore, has no effect on gut flora. It is present for brief periods at high concentrations in the urine and leads to repeated elimination of bacteria from the urine. Nitrofurantoin prophylaxis, therefore, does not lead to a change in vaginal or introital colonization with Enterobacteria. The bacteria colonizing the vagina remain susceptible to nitrofurantoin because of the lack of bacterial resistance in the faecal flora. *Adverse reactions*: include GI upset; chronic pulmonary reactions (pulmonary fibrosis); peripheral neuropathy; allergic reactions (angioedema, anaphylaxis, urticaria, rash and pruritus); peripheral neuropathy; rarely: blood dyscrasias (agranulocytosis, thrombocytopenia, aplastic anaemia), liver damage. Risk of an adverse reaction increases with age (particularly >50 years old)

- **Cefalexin** at 250 mg or less nightly is an excellent prophylactic agent because faecal resistance does not develop at this low dosage. *Adverse reactions*: GI upset; allergic reactions

- **Fluoroquinolones** (e.g. ciprofloxacin): short courses eradicate Enterobacteria from faecal and vaginal flora. *Adverse reactions to quinolones*: tendon damage (including rupture), which may occur within 48 h of starting treatment. The risk of tendon rupture is increased by the concomitant use of corticosteroids. Contraindicated in patients with a history of tendon disorders related to quinolone use. Discontinue quinolone immediately if tendonitis suspected (elderly patients are most prone to tendonitis). *Other adverse reactions*: GI upset; Stevens–Johnson syndrome; allergic reactions. Some hospitals do not allow the routine use of ciprofloxacin in an attempt to reduce the incidence of symptomatic *Clostridium difficile*.

Natural yoghurt

Applied to the vulva and vagina can help restore normal vaginal flora, thereby improving the natural resistance to recurrent infections.

Post-intercourse antibiotic prophylaxis

Sexual intercourse has been established as an important risk factor for acute cystitis in women, and women using the diaphragm have a significantly greater risk of UTI those using other contraceptive methods.[3] Post-intercourse therapy with antimicrobials such as nitrofurantoin, cefalexin, or trimethoprim, taken as a single dose, effectively reduces the incidence of re-infection.

Self-start therapy

Women keep a home supply of an antibiotic (e.g. trimethoprim, nitrofurantoin, or a fluoroquinolone) and start treatment when they develop symptoms suggestive of UTI.

1   Raz R, Stamm WE (1993) A controlled trial in intravaginal estriol in postmenopausal women with recurrent urinary tract infection. *N Engl J Med* **329**:753.

2   Nicolle LE, Ronald AR (1987) Recurrent urinary tract infection in adult women: diagnosis and treatment. *Infect Dis Clin North Am* **1**:793.

3   Fihn SD, Latham RH, Roberts P, *et al.* (1985) Association between diaphragm use and urinary tract infection. *JAMA* **254**:240.

Management of men and women with recurrent UTIs due to bacterial persistence

Investigations: these are directed at identifying the potential causes of bacterial persistence, outlined above:

- KUB X-ray to detect radio-opaque renal calculi
- Renal ultrasound to detect hydronephrosis and renal calculi. If hydronephrosis is present, but the ureter is not dilated, consider the possibility of a radio-opaque stone obstructing the pelviureteric junction (PUJ) or a PUJ obstruction (PUJO)
- Determination of post-void residual urine volume by bladder ultrasound
- IVU or CTU, where a stone is suspected, but not identified on plain X-ray or ultrasound
- Flexible cystoscopy to identify possible causes of recurrent UTIs, such as bladder stones, an underlying bladder cancer (rare), urethral or bladder neck stricture, or fistula.

Treatment: depends on the functional or anatomical abnormality that is identified as the cause of the bacterial persistence. If a stone is identified, this should be removed. If there is obstruction (e.g. bladder outlet obstruction, PUJO, detrusor-sphincter-dyssynergia in spinal injured patients), this should be corrected.

Urinary tract infection: general treatment guidelines

Antimicrobial drug therapy

The aim is to eliminate bacterial growth from the urine. Empirical treatment involves the administration of antibiotics according to the clinical presentation and most likely causative organism, before culture sensitivities are available (📖 see Table 6.3). Men are often affected by complicated UTI and may require longer treatments, as may patients with uncorrectable structural or functional abnormalities (e.g. in-dwelling catheters, neuropathic bladders).

Bacterial resistance to drug therapy

Organisms susceptible to concentrations of an antibiotic in the urine (or serum) after the recommended clinical dosing are termed 'sensitive', and those that do not respond are 'resistant'. Bacterial resistance may be intrinsic (e.g. Proteus is intrinsically resistant to nitrofurantoin), via selection of a resistant mutant during initial treatment, or genetically transferred between bacteria by R plasmids.

Definitive treatment

Once urine or blood culture results are available, antimicrobial therapy should be adjusted according to bacterial sensitivities. Underlying abnormality should be corrected if feasible (i.e. extraction of infected calculus; removal of catheter; nephrostomy drainage of an infected, obstructed kidney). Post-menopausal women may benefit from topical oestrogen treatment.

General preventative advice

Encourage a good fluid intake; cranberry juice; double voiding. In women: voiding before and after intercourse; wiping perineum from 'front to back' after voiding; avoid using bubble bath or washing hair in the bath in (as this affects the protective commensal organisms, the lactobacilli).

1 Naber KG, Bishop MC, Bjerklund-Johansen TE, *et al.* (2007). *Guidelines on the Management of Urinary and Male Genital Tract Infections.* European Association of Urology, http://www.eau.org.

Table 6.3 Recommendations for antimicrobial therapy[1]

Infection	Bacteria	Initial empirical drug	Duration
Acute, uncomplicated cystitis	E. coli, Klebsiella, Proteus, Staphylococcus	Trimethoprim/co-trimoxazole	3 days
		Quinolone (ciprofloxacin) or	3 days
		Nitrofurantoin	7 days
Acute, uncomplicated pyelonephritis	E. coli, Proteus, Klebsiella, other Enterobacteriacae, Staphylococcus	Quinolone	7–10 days
		Cephalosporin or Aminopenicillin with beta-lactamase inhibitor (amoxicillin/clavulanic acid)	
		Aminoglycoside (gentamicin)	
Complicated UTI	E. coli, Enterococcus, Pseudomonas, Staphylococcus	Quinolone Aminopenicillin with beta-lactamase inhibitor Cephalosporin	Continue for 3–5 days after elimination of underlying factor
Nosocomial* UTI	Staphylococcus, Klebsiella, Proteus	Carbapenem (meropenem) ± Aminoglycoside	
Acute complicated pyelonephritis	Enterobacter, Pseudomonas, Candida	For Candida: –Fluconazole –Amphotericin B	

*Nosocomial = hospital acquired.

These are general recommendations only; you should be guided by your local microbiology department whose recommendations will be based on local and regional bacterial sensitivities and resistance.

Upper urinary tract infection: acute pyelonephritis

Pyelonephritis is inflammation of the kidney and renal pelvis.

Presentation

Clinical diagnosis is based on the presence of fever, flank pain, and tenderness, often with an elevated white count. Nausea and vomiting are common. It may affect one or both kidneys. There are usually accompanying symptoms suggestive of a lower UTI (frequency, urgency, suprapubic pain, urethral burning or pain on voiding) responsible for the subsequent ascending infection to the kidney.

Differential diagnosis Includes cholecystitis, pancreatitis, diverticulitis, appendicitis.

Risk factors Females>males; vesicoureteric reflux (VUR); urinary tract obstruction; calculi; spinal cord injury (neuropathic bladder); diabetes mellitus; congenital malformation; pregnancy; in-dwelling catheters; urinary tract instrumentation.

Pathogenesis and microbiology Initially, there is patchy infiltration of neutrophils and bacteria in the parenchyma. Later changes include the formation of inflammatory bands extending from renal papilla to cortex, and small cortical abscesses. 80% of infections are secondary to *E. coli* (possessing P pili virulence factors). Other infecting organisms: Enterococci (*Streptococcus faecalis*), *Klebsiella*, *Proteus*, and *Pseudomonas*. Any process interfering with ureteric peristalsis (i.e obstruction) may assist in retrograde bacterial ascent from bladder to kidney.

Investigation and treatment

- For those patients who have a fever, but are not systemically unwell, outpatient management is reasonable. Culture the urine and start oral antibiotics according to your local antibiotic policy (which will be based on the likely infecting organisms and their likely antibiotic sensitivity). An option is oral ciprofloxacin, 500 mg bd for 10 days
- If the patient is systemically unwell, culture urine and blood, start intravenous (IV) fluids and IV antibiotics, again selecting the antibiotic according to your local antibiotic policy. Options include IV amoxicillin 1 g tds and gentamicin 3 mg/kg as a once-daily dose
- Arrange a KUB X-ray and renal ultrasound, to see if there is an underlying upper tract abnormality (such a ureteric stone), unexplained hydronephrosis, or (rarely) gas surrounding the kidney (suggesting emphysematous pyelonephritis)

- If the patient does not respond within 3 days to a regimen of appropriate IV antibiotics (confirmed on sensitivities), arrange a CTU (computed tomography urogram). Failure of response to treatment suggests possible pyonephrosis (i.e. pus in the kidney, which will only respond to drainage), a perinephric abscess (which again will only respond to drainage), or emphysematous pyelonephritis. The CTU may demonstrate an obstructing ureteric calculus that may have been missed on the KUB X-ray, and ultrasound may show a perinephric abscess. A pyonephrosis should be drained by insertion of a percutaneous nephrostomy tube. A perinephric abscess should also be drained by insertion of a drain percutaneously

- If the patient responds to IV antibiotics, change to an oral antibiotic of appropriate sensitivity when they become apyrexial (3–5 days after control of infection or after elimination of underlying problem), and continue this for approximately 10–14 days.

Pyonephrosis and perinephric abscess

Pyonephrosis

An infected hydronephrosis, where pus accumulates within the renal pelvis and calyces. It is associated with damage to the parenchyma, resulting in loss of renal function. The causes are essentially those of hydronephrosis, where infection has supervened (e.g. ureteric obstruction by stone, PUJ obstruction).

Presentation: patients with pyonephrosis are usually very unwell, with a high fever, flank pain, and tenderness.

Risk factors Stone disease, previous urinary tract infection, or surgery.

Investigation
- **KUB X-ray:** may show an air urogram (secondary to gas produced by infecting pathogens)
- **USS:** shows evidence of obstruction (hydronephrosis) with a dilated collecting system, fluid-debri levels or air in the collecting system
- **CT:** shows hydronephrosis, stranding of perinephric fat, and thickening of renal pelvis.

Treatment: intravenous fluids and antibiotics (as for pyelonephritis), with urgent percutaneous drainage (nephrostomy) or ureteric drainage (via ureteric catheter under endoscopic and X-ray guidance).

Perinephric abscess

Perinephric abscess develops as a consequence of extension of infection outside the parenchyma of the kidney in acute pyelonephritis or, more rarely, from haematogenous spread of infection from a distant site. The abscess develops within Gerota's fascia.

Risk factors: diabetes mellitus; obstructing ureteric calculus may precipitate development of the perinephric abscess.

Causes: perinephric abscesses are caused by *Staphylcoccus aureus* (gram +ve); *Escherichia coli*, and *Proteus* (gram –ves).

Presentation: patients present with fever, unilateral flank tenderness, and a ≥5-day history of milder symptoms. Failure of a seemingly straightforward case of acute pyelonephritis to respond to intravenous antibiotics within a few days also arouses suspicion that there is an accumulation of pus in or around the kidney, or obstruction with infection.

A flank mass with overlying skin erythema and oedema may be observed. Extension of the thigh (stretching the psoas) may trigger pain, and psoas spasm may cause a reactive scoliosis.

Investigation
- **Full blood count** shows raised white cell count
- **Urine analysis and cultures**
- **Blood cultures** are required to identify organisms responsible for haematogenous spread of infection (*Staph. aureus*)
- **USS or CT with contrast** can identify size, site and extension of retroperitoneal abscesses, and allow radiographically controlled percutaneous drainage of the abscess.

Treatment
Commence broad-spectrum intravenous antibiotics (i.e. aminoglycoside and aminopenicillin with beta-lactamase inhibitor) until culture sensitivities are available. Intravenous drugs should be used for 7–14 days, and followed by a course of oral antimicrobials until clinical review and re-imaging confirms resolution of infection. Drainage of the collection should be performed, either radiographically, or by formal open incision and drainage if the pus collection is large. Nephrectomy may be required for extensive renal involvement, or a non-functioning infected kidney.

Other forms of pyelonephritis

Emphysematous pyelonephritis

A rare, severe form of acute pyelonephritis caused by gas-forming organisms. It is characterized by fever and abdominal pain, with radiographic evidence of gas within and around the kidney (on plain radiography or CT; Fig. 6.1). It usually occurs in diabetics, and in many cases is precipitated by urinary obstruction by, for example, ureteric stones. The high glucose levels associated with poorly controlled diabetes provides an ideal environment for fermentation by *Enterobacteria*; carbon dioxide being produced during this process.

Presentation: severe acute pyelonephritis (high fever and systemic upset) that fails to respond within 2–3 days with conventional treatment in the form of intravenous (IV) antibiotics. Commonly caused by *E. coli*, less frequently by *Klebsiella* and *Proteus mirabilis*. On KUB X-ray, a crescent or kidney-shaped distribution of gas may be seen around the kidney. Renal ultrasonography often demonstrates strong focal echoes, indicating gas within the kidney. Intra-renal gas is seen on CT scan.

Management: patients with emphysematous pyelonephritis are usually very unwell and mortality is high. In selected cases, it can be managed conservatively, by IV antibiotics and fluids, percutaneous drainage, and careful control of diabetes. In those where sepsis is poorly controlled, emergency nephrectomy is required.

Xanthogranulomatous pyelonephritis

A severe renal infection usually (although not always) occurring in association with underlying renal calculi and renal obstruction. The severe infection results in destruction of renal tissue leading to a non-functioning kidney. *E. coli* and *Proteus* are common causative organisms. Macrophages full of fat become deposited around abscesses within the parenchyma of the kidney. The infection may be confined to the kidney or extend to the perinephric fat. The kidney becomes grossly enlarged and macroscopically contains yellowish nodules (pus), and areas of haemorrhagic necrosis. It can be very difficult to distinguish the radiological findings from a renal cancer on imaging studies such as CT. Indeed, in most cases the diagnosis is made after nephrectomy for what was presumed to be a renal cell carcinoma.

Presentation: acute flank pain, fever and a tender flank mass. Bacteria (*E. coli*, *Proteus*) may be found on culture urine. Renal ultrasonography shows an enlarged kidney containing echogenic material. On CT, renal calcification is usually seen within the renal mass. Non-enhancing cavities are seen, containing pus and debris. On radioisotope scanning, there may be some or no function in the affected kidney.

Management: on presentation these patients are usually commenced on antibiotics as the constellation of symptoms and signs suggest infection. When imaging studies are done, such as CT, the appearances usually suggest the possibility of a renal cell carcinoma, and therefore when signs of infection have resolved, the majority of patients will proceed to nephrectomy. Only following pathological examination of the removed kidney will it become apparent that the diagnosis was one of infection (xanthogranulomatous pyelonephritis), rather than tumour.

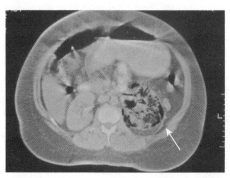

Fig. 6.1 CT scan demonstrating emphysematous pyelonephritis affecting the left kidney. Image kindly provided with permission from Professor S. Reif.

Acute pyelonephritis, pyonephrosis, perinephric abscess, and emphysematous pyelonephritis—making the diagnosis

Maintaining a degree of suspicion in all cases of presumed acute pyelone-phritis is the single most important thing in allowing an early diagnosis of complicated renal infection, such as a pyonephrosis, perinephric abscess, or emphysematous pyelonephritis, to be made. If the patient is very unwell, is diabetic, or has a history suggestive of stones, they may have something more than just a simple acute pyelonephritis. Specifically ask about a history of sudden onset of severe flank pain a few days earlier, suggesting the possibility that a stone passed into the ureter, with later infection supervening. Arranging a KUB X-ray and renal ultrasound in all patients with suspected renal infection will demonstrate the presence of hydronephrosis, pus, or stones.

Clinical indicators suggesting a more complex form of renal infection are length of symptoms prior to treatment, and time taken to respond to treatment. Most patients with uncomplicated acute pyelonephritis have been symptomatic for <5 days. Most with, for example, a perine-phric abscess have been symptomatic for >5 days prior to hospitalization. Patients with acute pyelonephritis became afebrile within 4–5 days of treatment with an appropriate antibiotic, whereas those with perinephric abscesses remain pyrexial.[1]

1 Thorley JD, Jones SR, Sanford JP (1974) Perinephric abscess. *Medicine* **53**:441.

Chronic pyelonephritis

In essence, this describes *renal scarring*, which may or may not be related to previous urinary tract infection (UTI). It is a radiological, functional or pathological diagnosis or description.

Causes

- Renal scarring due to previous infection
- Long-term effects of vesicoureteric reflux (with or without superimposed infection).

A child with reflux, particularly where there is reflux of infected urine, will develop reflux nephropathy (which if bilateral, may cause renal impairment or renal failure). If the child's kidneys are examined radiologically (or pathologically if they are removed by nephrectomy), the radiologist or pathologist will describe the appearances as those of 'chronic pyelonephritis'.

An *adult* may also develop radiological and pathological features of chronic pyelonephritis due to the presence of reflux or bladder outlet obstruction combined with high bladder pressures, again particularly where the urine is infected. This was a common occurrence in male patients with spinal cord injuries and detrusor sphincter dyssynergia before the advent of effective treatments for this condition.

Pathogenesis

Chronic pyelonephritis is essentially the end result of longstanding reflux (non-obstructive chronic pyelonephritis) or of obstruction (obstructive chronic pyelonephritis). These processes damage the kidneys leading to scarring, and the degree of damage and subsequent scarring is more marked if infection has supervened.

Presentation

Patients may be asymptomatic, or present with symptoms secondary to renal failure. Diagnosis is often from incidental findings during general investigation. There is usually no active infection.

Appearances on imaging

Scars can be 'seen' radiologically on a renal ultrasound, intravenous urogram (IVU), renal isotope scan, or a CT scan. The scars are closely related to a deformed renal calyx. Distortion and dilatation of the calyces is due to scarring of the renal pyramids. These scars typically affect the upper and lower poles of the kidneys, because these sites are more prone to intrarenal reflux. The cortex and medulla in the region of a scar is thin. The kidney may be so scarred that it becomes small and atrophic.

Management

Aim to investigate and treat any infection, prevent further UTI, and monitor and optimize renal function.

Complications

Renal impairment progressing to end-stage renal failure in bilateral cases (usually only if chronic pyelonephritis is associated with an underlying structural or function urinary tract abnormality).

Septicaemia

Bacteraemia is the presence of pathogenic organisms in the blood stream. This can lead to *septicaemia* or *sepsis*—the clinical syndrome caused by bacterial infection of the blood. This is confirmed by positive blood cultures for a specific organism, and accompanied by a systemic response to the infection known as the *systemic inflammatory response syndrome (SIRS)*. SIRS is defined by at least two of the following:

- Fever (>38°C) or hypothermia (<36°C)
- Tachycardia (>90 beats/min in patients not on beta-blockers)
- Tachypnoea (respiration >20 breaths/min, or P_aCO_2 <4.3 kPa, or a requirement for mechanical ventilation)
- White cell count >12,000 cells/mm^3, <4000 cells/mm^3 or 10% immature (band) forms.

Septicaemia is often accompanied by *endotoxaemia*—the presence of circulating bacterial endotoxins.

Severe sepsis or sepsis syndrome is a state of altered organ perfusion or evidence of dysfunction of one or more organs, with at least one of the following: hypoxaemia, lactic acidosis, oliguria, or altered mental status.

Septic shock is severe sepsis with hypotension,[1] hypoperfusion, and organ dysfunction. It results from gram +ve bacterial toxins or gram −ve endotoxins, which trigger release of cytokines (TNF, IL-1), vascular mediators, and platelets, resulting in vasodilatation (manifest as hypotension) and disseminated intra-vascular coagulation (DIC).

Refractory shock is defined as septic shock (lasting >1 h), which fails to respond to therapy.

Causes of urinary sepsis

In the hospital setting, the most common causes are the presence or manipulation of in-dwelling urinary catheters, urinary tract surgery (particularly endoscopic—TURP, TURBT, ureteroscopy, PCNL), and urinary tract obstruction (particularly that due to stones obstructing the ureter). Septicaemia occurs in approximately 1.5% of men undergoing TURP. Diabetic patients, patients in ICUs, and patients on chemotherapy and steroids are more prone to urosepsis.

Causative organisms in urinary sepsis: E. coli, enterococci (*Streptococcus faecalis*), staphylococci, *Pseudomonas aeruginosa*, *Klebsiella*, and *Proteus mirabilis*.

Management

The principles of management include early recognition, resuscitation, localization of the source of sepsis, early and appropriate antibiotic administration, and removal of the primary source of sepsis. From a urological perspective, the clinical scenario is usually a post-operative patient who has undergone TURP or surgery for stones. On return to the ward they become pyrexial, start to shiver (chills) and shake, and are tachycardic and tachypnoea (leading initially to respiratory alkalosis). They may be confused and oliguric. They may initially be peripherally vasodilatated (flushed appearance with warm peripheries). Consider the possibility of a non-urological source of sepsis (e.g. pneumonia). If there are no indications of infection elsewhere, assume the urinary tract is the source of sepsis.

Investigations

- **Urine culture:** an immediate gram-stain may aid in deciding which antibiotic to use
- **Full blood count:** the white blood count is usually elevated.
  The platelet count may be low—a possible indication of impending DIC
- **Coagulation screen:** this is important if surgical or radiological drainage of the source of infection is necessary
- **Urea and electrolytes** as a baseline determination of renal function, and C-reactive protein (CRP), which is usually elevated
- **Arterial blood gases** to identify hypoxia and the presence of metabolic acidosis
- **Blood cultures**
- **CXR**: looking for pneumonia, atelectasis, and effusions.

Depending on the clinical situation, a renal ultrasound may be helpful to demonstrate hydronephrosis or pyonephrosis, and CT urography (CTU) may be used to establish the presence or absence of a ureteric stone.

Treatment

- A (**A**irway), B (**B**reathing), C (**C**irculation)
- 100% oxygen via a face-mask
- Establish intravenous access with 2 wide-bore cannulae
- Intravenous crystalloid (e.g. normal saline) or colloid (e.g. Gelofusin®)
- Catheterize to monitor urine output
- Empirical antibiotic therapy (see below). This should be adjusted later when cultures are available
- If there is septic shock, the patient needs to be transferred to ICU. Inotropic support may be needed. Steroids may be used as adjunctive therapy in gram –ve infections. Naloxone may help revert endotoxic shock. Blood glucose is carefully controlled, and recombinant activated protein C has proven benefit in severe sepsis. This should all be done under the supervision of an intensivist
- Treat the underlying cause. Drain any obstruction and remove any foreign body. If there is a stone obstructing the ureter then either ask the radiologist to insert a nephrostomy tube to relieve the obstruction, or take the patient to the operating room and insert a JJ-ureteric stent. Send any urine specimens obtained for microscopy and culture.

---

1 Hypotension in septic shock is defined as a sustained systolic BP <90 mmHg, or a drop in systolic pressure of >40 mmHg for >1 h, when the patient is normovolaemic, and other causes have been excluded or treated.

Empirical treatment of septicaemia

This is 'blind' use of antibiotics based on an educated guess of the most likely pathogen that has caused the sepsis. Gram –ve aerobic rods are common causes of urosepsis (e.g. *E. coli*, *Klebsiella*, *Citrobacter*, *Proteus*, and *Serratia*). The enterococci (gram +ve aerobic non-haemolytic streptococci) may sometimes cause urosepsis. In urinary tract operations involving the bowel, anaerobic bacteria may be the cause of urosepsis, and in wound infections, staphylococci (e.g. *Staph. aureus* and *Staph. epidermidis*) are the usual cause.

Recommendations for treatment of urosepsis[1]

- A third-generation cephalosporin [e.g. intravenous (IV) cefotaxime or ceftriaxone]. These are active against gram –ve bacteria, but have less activity against staphylococci and gram +ve bacteria. Ceftazidime also has activity against *Pseudomonas aeruginosa*
- Fluoroquinolones (e.g. ciprofloxacin) are an alternative to cephalosporins. They exhibit good activity against enterobacteriaceae and *P. aeruginosa*, but less activity against staphylococci and enterococci. Gastrointestinal tract absorption of ciprofloxacin is good, so oral administration is as effective as IV
- Use metronidazole if there is a potential anaerobic source of sepsis
- If no clinical response to the above antibiotics, consider a combination of antipseudomonal penicillin and beta-lactamase inhibitor (i.e. pipera-cillin and tazobactam; trade name Tazocin®). This combination is active against enterobacteriaceae, enterococci, and *Pseudomonas*
- Aminoglycoside (i.e. gentamicin) is used in conjunction with other antibiotics. It has a relatively narrow therapeutic spectrum against gram –ve organisms. Close monitoring of therapeutic levels and renal function is important. It has good activity against enterobacteriaceae and *Pseudomonas*, with poor activity against streptococci and anaerobes, and therefore should ideally be combined with β-lactam antibiotics (i.e. meropenem) or ciprofloxacin.

If there is clinical improvement, treatment (IV) should continue for 3–5 days after the infection has been controlled (or complicating factor has been eliminated), followed by a course of oral antibiotics. Make appropriate adjustments when sensitivity results are available from urine cultures (which may take about 48 h).

Mortality rate: 13% with septicaemia alone; 28% with septicaemia and shock; 43% with septicaemia followed by septic shock.[2]

---

1 Naber KG, Bishop MC, Bjerklund-Johansen TE, *et al.* (2007). *Guidelines on the Management of Urinary and Male Genital Tract Infections.* European Association of Urology, www.eau.org

2 Bone RC, Fisher CJ Jr, Clemmer TP, *et al.* (1989) Sepsis syndrome: a valid clinical entity. Methyl-prednisolone Severe Sepsis Study Group. *Crit Care Med* **17**:389–93.

Fournier's gangrene

A necrotizing fascitis of the external genitalia and perineum primarily affecting males and causing necrosis and subsequent gangrene of infected tissues. Also known as spontaneous fulminant gangrene of the genitalia, it is a urological emergency.

Causative organisms

Culture of infected tissue reveals a combination of aerobic (*E. coli*, entero-cocci, *Klebsiella*) and anaerobic organisms (*Bacteroides*, *Clostridium*, micro-aerophilic streptococci), which are believed to grow in a synergistic fashion.

Predisposing factors

Diabetes mellitus, chronic alcohol excess, local trauma to the genitalia and perineum (e.g. zipper injuries to the foreskin, periurethral extravasa-tion of urine following traumatic catheterization or instrumentation of the urethra), and surgical procedures, such as circumcision, paraphimosis, peri-anal or perirectal infections.

Pathophysiology

Fournier's gangrene is usually related to an initial genitourinary tract infec-tion, skin trauma or from direct extension from a perirectal focus. Spread of infection is through local fascia (Buck's fascia in the penis; Dartos fascia in the scrotum; Colle's fascia in the perineal region, and Scarpa's fascia of the anterior abdominal wall). Infection produces tissue necrosis that can spread rapidly and pus produced by anaerobic pathogens (*Bacteroides*) produces the typical putrid smell.

Presentation

A previously well patient may become systemically unwell following a seem-ingly trivial injury to the external genitalia. Early clinical features include localized skin erythema, tenderness and oedema, sometimes with lower urinary tract symptoms (dysuria, difficulty voiding, urethral discharge). This progresses to fever and sepsis, with cellulitis and palpable crepitus in the affected tissues indicating the presence of subcutaneous gas produced by gas-forming organisms. As the infection advances, blisters (bullae) appear in the skin and, within a matter of hours, areas of necrosis may develop, which spread to involve adjacent tissues (e.g. lower abdominal wall).

Diagnosis

The diagnosis is a clinical one, and is based on awareness of the condition and a low index of suspicion. In early stages of disease, abdominal X-ray or scrotal USS may demonstrate the presence of air in tissues.

Management

Do not delay. Obtain intravenous access, take blood cultures, start intravenous fluids, and administer oxygen. Broad spectrum parenteral antibiotics are given immediately to cover both gram +ve and negative aerobes and anaerobes (e.g. combination of ampicillin with beta-lactamase inhibitor plus gentamicin plus clindamycin or metronidazole). Transfer the patient to theatre as quickly as possible for debridement of necrotic tissue (skin, subcutaneous fat). Extensive areas of tissue may have to be removed, but it is unusual for the testes or deeper penile tissues to be involved, and these can usually be spared. A suprapubic catheter is inserted to divert urine and allow monitoring of urine output. Repeated debridement to remove residual necrotic tissue may be required. Wound irrigation with hydrogen peroxide has been used, and where facilities allow, treatment with hyperbaric oxygen therapy may be beneficial.[1] Reconstruction can be contemplated when wound healing is complete.

Mortality is in the order of 20–30%. There is debate about whether diabetes increases the mortality rate.[2,3]

1   Pizzorno R, Bonini F, Donelli A, *et al.* (1997) Hyperbaric oxygen therapy in the treatment of Fournier's gangrene in 100 male patients. *J Urol* **158**:837–40.

2   Nisbet AA, Thompson IM (2002) Impact of diabetes mellitus on the presentation and outcomes of Fournier's gangrene. *Urology* **60**:775–79.

3   Chawla SN, Gallop C, Mydlo JH (2003) Fournier's gangrene: an analysis of repeated surgical debridement. *Eur Urol* **43**:572–75.

Peri-urethral abscess

Peri-urethral abscess can occur in patients with urethral stricture disease, in association with gonococcal urethritis, and following urethral catheterization. These conditions predispose to bacteria (gram –ve rods, enterococci, anaerobes, gonococcus) gaining access through Buck's fascia to the peri-urethral tissues. If not rapidly diagnosed and treated, infection (fascitis) can spread to the perineum, buttocks, and abdominal wall.

Presentation

The majority (90%) of patients present with scrotal swelling and a fever. ~20% will have presented with urinary retention, 10% with a urethral discharge, and 10% having spontaneously discharged the abscess through the urethra.

Management

Emergency treatment is required. The abscess should be incised and drained, a suprapubic catheter placed to divert the urine away from the urethra, and broad spectrum parenteral antibiotics commenced (gentamicin and cephalosporin) until antibiotic sensitivities are known. Any devitalized and necrotic tissue requires immediate surgical debridement.

Epididymitis and orchitis

Acute epididymitis is an inflammatory condition of the epididymis, often involving the testis, and caused by bacterial infection. It has an acute onset and a clinical course lasting <6 weeks, presenting with epididymal pain, swelling, and tenderness.

Pathogenesis

Infection ascends from the urethra or bladder. In sexually active men aged <35 years, the infective organism is usually *N. gonorrhoeae*, *C. trachomatis*, or coliform bacteria (causing a urethritis, which then ascends to infect the epididymis). In children and older men, the infective organisms are usually common uropathogens (i.e. *Escherichia coli*). *Mycobacterium tuberculosis* (TB) is a rarer cause—the epididymis feels like a 'beaded' cord (☐ see p. 210).

A rare, non-infective cause of epididymitis is the anti-arrhythmic drug amiodarone, which accumulates in high concentrations within the epididymis, causing inflammation.[1] It can be unilateral or bilateral, and resolves on discontinuation of the drug.

Presentation

Fever; testicular swelling; scrotal pain that may radiate to the groin (spermatic cord) and lower abdomen; erythema of scrotal skin; thickening of spermatic cord; reactive hydrocele; evidence of underlying infection (urethral discharge, symptoms of urethritis, cystitis, or prostatitis).

Differential diagnosis

- Testicular torsion is the main differential diagnosis. In torsion, pain and swelling are more acute and localized to the testis, whereas epididymitis is mainly preceded by infective symptoms with pain, tenderness and swelling tending to be confined to the epididymis.

If any doubt in diagnosis exists, exploration is the safest option. Although radionuclide scanning can differentiate between a torsion and epididymitis, this is not widely available. Colour Doppler ultrasound scan (USS), which provides a visual image of blood flow, can differentiate between a torsion and epididymitis, but its sensitivity for diagnosing torsion is only 80% (i.e. it 'misses' the diagnosis in 20% of cases). Its sensitivity for diagnosing epididymitis is about 70%.

- Torsion of testicular appendage
- Acute haemorrhage of testicular tumour
- Testicular trauma
- Mumps orchitis.

Investigation

Culture urine, any urethral discharge, and blood (if systemically unwell). Consider urethral swabs and scrotal USS.

Treatment

This consists of bed rest, analgesia, scrotal elevation and antibiotics. Until culture sensitivities are available, where *C. trachomatis* is a possible infecting organism, prescribe a 14-day course of doxycycline 100 mg twice daily. If gonorrhoeae is suspected or confirmed on a gram stain or culture of urethral swab, prescribe ciprofloxacin (500 mg bd for 14 days). For non-sexually transmitted infection related epididymitis, prescribe antibiotics empirically (until culture results are available) according to your local microbiology department advice. Our empirical antibiotic regimen is ciprofloxacin for 2 weeks. When the patient is systemically unwell, we admit them for intravenous cephalosporin and intravenous gentamicin (initially 3–5 mg/kg, then adjusted according to serum gentamicin concentration). When the patient becomes apyrexial, we change to oral ciprofloxacin for 2 weeks.

Complications of acute epididymitis

These include abscess formation, infarction of the testis, chronic pain, and infertility.

Chronic epididymitis is diagnosed in patients with long-term pain in the epididymis (± testicle). It can result from recurrent episodes of acute epididymitis. Clinically, the epididymis is thickened and may be tender. Treatment is with the appropriate antibiotics (guided by cultures), or epididymectomy in severe cases.

Orchitis is inflammation of the testis, although it often occurs with epididymitis (epididymo-orchitis). Causes include mumps; *M. tuberculosis*; syphilis; auto-immune processes (granulomatous orchitis). The testis is swollen and tense, with oedema of connective tissues and inflammatory cell infiltration. Treat the underlying cause.

Mumps orchitis occurs in 30% of infected post-pubertal males. It manifests 3–4 days after the onset of parotitis, and can result in tubular atrophy. 10–30% of cases are bilateral, and are associated with testicular atrophy and infertility.

1 Gasparich JP, Mason JT, Greene HL *et al.* (1984) Non-infectious epididymitis associated with amiodarone therapy. *Lancet* **2**:1211-12.

Prostatitis: epidemiology and classification

Definition: prostatitis is infection and/or inflammation of the prostate.

National Institute of Health Classification of prostatitis[1]

I   Acute bacterial prostatitis: acute infection
II   Chronic bacterial prostatitis: recurrent infection
III   Chronic pelvic pain syndrome: no infection detected
III_A   Inflammatory chronic pelvic pain syndrome (chronic non-bacterial prostatitis): white blood cells (wbc) in expressed prostatic secretions (EPS), post-prostatic massage urine (VB_3), or semen
III_B   Non-inflammatory chronic pelvic pain syndrome (prostatodynia): no wbc in EPS, VB_3, or semen
IV   Asymptomatic inflammatory prostatitis (histological prostatitis): detected by prostate biopsy or presence of wbc in prostatic secretions as an incidental finding.

Epidemiology

Estimated to affect 50% of men at some point in their lives. The overall prevalence of prostatitis is reported at 5–14%. Age groups at increased risk are 20–50 and >70 years old.

Pathophysiology

In all types of prostatitis, the tissue surrounding the prostatic acini (parenchyma) becomes infiltrated with inflammatory cells (lymphocytes).

Bacterial prostatitis: the most common infective pathogens are gram −ve enterbacteriaceae [*Escherichia coli* (80% of cases), *Pseudomonas aeruginosa*, *Klebsiella*, *proteus*, *Serratia*, *Enterobacter aerogenes*]. Both type 1 and P pili are important bacterial virulence factors that facilitate infection. 5–10% of infections are caused by gram +ve bacteria (*Staphylococcus aureus* and *saprophyticus*, *Streptococcus faecalis*). Acute bacterial prostatitis is often secondary to infected urine refluxing into prostatic ducts that drain into the posterior urethra. The resulting oedema and inflammation may then obstruct the prostatic ducts, trapping uropathogens and causing progression to chronic bacterial prostatitis in ~5%.

Inflammatory and non-inflammatory prostatitis: the underlying aetiology is likely to be multifactorial, with inflammatory, immunological, neuropathic and neuroendocrine mechanisms all playing a possible role in susceptible patients.

Special investigations

Segmented urine cultures A useful investigation for all prostatitis, as it helps to localize bacteria to a specific part of the urinary tract by sampling different parts of the urinary stream, with or without prostatic massage (which produces expressed prostatic secretions (EPS)). Where cultures are negative, increased leucocytes per high-powered field (>10) favour a diagnosis of inflammatory chronic pelvic pain syndrome.

- **VB$_1$:** first 10 mL of urine voided. Positive culture indicates urethritis or prostatitis
- **VB$_2$:** mid-stream urine. Positive culture indicates cystitis
- **VB$_3$:** first 10 mL of urine voided following prostatic massage. Positive culture indicates prostatitis
- **EPS:** Positive culture indicates prostatitis.

1 Krieger JN, Nyberg LJ, Nickel JC (1999) NIH consensus definition and classification of prostatitis. *JAMA* **282:**236–7.

Bacterial prostatitis

Acute bacterial prostatitis

Acute bacterial prostatitis is infection of the prostate associated with lower urinary tract infection and generalized sepsis.

Risk factors

Factors that predispose to genitourinary tract and then prostatic colonization with bacteria are:

- Urinary tract infection
- Acute epididymitis
- In-dwelling urethral catheters
- Transurethral surgery
- Intraprostatic ductal reflux
- Phimosis
- Prostatic stones (which can provide a nidus of infection for chronic prostatitis).

Presentation

Acute onset of fevers, chills, nausea, and vomiting; perineal and suprapubic pain; 'irritative' urinary symptoms (urinary frequency, urgency and dysuria); 'obstructive' urinary symptoms (hesitancy, strangury, intermittent stream, or urinary retention). Signs of systemic toxicity (fever, tachycardia, hypotension) may be present. Suprapubic tenderness and a palpable bladder will be present if there is urinary retention. On digital rectal examination the prostate is extremely tender.

Investigation

- Flow rate and post void residual urine measurement
- Urinalysis, urine culture ± cytology
- Segmented urine cultures
- NIH-CPSI questionnaire (National Institute of Health Chronic Prostatitis Symptom Index). This scores 3 main symptom areas: pain (location, frequency, severity); voiding (obstructive and irritative symptoms), and impact on quality of life.

Treatment

- **Antibiotics:** if the patient is systemically well use an oral quinolone (ciprofloxacin 500 mg bd) for 2–4 weeks. For a patient who is systemically unwell, intravenous antibiotics i.e. aminoglycoside (gentamicin) + 3rd generation cephalosporin (or ampicillin), and pain relief
- **Treat urinary retention:** where indicated use in-and-out catheterization; short periods of with an in-dwelling urethral catheter or suprapubic catheter.

Complications

Prostatic abscess

Failure to respond to this treatment regimen (i.e. persistent symptoms and fever while on antibiotic therapy) suggests the development of a prostatic abscess. The majority are due to *E. coli* infection. Risk factors include diabetes mellitus, immunocompromise, renal failure, transurethral instrumentation and urethral catheterization. A transrectal ultrasound or CT scan (if the former proves too painful) is the best way of diagnosing a prostatic abscess. This may be drained by a percutaneous or transurethral incision.

Chronic bacterial prostatitis

Caused by recurrent UTI. Chronic episodes of pain and voiding dysfunction may be a feature. DRE may show a tender, enlarged, and boggy prostate. A prolonged course of antibiotics is recommended. Consider continuing low dose prophylaxis in selected cases. Alpha-adrenoceptor blockers may provide some benefit. They act on the prostate and bladder neck α receptors, causing smooth muscle relaxation, improved urinary flow, and reduced intraprostatic ductal reflux.

Chronic pelvic pain syndrome

Chronic pelvic pain syndrome (CPPS)

Both inflammatory (III_A) and non-inflammatory (III_B) types present with >3 months history of localized pain (perineal, suprapubic, penile, groin or external genitalia); pain with ejaculation; mixed lower urinary tract symptoms (dysuria, frequency, urgency, poor flow) ± erectile dysfunction. Symptoms can be difficult to treat. They can recur over time and severely affect patient's quality of life. Younger men have a higher risk of suffering severe symptoms.

Evaluation

- **Uroflowmetry** and post void residual urine volume
- **NIH-CPSI questionnaire** (National Institute of Health Chronic Prostatitis Symptom Index). This scores 3 main symptom areas: pain (location, frequency, severity); voiding (obstructive and irritative symptoms), and impact on quality of life
- **Segmented urine cultures and expressed prostatic secretions (EPS)** These specimens may or may not reveal leucocytes, but for the diagnosis, EPS and post-prostatic massage urine (VB_3) cultures should not identify any bacteria
- **Urine and EPS cytology**
- **Urodynamics** Useful for further assessment of urinary symptoms and to assess for related problems, such as include hypertrophy or fibrosis of the bladder neck, external sphincter dyssynergia, urethral obstruction, and bladder overactivity.

Treatment

- **Antibiotics:** some benefit in patients presenting early with a new diagnosis of inflammatory CPPS, but they do not appear effective for long-standing, refractory chronic prostatitis/chronic pelvic pain syndrome
- **Alpha-adrenoceptor blockers:** again, only useful in newly diagnosed disease
- **Anti-inflammatory drugs:** NSAIDs, steroids
- **5-α-reductase inhibitors:** anti-androgens (i.e. finasteride) have the ability to reduce prostatic glandular tissue and improve intraductal reflux and symptoms in selected cases
- **Analgesics** (consider low dose tricyclic such as amitriptyline)
- **Muscle relaxants** (diazepam)
- **Prostatic massage:** 2/3 times per week for 6 weeks with antibiotic therapy
- **Biofeedback**
- **Supportive treatment** (counselling)
- **Sitz baths**
- **Diet modification:** avoiding caffeine, spicy foods and alcohol can help some patients
- **Microwave heat therapy:** only consider where severe symptoms are refractory to all treatments.

Painful bladder syndrome/interstitial cystitis (PBS/IC)

PBS/IC is a chronic, refractory bladder disorder characterized by urinary frequency, nocturia, urgency, and bladder pain. Glomerulations (petechiae) seen after bladder distension or Hunner's ulcers help confirm clinical suspicion. PBS/IC is a diagnosis of exclusion—other possible pathological causes should be excluded (e.g. drug, TB, or radiation-induced cystitis; OAB; see Table 6.4).

ICS definitions

Painful bladder syndrome (PBS): is 'the complaint of suprapubic pain related to bladder filling, accompanied by other symptoms such as increased daytime and night-time frequency in the absence of proven urinary infection or other obvious pathology'.[1]

Interstitial cystitis (IC): as above, with 'unspecified typical cystoscopic and histological features'.

Epidemiology

Predominantly affects females (female:male ratio is >5:1). Reported prevalence rates vary widely. Estimated female IC prevalence is 18 cases per 100,000 from European studies.[2] American data suggests higher rates of 52–67 per 100,000.[3]

Associated disorders

Allergies, irritable bowel syndrome, fibromyalgia, focal vulvitis, Sjögren's syndrome, and inflammatory bowel disease.

Pathogenesis

IC appears to be a multifactorial syndrome. Possible contributing factors include:

- **Mast cells:** frequently associated with the PBS/IC bladder, located around detrusor, blood vessels, nerves and lymphatics. Activated mast cells release histamine, causing pain, hyperaemia and fibrosis in tissues
- **Defective bladder epithelium:** an abnormal glycosaminoglycan (GAG) layer may allow urine to leak past the luminal surface, causing inflammation in muscle layers
- **Neurogenic mechanisms:** abnormal activation of sensory nerves causes release of neuropeptides, resulting in neurogenic inflammation
- **Reflex sympathetic dystrophy of the bladder:** excessive sympathetic activity
- **Bladder autoimmune response**
- **Urinary toxins or allergens**
- **Urine antiproliferative factor** (APF) is made by bladder urothelium. It inhibits bladder cell propagation, and may predispose susceptible individuals to PBS/IC following other bladder insults.

Table 6.4 NIDDK* diagnostic criteria for interstitial cystitis

Diagnosis criteria	1. Cystoscopic evidence of Hunner's ulcer or petechiae (glomerulations)
	2. Bladder/pelvic pain or urinary urgency
Exclusion criteria	1. Bladder capacity >350 mL, measured by awake cystometry
	2. Lack of urgency with a 150 mL injection in cystometry
	3. Uninhibited contractions during cystometry (i.e. OAB)
	4. <9 months from onset
	5. Absence of nocturia
	6. Symptoms improved by antibiotics, anticholinergic or antispasmodics
	7. Daytime voids <8
	8. Bacterial cystitis or prostatitis within 3 months
	9. Bladder or ureteral calculi
	10. Genital herpes
	11. Uterine, cervical, vaginal or urethral cancer
	12. Urethral diverticulum
	13. Cyclophosphamide or drug-induced cystitis
	14. Tuberculous cystitis
	15. Radiation cystitis
	16. Bladder tumour
	17. Vaginitis
	18. <18 years old

*NIDDK: National Institute of Diabetes and Digestive and Kidney Diseases.

1 Abrams P, Cardozo L, Fall M, *et al.* (2002) The standardisation of terminology of lower urinary tract function: report from the standardisation sub-committee of the International Continence Society. *Neurourol Urodyn* **21**:167–78.

2 Oravisto KJ (1975) Epidemiology of interstitial cystitis. *Ann Chir Gynaecol Fenn* **64(2)**:75–7.

3 Curhan GC, Speizer FE, Hunter DJ, *et al.* (1999) Epidemiology of interstitial cystitis: a population based study. *J Urol* **161**:549–52.

Evaluation

Exclude other causes for symptoms (see Table 6.4). History, examination (including pelvic in women and DRE in men), urinalysis, and culture. Symptom questionnaire, voiding diaries and urodynamics are useful to exclude OAB.

- **Cystoscopy:** 10% of patients may have pink ulceration of bladder mucosa (Hunner's ulcer). Under anaesthesia, the bladder should be distended twice (to 80–100 cmH$_2$O for 1–2 min), and then inspected for diffuse glomerulations (>10 per quadrant in ¾ bladder quadrants). Bladder biopsy is only indicated to rule out other pathologies. In conscious patients, bladder filling causes pain, and reproduces symptoms
- **Potassium sensitivity test:** instillation of KCl intravesically can provoke the pain and symptoms of PBS/IC. *Riedl's test:* the bladder is emptied, and filled with saline at 50 mL/min to the maximal capacity tolerated. Drain the bladder and record volumes. Repeat procedure using 0.2 M KCl. Volume saline − volume KCl/volume saline × 100 = % reduction. A reduction of ≥ 30% in bladder capacity with KCl indicates a defective GAG layer.

Treatment

- **Behavioural therapy:** avoiding foods that exacerbate symptoms (e.g. spicy foods, coffee, alcohol)
- **Oral medications:** tricyclics (amitriptyline) have anticholinergic, antihistamine and sedative effects; pentosanpolysulphate is an anti-inflammatory synthetic GAG analogue; cimetidine (H$_2$ histamine receptor anatagonist); hydroxyzine (H$_1$ antagonist); long-term analgesia (NSAIDs, paracetamol)
- **Repeated intravesical drug installation:** dimethyl sulphoxide (DMSO) ± local anaesthetic; GAG analogues (sodium hyaluronate); BCG; capsaicin, resiniferotoxin
- **Nerve stimulation:** transcutaneous electrical nerve stimulation (TENS); sacral nerve neuromodulation
- **Surgery:** considered only after failed conservative treatments Transurethral resection, laser coagulation, or diathermy of Hunner's ulcers and bladder hydrodistension may be beneficial, Bladder augmentation, or urinary diversion ± cystectomy may ultimately be required.

Note: definitions and terminology for PBS/IC have changed a number of times. The European Society for the Study of IC/BPS (ESSIC) suggests using the term 'Bladder Pain Syndrome' (BPS). NIDDK also refers to the collective conditions of IC/PBS/chronic prostatitis as 'Urological Chronic Pelvic Pain syndromes' (UCPPS).

Genitourinary tuberculosis

Tuberculosis (TB) of the genitourinary (GU) tract is caused by *Mycobacterium tuberculosis*. TB was formerly predominantly seen in Asian populations, but is now seen with increasing incidence in those from other ethnic groups. It has a higher incidence in males than females.

Pathogenesis

Primary TB: the primary granulomatous lesion forms in the mid to upper zone of the lung. It consists of a central area of caseation surrounded by epithelioid and Langhans' giant cells, accompanied by caseous lesions in the regional lymph nodes. There is early spread of bacilli via the bloodstream to the GU tract, but immunity rapidly develops, and the infection remains quiescent. Acute diffuse systemic dissemination of tubercle bacilli can result in symptomatic miliary TB.

Post primary TB: reactivation of infection is triggered by immune compromise (including HIV). It is at this point that patients develop clinical manifestations.

Effects on genitourinary tract

- **Kidney:** the most common site of extrapulmonary TB. Haematogenous spread causes granuloma formation in the renal cortex, associated with caseous necrosis of the renal papillae and deformity of the calyces, leading to release of bacilli into the urine. This is followed by healing fibrosis and calcification, which causes destruction of renal architecture and autonephrectomy
- **Ureters:** spread is directly from the kidney, and can result in stricture formation (vesicoureteric junction, pelviureteric junction, and mid-ureteric) and ureteritis cystica
- **Bladder:** usually secondary to renal infection, although iatrogenic TB can be caused by intravesical bacillus Calmette–Guérin (BCG) treatment given for bladder cancer. The bladder wall becomes oedematous, red and inflamed, with ulceration and tubercles (yellow lesions with a red halo). Disease progression causes fibrosis and contraction (resulting in a small capacity 'thimble' bladder; Fig. 6.2), obstruction, calcification and fistula formation
- **Prostate and seminal vesicles:** haematogenous spread causes cavitation and calcification, with palpable, hard feeling structures. Fistulae may form to the rectum or perineum
- **Epididymis:** results from descending renal infection or haematogenous spread. Features include a 'beaded' cord, which may be tender or asymptomatic, and is usually unilateral. Complications include abscess, spread of infection to the testis, and infertility
- **Penile:** rare manifestation transmitted from sexual contact or local contamination resulting in ulceration of the glans or a penile nodule. Biopsy confirms the diagnosis.

Presentation

Early symptoms include fever, lethargy, weight loss, night sweats, and UTI not responding to treatment. Later manifestations include lower urinary tract symptoms, haematuria, and flank pain.

Investigation

- **Urine:** at least 3 early morning urines (EMUs) are required for culture. A typical finding is sterile pyuria (leucocytes, but no growth). Ziehl-Neelsen staining will identify these acid- and alcohol-fast bacilli (cultured on Lowenstein-Jensen medium). Polymerase chain reaction (PCR) of urine where available is useful for TB detection
- **CXR and sputum**
- **Tuberculin skin test**
- **IVU:** findings include renal calcification, irregular calyces, infundibular stenosis, cavitation, pelviureteric and vesicoureteric obstruction, and a contracted, calcified bladder
- **Cystoscopy and biopsy.**

Treatment

An initial phase of 2 months of isoniazid, rifampicin, and pyrazinamide and ethambutol is followed by a continuation phase of 4 months of isoniazid and rifampicin. Longer treatments or modification of drugs is needed for complications and resistant organisms. Non-functioning, calcified kidney may need nephrectomy. Regular follow-up imaging with IVU is recommended to monitor for ureteric strictures, which may need stenting, nephrostomies, or ureteric reimplantation. Severe bladder disease may require surgical augmentation, urinary diversion or cystectomy and neobladder reconstruction. For epididymal involvement, epididymectomy ± orchidectomy is considered if pharmacotherapy fails or extensive disease is present.

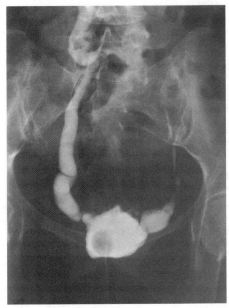

Fig. 6.2 Micturating cystourethrogram showing a contracted 'thimble' bladder and multiple ureteric strictures. Image kindly provided with permission from Professor S. Reif.

Parasitic infections

Schistosomiasis (bilharzia)

Urinary schistosomiasis is caused by a trematode (or fluke) called *Schistoma haematobium*. It occurs in Africa, Egypt, and the Middle East. Fresh water snails release the infective form of the parasite (cercariae), which can penetrate the skin and migrate to the liver (as schistosomules), where they mature. Adult flukes couple, migrate to vesical veins, and lay eggs (containing miracidia larvae), which leave the body by penetrating the bladder and entering the urine. The disease has two main stages: active (when adult worms are actively laying eggs) and inactive (when the adult has died and there is a reaction to the remaining eggs).

Clinical presentation

- 'Swimmer's itch' is the first clinical sign due to local inflammatory response from cercarial penetration (<24 h)
- Katayama fever (acute schistosomiasis), a generalized allergic reaction associated with onset of egg laying, which includes fever, urticaria, lymphadenopathy, hepatosplenomegaly and eosinophilia (3 weeks–4 months)
- Active inflammation phase when eggs are deposited, penetrate tissues and are excreted, resulting in haematuria, frequency, and terminal dysuria
- Chronic active phase is associated with low activity egg laying and excretion. It occurs after several years. Nephritic syndrome may develop due to deposition of immunoglobulin complex in renal glomeruli
- Chronic inactive phase (no viable eggs) may feature symptoms of obstructive uropathy.

Investigation

- Midday urine specimen may contain eggs (distinguished by having a terminal spine)
- Bladder and rectal biopsies (may identify eggs)
- Serology tests (ELISA)
- Cystoscopy identifies eggs in the trigone ('sandy patches')
- CT or IVU may show a calcified, contracted bladder, and obstructive uropathy
- USS demonstrates hydronephrosis and a thickened bladder wall.

Treatment

Praziquantel 20 mg/kg in 2 divided doses 4–6 h apart.

Complications

Obstructive uropathy, ureteric stenosis, renal failure, and bladder contraction, ulceration, or squamous cell carcinoma.

Hydatid disease

Infection occurs after ingestion of the dog parasite, *Echinococcus granulosus* (tapeworm). Sheep are the intermediate hosts. Cases occur in the Middle East, Australia, and Argentina. 3% affects the kidneys. Large cysts form, which can be asymptomatic or present with flank pain. A peripheral eosinophilia is seen, with a positive hydatid complement-fixation test. X-rays and CT scans show a thick-walled, fluid-filled spherical cyst with a calcified wall. Medical treatment is with albendazole. Where surgical excision is indicated, cysts can be first sterilized with formalin or alcohol. Praziquantel is also recommended preoperatively, or if cyst contents are spilt (which can provoke systemic anaphylaxis).

Genital filariasis

Lymphatic filariasis caused by *Wuchereria bancrofti* nematode infection is common in the tropics, and is transmitted by mosquitoes. Genitourinary manifestations, which may be delayed up to 5 years, include funiculoe-pididymitis, orchitis, hydrocele, scrotal and penile elephantitis, and lymph scrotum (oedema). Diagnosis is on thick film, serology, or biopsy. Medical treatment is with diethylcarbamazine. Surgical excision of fibrotic and oedematous tissue may be needed for genital elephantitis.

Phimosis

A condition where the contracted foreskin cannot be retracted behind the glans. A physiological phimosis is present at birth due to adhesions between the foreskin and glans. As the penis develops, epithelial debris (smegma) accumulates under the foreskin, causing gradual separation. 90% of foreskins are retractile at age 3.[1] Few persist into adulthood (<1% phimosis at age 17).[2] Recurrent balanitis in uncircumcised males can cause new phimosis.

Presentation

Usually asymptomatic. Inflammation or infection (balanitis) may cause bleeding, pain, or dysuria. Patients may describe ballooning of the foreskin on voiding, and an inability to fully retract the foreskin, which in sexually active men may also cause discomfort or skin trauma during sexual intercourse.

Treatment

Adults: if symptomatic, may require surgery with options of preputioplasty or circumcision (📖 see p. 714).

Children: older children with phimosis suffering infection (balanitis) can be treated with a course of topical 0.1% betamethasone (betnovate) cream, which acts to soften the phimosis and allow foreskin retraction. The recommendations are to avoid circumcision where possible.[1]

Indications for circumcision in children include phimosis associated with recurrent balanitis; balanitis xerotica obliterans (BXO); urinary tract infection (UTI) associated with an underlying abnormality (i.e. vesicoureteric reflux,[3] posterior urethral valves, neuropathic bladder dysfunction); recurrent UTI;[3] failed medical therapy for UTI; stone disease, and for religious reasons.

Contraindications to (neonatal) circumcision include the presence of hypospadias (± chordee or hooded foreskin), small penis, or large hernia or hydrocele (where repair after circumcision may cause a buried penis or secondary phimosis).

Complications of phimosis

- **Paraphimosis:** the foreskin is retracted behind the glans, but cannot be replaced again. An existing degree of phimosis and/or prolonged retraction produces a tight ring of tissue at the corona, leading to venous congestion, oedema and swelling of the glans, which can progress to arterial occlusion and necrosis (📖 see p. 518)
- **Recurrent balanitis**
- **Balanoposthitis:** severe balanitis where inflammatory secretions and pus are trapped in the foreskin by the phimotic band
- **Chronic inflammation**
- **Penile cancer (squamous cell carcinoma):** increased risk in uncircumcised males
- **Sexually transmitted infection:** increased risk (including HIV) in uncircumcised males.

1   Gairdner D (1949) The fate of the foreskin. A study in circumcision. *BMJ* **2**:1433–7.

2   Oster J (1968) Further fate of the foreskin. Incidence of preputial adhesions, phimosis, and smegma among Danish schoolboys. *Arch Dis Child* **43**:200–3.

3   Singh-Grewal D, Macdessi J, Craig J (2005) Circumcision for the prevention of urinary tract infection in boys: a systematic review of randomised trials and observational studies. *Arch Dis Child* **90**: 853–8.

Inflammatory disorders of the penis

(Table 6.5)

Balanitis and balanoposthitis

Balanitis is inflammation of the glans penis; balanposthitis is inflammation of the prepuce (foreskin). Causes include candidiasis, bacterial infection, irritant contact dermatitis, and local trauma. Increased risk with phimosis and uncircumcised males. Clinical features include pain, erythema, discharge, and voiding dysfunction. Treat any proven infection, instruct on good hygiene and avoid irritants. A short course of topical steroid cream (i.e. 0.1% bethamethasone) can be applied to improve retractability of the prepuce. Surgical options for recurrent infection include circumcision.

Lichen sclerosis et atrophicus

Chronic dermatitis which presents as itchy, flat-topped white papules that coalesce to form white patches. It commonly affects the genitalia (vulva and penis). On the penis it is called balanitis xerotica obliterans (BXO), which can result in urethral meatal stenosis and phimosis. It is a pre-malignant condition, although progression to squamous cell carcinoma is rare. Close follow-up is recommended, with biopsy if lesions change. General treatment includes topical steroids; clobetasol proprionate (0.05%) has proven beneficial in women. Men may require circumcision and urethral meatal dilatation.

Zoon's balanitis

Patients present with well-circumscribed, erythematous lesions (± erosions) up to 2 cm in diameter, which are only seen in uncircumcised males. It is usually asymptomatic, but may present with irritation, pain or discharge. The cause is unknown, but it appears to be plasma-cell mediated. Biopsy can help with diagnosis. Treatment is with circumcision.

Lichen planus

Presents as an itchy, papular rash. It consists of mauve papules, which have a flat top covered in white streaks (Wickham's striae). It affects flexor surfaces (wrists, elbows); genitalia (appearing as a white annular lesion on the glans penis); buccal mucosa; lumbar region and ankles. Erosions may occur on vulva and vagina causing pain. It is self-limiting, and usually resolves spontaneously. Topical steroids may be prescribed for symptomatic lesions.

Psoriasis

Chronic papulosquamous inflammatory skin disease, presenting with itchy pink plaques covered in silver-white scales in hair-bearing areas, and extensor surfaces (knees and elbows). It also causes pitting of the nails. Lesions may be guttate (raindrop-shaped), circinate (rings), or geographic. Genital psoriasis may involve the glans, which can be treated with topical emollients, and short courses of topical low-dose steroid creams.

Reiter's syndrome

The typical triad of symptoms is urethritis, conjunctivitis, and seronegative arthritis. Genital mainfestations include circinate balanitis (ring-shaped eroded lesions on the glans penis), which is self-limiting and responds well to topical steroid treatment.

Behçet's syndrome

An uncommon disorder of unknown cause characterized by painful genital (scrotum, prepuce, glans) and oral (aphthous) ulceration, polyarthritis, uveitis and neurological syndromes. Treatment of genital lesions is with topical steroids corticosteroids. Oral steroids or colchicine are used to treat the other features.

Table 6.5 Descriptions of skin lesions

Lesion	Description
Blister, bulla	Vesicle >1 cm
Crust	Lesion covered with drying exudate (serum, blood, pus)
Erosions	Loss of epidermis
Erythema	Redness of skin (usually blanches on pressure)
Macule	Flat, discrete lesion, different colour to surrounding skin <1 cm diameter
Maculo-papular	Raised spots different in colour to surrounding skin
Papule	Raised palpable lesion <0.5 cm
Patch	Macule >1 cm diameter
Plaque	Coalesced papules (larger, raised flat areas)
Pustule	Circumscribed pus-filled lesion
Nodule	Solid dermal or hypodermal lesion >0.5 cm
Scale	Flake of hard skin
Ulcer	Break in epithelium (+ superficial dermis)
Vesicle	Small fluid-filled lesion <1 cm

Urological neoplasia: pathology and molecular biology

Neoplasia (the formation and growth of a tumour) may be a **benign or malignant** process. Malignant neoplasms, characterized by local invasion of normal tissue or distant spread (metastasis) via lymphatic or vascular channels, may be **primary or secondary**. Neoplasms are considered to arise by clonal expansion of a single abnormal cell, through uncontrolled aberrant divisions. This cell may be **stem cell**, rather than a terminally-differentiated cell. An identifiable precursor lesion may exist.

Urological neoplasms most commonly arise from the lining epithelium of the genito-urinary tract. Benign epithelial neoplasms from glandular or transitional epithelium are respectively termed **adenoma** or **transitional cell papilloma**. Malignant epithelial neoplasms are **carcinomas**; they may be further characterized histologically by prefixing either **adeno** if the neoplasm is glandular, or **squamous cell** or **transitional cell** according to the epithelium from which it has arisen. Carcinomas arise from non-invasive epithelial lesions, some of which are identifiable histologically: in the bladder it is **flat carcinoma in situ (CIS)**, while in the prostate it is **prostatic intraepithelial neoplasia (PIN)**. **Connective tissue neoplasms** are described according to their components, adding benign (-oma) or malignant (-sarcoma) suffixes. For example, a benign neoplasm composed of blood vessels, fat and smooth muscle is an **angiomyolipoma**; a malignant neoplasm composed of smooth muscle is a **leiomyosarcoma**. Genitourinary sarcomas are rare, constituting 1% of all neoplasms.

There are exceptions: In the testis, the most common primary neoplasms arise from seminiferous tubules and are termed **germ cell tumours**. Rarely, primary malignant **lymphoma** can arise in the testis. In the kidney, the childhood **Wilm's tumour** arises from the embryonic mesenchyme of the metanephric blastema, while the benign **oncocytoma** is thought to arise from cells of the collecting ducts.

Secondary malignant neoplasms within urological tissues are uncommon; they may arise by direct invasion from adjacent tissues (for example, adenocarcinoma of the sigmoid colon may invade the bladder), or haematogenous metastasis from a distant site, such as the lung.

Urological neoplasia is a genetic disease: it may be **hereditary** or **sporadic**, depending on whether the genetic abnormalities are constitutional (germ-line) or somatic (acquired). Hereditary tumours tend to appear at a younger age than their sporadic counterparts, and are often multifocal, due to an underlying constitutional genetic abnormality. Tumour formation results from loss of the balance between cell division, and withdrawal from the cell-cycle by differentiation or programmed cell death (apoptosis). Signals regulating cell proliferation and interactions come from proteins, encoded by messenger RNA that is, in turn, transcribed from genomic DNA.

Genetic and epigenetic abnormalities may promote tumour development or growth in a number of ways:
- Activation (over-expression) of **oncogenes** encoding transcription factors e.g. c-myc
- Inactivation (reduced expression) of **tumour suppressor genes**, e.g. p53
- Over-expression of **peptide growth factors**, e.g. insulin-like growth factor type 1 or vascular endothelial growth factor
- *Promoter methylation or acetylation* of detoxification enzyme genes, e.g GSTP1

The diverse proteins encoded by **tumour suppressor genes** stabilize the cell, ensuring differentiation and a finite lifespan in which it performs its function. Inactivation of such genes by deletion or mutation may result in loss of this negative growth control. For example, the gene on chromosome 10q, PTEN, is a prostate tumour suppressor gene encoding a phosphatase that is active against protein and lipid substrates. It is present in normal epithelium, but is commonly reduced in prostate cancer due to allele loss of chromosome 10q. It inhibits one of the intracellular signalling pathways, PI3 kinase-Akt, that is essential for cell-cycle progression and cell survival. Inactivation of PTEN therefore promotes cell immortalization and proliferation.

Interest in the molecular genetics of urological neoplasia will lead to the development of screening tests for hereditary diseases, diagnostic or prognostic tumour profiling and new strategies for treatment.

Wilms' tumour (nephroblastoma)

This is a rare childhood tumour, affecting 1 in 10,000 children. It represents 80% of all genitourinary tumours affecting children under 15 years. Male and female are equally affected, 20% are familial and 5% are bilateral. 75% present under the age of 5 years.

Pathology and staging

Wilms' tumour is a soft pale grey tumour (it looks like brain). It contains blastema, epithelial, and connective tissue components.

Mutation or deletion of both copies (alleles) of the chromosome 11p WT-1 tumour suppressor gene result in tumourigenesis. The familial disease exhibits autosomal dominant inheritance, but is recessive at the cellular level. Affected family members harbour a germ-line WT-1 mutation, conferring susceptibility. One further 'hit' is required, while two 'hits' are required to cause the sporadic disease. This explains why hereditary Wilm's tumours tend to develop multifocally and at a slightly younger age than its sporadic counterpart.

Tumour staging relates to the relationship of the tumour to the renal capsule, excision margins, and local lymph nodes at nephrectomy, as well as the presence of soft tissue (typically lung) or bone metastases.

Presentation

90% have a mass, 33% complain of abdominal or loin pain, 30–50% develop haematuria, 50% are hypertensive, and 15% exhibit other anomalies, such as hemihypertrophy, aniridia, and cryptorchidism.

Investigations

The first-line investigation for a child with an abdominal mass or haematuria is ultrasound, which will reveal a renal tumour. Further diagnostic imaging and staging is obtained by CT, including the chest.

Treatment and prognosis

Children with renal tumours should be managed by a specialist paediatric oncology centre. Staging nephrectomy, with or without pre-operative or post-operative chemotherapy, remains the mainstay of treatment. The chemotherapy most frequently used is actinomycin D, vincristine, and doxorubicin. Survival is generally good, at 92% overall, ranging from 55 to 97%, according to stage and histology.

Neuroblastoma

The most common extracranial solid tumour of childhood. 80% are diagnosed <4 years old. The tumour is of neural crest origin; 50% occur in the adrenal gland and most of the remainder arise along the sympathetic trunks.

Presentation

Systemic symptoms and signs are common: fever, abdominal pain/distension, mass, weight loss, anaemia, and bone pain. Retro-orbital metastases may cause proptosis.

Imaging and staging

Ultrasound initially; CT of chest and abdomen. Calcification in tumour helps distinguish neuroblastoma from Wilms' tumour. MIBG scans are very sensitive for detection of neuroblastomas.

- *Stage 1:* tumour confined to organ of origin and grossly complete excision
- *Stage 2:* unilateral tumour with residual disease post-resection or lymphadenopathy
- *Stage 3:* tumour crossing midline or contralateral nodes
- *Stage 4:* metastatic disease beyond regional nodes; survival 6%
- *Stage 4S:* unilateral tumour with metastasis limited to liver, skin, or bone marrow; survival 77%.

Treatment and prognosis

Surgical excision; radiotherapy; combination chemotherapy, possibly with autologous bone marrow transplantation. Stage 4S tumours may resolve with little or no treatment. Prognosis is poor except for stages 1 and 4S disease.

Radiological assessment of renal masses

Abdominal **ultrasound scan (USS)** is the first-line investigation for a patient with loin pain or a suspected renal mass. The size resolution for renal masses is 1.5 cm, exhibiting variable echo patterns. Ultrasound may also detect renal cysts, most of which are simple: smooth-walled, round or oval, without internal echoes and complete transmission with a strong acoustic shadow posteriorly. If the cyst has a solid intracystic element, septations, an irregular or calcified wall, further imaging with **CT** is indicated. Bosniak developed the following radiological classification of renal cysts:

- **I:** uncomplicated simple (see above criteria); benign; no follow-up if asymptomatic
- **II:** minimally-complicated; septa, calcification, hyperdense (contain blood); benign, but require radiological follow-up
- **III:** complicated; irregular margin, thickened septa, thick irregular calcification; indeterminate, surgical exploration indicated unless there is history of trauma or infection
- **IV:** large, irregular cyst margins with solid components internally; cystic renal carcinoma until proved otherwise; surgery required.

If a renal mass is detected by USS, a thin slice or helical *CT scan* before and after IV contrast is the most important investigation for characterization and staging. In general, any solid enhancing renal mass is considered a renal cell carcinoma (RCC) until proven otherwise. Even relatively avascular renal carcinomas enhance by 10–25 *Hounsfield units. Occasionally, an isodense but enhancing area of kidney is demonstrated: this is termed 'pseudotumour' and may correspond to a harmless hypertrophied cortical column (of Bertin) or dysmorphic segment. CT may mislead with respect to liver invasion (rare) due to 'partial volume effect'; real-time ultrasound is more accurate. Lymphadenopathy >2 cm is invariably indicative of metastasis.

MRI with gadolinium contrast may be used for imaging the inferior vena cava (IVC), locally-advanced disease, renal insufficiency or for patients allergic to iodinated contrast. Doppler ultrasound may also evaluate IVC tumour thrombus. **Renal arteriography** is seldom used in the diagnostic setting, but may be helpful to delineate the number and position of renal arteries in preparation for nephron-sparing surgery or surgery for horseshoe kidneys.

Ultrasound or CT-guided **fine needle aspiration (FNA)** or **needle biopsy** in the investigation of renal masses is of limited value because of the accuracy of modern cross-sectional imaging, false-negative biopsy results (5-15%), plus risks of haemorrhage (5%) and tumour spillage (rare). FNA is useful for aspiration of renal abscess or infected cyst, or to diagnose suspected lymphoma or metastatic lesions. In certain circumstances a needle biopsy is indicated, for example, a histological diagnosis may be required prior to entering inoperable patients into clinical trials of systemic therapies.

Table 7.1 shows a practical radiological classification of renal masses.

Table 7.1 A classification of renal masses by radiographic appearance

Simple cyst	Complex cyst	Fatty mass	Others (excluding rarities)
Cyst	Renal carcinoma	Angiomyolipoma	Renal cell carcinoma
Multiple cysts	Cystic nephroma	Lipoma	Metastasis
Parapelvic cyst	Haemorrhagic cyst	Liposarcoma	Lymphoma
Calyceal diverticulum	Metastasis		Sarcoma
	Wilms' tumour		Abscess
	Infected cyst		Tuberculosis
	Lymphoma		Oncocytoma
	Tuberculosis		Xanthogranulomatous pyelonephritis
	Renal artery aneurysm		Phaeochromocytoma (adrenal)
	Arterio-venous malformation		Wilms' tumour
	Hydrocalyx		Transitional cell carcinoma

*Hounsfield units are a measure of X-ray attenuation applied to CT scanning: 1000 units equates with air, 0 units equates with water and +1000 equates with bone.

It has been suggested that abdominal USS could be used as a *screening* test for early detection and treatment of RCC; this has been piloted in Germany and Japan. While there is currently no plan for population screening in the UK, it would be appropriate to offer USS to high-risk individuals, such as relatives of VHL syndrome patients.

Benign renal masses

The most common (70%) are *simple cysts*, present in >50% of >50 year olds. Rarely symptomatic, treatment by aspiration or laparoscopic de-roofing is seldom considered.

Most benign renal tumours are rare; the two most clinically important are *oncocytoma* and *angiomyolipoma*.

Oncocytoma

This is uncommon, accounting for 3–7% of renal tumours. Males are twice as commonly affected as females. They occur simultaneously with renal cell carcinoma in 7–32% of cases.

Pathology

Oncocytomas are spherical, capsulated, brown/tan-colour, mean size 4–6 cm. Half contain a central scar. They may be multifocal and bilateral (4–13%) and 10–20% extend into perinephric fat. Histologically, they comprise aggregates of eosinophillic cells, packed with mitochondria. Mitoses are rare and they are considered benign, not known to metastasize. There is often loss of the Y chromosome.

Presentation

Oncocytomas often (83%) present as an incidental finding, or with loin pain or haematuria.

Investigations

Oncocytoma cannot often be distinguished radiologically from RCC; they may co-exist with RCC. Rarely, they exhibit a 'spoke-wheel' pattern on CT scanning, caused by stellate central scar. Percutaneous biopsy is not usually recommended, since there is often continuing uncertainty about the diagnosis.

Treatment

Radical or partial nephrectomy is indicated, as for renal carcinoma. Minimally-invasive techniques such as radiofrequency ablation (RFA) or high-intensity focused ultrasound (HIFU) could be considered for smaller tumours. No follow-up is necessary.

Angiomyolipoma (AML)

80% of these benign clonal neoplasm (hamartoma) occur sporadically, mostly middle-aged females. 20% are in association with tuberous sclerosis (TS), an autosomal dominant syndrome characterized by mental retardation, epilepsy, adenoma sebaceum, and other hamartomas. 50% of TS patients develop AMLs, mean age 30 years, 66% female, frequently multifocal and bilateral.

Pathology

AML is composed of blood vessels, smooth muscle, and fat. They are always considered benign, although extrarenal AMLs have been reported in venous system and hilar lymph nodes. Macroscopically, it looks like a well-circumscribed lump of fat. Solitary AMLs are more frequently found in the right kidney.

Presentation

AMLs frequently present as incidental findings (>50%) on ultrasound or CT scans. They may present with flank pain, palpable mass, or painless haematuria. Massive and life-threatening retroperitoneal bleeding occurs in up to 10% of cases (Wunderlich's syndrome).

Investigations

Ultrasound reflects from fat; hence, a characteristic bright echo-pattern. This does not cast an 'acoustic shadow' beyond, helping to distinguish an AML from a calculus. CT shows fatty tumour as low-density (Hounsfield units <10) in 86% of AMLs. If the proportion of fat is low, a definite diagnosis cannot be made. Measurement of the diameter is relevant to treatment.

Treatment

In studies, 52–82% of patients with AML >4 cm are symptomatic compared with only 23% with smaller tumours. Therefore, asymptomatic AMLs can be followed with serial ultrasound if <4 cm, while those bleeding or >4 cm, should be treated surgically. Emergency nephrectomy or selective renal artery embolization may be life-saving. In patients with TS, in whom multiple bilateral lesions are present, conservative treatment should be attempted. HIFU could be considered for asymptomatic tumours.

Renal cell carcinoma: pathology, staging, and prognosis

RCC is adenocarcinoma of the renal cortex, believed to arise from proximal convoluted tubule. Usually tan coloured and solid, 7–20% are multifocal, 10–20% contain calcification, and 10–25% contain cysts or are predominantly cystic. Rarely grossly infiltrative, they are usually circumscribed by a pseudocapsule of compressed tissue.

Spread is by: direct extension to adrenal gland (7.5% in tumours >5 cm), through the renal capsule, into renal vein (5% at presentation), inferior vena cava (IVC), right atrium; by lymphatics to hilar and para-aortic lymph nodes; haematogenous to lung (75%), bone (20%), liver (18%), and brain (8%).

Histological classification of RCC

- **Conventional** (80%); arise from the proximal tubule; highly vascular; cells clear (glycogen, cholesterol) or granular (eosinophillic cytoplasm, mitochondria)
- **Papillary** (10–15%), papillary, tubular and solid variants, 40% multifocal; small incidental tumours could equate with Bell's legendary 'benign adenoma'
- **Chromophobe** (5%), arises from the cortical portion of the collecting duct; possess a perinuclear halo of microvesicles
- **Collecting duct (Bellini)** rare, young patients, poor prognosis
- **Medullary cell** rare, arises from calyceal epithelium; young black sickle-cell sufferers; poor prognosis.

The term '**sarcomatoid**' is used to describe an infiltrative poorly-differentiated variant of any type.

Genetic changes associated with RCC are described on p. 245. RCC is an unusually immunogenic tumour, expressing numerous antigens (e.g. RAGE-1, MN-9). Reports of spontaneous regression, prolonged stabilization and complete responses to immunotherapy support this. Tumour infiltrating lymphocytes are readily obtained from RCCs including T-helper, dendritic, natural killer, and cytotoxic T cells. RCC is also unusually vascular, over-expressing angiogenic factors, principally VEGF, but also basic FGF and TGF-β.

Grading is by the *Fuhrman system* (1 = well-differentiated; 2 = moderately-differentiated; 3 and 4 = poorly-differentiated) based on nuclear size, outline, and nucleoli. It is an independent prognostic factor.

Staging is by the TNM classification following histological confirmation of the diagnosis (Fig 7.1 and Table 7.2). All rely upon physical examination and imaging, the pathological classification (prefixed 'p') corresponds to the TNM categories. *Staging is the most important prognostic indicator for RCC.*

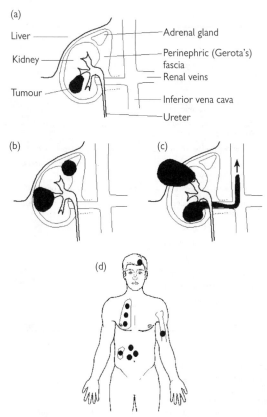

Fig. 7.1 Renal cell carcinoma staging. (a) Primary tumour limited to kidney (T1/T2). (b) Primary tumour invading perinephric fascia or adrenal gland (T3a). (c) Primary tumour extends into renal veins or IVC below diaphragm (T3b); above diaphragm/ into right atrium (T3c); outside perinephric fascia (e.g. into liver, bowel, or posterior abdominal wall) (T4). (d) N and M staging: multiple para-aortic/para-caval nodes; pulmonary, bone, or brain metastases (T1–4N2M1).

Table 7.2 2002 TNM staging of RCC

Tx	Primary tumour cannot be assessed
T0	No evidence of primary tumour
T1	Tumour 7cm or less, limited to the kidney
	a <4 cm
	b 4–7 cm
T2	Tumour >7 cm, limited to the kidney
T3	Tumour extends outside the kidney, but not beyond Gerota's (perinephric) fascia
	a Tumour invades renal sinus, adrenal gland or perinephric fat
	b Tumour grossly extends into renal vein or its segmental branches, or sub-diaphragmatic IVC
	c Tumour grossly extends into supra-diaphragmatic IVC or heart
T4	Tumour directly invades beyond Gerota's fascia into surrounding structures, e.g. liver
Nx	Regional (para-aortic) lymph nodes cannot be assessed
N0	No regional lymph node metastasis
N1	Metastasis in a single node
N2	Metastasis in 2 or more nodes
Mx	Distant metastasis cannot be assessed
M0	No distant metastasis
M1	Distant metastasis present

Prognosis Factors for RCC survival include:
- TNM stage grouping (below)
- Fuhrman Grade
- Performance status and systemic symptoms
- Molecular factors (under investigation: VEGF, HIF-1, p53, gene expression profiling).

RCC: 5-year survival
- **Organ-confined T1 (TNM stage I):** 70–94% (depends on grade)
- **Organ-confined T2 (TNM stage II):** 65–75%
- **Locally-advanced T3 (TNM stage III):** 40–70% (25% with IVC wall invasion)
- **N1 (TNM stage III):** 40–70%
- **Locally-advanced T4, N2, or M1 (TNM stage IV):** 10–40%.

A prognostic nomogram has been developed to predict 5-year probability of treatment failure for patients with newly-diagnosed RCC. It is available for download at: http://www.mskcc.org/mskcc/html/6156.cfm

Renal cell carcinoma (RCC): epidemiology and aetiology

RCC, also known as hypernephroma (since it was erroneously believed to originate in the adrenal gland), clear cell carcinoma, and Grawitz tumour, is an adenocarcinoma. It is the commonest of renal tumours, accounting for 85% of renal malignancies and 2% of all cancers. In the UK the incidence is rising, with 7044 patients diagnosed in 2005 (compared with 3676 patients in 1999) and 3580 deaths. RCC is the most lethal of all urological tumours, approximately 50% of patients dying of the condition. Incidence has increased since the 1980s when ultrasound was introduced to investigate non-specific abdominal symptoms, though the mortality has remained unaffected. It occurs in sporadic (common) and hereditary (rare) forms.

Aetiology

Males are affected 1.5 times as commonly as females; peak incidence of sporadic RCC is between 60–70 years of age.

Environmental

Studies have shown associations with urban dwelling, low socio-economic status, tobacco chewing and smoking cigarette, pipe, or cigar (1.4-2.3-fold risk), renal failure and dialysis (30-fold risk), obesity, hypertension (1.4-2-fold risk), asbestos exposure, the analgesic phenacitin, thorium dioxide. Nutrition is considered important: Asian migrants to Western countries are at increased risk of RCC; vitamins A, C, E and fruit/vegetable consumption are protective. Anatomical risk factors include polycystic and horseshoe kidneys.

Genetic

von Hippel Lindau (VHL) syndrome: 50% of individuals with this autosomal dominant syndrome, characterized by phaeochromocytoma, renal and pancreatic cysts and cerebellar haemangioblastoma, develop RCC, often bilateral and multifocal. Patients typically present in 3rd, 4th, or 5th decades. VHL syndrome occurs due to loss of both copies of a tumour suppressor gene at chromosome 3p25–26; this and other genes on 3p are also implicated in causing most sporadic RCC's. Inactivation of the VHL gene leads to effects on gene transcription, including dysregulation of hypoxia inducible factor 1 (HIF-1), an intracellular protein that plays an important role in the cellular response to hypoxia and starvation. This results in up-regulation of vascular endothelial growth factor (VEGF), the most prominent angiogenic factor in RCC, explaining why some RCC's are highly vascular.

A papillary variant of RCC also has an autosomal dominant familial component, characterized by trisomy 7 and 17, with activation of the c-MET proto-oncogene. c-MET is the receptor tyrosone kinase for hepatocyte growth factor, which regulates epithelial proliferation and differentiation in a wide variety of organs, including the normal kidney.

Renal cell carcinoma (RCC): presentation and investigation

More than 50% of RCC are now detected incidentally on abdominal imaging, carried out to investigate vague or unrelated symptoms. Thus, the stage at diagnosis of RCC is lower than it was in the pre-ultrasound era.

Presentation

History: of the symptomatic RCC's diagnosed, 50% of patients present with haematuria, 40% with loin pain, 30% of patients notice a mass, and 25% have symptoms or signs of metastatic disease, including bone pain, night sweats, pyrexia of unknown origin, fatigue, weight loss, and haemoptysis. Less than 10% of patients exhibit the classic triad of haematuria, pain and abdominal mass. Less common presenting features include acute varicocoele, due to obstruction of the testicular vein by tumour within the left renal vein (5%), and lower limb oedema due to venous obstruction. Paraneoplastic syndromes due to ectopic hormone secretion by the tumour occur in 30% of patients; these may be associated with any disease stage (Table 7.3).

Table 7.3 Paraneoplastic syndromes

Syndrome associated with RCC	Cause
Anaemia	Haematuria, chronic disease
Polycythaemia	Ectopic secretion of erythropoeitin
Hypertension (25%)	Ectopic secretion of renin, renal artery compression, or A-V fistula
Hypoglycaemia	Ectopic secretion of insulin
Cushing's	Ectopic secretion of ACTH
Hypercalcaemia (10–20%)	Ectopic secretion of parathyroid hormone-like substance
Gynaecomastia, amenorrhoea, reduced libido, baldness	Ectopic secretion of gonadotrophins
Stauffer's syndrome: hepatic dysfunction, fever, anorexia	Unknown; resolves in 60–70% of patients post-nephrectomy

Clinical examination may reveal abdominal mass, cervical lymphadenopathy, non-reducing varicocoele, or lower limb oedema (both suggestive of venous involvement).

Investigations

Radiological evaluation of haematuria, loin pain and renal mass is described on p. 228 together with discussion of needle biopsy of renal masses. Urine cytology and culture should be normal. Full blood count may reveal polycythaemia or anaemia. Serum creatinine and electrolytes, calcium, and liver function tests are essential.

When RCC is diagnosed radiologically, staging chest CT will follow, and bone scan if clinically indicated. Any suggestion of renal vein or IVC involvement on CT may be further investigated with Doppler USS or MRI. Angiography may be helpful in planning partial nephrectomy or surgery for horseshoe kidneys. Contralateral kidney function is assessed by uptake and excretion of CT contrast and the serum creatinine. If doubt persists, an isotope renogram is obtained.

Localized renal cell carcinoma: surgical treatment I

Surgery is the mainstay of treatment for RCC. Increases in diagnosis of smaller early-stage RCC and the concept of cytoreductive surgery for advanced disease has impacted on surgical treatment strategies of the disease, while reduction in mortality remains elusive.

Radical nephrectomy

With the exceptions discussed below, removal of the tumour-bearing kidney remains the gold standard curative treatment of localized RCC. There is currently no evidence to favour a specific surgical approach. In the case of upper pole or T2 tumours, adrenalectomy is also necessary.

Open approach: this may in future be practised only for large or locally-advanced RCCs. The aim is to excise the kidney with Gerota's fascia, perhaps with ipsilateral adrenal gland (tumours >5 cm) and regional nodes (controversial), removing all tumour with adequate surgical margins. Surgical approach is transperitoneal (good access to hilar vessels) or thoraco-abdominal (for very large or T3c tumours). Following renal mobilization (avoiding tumour manipulation), the ureter is divided; ligation and division of the renal artery or arteries should ideally take place prior to ligation and division of the renal vein to prevent vascular swelling of the kidney. If present, excision of hilar or para-aortic/para-caval lymph nodes will improve pathological tumour staging. Complications include mortality up to 2% from bleeding or embolism of tumour thrombus; bowel, pancreatic, splenic, or pleural injury.

Laparoscopic approach: now considered by many to be the gold standard approach for T1 (<7 cm) RCC's. It is expected that laparoscopic nephrectomy will become a widely-distributed treatment option in centres offering laparoscopic expertise. Approaches are either transperitoneal or retroperitoneal. The specimen is removed whole or morselated in a bag through an iliac incision. Advantages over open surgery include less pain, reduced hospital stay and quicker return to normal activity. Morbidity is reported in 8–38% of cases, including pulmonary embolism and poorly-understood effects on renal function. Long-term (10-year) results are not yet available, but 5-year disease-specific survival (>90% for T1 tumours) are equivalent to those obtained by open surgery.

Localized disease: partial nephrectomy

Nephron-sparing surgery is indicated as follows:
- **Absolute:** tumour in single functioning kidney
- **Relative:** multifocal or bilateral tumours, particularly if the patient has VHL syndrome, aiming to avoid renal replacement therapy
- **Elective:** T1 (up to 7 cm) tumours with a normal contralateral kidney, unless the tumour is close to the pelvicalyceal system.

3-dimentional CT reconstructions provide the surgeon with preoperative identification of the arterial anatomy. Open transperitoneal or loin approaches are used. The renal artery is clamped and the kidney packed with crushed ice to avoid warm ischaemia. Generally, results are comparable with open surgery. If the surgical margin is clear of tumour, the depth of the margin does not influence risk of local recurrence (up to 10%). Specific complications include urinary leak from the collecting system and hyperfiltration renal injury, which may eventually require renal replacement therapy: proteinuria is a prognostic sign.

Laparoscopic partial nephrectomy may become a standard approach in centres with great expertise, for small peripheral RCC. Oncological outcomes data are awaited. Complications disadvantaging the approach include a longer (up to 30 min) warm ischaemia time, and increased per-operative complications.

Post-operative follow-up aims to detect local or distant recurrence, to permit additional treatment if indicated; incidence is 7% for T1N0M0 RCC, 20% for T2N0M0, and 40% for T3N0M0. After partial nephrectomy, concern will also focus on recurrence in the remnant kidney. There is no consensus regarding the optimal regime, typically stage-dependent 6-monthly clinical assessment, and annual CT imaging of chest and abdomen for 3–10 years.

A nomogram combining prognostic factors for prediction of 5-year recurrence risk following surgery can be downloaded at: http://www.mskcc.org/mskcc/html/6156.cfm.

Renal cell carcinoma: surgical treatment II

Localized RCC: lymphadenectomy

Lymph node involvement in RCC is a poor prognostic factor. Incidence ranges from 6% in T1–2 tumours, 46% in T3a, and 62–66% in higher stage disease. Lymphadectomy at time of nephrectomy may add prognostic information, especially if there is obvious lymphadenopathy, but therapeutic benefit remains unclear. Formal lymphadenectomy adds time and increases blood loss, while nodes are clear in about 95% of cases.

Localized RCC: adjuvant therapy

No adjuvant therapy has been shown to improve survival after nephrectomy.

Localized RCC: treatment of local recurrence

Although uncommon, if there is local recurrence in the renal bed after radical nephrectomy, surgical excision remains the preferred treatment choice, provided there are no signs of distant disease. Local recurrence is more common after partial nephrectomy, where it can be treated by a further partial, or total nephrectomy.

Localized RCC: alternatives to surgery

Embolization: indicated for patients with gross haematuria who are unfit for curative surgery.

Observation: small (<3 cm) solid well-marginated renal masses may be safely followed with repeat scans in elderly or unfit individuals; growth is slow and metastasis rare.

Cryosurgery: performed using intra-operative ultrasound by open, percutaneous or laparoscopic routes, this is under evaluation as a nephron-sparing treatment option.

High intensity focused ultrasound: this minimally-invasive treatment, delivered percutaneously, is under evaluation as a nephron-sparing treatment option.

Image-guided radiofrequency ablation: this minimally-invasive treatment, delivered by extracorporeal or laparoscopic routes, is under evaluation as a nephron-sparing treatment option.

Locally-advanced RCC

Disease involving the IVC, right atrium, liver, bowel, or posterior abdominal wall demand special surgical skills. In appropriate patients, an aggressive surgical approach involving a multidisciplinary surgical team to achieve negative margins appears to provide survival benefit.

Adjuvant treatment—radiotherapy: early studies suggested a role for preoperative RT, although recent studies have failed to show a survival benefit for either pre- or postoperative RT. It may retard growth of residual tumour after nephrectomy.

Immunotherapy: randomized trials of adjuvant tumour vaccination are ongoing, for patients with positive nodes, surgical margins and venous invasion.

Metastatic RCC

Nephrectomy has long been indicated for symptom palliation (pain, haematuria) in patients with metastatic RCC (if inoperable, arterial embolization can be helpful) and is also performed prior to systemic therapy if appropriate. A median survival benefit of 10 months for patients with good performance status treated with cytoreductive nephrectomy prior to immunotherapy (interferon-α) has been reported.

Resection of a solitary metastasis is an option for a small number of patients, usually a few months after nephrectomy to ensure the lesion remains solitary.

Renal cell carcinoma: management of metastatic disease

Approximately 25% of patients with RCC have metastatic disease at presentation; 30% progress subsequently to this stage following nephrectomy. The prognosis is poor (p. 234), although good performance status, tumour nephrectomy, single organ site of metastatis, solitary metastasis, normal serum calcium, and absence of tumour thrombus are factors associated with an improved prognosis.

Surgery: despite the rare possibility of spontaneous metastatic regression following nephrectomy, it was rarely undertaken except to relieve local symptoms of pain or haematuria. The role of nephrectomy in metastatic RCC is discussed on p. 241

Metastasectomy may be of benefit to the 1.5–3% of patients who develop a solitary metastasis (particularly in lung, adrenal, or brain) following nephrectomy.

Signal-transduction inhibitors

As discussed earlier (p. 235) most RCC's are highly angiogenic, so should be good therapeutic targets for angiogenesis inhibitors. Via its cell-surface receptor (VEGFR), vascular endothelial growth factor (VEGF) is a pro-angiogenic peptide growth factor that activates the PI3kinase/AKT signal transduction pathway, which is one of 3 major receptor tyrosine-kinase (RTK) signalling pathways. VEGF is over-expressed in most sporadic RCC as a result of HIF-1 over-expression, caused by inactivation of the VHL tumour suppressor gene. In randomized trials, two oral multi-RTK inhibitors sunitinib and sorafenib, have recently been shown to prolong progression-free survival in metastatic RCC patients by 3–6 months compared with interferon alpha (IFNα) or placebo, respectively. The patients in the sorafanib trial were already resistant to immunotherapy. Complete responses were rare, partial responses modest (10–36%), but comparatively more patients enjoyed stable disease.[1,2] Both drugs were well-tolerated with fewer withdrawals due to serious adverse events compared with patients receiving immunotherapy. A further randomized trial demonstrated a >3-month survival advantage of temsirolimus, an inhibitor of cytoplasmic mTOR kinase (a downstream component of the same pathway) in metastatic RCC patients compared with IFNα.[3] These, together with other targeted therapies under development, represent a major new advance in the 1st and 2nd line treatment of metastatic RCC.

Immunotherapy

The immunogenicity of RCC is discussed on p. 232. The first cytokines to be used therapeutically, to activate anti-tumour immune response, were interferons and subsequently interleukin-2 (IL-2). Randomized studies in the 1990s demonstrated modest response rates (10–20%) after *systemic immunotherapy* using these cytokines alone and in combination; toxicity could be severe. Responses were more likely in patients with good performance status, prior nephrectomy and small-volume metastatic burden. An MRC trial of interferon-α versus medroxyprogesterone demonstrated a 2.5-month survival advantage in the immunotherapy group. The use of immunotherapy has been overshadowed recently by the development of RTK inhibitors.

Hormone therapy and chemotherapy: little role in RCC due to high multi-drug resistance P glycoprotein expression.

Radiotherapy: useful for palliation of metastatic lesions in bone and brain, and in combination with surgery for spinal cord compression.

Palliative care

Steroids (e.g. dexamethazone 4 mg qds) improve appetite and mental state, but are unlikely to impact on tumour growth. The involvement of multi-disciplinary uro-oncology, palliative and primary care teams is essential to support these patients and their relatives.

1 Motzer *et al.* (2007) Sunitinib versus Interferon Alpha in metastatic renal-cell carcinoma *NEJM*, **356:**115–24.

2 Escudier *et al.* (2007) Sorafenib in advanced clear-cell renal-cell carcinoma *NEJM*, **356:**125–34.

3 Hudes *et al.* (2007) Temsirolinus, Interferon Alfa, or both for advanced renal-cell carcinoma *NEJM*, **356:**2271–80.

Transitional cell carcinoma (TCC) of the renal pelvis and ureters

Transitional cell carcinoma (TCC) accounts for 90% of upper urinary tract tumours, the remainder being benign inverted papilloma, fibro-epithelial polyp, squamous cell carcinoma (associated with longstanding staghorn calculus disease), adenocarcimona (rare), and various rare non-urothelial tumours, including sarcoma.

TCC of the renal pelvis: uncommon, accounting for 10% of renal tumours and 4% of all TCC. *Ureteric TCC* is rare, accounting for only 1% of all newly-presenting TCC. Half are multifocal; 75% located distally, while only 3% are located in the proximal ureter.

Risk factors are similar to those of TCC in the bladder (p. 248).

- **Males** are affected three times as commonly as females
- Incidence increases with **age**
- **Smoking** confers a two-fold risk and there are various occupational causes
- TCC does not have a genetic hereditary form, although there is a high incidence of upper tract TCC in families from some villages in Balkan countries ('**Balkan Nephropathy**') that remains unexplained.

Pathology and staging

The tumour usually has a papillary structure, but occasionally solid. It is bilateral in 2–4%. It arises within the renal pelvis, less frequently in one of the calyces or ureter. Histologically, features of TCC are present, described below. Staging is by the TNM classification. Spread is by:

- Direct extension, including into the renal vein and vena cava
- Lymphatic spread to para-aortic, para-caval and pelvic nodes
- Blood-borne spread most commonly to liver, lung, and bone.

Presentation

- Painless total haematuria (80%)
- Loin pain (30%), often caused by clots passing down the ureter ('clot colic')
- Asymptomatic when detected, associated with synchronous bladder TCC (4%).

At follow-up, approximately 50% of patients will develop a metachronous bladder TCC and 2% will develop contralateral upper tract TCC.

Investigations

Ultrasound is excellent for detecting the more common renal parenchymal tumours, but not sensitive in detecting tumours of the renal pelvis or ureter.

Diagnosis is usually made on urine cytology *and* CTU or IVU, respectively, revealing malignant cells and a filling defect in the renal pelvis or ureter. If doubt exists, selective ureteric urine cytology, retrograde ureteropyelography, or flexible uretero-renoscopy with biopsy are indicated.

If ultrasound and cystoscopy are normal during the investigation of haematuria, an IVU or CTU is recommended. Staging imaging is obtained by contrast-enhanced abdominal CT, chest X-ray, and occasionally isotope bone scan.

Staging is by the TNM (1997) classification (Table 7.4) following histo-logical confirmation of the diagnosis. All rely upon physical examination and imaging, the pathological classification corresponding to the TNM categories.

Table 7.4 TNM staging of carcinomas of the renal pelvis and ureter

Tx	Primary tumour cannot be assessed
T0	No evidence of primary tumour
Ta	Non-invasive papillary carcinoma
Tis	Carcinoma *in situ*
T1	Tumour invades subepithelial connective tissue
T2	Tumour invades muscularis propria
T3	Tumour invades beyond muscularis propria into perinephric or periureteric fat or renal parenchyma
T4	Tumour invades adjacent organs or through kidney into perinephric fat
Nx	Regional (para-aortic) lymph nodes cannot be assessed
N0	No regional lymph node metastasis
N1	Metastasis in a single lymph node up to 2 cm
N2	Metastasis in a single lymph node 2–5 cm, or multiple nodes up to 5 cm
N3	Metastasis in a single lymph or multiple nodes >5 cm
Mx	Distant metastasis cannot be assessed
M0	No distant metastasis
M1	Distant metastasis present

Treatment and prognosis

If staging indicates non-metastatic disease in the presence of a normal contralateral kidney, the gold standard treatment with curative intent is nephro-ureterectomy, open or laparoscopic:

The open approach uses either a long transperitoneal midline incision or separate loin and iliac fossa incisions. The entire ureter is taken with a cuff of bladder, because of the 50% incidence of subsequent ureteric stump recurrence.

The laparoscopic approach focuses on mobilizing the kidney and upper ureter extraperitoneally; the lower ureter with bladder cuff is dissected via a Gibson-type open incision, through which the entire specimen is retrieved. As for laparoscopic nephrectomy, benefits include reduced post-operative pain and faster recovery. Tumour spillage and port-site metas-tases are theoretical hazards. Long-term results are as yet unavailable, but are expected to show equivalence with the open approach.

Follow-up should include annual cystoscopy and CTU or IVU to detect metachronous TCC development.

For patients with a single functioning kidney, bilateral disease or those who are unfit, percutaneous or ureterorenoscopic resection or ablation of the tumour are the minimally-invasive options. Topical chemotherapy (for example, mitomycin C) may subsequently be instilled through the nephrostomy or ureteric catheters. This nephron-sparing approach is less likely to be curative than definitive surgery.

Systemic combination chemotherapy for unresectable or metastatic disease using cyclophosphamide, methtrexate, and vincristine is associated with a 30% total or partial response at the expense of moderate toxicity.

Palliative surgery or ***arterial embolization*** may be necessary for troublesome haematuria. Radiotherapy is generally ineffective.

5-year survival
- Organ-confined   T1,2   60–100%
- Locally-advanced   T3,4   20–50%
- Node-positive   N+   15%
- Pulmonary, bone metastases M+   10%.

Bladder cancer: epidemiology and aetiology

Bladder cancer is the second most common urological malignancy, accounting for 4734 UK deaths in 2004. This represents 3% of all cancer deaths. UK incidence is approximately 11,000 per year, indicating that the majority of patients have curable or controllable disease.

Risk factors

- **Men** are 2.5 times more likely to develop the disease than women, the reasons for which are unclear, but may be associated with greater urine residuals in the bladder
- **Age** increases risk, most commonly diagnosed in the 8th decade and rare below age 50 years
- **Smoking** is the major cause of bladder cancer in the developed world. Smokers have a 2–5-fold risk of developing bladder cancer, subsequent recurrences and higher mortality compared with non-smokers. Estimates suggest that 30–50% of bladder cancer is caused by smoking. Cigarette smoke contains the carcinogens 4-aminobiphenyl (4-ABP) and 2-naphthylamine. Slow hepatic acetylation (detoxification) of 4-ABP by N-acetyltransferase and glutathione S-transferase M1 (GSTM1), or induction of the cytochrome p-450 1A2 demethylating enzyme appear to increase urothelial carcinogenic exposure. There is a slow (20-year) risk reduction following cessation of smoking
- **Occupational exposure** to carcinogens, in particular aromatic hydrocarbons like aniline (□ see Fig. 7.2), is a recognized cause of bladder cancer. Examples of 'at risk' occupations are shown in Table 7.5. A latent period of 25–45 years exists between exposure and carcinogenesis
- **Environmental carcinogens** found in urine are the major cause of bladder cancer
- **Chronic inflammation of bladder mucosa:** bladder stones, long-term catheters and notoriously the ova of *Schistosoma haematobium* (bilharziasis) are implicated in the development of squamous cell carcinoma of the bladder
- **Drugs:** phenacitin and cyclophosphamide
- **Race:** black people have a lower incidence than white people, but inexplicably they appear to carry a poorer prognosis
- **Pelvic radiotherapy.**

No evidence for a hereditary genetic aetiology exists, although many somatic genetic abnormalities have been identified. The most common cytogenetic abnormality is loss of chromosomes 9p, 9q, 11p 13q and 17q. Activation/amplification of oncogenes (p21 ras, c-myc, c-jun, erbB-2), inactivation of tumour suppressor genes (p53 mutations appear to worsen survival after treatment, retinoblastoma, p16 cyclin-dependent kinse inhibitor) and increased expression of angiogenic factors (for example, vascular endothelial growth factor, VEGF) are reported in transitional cell carcinomas.

Table 7.5 Occupations associated with TCC

Rubber manufacture e.g. tyres or electric cable
Paint and dye manufacture
Fine chemical manufacture e.g. auramine
Gas and tar manufacture
Iron and Aluminium processing
Hairdressers
Leather workers
Plumbers
Painters
Drivers exposed to diesel exhaust

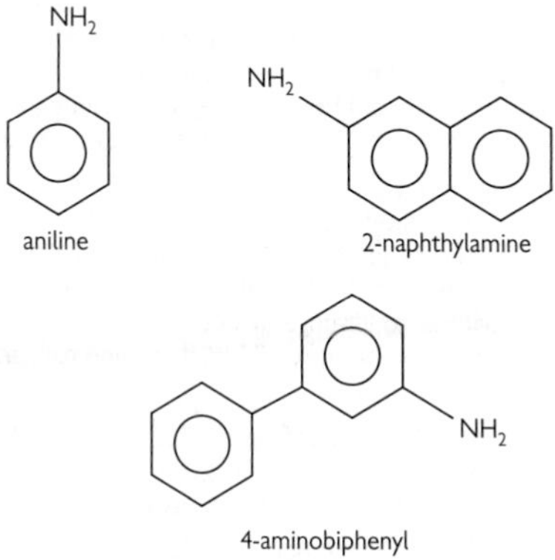

Fig. 7.2 Carcinogens known to increase risk of bladder cancer.

Bladder cancer: pathology and TNM staging

Benign tumours of the bladder, including inverted urothelial papilloma and nephrogenic adenoma, are uncommon.

The vast majority of primary bladder cancers are malignant and epithelial in origin:

- >90% are transitional cell carcinoma (TCC)
- 1–7% are squamous cell carcinoma (SCC)
- 75% are SCC in areas, where schistosomiasis is endemic
- 2% are adenocarcinoma
- Rarities include phaeochromocytoma, melanoma, lymphoma, and sarcoma arising within the bladder muscle
- Secondary bladder cancers are mostly metastatic adenocarcinoma from gut, prostate, kidney, or ovary.

Tumour spread is:

- **Direct** tumour growth to involve the detrusor, the ureteric orifices, prostate, urethra, uterus, vagina, perivesical fat, bowel, or pelvic side-walls
- **Implantation** into wounds/percutaneous cather tracts
- **Lymphatic** infiltration of the iliac and para-aortic nodes
- **Haematogenous** most commonly to liver (38%), lung (36%), adrenal gland (21%), and bone (27%). Any other organ may be involved.

Histological grading has traditionally (1973 WHO Classification) been divided into: well-, moderately-, and poorly-differentiated (abbreviated to G1, G2, and G3, respectively). Most clinical trials and guidelines are based on this classification. The (unvalidated) 2004 WHO grading uses cytological and architectural criteria to distinguish between papillary urothelial neoplasms of low malignant potential (PUNLMP), low-, and high-grade urothelial carcinomas.

Staging is by the TNM (1997) classification (📖 Fig. 7.3 and Table 7.6). All rely upon physical examination and imaging, the pathological classification (prefixed 'p') corresponding to the TNM categories.

TCC may be single or multifocal. Because 5% of patients will have a synchronous upper tract TCC and metachronous recurrences may develop after several years, the urothelial 'field-change' theory of polyclonality has been favoured over the theory of tumour monoclonality with transcoelomic implantation (seeding).

Primary TCC is considered clinically as superficial or muscle-invasive:

- 70% of tumours are papillary, usually G1 or G2, exhibiting at least seven transitional cell layers covering a fibro-vascular core (normal transitional epithelium has approximately 5 cell layers). Papillary TCC is usually superficial, confined to the bladder mucosa (Ta) or submucosa (T1). 10% of patients subsequently develop muscle-invasive or metastatic disease. However, a subset of superficial TCC, G3T1 tumours, are more aggressive with 40% subsequently upstaging.

- 10% of TCC have mixed papillary and solid morphology and 10% are solid. These are usually G3, half of which are muscle-invasive at presentation.
- 10% of TCC is flat carcinoma *in situ* (CIS). This is poorly-differentiated carcinoma, but confined to the epithelium and associated with an intact basement membrane. 50% of CIS lesions occur in isolation; the remainder occur in association with muscle-invasive TCC. CIS usually appears as a flat red velvety patch on the bladder mucosa; 15–40% of such lesions are CIS, the remainder being focal cystitis of varying aetiology. The cells are poorly cohesive, up to 100% of patients with CIS exhibiting positive urine cytology, in contrast to much lower yields (17–72%) with G1/2 papillary TCC. 40–83% of untreated CIS lesions will progress to muscle-invasive TCC, making CIS the most aggressive form of superficial TCC.

5% of patients with G1/2 TCC and at least 20% with G3 TCC (including CIS) have vascular or lymphatic spread. Metastatic lymph node disease is found in: 0% Tis; 6% Ta; 10% T1; 18% T2 and T3a; 25–33% T3b and T4 TCC.

Squamous cell carcinoma is usually solid or ulcerative and muscle-invasive at presentation. SCC accounts for only 1% of UK bladder cancers. SCC in the bladder is associated with chronic inflammation and urothelial squamous metaplasia, rather than CIS. In Egypt, 80% of SCC is induced by the ova of *Schistosoma haematobium*. 5% of paraplegics with long-term catheters develop SCC. Smoking is also a risk factor for SCC. The prognosis is better for bilharzial SCC than for non-Bilharzial disease, probably because it tends to be lower-grade and metastases are less common in these patients.

Adenocarcinoma is rare, usually solid/ulcerative, G3 and carry a poor prognosis. One-third originate in the urachus, the remnant of the allantois, located deep to the bladder mucosa in the dome of the bladder. Adenocarcinoma is a long-term (10–20+ year) complication of bladder exstrophy and bowel implantation into the urinary tract, particularly bladder substitutions and ileal conduits after cystectomy. There is association with cystitis glandularis, rather than CIS. Secondary adenocarcinoma of the bladder may arise as discussed above (see Table 7.6).

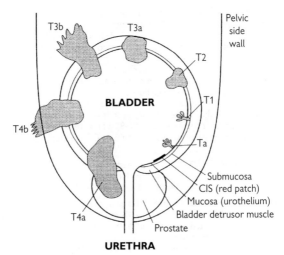

Fig. 7.3 The T staging of bladder cancer.

Table 7.6 TNM staging of bladder carcinoma

Tx	Primary tumour cannot be assessed
T0	No evidence of primary tumour
Ta	Non-invasive papillary carcinoma
Tis	Carcinoma *in situ*
T1	Tumour invades subepithelial connective tissue
T2	Tumour invades muscularis propria (detrusor):
	a inner half; T2b outer half
T3	Tumour invades beyond muscularis propria into perivesical fat:
	a microscopic
	b macroscopic
T4	a tumour invades any of: prostate, uterus, vagina, bowel
	b tumour invades pelvic or abdominal wall
Nx	Regional (iliac and para-aortic) lymph nodes cannot be assessed
N0	No regional lymph node metastasis
N1	Metastasis in a single lymph node up to 2 cm in greatest dimension
N2	Metastasis in a single lymph node 2–5 cm or multiple nodes up to 5 cm
N3	Metastasis in a single lymph or multiple nodes >5 cm in greatest dimension
Mx	Distant metastasis cannot be assessed
M0	No distant metastasis
M1	Distant metastasis present

Bladder cancer: presentation

Symptoms

- The commonest presenting symptom (85% of cases) is **painless macroscopic haematuria**. Haematuria may be initial or terminal if the lesion is at the bladder neck or in the prostatic urethra. 34% of patients >50 years and 10% <50 years with macroscopic haematuria have bladder cancer. A history of smoking or occupational exposure is relevant
- **Asymptomatic microscopic haematuria** found on routine urine stick-testing account for an important minority of presentations. Up to 16% of females and 4% of males have stick-test haematuria: less than 5% of those <50 years and 7–13% of those >50 years will have a malignancy
- **Filling-type lower urinary tract symptoms**, such as urgency or suprapubic pain. There is almost always microscopic or macroscopic haematuria. This so-called 'malignant cystitis' is typical in patients with CIS.
- More advanced cases may present with **lower-limb swelling** due to lymphatic/venous obstruction, bone pain, weight loss, anorexia, confusion and anuria (renal failure due to bilateral ureteric obstruction)
- Recurrent **urinary tract infections and pneumaturia** due to malignant colovesical fistula, though less common than benign causes (diverticular and Crohn's disease)
- **Pain** is unusual, even if the patient has obstructed upper tracts, since the obstruction and renal deterioration arise gradually
- Urachal adenocarcinomas may present with a blood or mucus **umbilical discharge** or a deep sub-umbilical mass.

Signs

General examination may reveal pallor, indicating anaemia due to blood loss or chronic renal impairment. Abdominal examination may reveal a suprapubic mass in the case of locally-advanced disease; digital rectal examination may reveal a pelvic mass above or involving the prostate.

Although the likelihood of diagnosing bladder cancer in patients <50 years is low, all patients with these presenting features should be investigated (p. 256).

Bladder cancer: diagnosis and clinical staging

Investigation of haematuria

After a urinary tract infection has been excluded or treated, ALL patients with persistent microscopic (2 out of 3 dipstick tests, or >10 red cells per high-power field) or macroscopic haematuria require investigation of their upper tracts, bladder and urethra. CT urography (CT-KUB with and without IV contrast) or IVU *plus* flexible cystoscopy *plus* urine cytology are the first-line investigations. CTU before and after IV contrast is becoming the standard radiological investigation of haematuria. It is faster and more sensitive than ultrasound or IVU in the detection of renal (parenchymal and urothelial) and ureteric tumours. However, it carries a higher radiation dose and is more expensive. CTU also detects some bladder tumours, but may over-call bladder wall hypertrophy as tumour and will miss flat CIS and urethral pathology, so it cannot replace cystoscopy. If there is hydronephrosis in association with a bladder tumour, it is likely that the tumour is causing the obstruction to the distal ureter. This tends to be caused by muscle-invasive disease rather than superficial TCC.

In younger (<50 years) patients with microscopic haematuria, imaging of the upper tract may be carried out with ultrasound to reduce radiation dose.

If all investigations are normal, consideration should be given to nephrological disorders that may cause haematuria, such as glomerulonephritis. Cross-referral to a renal physician is advised in patients with persisting microscopic haematuria, especially those with associated proteinuria or hypertension.

Patients with predominantly filling-type LUTS, suprapubic pain or recurrent UTI/pneumaturia should also have urine cytology and cystoscopy.

Urine cytology

Examination of voided urine for exfoliated cells is most sensitive (90–100%) in patients with high-grade TCC and CIS, anywhere in the urinary tract. It is costly, and less than 1% of cancers are detected by cytology alone when other investigations are normal. False-negative cytology is frequent (40–70%) in patients with papillary TCC, while false-positive cytology can arise due to infection, inflammation, stones, instrumentation and intravesical instillations, such as chemotherapy.

Urine molecular markers

ELISA tests for detecting tumour-specific urinary markers, such as bladder tumour antigen or nuclear matrix protein 22 (Nmp-22) tend to have greater sensitivity, but reduced specificity for detecting TCC, compared with urine cytology. The absence of clinical trials and the costs involved mean that it is unclear whether these tests, alone or in combination, may replace any of the standard investigations for haematuria.

Staging of bladder cancer

- **Transurethral resection of bladder tumour (TURBT)** usually provides definitive histological diagnosis (see p. 258). This is undertaken under general or spinal anaesthesia; bimanual examination is mandatory before and after bladder tumour resection, to assess size, position and mobility. The pathologist should report on the tumour type, grade and stage; in particular, the presence or absence of muscularis propria should be noted, since its absence will preclude reliable T staging. Red patches are biopsied separately; the prostatic urethra is biopsied if radical reconstructive surgery is under consideration. Care is taken in resecting tumours at the dome, since intraperitoneal bladder perforation may occur, especially in women with thin-walled bladders

- **Staging investigations** are usually reserved for patients with biopsy-proven muscle-invasive bladder cancer, unless clinically indicated, since superficial TCC and CIS are rarely associated with metastases
- **Pelvic CT or MRI** may demonstrate extra-vesical tumour extension, upper tract obstruction or iliac lymphadenopathy, reported if >8 mm in maximal diameter. T stage correlation with pathological findings at cystectomy is 65–80%. Both modalities will miss microscopic nodal disease in 70% of cases
- **Chest X-ray**
- **Isotope bone scan** (positive in 5–15% of patients with muscle-invasive TCC) is obtained in cases being considered for radical treatment
- Staging **lymphadenectomy** (open or laparoscopic) may be indicated in the presence of CT-detected pelvic lymphadenopathy if radical treatment was under consideration
- **Ultrasound** scanning is used for detection of liver metastases if the serum liver function is abnormal: albumin indicates the nutritional status of the patients; alkaline phosphatase is not a reliable marker for bone disease in bladder cancer patients.

Management of superficial TCC: surgery and recurrence

Transurethral resection of bladder tumour (TURBT)

The diagnostic role of TURBT has been discussed on p. 256. As a primary treatment, a visually-complete tumour resection is adequate for 70% of newly-presenting patients with Ta/T1 superficial disease. The remaining 30% of patients experience early recurrence, 15% with upstaging. Because of this, it is standard care that all new patients receive adjuvant treatment. Complications are uncommon, including bleeding, sepsis, bladder perforation, incomplete resection, and urethral stricture.

Alternatives to TURBT

Transurethral cystodiathermy or laser are accepted, quicker, and less morbid procedure for ablating small superficial recurrences when obtaining tissue for histology is not considered necessary.

Fluorescence cystoscopy uses blue light in combination with a porphyrin-based photosensitizer, (hexi)-aminolevulinic acid (HAL). This can reveal CIS lesions and developing papillary tumours, which cannot be seen using standard white light for tumour detection and resection. This technique is gaining popularity, but is expensive and is not yet widespread in routine clinical practice.

Follow-up after TURBT

2nd resection: an early repeat TUR (within 2–6 weeks) should be undertaken (a) if the first resection was incomplete, (b) when the pathologist reports that the resected specimen contains no muscularis propria, or (c) if a high-grade, but apparently non-invasive Ta or T1 tumour has been reported, since 10% of these G3pT1 tumours are understaged T2 tumours. This strategy reduces recurrences and improves prognosis.

In the absence of these indications for 2nd resection, review cystoscopy is perform at 3 months. If this demonstrates recurrence, 70% will recur further. If not, only 20% will recur further. If the bladder is clear at follow-up, subsequent cystoscopies are performed under local anaesthetic at 6 months and, thereafter, annually for 5 years (patients with low-risk TCC) or until the patient is no longer fit to undergo treatment (patients with high-risk disease).

Patients with G3T1, TCC, and CIS are at significantly higher risk of recurrence, and 40% subsequently upstage. Some patients experience persistent symptomatic multifocal G1/2, Ta/1 recurrent TCC, demanding frequent follow-up procedures. In these circumstances, adjuvant treatment is indicated (📖 see p. 262).

There is no accepted protocol for upper tract surveillance in patients with a history of bladder TCC, although EAU guidelines[1] recommend yearly IVU for patients with high-risk disease.

Predicting recurrence and progression in Ta/T1 TCC

A scoring system based on the following factors has been developed (by the EORTC)[2]:
- Number of tumours (1 vs. 2–7 vs. 8 or more)
- Tumour size (<3 vs. >3 cm)
- Prior recurrence (<1 vs. >1 per year)
- T stage (Ta vs. T1)
- Tumour grade (G1 vs. G2 vs. G3)
- Presence of CIS.

This system divides superficial tumours into those at low-risk (50%), intermediate-risk (35%), or high-risk (15%) of recurrence and progression. Scoring tables and risk calculators are available at: http://www.eortc.be/tools/bladdercalculator/

Table 7.7 summarizes the management of bladder cancer stage-by-stage.

1 *European Association of Urology Guidelines*, 2008. Available at www.uroweb.org/professional-resources/guidelines.

2 Sylvester RJ et al. (2006) Predicting recurrence and progression in individual patients with stage Ta T1 bladder cancer using EORTC risk tables: a combined analysis of 2596 patients from seven EORTC trials. *Eur Urol* **49**:466–77.

Table 7.7 A summary of the management of bladder cancer

Histology	Risk of recurrence post- TURBT	Risk of stage progression	Further treatment	Urological Follow-up
G1/2, Ta/1, TCC	30%	10–15%	Immediate post-operative single dose intravesical chemotherapy	Review cystoscopies, commencing 3 months
Recurrent multifocal G1/2, Ta/1 TCC	70%+	10–15%	Intravesical chemotherapy ×6 weekly doses	Review cystoscopies, commencing 3 months
G3, Ta/T1 TCC	80%	40%	2nd resection; Intravesical BCG ×6 weekly doses; consider cystectomy for recurrence	Review cystoscopies, commencing 6–12 weeks
CIS (carcinoma in situ, severe intraepithelial dysplasia)	80%	40%	Intravesical BCG ×6 weekly doses +/- maintenance; Consider cystectomy for recurrence	Cystoscopies + biopsy and cytology commencing 3 months
pT2/3, N0, M0 TCC, SCC or adenocarcinoma	Usually TUR is incomplete	N/a	Cystectomy or radiotherapy ± neo-adjuvant chemotherapy or palliative TURBT (unfit)	Cystoscopies if bladder is preserved. Urethral washings for cytology.
T4 or metastatic TCC, SCC or adenocarcinoma	Usually TUR is incomplete	N/a	Systemic chemotherapy; multidisciplinary team symptom palliation	Palliative treatment for local bladder symptoms

Superficial TCC: adjuvant treatment

Intravesical chemotherapy (e.g. mitomycin C [MMC] 40 mg in 50 ml saline) is used for G1-2, Ta, or T1 tumours and recurrent multifocal TCC. MMC is an antibiotic chemotherapeutic agent that inhibits DNA synthesis. In experimental studies, it may cause regression of small papillary TCC, so it should be cytotoxic for microscopic residual disease post-TURBT. A meta-analysis of seven randomized trials[1] has shown that a single dose given within 24 h of first TURBT significantly (40%+) reduces the likelihood of tumour recurrence compared with TURBT alone. This risk reduction is equivalent to weekly instillations for 6 weeks commencing up to 2 weeks post-TURBT. However, intravesical chemotherapy has never been shown to prevent progression to muscle-invasion and has no impact upon survival. It is administered via a urethral catheter, is held in the bladder for 1 h and should not be used if bladder perforation is suspected.

Toxicity of MMC: 15% patients report transient filling-type LUTS; occasionally a rash develops on the genitals or palms of the hands, so treatment must be stopped. Systemic toxicity is rare with MMC.

Other intravesical chemotherapy agents included doxorubicin and epirubicin.

Intravesical Bacille Calmette–Guérin (BCG) is an attenuated strain of *Mycobacterium bovis*. Commercially-available strains include Pasteur, Connaught, and Tice. It acts as an immune stimulant, up-regulating cytokines, such as IL-6 and IL-8 in the bladder wall, activating immune effector cells.

BCG produces complete responses in 60–70% of patients, compared with TURBT alone. 30% do not respond and 30% of responders relapse within 5 years. It is as effective as chemotherapy for adjuvant treatment of low- and intermediate-risk G1/2,Ta/1 TCC, therefore is not often used (except as second-line) because of the additional toxicity. In high-risk patients, with multiple G2T1, G3Ta/T1 or CIS, the benefit of BCG over chemotherapy in reducing risk of recurrence is clear and it is standard care. BCG is given as a 6-week course for G3T1 TCC and for CIS, starting at least 2 weeks post-TURBT. It is administered via a urethral catheter, 80 mg in 50 ml saline and retained in the bladder for 1 h. For recurrent G3T1 TCC or CIS, a second course of BCG may be offered, 50% will respond. Otherwise proceed without delay to radical cystectomy. The latter has a cure rate of 90%.

A meta-analysis of 24 trials has demonstrated that BCG reduces risk of stage progression (to muscle-invasion) by 27%, based on a median follow-up of 2.5 years.[2] This effect was only seen in patients who received maintenance BCG (e.g. 30 treatments over 3 years after the initial 6-week induction), the optimal dose and schedule of which remains unclear.

Although less expensive and more effective, BCG is more toxic than intravesical chemotherapy, causing cystitis symptoms in >90% patients and low-grade fever with myalgia in 25%. Up to 6% of patients develop a high persistent fever, requiring antituberculous therapy for up to 6 months with isoniazid and pyridoxine, or standard triple therapy (rifampicin, isoniazid, and ethambutol) in critically-ill patients. Death due to BCG sepsis, granulomatous prostatitis, and epididymo-orchitis are rarely reported complications.

Contraindications to intravesical BCG include:

- Immuno-suppressed patients
- Pregnant or lactating women
- Patients with haematological malignancy
- Following traumatic catheterization.

Cystoscopy too early after BCG can appear alarming, due to generalized inflammatory response. Review cystoscopy and biopsy 3 months after BCG may still reveal chronic granulomatous inflammation.

1 Sylvester RJ et al. (2004) A single immediate postoperative instillation of chemotherapy decreases the risk of recurrence in patients with stage TaT1 bladder cancer: a meta-analysis. J Urol **171**:2186–90.

2 Sylvester RJ et al. (2002) Intravesical BCG reduces the risk of progression in patients with superficial bladder cancer: a combined analysis of results of published clinical trials. J Urol **168**:1964–70.

Muscle-invasive bladder cancer: surgical management of localized (pT2/3a) disease

This is a dangerous disease; untreated, the 5-year survival is 3%. Management of patients with invasive bladder cancer requires a multidisciplinary team approach, involving case-by-case discussion between the urological surgeon, radiotherapist, and medical oncologist. In the absence of prospective randomized trials comparing the surgical and non-surgical treatments, there are a number of options for a patient with newly-diagnosed confined muscle-invasive bladder cancer.

Bladder preserving

- Radical transurethral resection of bladder tumour (TURBT) plus systemic chemotherapy: little data, not mainstream
- Palliative TURBT ± palliative radiotherapy (RT): for elderly/unfit patients
- Partial cystectomy ± neo-adjuvant systemic chemotherapy
- TURBT plus definitive RT (🕮 see p. 268): poor options for squamous and adenocarcinoma as they are seldom radiosensitive.

Radical cystectomy

- Ileal conduit urinary diversion
- Ureterosigmoidostomy urinary diversion
- Continent urinary diversion
- ± Neo-adjuvant chemotherapy: some evidence of benefit (🕮 see p. 270)
- ± Neo-adjuvant RT: no evidence of benefit (🕮 see p. 270).

Partial cystectomy is a good option for well-selected patients with small solitary disease located near the dome and for urachal carcinoma. Morbidity is less than with radical cystectomy and diversion is not required. The surgical specimen should be covered with perivesical fat, with a 1.5 cm margin of macroscopically normal bladder around the tumour. There should be no biopsy evidence of CIS elsewhere in the bladder. The bladder must be closed without tension and catheterized for 7–10 days to allow healing. Subsequent review cystoscopies are mandatory to ensure no tumour recurrence.

Radical cystectomy with urinary diversion

This is the most effective primary treatment for muscle-invasive TCC, SCC and adenocarcinoma, and can be performed as salvage treatment if RT has failed. It is also a treatment for G3T1 TCC and CIS, refractory to BCG. Any ureteric obstruction caused by the primary tumour will be relieved by the concomitant urinary diversion. However, this is a major undertaking for the patient and surgeon, requiring support from cancer specialist nurse, stomatherapist, or continence advisor.

The procedure: through a midline abdominal transperitoneal approach, a bilateral pelvic lymphadenectomy is undertaken. The extent of lymphadenectomy ranges from limiting dissection to the obturator fossa to extending the dissection up to the aortic bifurcation. Studies have suggested a survival advantage to the extended approach, provided the primary cancer is stage T2 or less. The findings of frozen section histology may influence the decision to proceed in some cases. The entire bladder is then excised along with perivesical fat, vascular pedicles, and urachus, plus the prostate/seminal vesicles or anterior vaginal wall. The anterior urethra is not excised unless there is prior biopsy evidence of tumour at the female bladder neck or prostatic urethra (when recurrence occurs in 37%). The ureters are divided close to the bladder, ensuring their disease-free status by frozen-section histology if necessary, and anastamosed into the chosen urinary diversion (📕 see p. 272).

Some centres are pioneering laparoscopic cystectomy. Potential advantages include less blood loss, less post-operative analgesia requirement and faster recovery time. However, long operating times and technical considerations may limit widespread adoption of this approach.

Major complications affect 25% of cystectomy patients. These include perioperative death (1.2%), re-operation (10%), bleeding, thromboembolism, sepsis, wound infection/dehiscence (10%), intestinal obstruction, or prolonged ileus (10%) cardio-pulmonary morbidity, and rectal injury (4%). Erectile dysfunction is likely after cystectomy due to cavernosal nerve injury.

The complications of urinary diversion are discussed on p. 272.

Postoperative care

- Many patients will spend the first 24 h in the high-dependence unit or ITU
- Daily clinical evaluation, including inspection of the wound (and stoma if present), plus monitoring of blood count and creatinine/electrolytes, is mandatory
- Broad-spectrum antimicrobial prophylaxis and thrombo-embolic prophylaxis with TED stockings, pneumatic calf compression and subcutaneous heparin are standard
- Mobilization after 24 h is ideal
- Chest physiotherapy and adequate analgesia is especially important in smokers and patients with chest co-morbidity
- Oral intake is restricted until bowel sounds are present; patients may require parenteral nutrition in the presence of gastro-intestinal complications
- Drains are usually sited in the pelvis and near the uretero-diversion anastamosis; ureteric catheters pass from the renal pelvis through the diversion and exit percutaneously; a catheter drains the diversion (except in the case of ileal conduit) exiting urethrally or suprapubically
- Most patients stay in hospital 10–14 days.

Salvage radical cystectomy is technically a more difficult and slightly more morbid procedure. Relatively few patients who have failed primary RT are suitable for this second chance of a cure; these are fit patients with mobile clinically-localized disease.

Efficacy of radical cystectomy

Failure to cure may result from inadequate excision of the primary tumour, or presence of metastases. Pathological upstaging of the primary can occur in up to 40% of cases. Lymph node metastases occur in 10% of T1 and up to 33% of T3–4 cancers. The use of neo-adjuvant chemotherapy in muscle-invasive disease is discussed on p. 266.

5-year survival rates for cystectomy alone are as follows:

- Stage T1/CIS   90%+
- Stages T2,T3a   55–63%
- Stage T3b   31–40%
- Stage T4a (into prostate)   10–25%
- Stage TxN1-2   30%
- Salvage T0   70%
- Salvage T1   50%
- Salvage, T2, 3a   25%

Invasive bladder cancer: radical radiotherapy and palliative treatment

Management of patients with invasive bladder cancer requires a multi-disciplinary team approach, involving case-by-case discussion between the urological surgeon, radiotherapist, and medical oncologist, with support from the pathologist, radiologist, and cancer specialist nurse.

Radical external beam radiotherapy (RT) is a good option for treating muscle-invasive (pT2/3/4) TCC in patients who are unfit or unwilling to undergo cystectomy, but who still wish to have the chance of cure. Typically, a total dose of 66 Gray is administered in 30 fractions over 6 weeks. The target field comprises the bladder only, with a 1.5-cm safety margin to allow for movement.

The 5-year survival rates, at 40–60%, are inferior to those of cystectomy, but the bladder is preserved and the complications are less significant. Higher-grade tumours tend to do less well, perhaps because of the undetected presence of disease outside the field of irradiation. Beyond this, prediction of radiotherapy response remains difficult, relying on follow-up cystoscopy and biopsy. Local recurrence occurs in approximately 30% of patients. There may be a small benefit in the use of neo-adjuvant or adjuvant cisplatin-based combination chemotherapy with RT in locally-advanced (pT3b/4) disease (📖 see p. 271).

Interstitial brachytherapy using caesium or iridium sources can be used to treat small T2 TCC in combination with RT and bladder-preserving surgery. Use of this technique is not widespread.

CIS, SCC, and adenocarcinoma are poorly sensitive to radiotherapy. There is no advantage in giving pre-cystectomy RT for invasive TCC.

Complications occur in 70% of patients, self-limiting in 95% of cases. These include radiation cystitis (filling LUTS and dysuria) and proctitis (diarrhoea and rectal bleeding), usually lasting only a few months. Refractory radiation cystitis and haematuria may rarely require desperate measures such as intravesical alum, formalin, hyperbaric oxygen, iliac artery embolization, or even palliative cystectomy.

Efficacy of RT

5-year survival rates are as follows:
- Stage T1   35%
- Stages T2   40%
- Stage T3a   35%
- Stage T3b,T4   20%
- Stage TxN1-2   7%

If disease persists or recurs, salvage cystectomy may still be successful in appropriately-selected patients, 5-year survival rates 30–50% (p. 265). Otherwise, cytotoxic chemotherapy (p. 271) and palliative measures may be considered

Palliative treatment

RT (30 Gray) is effective for *metastatic bone pain* or to palliate symptomatic local tumour (40–50 Gray).

Intractable haematuria may be controlled by intravesical formalin or alum, hyperbaric oxygen, bilateral internal iliac artery embolization or ligation, or palliative cystectomy.

Ureteric obstruction may be relieved by percutaneous nephrostomy and antegrade stenting (p. 340).

Involvement of a palliative care team can be very helpful to the patient and family.

Muscle-invasive bladder cancer: management of locally-advanced and metastatic disease

Management of patients with invasive bladder cancer requires a multi-disciplinary team approach, involving case-by-case discussion between the urological surgeon, radiotherapist, and medical oncologist, with support from the pathologist, radiologist, and cancer specialist nurse.

Locally-advanced bladder cancer (pT3b/4)

Many patients treated with primary cystectomy or radiotherapy (RT) with curative intent succumb to metastatic disease due to incomplete tumour excision or micrometastases. Up to 50% of patients develop metastases, mostly at distant sites. At this stage, the 5 years survival is only 25%. There is interest in augmenting primary treatment in an effort to improve outcomes.

Neo-adjuvant and adjuvant *RT*

Randomized studies have suggested improvements in local control using RT prior to cystectomy, but no survival benefit has been demonstrated. The rationale for post-cystectomy RT is that patients with proven residual or nodal disease may benefit from loco-regional treatment. However, it leads to unacceptably high morbidity and has no demonstrable advantages. Post-treatment bowel obstruction occurs 4.5 times more commonly in RT patients.

Adjuvant cystectomy

Two studies have demonstrated an improvement in local control and a survival advantage when treating locally-advanced disease with cystectomy after RT, compared with RT alone. However, this treatment strategy does not happen in current UK practice, probably due to the increased morbidity of surgery in this setting.

Neo-adjuvant chemotherapy with cystectomy

Preoperative chemotherapy could be given to operable patients with T2–T4a disease. It could theoretically downstage the disease and treat micrometastases before the patient was debilitated by surgery. A meta-analysis of 10 trials[1] has suggested a 5% 5-year survival advantage with the use of cisplatin-based combination chemotherapy prior to cystectomy compared with cystectomy alone. The absolute gain was the same regardless of stage: 55–60% for T2, 40–45% for T3, and 25–30% for T4 patients. The relative gain was therefore greater for higher stage patients. One randomized trial demonstrated a median survival of advantage of 30 months in the group treated with neo-adjuvant combination chemotherapy compared with the group receiving cystectomy alone. This treatment should be discussed with suitable patients suspected of having locally-advanced or micrometastatic disease, prior to cystectomy.

Adjuvant chemotherapy

The rationale for post-cystectomy chemotherapy is that patients with proven residual or nodal disease may benefit from systemic treatment. Trials have been hampered by protocol problems, small numbers, surgical complications interfering with treatment and difficulty in assessing response in the absence of measurable disease. However, 2 out of 4 studies have shown a survival benefit of almost 2 years in the treated groups, using cisplatin-based regimes.

Neo-adjuvant or adjuvant chemotherapy with RT

While controversial, neo-adjuvant cisplatin-based combination chemotherapy with bladder preservation has been demonstrated to produce 5-year survival rates of 42–63% when RT was used as definitive treatment. This may be offered to patients suspected of having locally-advanced disease after clinical examination and staging imaging.

Metastatic bladder cancer

Systemic chemotherapy

This modality is recommended for patients with unresectable, diffusely metastatic measurable disease. Combination therapy is more effective than single-agent treatment. A complete response is seen in 20% of patients given methotrexate, vinblastine, adriamycin, and cisplatin (MVAC), although 20% of patients develop neutropaenia and 3% die of sepsis. Long-term disease-free survival is rare. Most UK centres are using cisplatin, methotrexate, and vinblastin (CMV). Gemcitaobine, a relatively new antimetabolite agent, has been used alone and in combination with cisplatin, with complete responses reported in 25–40% of patients. Another new class of agents, taxanes paclitaxel and docetaxel, are microtubule disassembly inhibitors. Responses range from 25 to 80% using these agents alone or in combination.

Prognostic factors predicting response to chemotherapy include alkaline phosphatize, age >60 years, performance status, and visceral metastases. Depending on the number of factors, median survival varies from 9 to 30 months[2]. In future, molecular markers such as tumour p53 status may be shown to predict chemosensitivity.

Radiotherapy

Roles for RT include palliation of metastatic pain; spinal cord compression.

Surgery

There is no surgical role in treatment of extravesical metastatic disease.

1   Vale C et al. (2003) Advanced bladder cancer meta-analysis collaboration. Neo-adjuvant chemotherapy in invasive bladder cancer: a systematic review and meta-analysis. *Lancet* **361:** 1927–34.

2   Bajorin DF et al. (1999) Long-term survival in metastatic transitional cell carcinoma and prognostic factors predicting outcome of therapy. *J Clin Oncol* **17:**3173–81.

Bladder cancer: urinary diversion after cystectomy

The choice of urinary diversion requires consideration of both clinical and quality of life (QOL) issues. Patients planned for cystectomy should be informed of the possible options. Contra-indications to the continent reconstructive procedures include debilitating neurological and psychiatric illness, short life expectancy, and impaired renal or liver function. These patients must be motivated and able to perform intermittent self-catheterization (ISC). Contra-indications to orthotopic neobladder include tumour in the prostatic urethra, widespread CIS, and urethral stricture disease.

The majority of patients report good overall QOL following urinary diversion. The reconstructive procedures were expected to be better for social functioning compared with the ileal conduit: most QOL studies have not shown significant differences, although patients with continent diversions generally score more favourably in terms of body image, social activity, and physical function.

Ureterosigmoidostomy

The oldest form of urinary diversion, wherein the ureters drain into the sigmoid colon, either in its native form, or following detubularization and reconstruction into a pouch (Mainz II). This diversion requires no appliance (stoma bag, catheter), so remains popular in developing countries. In recreating a 'cloaca', the patient may be prone to upper UTI with the risk of long-term renal deterioration, metabolic hyperchloraemic acidosis, and loose frequent stools. The low-pressure and capacious Mainz II pouch reduces these complications.

Ileal conduit

This was developed in 1950 and remains the most popular form of urinary diversion in the UK. 15 cm of subterminal ileum is isolated on its mesentery, the ureters are anastomosed to the proximal end. The distal end is brought out in the right iliac fossa as a stoma. The native ileum is anastomosed to gain enteral continuity.

Complications of ileal conduit are:

- Prolonged ileus
- Urinary leak
- Enteral leak
- Pyelonephritis
- Uretero-ileal stricture
- Stoma problems (20% 0—skin irritation, stenosis and parastomal hernia
- Upper tract dilatation (30%).

Patients require stomatherapy support and some find difficulty in adjusting their lifestyle to cope with a stoma-bag. Metabolic complications are uncommon.

In post-RT salvage patients, a jejunal or colonic conduit is used because of concerns about the healing of radiation-damaged ileum. The conduit may be brought out in the upper abdomen and patients require careful electrolyte monitoring due to sodium loss and hyperkalaemia.

Continent diversion

The advantage is the absence of an external collection device. There are two types of continent diversion:

A **continent pouch** is fashioned from 60 cm of detubularized ileum or right hemicolon. The ureters drain into this low-pressure balloon-shaped reservoir, usually through an anti-reflux submucosal tunnel. This is drained by the patient via a continent catheterizable stoma, such as the appendix or uterine tube (the Mitrofanoff principle) brought out in the right iliac fossa.

A similarly-constructed pouch may be anastomosed to the patient's urethra to act as an orthotopic neobladder, so that natural voiding can be established and no stoma is necessary. Patients void by relaxing their external sphincter and performing a Valsalva. This neobladder should require no catheter, unless the pouch is too large* and fails to empty adequately. In this case, the patient must be prepared to perform ISC.

Popular ileal pouches include those of Studer (Fig. 7.4), Camey II and Kock. Ileo-caecal pouches include the Indiana and Mainz I. Which one is chosen often comes down to the surgeon's preference; they carry similar complication risks. Previously irradiated bowel can safely be used to form pouches, though complications are more likely.

Complications relating to pouches and neobladders are divided into early (12%) and late (37%). They include:

- Urinary leakage and peritonitis
- Pelvic abscess
- Stone formation
- Catheterizing difficulties and stomal stenosis
- Urinary incontinence and nocturnal enuresis (particularly with neobladders)
- Pouch-ureteric reflux and UTI
- Uretero-pouch anastomotic stricture
- Late neobladder rupture.

Metabolic abnormalities include early fluid and electrolyte imbalances; later, urinary electrolyte absorption may cause hyperchloraemic acidosis, and loss of small bowel may result in vitamin B12 deficiency. Metabolic acidosis is less likely in patients with normal renal function; treatment is with sodium bicarbonate and potassium citrate. Annual B12 monitoring should be undertaken with supplementation if necessary.

Adenocarcinoma may develop (5%) in intestinal conduit, neobladder, or sigmoid colon mucosa in the long-term, due to the carcinogenic bacterial metabolism of urinary nitrosamines. This tends to occur near to the inflow of urine. It is therefore advisable to perform annual visual surveillance of urinary diversions after 10 years. If the urethra is *in situ*, annual urethroscopy and cytology is important.

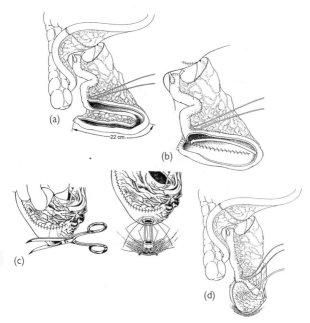

Fig. 7.4 (a) The distal 40–44 cm of resected ileum opened along the antimesenteric border with scissors. Spatulated ureters are anastomosed end to side with 4-0 running suture on either side of proximal end of afferent tubular ileal limb. Ureters are stented. (b) The two medial borders of the U-shaped, opened distal ileal segment are oversewn with a single layer seromuscular continous suture. The bottom of the U is folded between the two ends of the U. (c) Before complete closure of the reservoir, a 8–10 mm hole is cut into the most caudal part of the reservoir (left). Six sutures are placed between the seromuscular layer of the anastomotic area of the reservoir and the membraneous urethra (right). An 18F urethral catheter is inserted. (d) Before complete closure of the pouch, a cystostomy tube is inserted and brought out suprapubically adjacent to the wound. (Reproduced with permission from Studer et al. 1996).[1]

1 Studer UE, Danuser H, Hochreiter W, et al. (1996) Summary of 10 years experience with an ileal low-pressure substitute combined with an afferent tubular isoperistaltic segment. *World J Urol* **14**:29–39.

Prostate cancer: epidemiology and aetiology

Hormonal factors and diet

Growth of prostate cancer (PC), like benign prostatic epithelium, is largely under the promotional influence of testosterone and its potent metabolite, dihydrotestosterone. Androgen ablation by orchidectomy results in programmed epithelial cell death (apoptosis) and involution of the prostate. PC is not seen in eunuchs or people with congenital deficiency of 5α-reductase. Response to LH–RH analogue therapy in the treatment of patients with PC may be sub-optimal if the serum testosterone is not suppressed to castrate levels (<50 nmol/l). Oestrogens, including phyto-oestrogens found in foodstuffs used in Asian and Oriental cuisine, have a similar negative growth effect on PC. This may explain why these races rarely develop the clinical disease or die of prostate cancer.

Other dietary inhibitors of PC growth include vitamins E and D, the anti-oxidant lycopene (present in cooked or processed tomatoes), pomegranate, legumes, and the trace element selenium. Obesity does not confer increased risk of PC diagnosis, but appears to be associated with more aggressive disease. High charred meat and alpha-linolenic acid consumption are associated with increased risk, while linoleic acid appears protective. (Ⓜ see also p. 280.)

Other risk factors

Age is an important risk factor for development of histological PC, the disease being rare below 40 years and becoming increasingly common with rising age, according to post-mortem studies. Prevalence of PC rises from 29% in the fifth decade to 67% in the ninth decade. This is paralleled 20 years earlier by the presence of prostatic intraepithelial neoplasia (PIN), the accepted pre-malignant lesion. However, most prostate cancer does not become clinically-recognized or life-threatening. 75% of prostate cancers are diagnosed in men >65 years, although the incidence amongst men aged 50–59 has trebled since the 1970s.

Geographic variation, the disease is more common in Western nations, particularly Scandinavian countries (where low sunlight and Vitamin D synthesis may be implicated) and North America. The disease is rare in Asia and the Far East, but US migrants from Asia and Japan have a 20-fold increased risk. This suggests an environmental aetiology, such as the Western diet, may be important.

Race: Black men are at greatest risk, then Caucasians; Asians, and Oriental races develop PC uncommonly unless they migrate to the West. The world's highest incidence is among African Americans and Jamaicans, although there are scant data available regarding native African men. A recent study suggests that African Europeans are at 3 times risk of developing PC compared with white men, although the risk of PC death is similar.

Family history: 5% of prostate cancers are believed to be inherited. Hereditary prostate cancer tends to occur in younger (<60 years) men who have a family history; genetic abnormalities on chromosomes 1q (HPC1 locus), 8p (MSR-1 locus), Xp, and Y, as well as mutations of the

BRCA2 gene are reported. The risk of a man developing PC is doubled if there is one affected first-degree relative and is 4-fold if there are two. Men without sons are at greater risk than those that have fathered sons.

Some controversy surrounds the possible increased risk of developing PC conferred by sexual activity, infectious agents and vasectomy. The balance of data and opinion go against these putative risk factors at present. Exposure to cadmium has been suggested to raise the risk of PC, but no new data have been forthcoming since the 1960's. High alcohol intake appears to be associated with increased risk, while smoking does not. However, smoking appears to increase the risk of fatal PC.

Prostate cancer: incidence, prevalence, and mortality

Incidence

The diagnosis of prostate cancer (PC) is on the increase, probably as a result of increasing use of serum PSA testing for both symptomatic and asymptomatic men, and the use of more extensive prostatic biopsy protocols. PC is the most commonly diagnosed male cancer (excluding skin) in the UK and USA. In 1999, 24,714 men were diagnosed with prostate cancer in the United Kingdom, mean age 72 years; by 2002 this had increased to 31,923. The lifetime risk of a man being diagnosed with PC is 1 in 12. Risk factors and aetiology are discussed on p. 276–7.

Prevalence

While the incidence of PC continues to rise (now approximately 8% of all men) the true prevalence of the disease is highlighted by post-mortem studies carried out on men who died of unrelated causes. These have demonstrated histological evidence of PC in 10% of men in their third decade, 34% in the fifth decade to 67% in the ninth decade. Much of this 'latent' or clinically-insignificant prostate cancer may be detected by PSA screening and treated unnecessarily at the older end of the age spectrum.

Mortality

It is estimated that 3% of men die of PC. In 2004, 10,209 deaths were attributed to prostate cancer in the UK, the second most common (13% of all) form of male cancer death. This compares with 8524 deaths due to colorectal cancer and 20,384 due to lung cancer. Because most deaths occur in men over 75 years old, however, the number of years of life lost per prostate cancer death is very low compared with less common cancers.

Mortality increased slowly in the UK and USA during the 1970s and 80s, peaking in 1990 at 3% per year. However, in 1991, mortality started to decrease in the USA by 2% per year. In the UK too there was a small reduction in mortality, which stabilized at the turn of the century. This could have been due to changes in the way death certificates were written, or treatment: perhaps earlier use of hormone therapy for advanced disease or increased treatment of localized disease carried out in the 1990s.

Survival rates for prostate cancer have been improving for more than 20 years. The detection of a greater proportion of latent, earlier, slow growing tumours has had a beneficial effect on survival rates. The relative 5-year survival rate for men diagnosed in England in 2000–2001 was 71% compared with only 31% for men diagnosed in 1971–1975. Indeed, it has been suggested that PC patients have an overall improved life expectancy due to more intensive concomitant healthcare received.

Prostate cancer: prevention, complementary, and alternative therapies

The fact that as many as 32% of men in their fifth decade have histological prostate cancer (PC), even though the disease is rarely detected clinically below the age of 50 years suggests opportunity for preventative strategies.

Dietary intervention

There are much epidemiological and laboratory data supporting dietary interventions, though randomized prospective trial are awaited.

High fat diets, particularly those rich in saturated fat and omega-6 fatty acids, are linked to increased risk of prostate cancer diagnosis.

Soy products contain phyto-oestrogens including the isoflavone genistein. Genistein is a natural inhibitor of tyrosine kinase receptors and inhibits PC cell lines. Chinese Americans have a 24-fold risk of developing prostate cancer compared with native Chinese, perhaps due to a difference in their respective diets.

Lycopene, present in cooked tomatoes and tomato products, is considered to reduce risk of PC progression and inhibits cell lines.

Selenium supplementation (0.2 mg/day = 2 brazil nuts) was shown to reduce the risk of developing PC in a melanoma prevention trial. Selenium is a trace element required as an antioxidant. It is found in relatively low concentration in European soil, and can be assayed using toe-nail clippings.

Vitamin E supplementation was shown to reduce the incidence of PC in Finnish smokers. It is an antioxidant. A randomized prospective study (SELECT) has recently shown no reduction in the risk of developing PC using Vitamin E supplements either alone or in combination with Selenium.

Vitamins A (retinoids) and D both inhibit growth of PC cell lines and vitamin D receptor polymorphisms appear to predispose certain individuals to prostate cancer.

Pomegranite juice appears to reduce PSA doubling time relapse following radical prostatectomy.

A pan-European study of large consumers of *vegetables* (for example, vegetarians) did not exhibit a reduced incidence of PC. However, one portion per week of cruciform vegetables, including broccoli, reduces the incidence of PC by 40%. Other beneficial dietary ingredients include turmeric and black pepper.

Studies from UK, Europe and the USA have shown that 25-40% of PC patients are taking some form of complementary therapy, most without informing their doctor. These can occasionally be harmful: for example, a 'Chinese herb' mixture called PC-SPES, now withdrawn, frequently caused thromboembolism.

Smoking has been shown in population studies to be significantly associated not with prostate cancer diagnosis, but fatal PC. No definite link exists between vasectomy or sexual activity and prostate cancer. Studies have suggested an increased risk associated with early sexual activity and a reduced risk associated with frequent masturbation, but these require substantiation. Similarly, a protective effect of regular physical exercise on PC has been suggested by small laboratory and prospective clinical studies.

Chemoprevention with anti-androgens

Given that most prostate cancer is initially an androgen-dependent disease, interest in its prevention has focussed on anti-androgens. While non-steroidal anti-androgens would have unacceptable side-effects and cost, the 5-α reductase inhibitors could be feasible chemoprevention agents. The Prostate Cancer Prevention Trial[1] recruited 18,000 men who had no clinical or biochemical evidence of prostate cancer. They were randomized to placebo or finasteride 5 mg daily for up to 7 years. The men were offered biopsy if they developed a rising PSA, an abnormality on DRE, or at end of study. Prostate cancer was detected in 24 and 18% of participants in placebo and finasteride arms, respectively, suggesting that finasteride reduces the risk of developing prostate cancer by 25%. However, Gleason 7+ cancers were significantly more frequent in the finasteride arm. While this could be due to the effect of the 5ARI on tissue architecture, or a selection artefact due to gland shrinkage, there is as yet no licence for prescribing 5ARI's for PC prevention. The REDUCE study to assess the chemopreventative effects of dutasteride is in progress.

1 Thompson IM *et al*, (2003) The influence of Finasteride on the development of prostate cancer. *NEJM* **349**:215–24.

Prostate cancer: pathology— adenocarcinoma

By far the most common (>95%) prostatic malignancy is adenocarcinoma, carcinoma of the acinar or ductal epithelium. The basal cell layer is absent and the basement membrane is breached by the malignant cells which invade into the prostatic fibromuscular stroma. Macroscopically, they tend to be hard and white, though a soft mucin-producing variety exists. The prostatic urethra, ducts or stroma may be invaded by transitional cell carcinoma of the bladder (☐ see p. 250 and 342 'Bladder Cancer Pathology' and 'Urethral Cancer'). Prostatic sarcomas, most common of which is the rhabdomyosarcoma, are rare, but may be seen in childhood. Secondary deposits (metastases) from other sites are rare.

Adenocarcinoma of the prostate

Most (75%) adenocarcinomas are located in the peripheral zone and most (85%) are multifocal. The mean number of cancers in a radical prostatectomy specimen is seven. 20% arise from the transition zones and 5% from the embryologically-distinct central zone. The tumour spreads locally through the flimsy prostatic capsule (this is absent at the apex and base of the gland) into surrounding tissue, at which time it is termed 'locally-advanced'. The disease may involve the urethral sphincter, corpora of the penis, seminal vesicles, or trigone of the bladder including the distal ureters, but rarely invades through Denonvilliers fascia to involve the rectum. Local spread is often along the course of autonomic nerves, so-called perineural invasion. The most frequent sites of metastasis are internal iliac lymph nodes and bone; although lung, liver, testis, and brain are not common metastatic sites. Bone metastases are characteristically sclerotic, rarely lytic. The axial skeleton (spine, ribs, and pelvis) are most commonly affected, followed by the proximal long bones, clavicles, and the skull.

Prostate cancer is a complex disease, exhibiting genetic, as well as morphological heterogeneity, increasing with stage and grade. Epigenetic changes, such as inactivating hypermethylation of the detoxifying enzyme *GSTP1* gene are observed in 90% of prostate cancers and 70% of PIN lesions, suggesting this may be an early event in carcinogenesis. Up to 50% of cancers carry a rearrangement of chromosome 21, whereby a translocation results in the fusion of an androgen-dependent protease TMPRSS2 and the ERG transcription factor (which then itself becomes androgen-dependent). It is postulated that this rearrangement could be an early step in prostate tumourigenesis. Frequent changes include somatic loss of alleles on chromosomes 16 and 18, inactivation of tumour suppressor genes pTEN (chromosome 10q) and MSR-1 (chromosome 8p), p53 (chromosome 17p) and activation of c-myc and bcl-2 protooncogenes. Interest is also focused on the potential tumourigenic role of a subset of prostatic basal epithelial cells that are thought to be immortal, undifferentiated stem cells.

Prostate cancer grading

Adenocarcinoma of the prostate is graded using the Gleason system (Fig. 7.5). Microscopically, adenocarcinoma is graded 1–5 according to its gland-forming differentiation at relatively low magnification. Cytological features play no part in this grading system. Since most PCs are multi-focal and heterogeneous, allowance is made by adding the two dominant grades to give a score between 2 and 10. If only one pattern is observed, the grade is doubled. The system is used with needle biopsies, TURP, and radical prostatectomy specimens.

Gleason scores 2–4 are considered well-differentiated; 5–7 are moderately-differentiated and 8–10 are poorly-differentiated. In practice, 75% of PC is graded 5, 6, or 7, 10% are graded 2–4 and 15% are graded 8–10. Among expert pathologists there is good inter-observer reproducibility with Gleason scoring. However, scores assigned to needle biopsies are rarely less than 3 + 3 = 6, since grades 1 and 2 are rarely if ever observed. In 30–40% of cases, needle biopsy scores are lower than those assigned to the subsequent radical prostatectomy specimen, while overgrading by needle biopsy is uncommon (5%).

The importance of the Gleason score is that it correlates well with prognosis, stage for stage, however the patient is managed. Indeed, it remains the most important prognostic indicator following radical curative treatment. Cancers of the same Gleason score have a worse prognosis if the predominant grade is higher (for example, 4 + 3 = 7 is worse than 3 + 4 = 7). Some men with low-grade tumours develop high-grade tumours after several years. This is probably due to clonal expansion of high-grade cells, rather than de-differentiation of low-grade tumour cells. In general, large volume tumours are more likely to be high-grade than low volume tumours, but occasionally exceptions are seen.

Finally, caution must be taken when Gleason-scoring tissue that has been subject to certain interventions, including radiotherapy and androgen deprivation therapy. It is recognized that prostate cancers treated with androgen ablation exhibit changes similar to those seen in cancers of Gleason score 8–10. It is possible that treatment of BPH with 5-alpha reductase inhibitors could adversely affect the Gleason score of cancer present in the gland. Pathologists are therefore keen to know relevant clinical details and are reluctant to provide Gleason scores for such patients.

Other prognostic indicators

As well as Gleason score, tumour stage and PSA level are independent predictors of PC prognosis. Tissue molecular markers, such as over-expression of p53, have been shown to correlate with adverse outcome following radical prostatectomy.

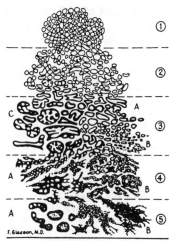

Fig. 7.5 A diagrammatic representation of the Gleason grading system for prostrate cancer. The grade depends on the structure of the prostatic glands and their relationship to the stromal smooth muscle.

Prostate cancer: staging and imaging

Tumour staging uses the TNM classification (Fig. 7.6 and Table 7.8). As with all cancer, prostate cancer staging may be considered clinical (prefixed with 'c') or pathological (prefixed with 'p'), dependent on available data.

T stage is assessed by digital rectal examination (📖 see Fig. 7.4) and imaging (TRUS, MRI). Imaging resolution limits reliability in detection of multi-focal and microscopic extraprostatic disease. Only 60% of cancers are visible on TRUS and only 40% of pT3 tumours will be detected. Using MRI, prediction of extra-prostatic extension and seminal vesicle involvement has 50–84% sensitivity and 22–95% specificity. Recent prostatic biopsy may also confuse the interpretation of MRI images, particularly regarding the seminal vesicles. Endorectal MRI appears more accurate for T staging than surface MRI or CT. Seminal vesicle biopsy may be carried out in cases considered at high-risk of seminal vesicle involvement.

N stage is assessed by imaging (MRI) or biopsy as necessary. Pelvic lymphadenectomy is the gold-standard assessment of N stage. This commonly involves bilateral excision of the obturator nodes, though 'extended' dissection including the external and common iliac nodes is popular in some centres which report higher positivity rates. MRI or CT scanning can image enlarged nodes; radiologists report nodes of >8mm in maximal diameter. However, nodes larger than this often contain no cancer, while micrometastases may be present in normal-sized nodes. Sensitivity ranges from 0 to 70%, with a positive predictive value of only 50%. In practice, MRI pelvic imaging is restricted to intermediate and high-risk patients (cT3; PSA >10; Gleason 7 or higher).

There is interest in the ProstascintTM (Indium-111 capromab-pendatide immunoscintigraphy) and lymphotropic nanoparticle-enhanced MRI for improving imaging N-staging.

M stage is assessed by physical examination, imaging (MRI 'marrow screen' or isotope bone scan, chest radiology) and biochemical investigations (including creatinine and alkaline phosphatize, which is elevated in 70% of metastatic bone disease). MRI marrow screening is more sensitive than isotope bone scintigraphy, though more expensive. In practice, bone imaging is not carried out unless there is a major component of Gleason pattern 4 in the biopsies, a PSA >20 ng/mL, or a clinical indication. PSA >100 ng/mL predicts metastatic disease in almost 100%.

Partin's nomograms, based on >5000 radical prostatectomies, are widely used to help predict pathological T and N stage by combining clinical T stage, PSA, and biopsy Gleason score. (Table 7.9 modified from Partin AW *et al.*[1]) However, it is recognized that N staging is under-estimated because lymphadenectomies were confined to the obturator fossa.

Higher pathological stage (i.e. pT3 disease) found at radical prostatectomy may also be predicted by: higher percentages (>66%) of positive biopsies; cancer invading adipose in the biopsies (there is no fat in the prostate) and the presence of perineural cancer invasion within the prostate.

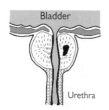

T1

Early (non-palpable) prostate
cancer only detectable under
the microscope; found at
TURP or by needle biopsy

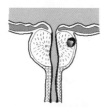

T2

Early (palpable) prostate
cancer—still confined to
the capsule

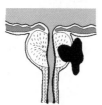

T3

Locally advanced prostate
cancer—into peri prostate
fat or seminal vesicles

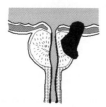

T4

Locally advanced prostate
cancer—invading the
bladder, rectum, penile
urethra, or pelvic side wall

Fig. 7.6 The T stages of prostate cancer.

Table 7.8 TNM (1992) staging of adenocarcinoma of the prostate

T0	No tumour (pT0 if no cancer found by histological examination)
Tx	T stage uncertain
T1	a Cancer non-palpable on digital rectal examination, present in <5% of TURP specimen (in up to 18% of TURPs)
	b Cancer non-palpable on digital rectal examination, present in >5% of TURP specimen
	c Cancer non-palpable on digital rectal examination, present in needle biopsy taken because of elevated PSA
T2	a Palpable tumour, feels confined, in < half of one 'lobe' on digital rectal examination
	b Palpable tumour, feels confined, in > half of one 'lobe' on digital rectal examination
	c Palpable tumour, feels confined, in both 'lobes' on digital rectal examination
T3	a Palpable tumour, locally-advanced into periprostatic fat, uni- or bilateral, and mobile on digital rectal examination
	b Palpable tumour, locally-advanced into seminal vesicle(s) on digital rectal examination
T4	a Palpable tumour, locally-advanced into adjacent structures, feels fixed on digital rectal examination
	b Palpable tumour, locally-advanced onto pelvic side-wall, feels fixed on digital rectal examination
Nx	Regional lymph not assessed
N0	No regional lymph node metastasis
N1	Tumour involves regional (pelvic) lymph nodes
Mx	Distant metastases not assessed
M0	No distant metastasis
M1a	Non-regional lymph nodes
M1b	Tumour metastasis in bone
M1c	Tumour metastasis in other sites

There is no provision in the T staging for suspected *local recurrence following radical prostatectomy* since the primary tumour has been removed. A nodule is occasionally palpable by DRE and current imaging is unhelpful and not recommended unless the PSA is >7ng/mL. Recently, [11C]-choline PET/CT imaging has been reported to detect local and node recurrence even when PSA <2.5ng/mL.

1 Partin AW, Mangold LLA, Lamm DM, *et al.* (2001) Contemporary update of prostate cancer staging nomograms (Partin Tables) for the new millennium. *Urology* **58**(b) 843.

Table 7.9 Combination of prostate-specific antigen, clinical stage, and Gleason score to predict pathological stage of localized prostate cancer. (Adapted with permission from Elsevier:[1])

PSA range (ng/mt)	Pathologic stage	Clinical stage T1c (nonpalpable, PSA elevated)				
		Gleason score				
		2–4	5–6	3+4=7	4+3=7	8–10
0–25	Organ confined	95 (89–99)	90 (88–93)	79 (74–85)	71 (62–79)	66 (54–76)
	Extraprostatic extension	5 (1–11)	9 (7–12)	17 (13–23)	25 (18–23)	28 (20–38)
	Seminal vesicle (+)	—	0 (0–1)	2 (1–5)	2 (1–5)	4 (1–10)
	Lymph node (+)	—	—	1 (0–2)	1 (0–4)	1 (0–4)
2.6–4.0	Organ confined	92 (82–98)	84 (81–86)	68 (62–74)	58 (48–67)	52 (41–63)
	Extraprostatic extension	8 (2–18)	15 (13–18)	27 (22–33)	37 (29–46)	40 (31–50)
	Seminal vesicle (+)	—	1 (0–1)	4 (2–7)	4 (1–7)	6 (3–12)
	Lymph node (+)	—	—	1 (0–2)	1 (0–3)	1 (0–4)
4.1–6.0	Organ confined	90 (78–98)	80 (78–83)	63 (58–83)	52 (43–60)	46 (36–56)
	Extraprostatic extension	10 (2–22)	19 (16–21)	32 (27–36)	42 (35–50)	45 (36–54)
	Seminal vesicle (+)	—	1 (0–1)	3 (1–5)	3 (1–6)	5 (3–9)
	Lymph node (+)	—	0 (0–1)	2 (1–3)	3 (1–5)	3 (1–6)

Key PSA = prostate-specific antigen.

(Continued)

Table 7.9 Combination of prostate-specific antigen, clinical stage, and Gleason score to predict pathological stage of localized prostate cancer. (Continued).

PSA range (ng/mt)	Pathologic stage	Clinical stage T1c (nonpalpable, PSA elevated)				
		Gleason score				
		2–4	5–6	3+4=7	4+3=7	8–10
6.1–10.0	Organ confined	87 (73–97)	75 (72–77)	54 (49–59)	43 (35–51)	37 (28–46)
	Extraprostatic extension	13 (3–27)	23 (21–25)	36 (32–40)	47 (40–54)	48 (39–57)
	Seminal vesicle (+)	–	2 (2–3)	8 (6–11)	8 (4–12)	13 (8–19)
	Lymph node (+)	–	0 (0–1)	2 (1–3)	2 (1–4)	3 (1–5)
>10.0	Organ confined	80 (61–95)	62 (58–64)	37 (32–42)	27 (21–34)	22 (16–30)
	Extraprostatic extension	20 (5–39)	33 (30–36)	43 (38–48)	51 (44–59)	50 (42–59)
	Seminal vesicle (+)	–	4 (3–5)	12 (9–17)	11 (6–17)	17 (10–25)
	Lymph node (+)	–	2 (1–3)	8 (5–11)	10 (5–17)	11 (5–18)
		Clinical stage T2a (palpable <½ of one lobe)				
0–2.5	Organ confined	91 (79–98)	81 (77–85)	64 (56–71)	53 (43–63)	47 (35–59)
	Extraprostatic extension	9 (2–21)	17 (13–21)	29 (23–36)	40 (30–49)	42 (32–53)
	Seminal vesicle (+)	–	1 (0–2)	5 (1–9)	4 (1–9)	7 (2–16)
	Lymph node (+)	–	0 (0–1)	2 (0–5)	3 (0–8)	3 (0–9)
2.6–4.0	Organ confined	85 (69–96)	71 (66–75)	50 (43–57)	39 (30–48)	33 (24–44)
	Extraprostatic extension	15 (4–31)	27 (23–31)	41 (35–48)	52 (43–61)	53 (44–63)
	Seminal vesicle (+)	–	2 (1–3)	7 (3–12)	6 (2–12)	10 (4–18)
	Lymph node (+)	–	0 (0–1)	2 (0–4)	2 (0–6)	3 (0–8)

PSA					
4.1–6.0	Organ confined	81 (63–95)	66 (62–70)	44 (39–50)	33 (25–41)	28 (20–37)
	Extraprostatic extension	19 (5–37)	32 (28–36)	46 (40–52)	56 (48–64)	58 (49–66)
	Seminal vesicle (+)	–	1 (1–2)	5 (3–8)	5 (2–8)	8 (4–13)
	Lymph node (+)	–	1 (0–2)	4 (2–7)	6 (3–11)	6 (2–12)
6.1–10.0	Organ confined	76 (56–94)	58 (54–61)	35 (30–40)	25 (19–32)	21 (15–28)
	Extraprostatic extension	24 (6–44)	37 (34–41)	49 (43–54)	58 (51–66)	57 (48–65)
	Seminal vesicle (+)	–	4 (3–5)	13 (9–18)	11 (6–17)	17 (11–26)
	Lymph node (+)	–	1 (0–2)	3 (2–6)	5 (2–8)	5 (2–10)
>10.0	Organ confined	65 (43–89)	42 (38–46)	20 (17–24)	14 (10–8)	11 (7–15)
	Extraprostatic extension	35 (11–57)	47 (43–52)	49 (43–55)	55 (46–64)	52 (41–62)
	Seminal vesicle (+)	–	6 (4–8)	16 (11–22)	13 (7–20)	19 (12–29)
	Lymph node (+)	–	4 (3–7)	4 (9–21)	18 (10–27)	17 (9–29)
Clinical stage T2a (palpable <½ of one lobe, not on both lobes)						
0–2.5	Organ confined	88 (73–97)	75 (69–81)	54 (46–63)	43 (33–54)	37 (26–49)
	Extraprostatic extension	12 (3–27)	22 (17–28)	35 (28–43)	45 (35–56)	46 (35–58)
	Seminal vesicle (+)	–	2 (0–3)	6 (2–12)	5 (1–11)	9 (2–20)
	Lymph node (+)	–	1 (0–2)	4 (0–10)	6 (0–14)	6 (0–16)
2.6–4.0	Organ confined	80 (61–95)	63 (57–69)	41 (33–48)	30 (22–39)	25 (17–34)
	Extraprostatic extension	20 (5–39)	34 (28–40)	47 (40–55)	57 (47–67)	57 (46–68)
	Seminal vesicle (+)	–	2 (1–4)	9 (4–15)	7 (3–14)	12 (5–22)
	Lymph node (+)	–	1 (0–2)	3 (0–8)	4 (0–12)	5 (0–14)

Key PSA = prostate-specific antigen.

(Continued)

Table 7.9 Combination of prostate-specific antigen, clinical stage, and Gleason score to predict pathological stage of localized prostate cancer. (Continued).

PSA range (ng/mt)	Pathologic stage	Clinical stage T2a (palpable ≤½ of one lobe, not on both lobes)				
		Gleason score				
		2–4	5–6	3+4=7	4+3=7	8–10
4.1–6.0	Organ confined	75 (55–93)	57 (52–63)	35 (29–40)	25 (18–32)	21 (14–29)
	Extraprostatic extension	25 (7–45)	39 (33–44)	51 (44–57)	60 (50–68)	59 (49–69)
	Seminal vesicle (+)	—	2 (1–3)	7 (4–11)	5 (3–9)	9 (4–16)
	Lymph node (+)	—	2 (1–3)	7 (4–13)	10 (5–18)	10 (4–20)
6.1–10.0	Organ confined	69 (47–91)	49 (43–54)	26 (22–31)	19 (14–25)	15 (10–21)
	Extraprostatic extension	31 (9–53)	44 (39–49)	52 (46–58)	60 (52–68)	57 (48–67)
	Seminal vesicle (+)	—	5 (3–8)	16 (7–20)	13 (7–20)	19 (11–29)
	Lymph node (+)	—	2 (1–3)	6 (4–10)	8 (5–14)	8 (4–16)
>10.0	Organ confined	57 (35–86)	33 (28–38)	14 (11–17)	9 (6–13)	7 (4–10)
	Extraprostatic extension	43 (14–65)	52 (46–56)	47 (40–53)	50 (40–60)	46 (36–59)
	Seminal vesicle (+)	—	8 (5–11)	17 (12–24)	13 (8–21)	19 (12–29)
	Lymph node (+)	—	8 (5–12)	22 (15–30)	27 (16–39)	27 (14–40)
		Clinical stage T2c (palpable on both lobes)				
0–2.5	Organ confined	86 (71–97)	73 (63–81)	51 (38–63)	39 (26–54)	34 (21–48)
	Extraprostatic extension	14 (3–29)	24 (17–33)	36 (26–48)	45 (32–59)	47 (33–61)
	Seminal vesicle (+)	—	1 (0–4)	5 (1–13)	5 (1–12)	8 (2–19)
	Lymph node (+)	—	1 (0–4)	6 (0–18)	9 (0–26)	10 (0–27)

PSA						
2.6–4.0	Organ confined	78 (58–94)	61 (50–70)	38 (27–50)	27 (18–40)	23 (14–34)
	Extraprostatic extension	22 (6–42)	36 (27–45)	48 (37–59)	57 (44–70)	57 (44–70)
	Seminal vesicle (+)	—	2 (1–5)	8 (2–17)	6 (2–16)	10 (3–22)
	Lymph node (+)	—	1 (0–4)	5 (0–15)	7 (0–21)	8 (0–22)
4.1–6.0	Organ confined	73 (52–93)	55 (44–64)	31 (23–4)	21 (14–31)	18 (11–28)
	Extraprostatic extension	27 (7–48)	40 (32–50)	50 (40–60)	57 (43–68)	57 (43–70)
	Seminal vesicle (+)	—	2 (1–4)	6 (2–11)	4 (1–10)	7 (2–15)
	Lymph node (+)	—	3 (1–7)	12 (5–23)	16 (6–32)	16 (5–33)
6.1–10.0	Organ confined	67 (45–91)	46 (36–56)	24 (17–32)	16 (10–24)	13 (8–20)
	Extraprostatic extension	33 (9–55)	46 (37–55)	52 (42–61)	58 (46–69)	56 (43–69)
	Seminal vesicle (+)	—	5 (2–9)	13 (6–23)	11 (4–21)	16 (6–29)
	Lymph node (+)	—	3 (1–6)	10 (5–18)	13 (6–25)	13 (5–26)
>10.0	Organ confined	54 (32–85)	30 (21–38)	11 (7–17)	7 (4–12)	6 (3–10)
	Extraprostatic extension	46 (15–68)	51 (42–60)	42 (30–55)	43 (29–59)	41 (27–57)
	Seminal vesicle (+)	—	6 (2–12)	13 (6–24)	10 (3–20)	15 (5–28)
	Lymph node (+)	—	13 (6–22)	33 (18–49)	38 (20–58)	38 (20–59)

Key PSA = prostate-specific antigen.

Prostate cancer: clinical presentation

Since the widespread use of serum PSA testing, the majority of patients have non-metastatic disease at presentation. Shown below are possible presentations, grouped by disease stage.

Localized prostate cancer (T1–2)

- Asymptomatic; detected in association with elevated or rising serum PSA or incidental abnormal digital rectal examination (DRE)
- Lower urinary tract symptoms (in most cases due to co-existing benign hyperplasia causing bladder outflow obstruction)
- Haematospermia
- Haematuria (probably in most cases due to co-existing benign hyperplasia)
- Perineal or voiding discomfort (probably due to co-existing prostatitis).

Locally-advanced cancer (T3–4)

- Asymptomatic, as above
- Lower urinary tract symptoms
- Haematospermia
- Haematuria
- Perineal or voiding discomfort
- Symptoms of renal failure/anuria due to ureteric obstruction
- Malignant priapism (rare)
- Rectal obstruction (rare).

Metastatic disease (N+, M+)

- Asymptomatic ('occult disease'), as above
- Swelling of lower limb(s) due to lymphatic obstruction
- Anorexia, weight loss
- Bone pain, pathological fracture
- Neurological symptoms/signs in lower limbs (spinal cord compression)
- Anaemia
- Dyspnoea, jaundice, bleeding tendency (coagulopathy).

A note about the DRE

Since most prostate cancers arise in the peripheral, posterior part of the prostate, they should be palpable on DRE. An abnormal DRE is defined by asymmetry, a nodule, or a fixed craggy mass. Approximately 50% of abnormal DRE's are associated with prostate cancer, the remainder being caused by benign hyperplasia, prostatic calculi, chronic prostatitis, or post-radiotherapy change. Only 40% of cancers diagnosed by DRE will be organ-confined. The fact that an abnormal DRE in the presence of a 'normal' PSA (<4.0 ng/mL) carries a 30% chance of predicting prostate cancer underlines it's important role in clinical practice.

Prostate cancer screening

By early detection and treatment, population screening of men aged between 50 and 70–75 years using PSA ± DRE may reduce the significant mortality and morbidity caused by prostate cancer. Proponents of screening say these acceptable and relatively inexpensive evaluations will detect clinically-significant, but curable (organ-confined) disease. The lead-time, estimated at 9–12 years, between the screened diagnosis and the clinical diagnosis due to symptoms, should enable more organ-confined cancers to be diagnosed and cured. However, because of the low specificity of PSA (40%) and the high prevalence of latent prostate cancer, those against screening argue that many men would suffer unnecessary anxiety, biopsies, over-diagnosis, and over-treatment. Added to this, the treatments have morbidity and cost to the healthcare system. Mathematical models suggest fewer men screened in their sixth decade would be over-diagnosed compared with those in their 7th or 8th decade: younger men have potentially more to gain in terms of life expectancy. It is also estimated that the number of screen-detected cancers needed to treat to save one life could be as many as 100.

From an academic point of view, prostate cancer fails to fulfil most of the 10 screening criteria set out by Wilson and Jungner, including a lack of clear understanding of the disease's natural history.

UK population screening studies have diagnosed prostate cancer in 2–3% of men tested, the vast majority diagnosed with localized disease. A large non-randomized study over a 6-year period from Tyrol, Austria, demonstrated an 80% reduction in the diagnosis of metastatic disease and a 30% reduction in the expected mortality due to prostate cancer. Conversely, a cohort comparison between biopsy and treatment rates in Seattle and Connecticut showed that diagnosis and interventions were more prevalent in Seattle, and yet the mortality rates were similar in the two States.

The results of pivotal European and North American randomized trials are awaited, due in 2009. Survival and quality of life are the key outcome measures. Currently there is little support for a prostate cancer screening programme in the UK, although the Department of Health recommends that asymptomatic men requesting screening should be counselled prior to being screened, the so-called 'risk management programme'. A large UK multicentre study, PROTECT, is under way that aims to address both the screening question and the treatment of screen-detected disease. Starting in 2001 and with 260,000 men now recruited, results are not expected until 2013.

Prostate cancer: prostate specific antigen (PSA)

See p. 47 for an introduction to the serum PSA test. Until the development of commercial serum PSA assays in the late 1980s, the only serum marker for prostate cancer was acid phosphatase. This was highly specific for prostate cancer metastatic to bone, but lacked sensitivity in detecting less advanced disease and was normal in >20% patients with bone metastases. Prior to the PSA era, most men with newly-diagnosed prostate cancer had advanced incurable disease. PSA has revolutionized the diagnosis and management of prostate cancer, although it's use in screening and early detection remain controversial. The predictive values of PSA and digital rectal examination (DRE) for diagnosing prostate cancer in biopsies are shown in Table 7.10. A sophisticated PC predictor, which also considers family history, race and previous negative biopsy, is available online at: http://www.compass.fhcrc.org/edrnnci/bin/calculator/main.asp?t=prostate &sub=disclaimer&v=prostate&m=&x=Prostate%20Cancer

In addition to its use as a serum marker for the diagnosis of prostate cancer, PSA elevations may help in staging, counselling, and monitoring prostate cancer patients. Here are some examples:

- PSA generally increases with advancing stage and tumour volume, although a small proportion of poorly-differentiated tumours fail to express PSA
- PSA is used, along with clinical (DRE) T stage and Gleason score to predict pathological tumour staging and outcome after radical treatments using statistically-derived nomograms and artificial neural networks
- >50% of patients have extra-prostatic disease if PSA >10ng/mL
- Less than 5% of patients have obturator lymph node metastases and only 1% have bone metastases shown by isotope scintigraphy if PSA <20 ng/mL
- 66% of patients have lymphatic involvement and 90% have seminal vesicle involvement if PSA >50 ng/mL
- PSA should be undetectable (<0.1 ng/mL in many laboratories) following radical prostatectomy for gland-confined disease
- PSA rise after radical prostatectomy precedes the development of metastatic disease by a mean time of 8 years
- PSA falls to within the normal range in 80% of patients with metastatic disease within 4 months of starting androgen ablation therapy; the PSA rises in a mean time of 18 months after starting hormone therapy, signalling progressing disease.

Table 7.10 The predictive value of PSA and DRE for biopsy diagnosis of prostate cancer

PSA (ng/mL)	0.1–1.0	1.1–2.5	2.6–4.0	4–10	>10
DRE normal	1%	5%	15%	25%	>50%
DRE abnormal	5%	15%	30%	45%	>75%

PSA is prostate-specific, but sadly not prostate cancer-specific. Other causes of elevated serum PSA are shown in Table 7.11, the most common of which is benign prostatic hyperplasia.

Table 7.11 Conditions excluding prostate cancer which cause elevated PSA

Cause of elevated PSA	Minor elevation <1.0 ng/mL	Intermediate elevation 1.0–20 ng/mL	Major elevation 20–100 ng/mL
Benign hyperplasia	√	√	
Urinary tract infection		√	√
Acute prostatitis		√	√
Chronic prostatitis	√	√	
Retention/ catheterization		√	
Biopsy, TURP		√	√
Ejaculation, DRE	√		

In the presence of infection or instrumentation, PSA should be requested at least 28 days after the event, to avoid a false-positive result, which may cause unnecessary anxiety. Ideally, PSA should not be requested within 2 days of ejaculation or DRE, but in practice it makes negligible difference to the result.

PSA derivatives and kinetics: free-to-total, density, velocity, and doubling time

Measurement of the *free-to-total PSA ratio* increases the specificity of total PSA because the ratio is lower in men with prostate cancer (PC) than in men with benign hyperplasia. This may be helpful in deciding whether to re-biopsy a patient with previous benign biopsies. While overall a man with a normal DRE and a PSA of 4–10 ng/mL has a 25% risk of prostate cancer (see Table 7.9), this risk rises to 60% if the F:T ratio is 10% and falls to 10% if his ratio is >25%. The F:T ratio may also be useful in the total PSA range 2.5–4 ng/mL. Chronic prostatitis may also cause a reduced F:T ratio. An important limitation of this investigation is the instability of free PSA. The serum must be assayed within 3 h or frozen at −20°C, otherwise the free component reduces and a low ratio will be reported. Assays measuring the more stable complex PSA concentration are developed but their place in clinical practice has not been defined.

Consideration may be given to the prostate volume, since large benign prostates are the most common cause of mildly elevated PSA. Serum PSA/prostate volume = *PSA-density*. Various cut-off densities have been proposed to raise the specificity of total PSA in the prediction of PC diagnosis by biopsy, for example >0.15. If the diagnosis of PC is made, PSAD >0.19 predicts pT3 and high grade disease in 50% of cases.

Short-term variations in serum PSA occur, the cause of which may be technical or physiological. Over longer-term, the PSA tends to rise slowly (<0.3 ng/mL/year) due to BPH and faster due to prostate cancer. The rate of rise per year is the *PSA velocity*. A landmark study demonstrated a PSA velocity >0.75 ng/mL/year in PSA range 4–10 ng/mL, consistent over at least 18 months, is suggestive of the presence of PC. Only 5% of men without cancer exhibited such a velocity. A PSA velocity >20% per year should also prompt the recommendation of a biopsy, although a slower velocity does not exclude the presence of cancer. It has been shown that a PSA velocity of >2 ng/mL/year in the year prior to radical curative treatment of PC is associated with a poorer cancer outcome.

PSA doubling time (PSADT) is the time it takes for the PSA to double. It is calculated with the formula: PSADT = log2 × dT/(logB − logA)—A & B are the initial (A) and final (B) PSA measurements, and dT is the time difference between the calendar dates of the two PSA measurements. PSADT may be the best indicator of the likely presence of PC or the rate of disease progression. Several serial measurements reduce confounding physiological variability. Not always easy to calculate, PSADT can be obtained online at www.pcngcincinnati.org/psa/index.htm. PSADT is increasingly being used to drive clinical management. Examples include: <5 years should raise suspicion of the presence of prostate cancer; <3 years should drive recommendation to treat a patient on active surveillance; 12 ± 6 months should drive recommendation of salvage local treatment; <6 months should drive recommendation of hormone therapy following radical treatment.

Counselling before PSA testing

Counselling is mandatory before offering a PSA and DRE to asymptomatic men, particularly to highlight the potential disadvantages of having an abnormal result. These must be weighed up against the potential benefit of having clinically-significant prostate cancer (PC) diagnosed at an earlier stage than it would have been without these evaluations. There is currently no clear evidence of benefit by screening for PC (📖 see p. 295). This forms the basis of the UK Department of Health NHS PC Risk Management Programme (2002), whereby only men requesting the investigations and who have been appropriately counselled should be tested. Such counselling is less fundamental when investigating a symptomatic patient, because a diagnosis of prostate cancer could alter his clinical management. However, all patients should be informed when PSA testing is being recommended.

The following points should be used in counselling *asymptomatic* men:
- Cancer will be identified in <5% men screened
- Sensitivity is 80%: a false negative result is possible
- Specificity is 40–50%: a false positive result is possible
- Prostatic biopsy is uncomfortable and carries a 1% risk of sepsis or significant bleeding
- Repeat biopsy may be recommended (previous PIN, ASAP or rising PSA)
- Treatment may not be necessary
- Treatment may not be curative
- Treatment-related morbidity could lead to a diminished quality of life.

Prostate cancer: other diagnostic markers

Given the limitations of PSA discussed on p. 297, there is considerable ongoing effort to identify better diagnostic markers in both serum and first-voided urine following a DRE. These are mostly the RNA or protein products of genes commonly over-expressed in prostate cancer tissue.

The most promising of these, already commercially available, is the **Prostate Cancer Antigen 3 (PCA3)** assay. This gene is over-expressed in 95% of PCs, though its function is unclear. RNA transcripts are amplified and detected from urine sediment. Specificity for PC diagnosis is improved compared with serum PSA alone, although sensitivity of 60% (i.e. 40% false negative results) remains an issue when advising patients whether or not to undergo prostate biopsies. In future, sensitivity could be improved by combining detection of PCA3 with other urinary markers, for example the TMPRSS2-ERG fusion transcript (🕮 see p. 282).

- **Osteoprotegerin** (OPG) is an osteoclastogenesis regulator, over-expressed in prostate cancer bone metastases and serum compared with primary cancer cells (sensitivity 88%; specificity 93%). OPG is currently under evaluation as a serum marker for bone metastasis
- **Telomerase** stops natural telomere shortening and is produced by immortal cells. Increased expression is observed in 90% prostate cancers and PIN, and is detectable in prostatic fluid and biopsies
- **Bone morphogenetic proteins** are involved in new bone formation and organ development. BMP-6 mRNA over-expression is observed in 95% of metastatic PCs, yet only in 25% localized PC and 29% non-prostate cancers. An assay is not yet developed for testing on body fluids
- **A-methylacyl-CoA racemase** (AMACR) immunohistochemical over-expression is 97% sensitive and 100% specific for PC diagnosis in needle biopsies. It is used routinely by histopathologists. Efforts are ongoing to develop AMACR assay for testing on body fluids
- Promotor hypermethylation of reducing enzyme **glutathione-S-transferase P1** (GSTP1) is the commonest epigenetic abnormality in prostate cancer, inactivating its transcription in 90% PCs and 70% of PIN lesions. Methylated GSTP1 DNA is detectable in both urine and serum
- **Human Kallikrein 2** (hK2) is a member of same protease family as PSA (which is also known as hK3), bearing 78% sequence homology. hK2 is expressed almost exclusively by prostatic epithelium, in lesser quantity than PSA. It is relatively over-expressed in PIN and higher Gleason score cancers. The ratio of hK2:PSA mRNA in urinary sediments may help to distinguish aggressive or advanced cancers.

Prostate cancer: transrectal ultrasonography and biopsies

The most common diagnostic modality for prostate cancer is transrectal ultrasonography (TRUS) with guided biopsies (Fig. 7.7). TRUS provides imaging of the prostate and seminal vesicles using a 7.5 MHz biplane rectal probe measuring approximately 1.5 cm in diameter. Most patients find the procedure uncomfortable, some painful. It takes about five minutes and is undertaken on an outpatient basis with some form of anaesthetic. Ultrasound-guided peri-prostatic injection of local anaesthetic is the gold standard; peri-anal GTN paste or inhalation of nitrous oxide/air (Entonox) are alternatives. A DRE precedes insertion of the probe. If biopsies are planned, an antiseptic rectal wall cleansing is also undertaken using, for example, aqueous iodine on a sponge-stick. Broad-spectrum antimicrobials are given before and after the procedure, typically for 48 h although this is not standardized.

Transrectal ultrasonography can image the outline of the prostate, cysts, abscesses, and calcifications within the prostate. Hypo- and hyper-echoic lesions in the peripheral zone may be due to prostate cancer or inflammatory conditions, although most prostate cancers are iso-echoic and are not 'seen'.

Indications for transrectal ultrasonography alone

- Estimation of prostate volume [mL] = anteroposterior distance (cm) × width (cm) × sagittal length (cm) × 0.52
- Male infertility with azospermia, to look for seminal vesicle and ejaculatory duct obstruction due to calculus or Müllerian cyst
- Suspected prostatic abscess (can be drained by needle aspiration)
- Investigation of chronic pelvic pain, looking for prostatic cyst or calculi.

Indications for transrectal ultrasonography with biopsies

The 2008 UK NICE guidelines stress the importance of discussing the risks and benefits of biopsy, individual risk factors, the use of nomograms to predict results (see p. 307) and allowing time for decision-making before proceeding.

- An abnormal DRE and/or an elevated PSA (exceptions include very elderly men with massively elevated PSA and abnormal DRE, or those in whom a TURP is indicated for BOO with severe LUTS/retention where histology will be obtained)
- Previous biopsies showing isolated PIN or ASAP
- Previous biopsies normal, but PSA rising or DRE abnormal
- To confirm viable prostate cancer following a treatment if salvage treatment is being considered.

Biopsy protocol

Systematic 18 g trucut needle biopsies are taken, including any palpable or sonographic target lesion. The traditional sextant protocol (a parasagittal base, mid-gland, and apex from each side) has been superseded by 8, 10, or 12 biopsies, adding samples from the far lateral peripheral zones (Fig. 7.8). Studies have demonstrated these extra biopsies detect up to 15% more cancers. Relating the number of biopsies to the prostatic volume seems logical; attempts have been made to optimize this concept, for example, the Vienna nomogram (Table 7.12).[1]

Table 7.12 The Vienna Nomogram: optimal number of cores on TRUS-guided prostate biopsy

Prostate volume on TRUS, mL	Patient age (years)			
	<50	50–60	60–70	>70
20–29	8	8	8	6
30–39	12	10	8	6
40–49	14	12	10	8
50–59	16	14	12	10
60–69	–	16	14	12
≥70	–	18	16	14

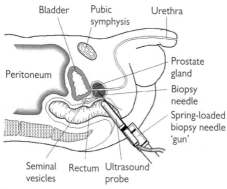

Fig. 7.7 Transrectal ultrasound scanning (TRUS). An ultrasound probe is inserted into the rectum to guide the biopsy needle into the correct position so that several core biopsies can be taken from different areas of the prostate.

---

1 Remzi M, et al. (2005) The Vienna nomogram: validation of a novel biopsy strategy defining the optimal number of cores based on patient age and total prostate volume. J Urol **174**:1256–60

Additional biopsies of each transition zone may be taken if a transition zone cancer is suspected, or if a patient is undergoing repeat biopsies due to a rising PSA. If repeated biopsies fail to diagnose cancer in the setting of a persistently rising PSA, *'saturation' needle biopsies* (between 20 and 30) may be taken transrectally or transperineally using a template device under general anaesthesia. Alternatively, some advocate resorting to *transurethral resection biopsies*, especially if the patient has a degree of bladder outflow obstruction.

Seminal vesicles biopsies occasionally add staging information if they are abnormal on DRE, TRUS, or MRI.

Complications of prostatic biopsy

- Occasional vaso-vagal 'fainting' immediately after the procedure
- 0.5% risk of septicaemia, which may be life-threatening
- 0.5% risk of significant rectal bleeding; this may require pressure by DRE using a swab soaked in vasoconstricting 1:10,000 adrenaline
- 0.5% risk of clot urinary retention
- Likely mild haemospermia or haematuria, for up to 3 weeks.

Note: it is not safe to biopsy a warfarinized patient; biopsying patients on low-dose aspirin remains controversial, but is not at present considered unsafe. Other anti-platelet drugs (e.g. clopidogrel) are usually stopped for 10 days prior.

It is important, too, that the patient understands that negative biopsies do not exclude the possibility of prostate cancer, and that a positive result will not necessarily result in the recommendation of immediate treatment.

Prostate cancer may also be diagnosed by TURP histology or clinically (without histology) in certain circumstances. For example, it could be viewed as unnecessarily invasive to biopsy a frail elderly patient with a craggy hard prostate and a PSA of >100 ng/mL prior to commencing palliative hormone therapy.

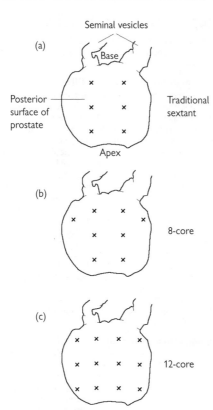

Fig. 7.8 Biopsy protocols.

Pathology: suspicious lesions

Two histological lesions are currently regarded as either pre- or peri-malignant. They are prostatic intraepithelial neoplasia and atypical small acinar proliferation.

Prostatic intraepithelial neoplasia (PIN)

PIN consists of architecturally benign prostatic acini and ducts lined by cytologically atypical cells. The basal cell layer is present, although the basement membrane may be fragmented (diagram). PIN was formerly known as ductal dysplasia or reported by pathologists as 'suspicious for cancer'. PIN was classified into low-grade (mild) and high-grade (moderate to severe) forms, based on the presence of prominent nucleoli. Subsequently pathologists have agreed to report only high-grade PIN, since low-grade PIN reporting is very subjective and has no prognostic value. On the other hand, high-grade PIN is believed to be a precursor for intermediate or high-grade prostate cancer. PIN is reported in 5–10% of prostate needle biopsies. It does not appear to affect the serum PSA value. The site of the PIN is not indicative of the site of subsequently diagnosed cancer, nor is PIN always present in a prostate containing cancer. When found in sextant prostate biopsies carries a 30–40% prediction of prostate cancer at subsequent biopsy. However, with the widespread use of more extensive biopsy protocols, the significance of isolated PIN has become less clear, with some studies reporting a positive re-biopsy rate that is equal or lower to the first-time cancer detection risk.

It is usual practice to recommended repeat systematic biopsies if PIN is reported in needle biopsy or TURP, though some authorities are favouring further PSA surveillance.

Atypical small acinar proliferation (ASAP)

This histopathological lesion reported by pathologists on needle biopsies as 'suspicious for cancer' must be taken seriously. The focus containing small acini is typically small, averaging 0.4 mm diameter. Acini are lined with cytologically abnormal epithelial cells and may exhibit atrophic features. The columnar cells have prominent nuclei containing nucleoli, while the basal layer is focally absent, according to high molecular weight cytokeratin immunostaining. PIN may be present in the same sample. Studies have shown ASAP in needle biopsies predict cancer at subsequent biopsy in over 40% of cases.

Currently it is recommended that immediate repeat systematic biopsies should be performed if isolated ASAP is reported on needle biopsy or TURP.

Prostate cancer: general considerations before treatment (modified from the 2008 UK NICE Guidance)

Once a diagnosis of prostate cancer has been made, it is essential to discuss the implications and management options with the patient, and any relative or friend he wishes to involve.

Treatment may or may not be appropriate; it may be given with curative or palliative intent.

If treatment is not recommended, explain the advantage and disadvantages to help the patient understand why he is not being treated.

Before starting treatment, inform the patient that it *may* result in:

• Altered physical appearance
• Altered sexual experience
• Loss of sexual function, ejaculation, and fertility
• Changes in urinary or bowel function
• Other common side-effects or complications.
  Offer the patient:
• Support in decision-making, access to written material and specialist nurse services
• Ongoing access to erectile dysfunction services if necessary
• Ongoing access to specialist psychosexual services if necessary
• A urological assessment is lower urinary tract symptoms are present
• Sperm storage (if appropriate).

Assess the risk category[1] applicable to men with clinically-localized prostate cancer:

Risk	PSA (ng/mL)		Gleason score		Clinical stage by DRE
Low	<10	and	≤ 6	and	T1–T2a
Intermediate	10–20	or	7	or	T2b–T2c
High	>20	or	8–10	or	T3–4

Low-risk is defined as <25% chance of relapse following radical treatment.

Intermediate-risk is defined as 25–50% chance of relapse after radial treatment.

High-risk is defined as >50% chance of relapse after radical treatment.

---

1 D'Amico AV *et al.* (1998). Biochemical outcome after radical prostatectomy, external beam radiotherapy or interstitial radiation therapy for clinically localised prostate cancer. *JAMA* **280**: 969–74.

Management of localized prostate cancer: watchful waiting and active surveillance

It can be understood from incidence and mortality data that the statement 'more men die with prostate cancer (PC) than because of it' is correct. This is because most PCs are slow-growing and the majority of men diagnosed are >70 years, often with competing morbidities. This forms the basis for 'watchful waiting' (WW), by deferring hormone therapy until the development of metastatic disease for some men diagnosed with non-metastatic prostate cancer.

The risks of developing metastatic disease and of death due to prostate cancer after 10–15 years of WW can be considered using published data, according to biopsy grade. Table 7.13 summarizes the data. Fig. 7.9 shows survival and cumulative mortality from prostate cancer and other causes up to 20 years after diagnosis, stratified by age at diagnosis and Gleason score.[1]

Selection of patients for watchful waiting

Watchful waiting is the best option for patients with localized prostate cancer and:
- Gleason score 2–4 disease at any age
- Gleason score 5 and 6 disease in elderly or unfit men, with life expectancy considered to be <10 years, for whom radical curative treatment would not be contemplated
- Stage T1a disease with normal PSA (only 17% T1a patients will progress compared with 68% with T1b).

However, WW should be considered/discussed with all who have Gleason score <7, when small-volume disease is predicted by DRE and biopsies.

Watchful waiting protocols

Most men with localized prostate cancer on WW are seen every 6 months for clinical history, examination including a DRE and a serum PSA test (before or after DRE). If the disease progresses during follow-up, palliative treatment (for example, androgen ablation therapy) is recommended. The threshold for treatment was traditionally when symptoms and signs of advanced disease appeared, for example back pain and metastases on bone scan. However, the use of PSA kinetics (velocity, doubling time), the evidence of benefit with earlier use of hormone therapy and involvement of patient choice have driven earlier thresholds for treatment. Hence, an asymptomatic patient with a rising PSA may choose whether to treat his disease and accept the side-effects, or whether to maintain his current quality-of-life, while leaving the disease untreated.

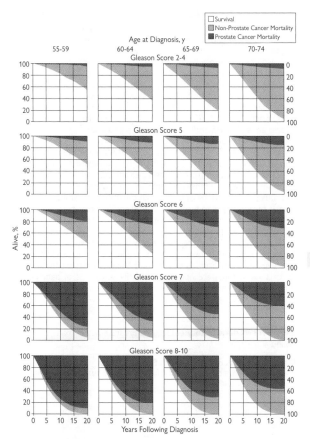

Fig. 7.9 The survival and cumlative mortality from prostate cancer (dark upper band) and other causes (light lower band) up to 20 years after diagnosis stratified by age at diagnosis and Gleason score. The percentage of men alive can be read from the left-hand scale; the percentage of men who have died can be read from the right-hand scale. Reproduced with permission from Albertsen PC, et al. (2005) p. 310.[1]

Active surveillance (AS)

With increasing numbers of low-risk cancers being diagnosed, there is concern that we are over-treating clinically-insignificant disease, leading to unnecessary loss of quality of life for patients and consumption of health-care resources. This may become even more important an issue with the possible introduction of population-based screening. AS has a different goal from WW, which is to identify and treat with curative intent localized cancers that are demonstrably progressing, whilst avoiding over-treatment for the majority.

A Canadian study of 299 men with low-risk PC has reported 65% of patients are still on AS after mean follow-up of 8 years.[2] Other studies are ongoing in the UK and Europe.

The 2008 UK NICE Guidelines recommend AS as the 'preferred' option for men with low-risk (stage T1c–T2a and Gleason score ≤6, and PSA <10 ng/mL) disease who might be considered for curative treatment. These men undergo more intensive evaluations than WW: PSA testing every 3 months (for velocity or doubling time calculation), DRE 6-monthly and 2-yearly repeat biopsy to assess for upgrading. PSA velocity >1 ng/mL/year and doubling times <3 years are currently considered evidence of progression, which prompt the recommendation of curative treatment.

The risk with AS is that the disease may progress beyond the possibility of cure. An initial PSA density <0.15 may predict PSA progression and need for active treatment. Randomized trials of AS versus immediate treatment (RP or radiotherapy) are needed to identify subgroups of patients who could most benefit from AS or immediate treatment, and to rigorously compare the cost benefits of each.

Table 7.13 Natural history of localized prostate cancer managed with no initial treatment

Biopsy grade	% Risk of metastasis (10 years)	% Risk of prostate cancer death (15 years)	Estimated lost years of life
2–4	19	4–7	<1 year
5	42	6–11	4
6	42	18–30	4
7	42	42–70	5
8–10	74	56–87	6–8

1 Albertsen PC *et al.* (2005) 20 year outcomes following conservative management of clinically localized prostate cancer *JAMA* **293**:2095–101.

2 Klotz L. (2006) *Urol Oncol Semin Orig Invest* **24**:46–50.

Management of localized prostate cancer: radical prostatectomy

Radical (total) prostatectomy (RP) is excision of the entire prostate including the prostatic urethra, with the seminal vesicles. First described by Young in 1905, anatomical studies and modifications in the 1980s lead by Patrick Walsh gained it's acceptance as the gold standard curative treatment for localized PC. Following excision of the prostate, reconstruction of the bladder neck and vesico-urethral anastomosis completes the procedure.

RP may be performed by open retropubic, open perineal, manual or robot-assisted laparoscopic approaches. The perineal approach does not allow a simultaneous pelvic lymph node dissection.

RP is indicated for the treatment (with curative intent) of fit men with localized prostate cancer whose life expectancy exceeds 10 years. Patients with Gleason score 2–4 disease appear to do as well in the long-term with surveillance as with treatment. The 2008 UK NICE Guidelines recommend RP for high-risk disease (PSA ≥20 or Gleason score ≥8 or cT3) only if there is a 'realistic prospect of long-term disease control', and for low-risk disease (PSA <10 and Gleason score ≤6 and cT1–2) is active surveillance is offered and declined. The surgeon should take part in multidisciplinary team discussion of each case. The patient should consider all available treatment options and the complications of RP before proceeding.

Advantages of the open procedure include relatively low major complication rates, low cost, and short operating time.

Steps in open RP

- The patient is under anaesthetic, catheterized and positioned supine with the middle of the table 'broken' to open up the entry to the pelvis
- Through an 8 cm lower midline incision, staying extraperitoneal, the retropubic space is opened
- Obturator fossa lymphadenectomy is undertaken if the PSA >10 or the Gleason score is 7 or higher; extended lymphadenectomy may be carried out in high-risk patients; frozen-section histology is rarely requested
- Incisions in the endopelvic fascia on either side allow access to the prostatic apex and membranous urethra
- Division and haemostatic control of the dorsal vein complex passing under the pubic arch allows access to the membranous urethra, which is divided at the prostatic apex
- The prostate is mobilized retrogradely from apex to base, taking Denonvilliers fascia on its posterior surface
- If cavernous nerve-sparing is undertaken, the apical and posterior dissection is modified, as described below
- Denonvilliers fascia is incised at the prostatic base, allowing access to the vasa (divided) and seminal vesicles (excised)
- The bladder neck is divided, thereby freeing the prostate; the ureteric orifices are identified
- The bladder neck is reconstructed to the approximate diameter of the membranous urethra
- A sutured vesico-urethral anastomosis is stented by a 16Ch urethral catheter, typically for 10–14 days
- The wound is closed leaving a pelvic drain, typically for 24 h.

The 'interfascial' nerve-sparing modification aims to reduce the risk of postoperative erectile dysfunction, minimizing cavernosal nerve injury as they pass from the autonomic pelvic plexus on either side in the groove between prostate and rectum, during mobilization of the prostate. The outer layer of prostatic fascia is incised to allow these nerves to fall away from the prostatic fascia and capsule. This should not be attempted in the presence of palpable disease as it may compromise cancer control. Non nerve-sparing is therefore 'extrafascial' (Fig. 7.10). The tips of the seminal vesicles may also be spared in cases with low-risk of cancer involvement, potentially reducing bleeding and cavernosal nerve injury.

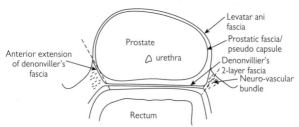

Fig. 7.10 Axial view of prostate fascial anatomy. The interfascial plane of dissection is shown on the left, while the extrafascial plane is shown on the right.

Laparoscopic radical prostatectomy (LRP) was pioneered in the late 1990s in a number of European centres. It is carried out transperitoneally or extraperitoneally, the latter having much in common with the open retropubic technique. Via five ports, with a 20–25° head-down tilt, extraperitoneal LRP is carried out in 12 steps shown below, with varying levels of difficulty (I–V).[1]

1. Trocar placement and dissection of the preperitoneal space: I
2. Pelvic lymphadenectomy: II
3. Incision of the endopelvic fascia and Dissection of the puboprostatic ligaments: I
4. Santorini plexus ligation: III
5. Anterior and lateral bladder neck dissection: II and dorsal bladder neck dissection: III
6. Dissection and division of vasa deferentia: III
7. Dissection of the seminal vesicles: III
8. Incision of the posterior Denonvillier's fascia- mobilization of the dorsal surface of the prostate from the rectum: III
9. Dissection of the prostatic pedicles: III
10. Nerve sparing procedure: V
11. Apical dissection, urethral division: IV
12. Urethrovesical anastomosis:
    • dorsal circumference (4, 5, 6, 7, 8 o'clock stitches): IV
    • 3 and 9 o'clock stitches: II
    • bladder neck closure, and 11 and 1 o'clock stitches: III.

The improved view has allowed a more precise 'intrafascial' nerve-sparing modification during mobilization of the gland, with dissection between the prostatic capsule and the inner layer of covering fascia (Fig. 7.10). In highly-experienced hands, laparoscopic RP operating times are comparable to those of open RP.

Robot-assisted LRP has gained popularity in the USA and a number of European centres. As with laparoscopic/endoscopic prostatectomy, it is minimally-invasive, with advantages of reduced bleeding, pain, and recovery time. Beyond this, the benefits remain uncertain in the absence of randomized trials. The training 'learning curve' is thought to be steeper than that of manual laparoscopy, because of the intuitive 'wristed' instrumentation of the *da Vinci*® surgical system. It is carried out using 6 ports, transperitoneally, starting at the bladder neck and working caudally. The surgeon sits at a remote consul, while the assistant stands with the robot 'cart' at the patient. The major disadvantage is cost, currently approximately £1M plus £100K annual maintenance. Medium and long-term oncological and functional outcomes are eagerly awaited, though the absence of these data are seemingly not slowing down the rapid ongoing proliferation of devices in the UK and Europe. Medium and long-term oncological and fuctional outcomes are eagerly awaited, though the absence of these data are seemingly not slowing down the rapid ongoing proliferation of devices in the UK and Europe.

1 Stolzenberg JU et al. (2005) Modular training per endoscopic extraperitoneal radical prostatectomy. *B J U Int* **96**:1022–7.

Postoperative routine course after RP

Day 1: mobilize, check FBC, C&E.

Day 2: free fluids and diet, drain removed, catheter care, encourage bowels.

Day 3: home.
Some surgeons discharge their patients on day 2, even if bowels have not moved.

Catheter time varies between 7 and 21 days; cystography is carried out if early removal (<7 days) is planned or if there has been a urine leak.

Complications of RP

General complications

Those of any major surgery (all rare, 1–2%): bleeding requiring re-operation and/or transfusion, infection, thromboembolism, and cardiac disturbance. These are minimized by attention to haemostasis, prophylactic antimicrobials, pneumatic calf compression, low-dose heparin postoperatively, and early mobilization. Chest infection may be prevented by physiotherapy and encouragement of deep breathing, especially in smokers. Postoperative death is estimated to occur 1 in 500 cases.

Specific complications: early

- Peroperative obturator nerve, ureteric or rectal injury (all rare <1%); these should be managed immediately if recognized: ureteric re-implantation; primary rectal closure with or without a loop colostomy
- Postoperative catheter displacement (rare); managed with careful replacement if within 48 h; if >48 h urethrography may reveal no anastomotic leak
- Postoperative urine or lymphatic leak (distinguished by dipstick glycosuria or creatinine concentration) through drains (occasional, 5%); managed by prolonged catheter and wound drainage; lymphatic leaks may require sclerotherapy with tetracycline.

Specific complications: late

- **Erectile dysfunction** (ED) affects 60–90% of patients; spontaneous erections can return up to 3 years post-operatively. Men >65 years or with pre-existing ED are more likely to suffer long-term. Nerve-sparing techniques improve outcomes. 40–70% respond to oral PDE5 inhibitors at 6 months, while others require intra-urethral or intracavernosal prostaglandin E1 treatments, a vacuum device or rarely a prosthesis
- **Incontinence (stress-type)** requiring >1 pad/day affects 5% of patients beyond 6 months; this is due to injury of the external urethral sphincter during division and haemostatic control of the dorsal vein complex. Predisposing factors include age >65 years and excessive bleeding. Pre-operative teaching of pelvic floor exercises helps to regain continence; peri-urethral bulking injections or implantation of an artificial urinary sphincter are occasionally necessary. Incontinence may also develop secondary to bladder neck stenosis or detrusor

instability; flow rates, post-void residual measurement, uro-dynamics, and cystoscopy may help
- **Bladder neck stenosis** affects 5% of patients. It typically presents 3–9 months postoperatively, patients complaining of poor flow and frequency/urgency of micturition. Predisposing factors include heavy bleeding, post-operative urinary leak and previous TURP. It is treated by endoscopic bladder neck incision and rarely becomes a recurrent problem.

In experienced hands, the complications of laparoscopic/endoscopic/ robot-assisted RP are comparable to those of open RP. On the learning curve, conversion to open RP and intraoperative major complications in 5–10% are cause for concern. Blood loss is significantly less, though transfusion rates are not. Earlier full recovery time (30 vs. 47 days) has been reported. ED is reduced to 49% at 48 months by the robot-assisted nerve-sparing technique.[1]

1 Menon M et al. (2007) Vattikuti Institute Prostatectomy: contemporary technique and analysis of results. *Eur Urol* **51**:648–58.

Prostate cancer: oncological outcomes of radical prostatectomy

While no randomized studies have compared RP outcomes with those of radiotherapy or brachytherapy, a randomized study comparing RP to WW has demonstrated, with a mean follow-up of just over 8 years, an overall and cancer-specific survival benefit, together 40 and 66% reductions in metastatic and local progression in favour of the RP group.[1] High-grade cancers were excluded from this trial, though non-randomized data suggest more patients with Gleason 7–10 localized disease survive 10 years following RP than with WW or radiotherapy.

Excellent long-term results are seen in well-selected patients following RP, particularly those with organ-confined disease and prior lower urinary tract symptoms due to bladder outflow obstruction. Serum PSA is measured a few days after RP, then 6-monthly; it should fall to <0.1 ng/mL. The 5-year outcomes of laparoscopic RP are similar to those of open RP. The 10-year PSA-progression rate following open RP, usually defined as a serum PSA > 0.2 ng/mL, is about 30%. Of these, 80% will fail within 3 years of RP. Without additional treatment, the time to development of clinical disease after PSA progression averages 8 years.[2] A 20-year clinical disease-free survival of 60% is reported.[3] Outcome correlates with: Gleason score; pre-operative PSA; pathological T stage and surgical margin status. Certain tissue markers, yet to be used routinely, may also predict PSA-progression, for example aberrant p53 expression in biopsy or RP specimen.[4]

Progression-free probabilities in four prognostic groups are shown in Table 7.14.[5] Probability of progression-free survival following radical prostatectomy can be predicted for individual patients using pre-operative or post-operative factors (PSA, stage, and Gleason score) using Kattan's nomograms (Fig. 7.11),[6,7] or estimated online, at: http://www.mskcc.org/mskcc/applications/nomograms/PostRadProstatectomy.aspx

Neo-adjuvant hormone therapy (hormone therapy given 3 months prior to RP) does not alter the PSA-progression rate, despite apparently reducing the incidence of positive surgical margins.

Management of biochemical relapse post-RP

The definition of rising PSA is controversial, though most agree >0.2 ng/mL.

DRE should be performed in case there is a nodule. Biopsy of the vesico-urethral anastomosis is not widely practised unless there is a palpable abnormality. Studies have shown that CT and bone scans are rarely helpful in searching for metastatic disease unless the PSA is >7 ng/mL.

Current management options include observation, pelvic radiotherapy or hormone therapy. A good response to pelvic radiotherapy is likely if:
- PSA rise is delayed > 1 year post-RP
- PSA doubling time > 10 months
- PSA is <1 ng/mL
- Low-grade and low-stage disease
- Radiation dose exceeds 64 Gy.

If the PSA never falls below 0.2, or it rises in the first year with a doubling time of less than 10 months, the response to pelvic radiotherapy is disappointing. It is likely in these circumstances that metastatic disease is present; hormone therapy is usually recommended: either non-steroidal anti-androgen monotherapy (for example bicalutamide 150 mg daily) or androgen deprivation. There are no comparative outcomes data in this clinical setting, so discussion focuses on the side-effects.

Table 7.14 Progression-free probabilities in four prognostic groups, by PSA and by margin status, following RP

Pathological stage	Progression-free 5 year (%)	Progression-free 10 year (%)
Gleason 2–6, T1–3, margin –ve	97	95
Gleason 2-6, T1–3, margin +ve OR Gleason 7, T1–3, margin –ve	86	72
Gleason 8–10, T1–2, margin +/–ve, OR Gleason 8–10, T3, Margin –ve OR Gleason 7–10, T3, margin +ve	62	41
Any LN +ve	37	13
PSA <4	91	
PSA 4–9.9	87	
PSA 10–19.9	70	
PSA 20–50	50	
Margin clear		81
Margin pos		36+

+Only 40–50% of patients with a positive surgical margin after RP develop a rising PSA.

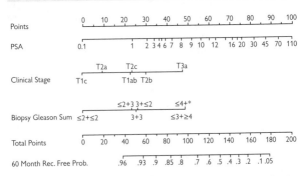

Instructions for Physician: Locate the patient's PSA on the PSA axis. Draw a line straight upwards to the Points axis to determine how many points towards recurrence the patient receives for his PSA. Rapeat this process for the Clinical Stage and Biopsy Gleason Sum axes, each time drawing straight upward to the Points axis. Sum the points achieved for each predictor and locate this sum on the Total Points axis. Draw a line straight down to find the patient's probability of remaining recurrence free for 60 months assuming he does not die of another cause first.

Note: This nomogram is not applicable to a man who is not otherwise a candidate for radical prostatctomy, You can use this only on a man who has already selected radical prostatectomy as treatment for his prostate cancer.

Instruction to Patient: "Mr. X, if we had 100 man exactly like you, we would expect between <predicated percentage from nomogram – 10%> and <predicated percentage + 10%> to remain free of their disease at 5 years following radical prostatectomy, and recurrence after 5 years is very rare."

© 1997 Michael W. Kattan and Peter T. Scardino
Scott Department of Urology

Fig. 7.11 A pre-operative nomogram per prostate cancer recurrence. Reproduced from Kattan.[6]

1   Bill-Axelson A et al. (2005) Radical prostatectomy versus watchful waiting in early prostate cancer. N Engl J Med **352**:1977–84.

2   Pound GR et al. (1999) Natural history of progression after PSA elevation following radical prostatectomy. J Am Med Ass **281**:1591–7.

3   Swanson GP et al. (2002) Long-term follow-up of radical rectropubic prostatectomy for prostate cancer. Eur Urol **42**:212–16.

4   Brewster S et al. (1999) Pre-operative p 53, bcl-2, CD44 and E-cad immunohistochemistry as predictors of biochemical recurrence after radical prostatectomy. J Urol **161**:1238–43.

5   Khan MA et al. (2003) Probability of biochemical recurrence by analysis of stage and margin status for localized prostate cancer. Urology **62**:866–71.

6   Kattan MW et al. (1998) A pre-operative nomogram for disease recurrence following radical prostatectomy. J Nat Cancer Institute **90**:766–71.

7   Kattan MW et al. (1999) Postoperative nomogram per disease recurrence after radical prostatectomy. J Clin Oncol **17**:1499–507.

Management of localized prostate cancer: radical external beam radiotherapy (EBRT)

Since the early 1980s advances in radiotherapy for localized prostate cancer have included the advent of linear accelerators, conformal, and intensity-modulated techniques to minimize toxicity to the rectum and bladder. EBRT is administered with curative intent to men with a life expectancy >5 years, accompanied by 24 months of neo-adjuvant/adjuvant androgen deprivation therapy in high-risk (Gleason ≥8) cases. A small, randomized study has demonstrated benefit in terms of progression and survival for patients treated with 6 months (2 months each of neo-adjuvant, concurrent and adjuvant) androgen ablation, in addition to radiotherapy, compared with radiotherapy alone.[1]

Indication: Clinically localized prostate cancer, Gleason score ≥6. Patients with Gleason score 2–5 disease appear to do as well with surveillance as with any other treatment at 15-year follow-up. The UK 2008 NICE Guidelines recommend low-risk cases (PSA <10 <u>and</u> Gleason score ≤6 <u>and</u> cT1–2) should first be offered active surveillance (controversial).

Contra-indications

- Severe lower urinary tract symptoms
- Inflammatory bowel disease
- Previous pelvic irradiation.

Protocol: the UK 2008 NICE Guidelines recommend conformal fractions (up to 2 Gy per treatment) amounting to a minimum dose of 74Gy.

Side-effects

- Transient moderate/severe filling-type LUTS (common, rarely permanent)
- Haematuria, contracted bladder 4–23%
- Moderate to severe gastro-intestinal symptoms, bloody diarrhoea, pain, rectal stenosis 3–32%
- Erectile dysfunction (ED) gradually develops in 30–50%
- The risk of a second solid pelvic malignancy is estimated to be 1 in 300, falling to 1 in 70 long-term survivors.

Outcomes of EBRT

Definitions of treatment failure: the 2005 Phoenix definition is the time at which the PSA rises by 2 ng/mL or more above the nadir. This has succeeded the complicated and flawed 1996 ASTRO (American Society of Therapeutic Radiation Oncologists) definition, which required 3 consecutive PSA increases above the nadir measured 4 months apart.

---

1 D'Amico AV *et al.* (2004) 6-month androgren supression plus radiation therapy vs. radiation therapy alone for patients with clinically-localised prostate cancer: a randomised controlled trial. *J Am Med Ass* **292**:821–7.

Pre-treatment prognostic factors: PSA, Gleason score, clinical stage, percentage of positive biopsies.

5-year biochemical disease-free (PSA failure-free) survival using 70 Gy is:
- 85% for **low-risk disease** (T1–2a and PSA <10 ng/mL and Gleason ≤6)
- 60% for **intermediate-risk disease** (T2b, or PSA 10–20, or Gleason 7)
- 40% for **high-risk disease** (T2c, or PSA >20 ng/mL, or Gleason 8–10).

Individual predictions of 5-year progression-free probability can be found online at: http://www.mskcc.org/mskcc/applications/nomograms/PreTreatment. aspx

Treatment of PSA relapse post-EBRT

Hormone therapy, either with anti-androgens or androgen deprivation, is currently the mainstay of treatment in this setting. However, local salvage treatments appear attractive, potentially offering another chance of cure if metastases cannot be demonstrated at repeat staging. Salvage radical prostatectomy is seldom undertaken because it is associated with highly morbidity and disappointing oncological outcomes. Other local salvage treatments include brachytherapy, cryotherapy and high-intensity focused ultrasound (HIFU) 📖 see p. 326). If salvage local treatment is under consideration, repeat prostatic biopsies should be taken to demonstrate viable tumour cells. This should be at least 18 months post-EBRT, because fatally-damaged cells may survive a few cell divisions.

Management of localized prostate cancer: brachytherapy (BT)

This is ultrasound-guided transperineal implantation of radioactive seeds, usually I125, into the prostate. It is currently popular, having failed in the 1970s, prior to transrectal ultrasonography. BT is minimally-invasive, requires general anaesthesia, and is completed in one or two stages. Either way, approximately 150 Gy is delivered, and this may be augmented by an EBRT boost. Another approach is to use Iridium192 wires, left for several hours *in situ* in a series of application, either before or after EBRT. The treatment is expensive due to the cost of the consumables.

Indications for BT: localized prostate cancer, cT1–2 and Gleason ≤7, and PSA < 20; life expectancy >5 years. The 2008 UK NICE Guidance suggests patients with low risk disease (PSA <10 *and* Gleason score ≤6 *and* cT1–2) should first be offered active surveillance and for those with intermediate risk disease, radical prostatectomy or conformal radiotherapy are preferred treatments.

Indications for BT with EBRT: T1–3, Gleason 7–8, PSA <20 prostate cancer.

Contraindications to BT: previous TURP (increases risk of incontinence); large volume prostate (>60 mL) causes difficulty with seed placement; moderate to severe lower urinary tract symptoms (risk of retention).

Complications
- Perineal haematoma (occasional)
- Lower urinary tract symptoms (common), due to prostatic oedema post-implant
- Urinary retention (5–20%)
- Incontinence (5%), particularly if TURP is required to treat urinary retention
- ED affects up to 50% of patients, gradual onset.

LH–RH analogues are often used to reduce prostatic volume prior to treatment.

Alpha-blockers are often used to treat LUTS and to improve the chance of successful trial without catheter in patients with urinary retention.

Outcomes of BT

PSA rises in the first 3 months post-implant, subsequently declines. As with EBRT, the ASTRO or Phoenix definitions (see p. 325) are used to define progression. Androgen-ablation is often used.

- 7-year biochemical progression-free survival (bPFS) for low-risk disease (cT1c-2a, Gleason <7, PSA <10 ng/mL) is 80–90%
- 7-year bPFS for moderate-risk disease (T2b, PSA 10–20 ng/mL, Gleason 7) is 70–80%
- 7-year bPFS for high-risk disease (T2c, PSA >20 ng/mL, Gleason >7) is 50–60%
- 10-year bPFS for low-risk disease is 60%.

Individual predictions of 5-year progression-free probability can be found online at: http://www.mskcc.org/mskcc/applications/nomograms/PreTreatment.aspx

Outcomes of BT plus EBRT (usually with androgen-ablation)

- 15-year bPFS for low-risk disease is 88%
- 15-year bPFS for moderate-risk disease is 80%
- 15-year bPFS for high-risk disease is 53%.

Comparisons of BT or BT plus EBRT with RP or EBRT alone

- There are no randomized studies
- In non-randomized comparisons, an age and tumour-matched radical prostatectomy series at 8 years yielded a progression-free survival of 98% (compared with 79% with BT)
- Outcome of BT appears inferior to EBRT and RP in men with PSA >10 and Gleason score 7–10.

Rising PSA post-BT

Salvage radical prostatetcomy, EBRT, cryotherapy, or HIFU are options if local recurrence is suspected; calculation of PSA doubling time, repeat biopsy and staging are necessary to select suitable cases. Whilst offering a further chance of cure, morbidity is higher with all, compared with their use in primary treatment (e.g. prostate-rectal fistula rates are 5% vs. 1% for primary cases). If metastatic disease is suspected or proven, further local treatment is unjustified.

Salvage brachytherapy following EBRT treatment failure is gaining popularity in some centres. Biochemical 5-year disease-free rates of 34–53% are reported, with moderate toxicity.

Management of localized and radio-recurrent prostate cancer: cryotherapy and high-intensity focused ultrasound

Minimally-invasive treatments for localized prostate cancer currently evolving are attractive to patients and their doctors. Proponents claim them to be alternatives to radical surgery or radiotherapy with shorter hospital stay, and less morbidity; also they are the only potentially curative options for 'salvage' treatment of organ-confined recurrent disease following radical radiotherapy.

Careful patient selection and training is important to achieve good results. No randomized outcomes data exist. The 2008 UK National Institute for Health and Clinical Excellence (NICE) guidance recommended that these technologies should be used only in the setting of a controlled clinical trial.

Whilst currently treating the entire prostate, these technologies may be suitable for **focal ablation** of tissue, such as strategy could reduce morbidity and cost, and is under investigation.

Cryotherapy

Transperineal ultrasound-guided placement of cryoprobes delivering Argon or liquid Nitrogen at temperature $-20°C$ to $-40°C$. When applied in two cycles of freeze-thaw, cellular necrosis occurs. The diameter of the ice-ball is monitored using ultrasound; precautions must be taken to protect the urethra, external sphincter and rectal wall, such as warming devices. An anaesthetic is required although this is a day-case procedure which can be repeated.

Results: PSA nadir is usually achieved within 3 months. 25–48% of men with localized disease achieve a PSA nadir of <0.1 ng/mL in 3 months, and 96% of men achieved PSA <0.2 ng/mL within 6 months. Positive biopsies are observed in 8–25% of patients after cryotherapy.

Complications: erectile dysfunction (40–80%); incontinence (4–27%); lower urinary tract symptoms due to urethral sloughing; pelvic pain; transient penile numbness; recto-urethral fistula (rare).

In the *salvage* setting, good short-term PSA responses are reported in 66% of men, at the expense of significant morbidity, including incontinence and urinary retention (70% each). In a contemporary UK series, 5-year freedom from PSA progression (ASTRO definition) was 73, 45, and 11% in low, medium and high risk patients respectively. Persistent incontinence developed in 13% of patients, while 1% developed recto-urethral fistula.

High-intensity focused ultrasound (HIFU)

HIFU allows the selective destruction of tissues at up to 4cm depth without damaging intervening structures, most importantly the rectal wall. Tissue is heated to the point of coagulative necrosis (over 85°C) by high-energy ultrasound transmitted to the prostate using a transrectal device. Numerous $6 \times 2 \times 2$ mm cigar-shaped lesions are produced, side by side to create a continuous volume in which the tissue is ablated. An anaesthetic is required although this is a day-case procedure, which can be repeated.

Results: from a large ($n = 463$) French series, PSA nadir is usually achieved within 4 months. 77% patients achieve PSA nadir 0.5 ng/mL or less. At 2-year median follow-up, 64% remained disease-free by the Phoenix definition.

Complications: erectile dysfunction (50%), urinary retention 8%, urethral stricture (10–25%), stress incontinence (2%), and recto-urethral fistula (1%).

Data for HIFU in the *salvage* setting are scarce. Good PSA responses are reported in 61% of men, with 38% remaining disease-free in a mixed group of patients. Morbidity is increased in the salvage treatment setting, recto-urethral fistula at 5%.

Another technology, ***photodynamic therapy***, is also under investigation.

Management of locally-advanced non-metastatic prostate cancer (T3–4 N0M0)

Radical prostatectomy is generally discouraged for men with cT3 disease in the UK. However, younger men with apparently non-metastatic mobile disease may benefit from surgery as part of a multi-modal treatment plan. Proponents accept that up to 80% will require additional treatment, but argue that 27% of cT3 cases are pathologically organ-confined. Cytoreductive surgery for true T3 disease could reduce morbidity from local progression and improve oncological outcome, while concurrent lymphadenectomy provides further staging information.

EBRT in combination with androgen deprivation therapy (ADT) has consistently demonstrated better outcomes compared with EBRT alone, which is associated with a 15–30% 10-year survival. In a European randomized study,[1] the ADT group received LH-RH analogues for 3 years starting at time of EBRT. The 5-year overall survival was 79% compared with 62% in the group treated with EBRT alone; the 5-year disease-free survival was 85% compared with 48%. There are potential advantages in starting ADT prior to EBRT, though the optimal timing and duration of therapy in this setting remains unclear. The 2008 UK NICE Guidance recommends neo-adjuvant and concurrent ADT for 3–6 months, increasing to a minimum of 2 years if the Gleason score ≥8.

Pelvic radiotherapy should be considered if risk of N+ disease >15%, according to the Roach formula: 2/3 PSA + (10 × [Gleason score − 6]).

Minimally-invasive treatments such as standard brachytherapy, HIFU and cryotherapy are not recommended outside clinical trials. High dose rate brachytherapy in combination with ADT is becoming popular, though long-term outcomes of trials are awaited.

Bisphosphonates are not currently recommended to prevent bone metastases.

Hormone therapy alone is an option for elderly patients or those unwilling to undergo EBRT. In this setting, a non-steroidal anti-androgen, such as bicalutamide 150mg daily, has equivalent efficacy to androgen deprivation by orchidectomy or LH-RH analogue, with potential advantages of reduced side-effects. However, counselling should include the point that hormone therapy is not a treatment offered with curative intent. A randomized trial of hormone therapy alone versus EBRT plus hormone therapy is in progress.

Watchful waiting is also an option for non-metastatic T3 disease in an elderly asymptomatic man, who may prefer to avoid side-effects of treatment.

Palliative treatment of locally-advanced disease

(□ See also p. 338) Palliative TURP, or medical therapy for LUTS, or urinary retention may be necessary. Incontinence can be a problem due to sphincter involvement, though bladder outflow obstruction and instability should be considered. A urinary convene sheath or catheter may be required. Patients may present in renal failure: percutaneous nephrostomy or ureteric stenting are occasionally necessary for bypassing ureteric obstruction. ADT in this setting may relieve this tumour compression of the distal ureters. Very rarely, a colostomy is necessary to bypass a rectal stenosis. Palliative EBRT may be useful for treatment of persistent prostatic haematuria or perineal pain.

1 Bolla M, et al. (2002) Long-term results with immediate androgen suppression and external irradiation in patients with locally-advanced prostate cancer (an EORTC study): phase III randomised trial. Lancet **360**: 103–108.

Management of advanced prostate cancer: hormone therapy I

Metastatic disease is the cause of nearly all prostate cancer-related death. Currently incurable, the 5-year survival is 25%. 10% survive <6 months, while <10% survive >10 years. The gold standard treatment is hormone therapy, with cytotoxic chemotherapy for progression and novel treatments (such as growth factor inhibitors, angiogenesis inhibitors, immunotherapy and gene therapy) in development. The concept of hormone therapy was realized in 1941 when Huggins and Hodges reported favourable symptomatic and biochemical (acid and alkaline phosphatase) responses in prostate cancer patients when castrated or given oestrogens.

Hormone dependence of prostate cancer

All prostate epithelial cells, with the exception of rare undifferentiated stem cells, are dependent on androgens and fail to grow or undergo programmed cell death (apoptosis) in their absence. Similarly, most previously untreated prostate cancer cells are dependent on androgens. In men, 95% of circulating androgen, mainly testosterone, is produced by the testicular Leydig cells under the influence of luteinizing hormone (LH). The anterior pituitary synthesizes LH, stimulated by hypothalamic LH-releasing hormone (LH–RH). The remaining 5% of circulating androgen is synthesized by the adrenal cortex from cholesterol, under the influence of pituitary ACTH. Testosterone is metabolized to the more potent dihydrotestosterone (DHT), by 5-α reductase (5AR) enzymes types 1 and 2. DHT binds cytoplasmic androgen receptor, which translocates to nucleus, there activating transcription of androgen-responsive genes, which drive the cell cycle or inhibit apoptosis.

Androgen deprivation results in a reduction in PSA and clinical improvement in >70% of patients. However, most patients with metastatic disease will still die within 5 years due to the emergence of **androgen-independent growth**. This may be due to selection of androgen-independent cell clones. The mean time to disease progression after androgen deprivation is 14 months in men with metastatic disease.

Prognostic factors

Predictors of poor hormone therapy response include:
• 5 metastatic lesions at presentation
• Elevated alkaline phosphatase at presentation
• Anaemia at presentation
• Poor performance status (level of activity) at presentation
• Low serum testosterone at presentation
• Failure of bone pain to improve within 3 months of treatment
• Failure of PSA to normalize (to <4 ng/mL) within 6 months of treatment (conversely a PSA nadir [= lowest value] of <0.1 ng/mL predicts a long-term response).

Management of advanced prostate cancer: hormone therapy II

Methods of androgen deprivation (androgen ablation) therapy (ADT)

- **Surgical castration:** bilateral orchidectomy
- **Medical castration:** luteinizing hormone-releasing hormone (LH–RH) agonists, oestrogens
- **Anti-androgen monotherapy (steroidal or non-steroidal):** androgen receptor blockade at target cell
- **Maximal androgen blockade (MAB):** medical or surgical castration plus anti-androgen
- **5-alpha reductase inhibition (5ARI)** with finasteride or dutasteride.

Both forms of castration have equivalent efficacy, so patients can be given the choice. Oestrogens are no longer used first-line, due to the significant cardiovascular morbidity observed when they were the only alternative to orchidectomy. MAB has a theoretical advantage over castration in blocking the effects of the adrenal androgens; significant clinical advantages (>5% improved 5-year survival) have not been demonstrated by trial meta-analyses. 5ARIs are not licensed for the treatment of prostate cancer, but may have a role in its prevention.

Bilateral orchidectomy

A simple procedure, usually carried out under general anaesthesia. Through a midline scrotal incision, both testes may be accessed. The tunica albuginea of each testis is incised and the soft tissue content is removed, after which the capsule is closed. The epidiymes and testicular appendages are preserved. Postoperative complications include scrotal haematoma or infection (both rare). Serum testosterone falls within 8 h to <0.2 nmol/L.

LH–RH analogues

LH–RH analogue were developed in the 1980s, giving patients an alternative to bilateral orchidectomy, with which they are considered clinically equivalent. They are given by subcutaneous or intramuscular injection, as monthly or 3-monthly depots. A 6-monthly formulation is expected. Examples include Goserelin, Triptorelin, and Leuprorelin acetates.

If the anterior pituitary is overwhelmed with an analogue of LH–RH, it switches off LH synthesis, although serum testosterone rises in the first 14 days due to a surge of LH. This can result in 'tumour flare', manifest in 20% patients by increased symptoms, including catastrophic spinal cord compression. To prevent this, cover with anti-androgens is recommended for a week before and two weeks after the first dose of LH-RH agonist. There is awareness that on occasions the serum testosterone level may not be suppressed at castrate by all LH–RH agonists.

An *LH-RH antagonist* is in development, which rapidly reduce serum testosterone, abolishing the issue of tumour flare.

Side-effects of bilateral orchidectomy and LH-RH agonists

- Loss of sexual interest and ED
- Hot flushes and sweats can be frequent and troublesome during work or social activity
- Weight gain
- Lethargy, fatigue
- Gynaecomastia
- Anaemia
- Cognitive changes, depression and memory loss
- Osteoporosis and pathological fracture (particularly of the hip) secondary to osteoporosis may occur in patients on long-term (>5 years) treatment. A single yearly dose of the bisphosphonate zoledronic acid appears to maintain bone mineral density, though the clinical advantage this may confer remains uncertain.

Anti-androgens

These are administered as tablets. Examples include bicalutamide (monotherapy dose is 150 mg daily or 50 mg daily for MAB in combination with LH-RH analogues or orchidectomy), flutamide and cyproterone acetate (CPA). The first two raise the serum testosterone slightly, so sexual interest and performance should be maintained although many such patients have pre-existing ED due to the advancing age and disease. Bone demineralization, lethargy, and cognitive changes are not seen with anti-androgens.

Anti-androgen monotherapy with bicalutamide 150 mg daily is less effective than ADT in treating metastatic disease, but equivalent for non-metastatic locally-advanced disease. Side-effects include frequent gynaecomastia, breast tenderness and occasional liver dysfunction. There are favourable reports of reduction or prevention of breast toxicity using tamoxifen 20 mg twice weekly. Flutamide at 250 mg tds also causes frequent GI upset.

At its full dose of 100 mg tds CPA is rarely used as monotherapy because it is less effective than ADT; it may cause reversible dyspnoea. At 50 mg bd, CPA may be helpful for prevention of castration-induced hot flushes.

Management of advanced prostate cancer: hormone therapy III

Monitoring treatment during ADT

Typically, patients will have baseline PSA, full blood count, renal, and liver function tests, a renal ultrasound and a bone scan. The PSA is repeated after 3 and 6 months, and 6-monthly thereafter until it rises. Liver function is checked 3-monthly if anti-androgen monotherapy is used. Physical examination, including DRE and serum renal function is checked on disease progression; imaging if clinically indicated.

While PSA is very useful as a marker for response and progression, 10% of patients show clinical progression without PSA rise. This may occur in anaplastic tumours that fail to express PSA.

Advice on exercise, diet, and treatment of erectile dysfunction is often sought by patients during treatment.

Immediate versus delayed hormone therapy

Traditionally hormone therapy was reserved for patients with symptomatic metastatic disease. Arguments against immediate use of hormone therapy focused on its side-effects and cost.

However, studies of patients with locally-advanced and metastatic disease have demonstrated slower disease progression and reduced morbidity when treated with androgen deprivation early (i.e. before the onset of symptoms). Improved survival has also been reported, in patients without bone metastases but including node-positive disease, when treated immediately. Subgroups of patients <70 years old, those with PSA doubling times <12 months and patients with baseline PSA >50 ng/mL appear to benefit most.

Trials have also demonstrated slower disease progression in patients given bicalutamide 150 mg daily (compared with placebo) for 2 years after treatment of high-risk locally-advanced prostate cancer with RP or RT. This benefit is not seen in patients managed by watchful waiting. The survival advantage for high-risk patients undergoing EBRT combined with ADT provides further evidence of benefit of immediate hormone therapy.

Intermittent hormone therapy

The potential advantages of stopping hormone therapy when the disease has remitted (PSA <4 ng/mL) then re-starting it when the PSA has risen again (to perhaps 10 or 20 ng/mL) are the reduced side-effects, thus improved quality of life during the off-treatment periods, and cost. These have been demonstrated in phase II trials. Of several ongoing phase III studies comparing long-term outcomes of intermittent versus continuous ADT or MAB, only one has so far reported equivalent survival at 5 years in men with locally-advanced or metastatic disease. None of the LH-RH agonists or anti-androgens are currently licensed for intermittent therapy, though it is already an option for patients who are intolerant of side-effects.

Management of advanced prostate cancer: androgen-independent (AI) and hormone-refractory (HR) disease

Second-line hormone therapy

When consecutive PSA rises from its nadir are observed or (uncommonly) if symptomatic progression occurs despite a favourable biochemical response to first-line hormone therapy, the disease has entered its AI phase. This may be due to proliferation of androgen-independent clones, androgen-receptor amplification, aberrant stimulation of androgen-dependent transcription pathways or a block to apoptosis induced by androgen withdrawal.

In these circumstances, especially with a rapid (<12 months) PSA doubling time, *second-line hormone therapy* is indicated. Most patients receiving anti-androgen monotherapy respond after switching to androgen ablation (orchidectomy or LH-RH analogue). If there is relapse during androgen ablation, 25% respond by adding an anti-androgen, for example, bicalutamide 50 mg daily, to establish maximal androgen blockade (MAB). If MAB was used from initiation of hormone therapy, withdrawal of the anti-androgen paradoxically elicits a favourable response in 25% of patients.

A further rise in PSA may require *third-line hormonal therapy*, such as the addition of oestrogens or corticosteroids. For example, diethylstilboestrol 1 mg daily with 75 mg aspirin for thromboembolic prophylaxis elicits a response in up to 60% of these patients. The mean duration of response is 4 months.

The prognostic factors for survival with AI disease are identical to the factors predicting response to hormone therapy (🕮 see p. 330), plus time from initiation of hormone therapy to initiation of chemotherapy and visceral metastasis status.

When the disease no longer responds to any hormonal therapy, including castrate serum testosterone, it has become HR. The mean survival at this point ranges from 9 months in the presence of extensive metastatic disease, to 27 months in asymptomatic patients without demonstrable metastases.

Cytotoxic chemotherapy

Systemic chemotherapy is offered to appropriate patients with HR metastatic disease, by the medical oncologist. Men with low-volume disease who have failed radical local treatment and hormone therapy are also candidates for chemotherapy. Frail and infirm patients with renal impairment or haematological abnormalities are unsuitable. Correction of renal and bone marrow dysfunction is necessary prior to treatment.

Symptom palliation

This is discussed in further detail on p. 338. Symptom improvements are reported with cytotoxic chemotherapy. In a randomized trial of mitoxantrone plus prednisolone versus prednisolone alone, 29% in the combination group experienced a reduction in pain and analgesic use compared with 12% in the prednisolone alone group. PSA response did not predict palliative response. In another study, docetaxel plus prednisolone produced a pain reduction in 35% compared with 22% of patients given mitoxantrone and prednisolone, resulting in improved quality of life scores.

Cancer control

Most single-agent cytotoxic chemotherapy trials define response as >50% decrease in PSA. Responses are reported in 20–40% of patients with haematological toxicity (especially neutropenia) for most agents. Better responses (up to 75%) reported with newer combination regimens (for example, estramustine phosphate plus docetaxel), but with greater toxicity. The median survival following chemotherapy ranges from 24 to 44 weeks. Results of two randomized studies comparing docetaxel with mitoxantrone plus prednisolone have shown a 2.4–3-month median survival advantage in favour of docetaxel. While there is interest is evaluating its use in earlier stage disease, docetaxel maintenance and salvage regimens using satraplatin are already in clinical use for progressing AI disease.

Novel therapies

Several phase I and II studies are underway to identify safe and effective treatments for AI disease, either alone or in combination with cytotoxic agents. Trials of tyrosine kinase receptor and endothelin-1 receptor antagonists, as well as cancer vaccines, have yielded disappointing results.

Palliative management of prostate cancer

Multidisciplinary involvement of the palliative care and acute pain teams is often necessary in the terminal phase of the illness, to optimize quality of life.

Pain is undoubtedly the most debilitating symptom of advanced prostate cancer. The pathogenesis of this pain is poorly understood, but there is known to be increased osteoclastic and osteoblastic activity. The table below categorizes the pain syndromes and their management. Androgen deprivation therapy is effective in newly-presenting disease. In hormone-refractory disease, the bisphosphonates (especially zoledronic acid) can reduce bone pain in up to 80% patients and the risk of skeletal complications, such as pathological fracture (Table 7.15).

Spinal cord compression

📖 see p. 341

Lower urinary tract symptoms/urinary retention

A TURP may be required for bladder outflow obstruction (BOO) or retention. Instrumentation can be difficult if there is a bulky fixed prostate cancer. The bladder may be contracted due to disease involvement, causing misery even after relief of BOO. This may perhaps respond to anticholinergic therapy. A long-term urethral or suprapubic catheter may be required for difficult voiding symptoms or recurrent retention.

Ureteric obstruction

This is a uro-oncological emergency. Locally-advanced prostate cancer and bladder cancer may cause bilateral ureteric obstruction. The patient presents either with symptoms and signs of renal failure, or anuric without a palpable bladder. Renal ultrasound will demonstrate bilateral hydronephrosis and an empty bladder. After treating any life-threatening hyperkalaemia, treatment options include bilateral percutaneous nephrostomies or ureteric stents. A clotting screen is required prior to nephrostomy insertion. Antegrade ureteric stenting following placement of nephrostomies is usually successful. Insertion of retrograde ureteric stents in this scenario is usually unsuccessful because tumour affecting the trigone obscures the ureteric orifices. Hormone therapy should be commenced if not previously used.

Unilateral ureteric obstruction is occasionally observed at presentation or on progression. Usually asymptomatic, this may be managed conservatively provided there is a normal contralateral kidney. Preservation of renal function becomes important if cytotoxic chemotherapy is being considered.

Table 7.15 Pain management

Pain type	Initial management	Other options
Focal bone pain	Medical: simple, NSAIDS, opiates Single-shot radiotherapy, 800 cGy (75% respond up to 6 months)	Surgical fixation of pathological fracture or extensive lytic metastasis
Diffuse bone pain	Medical: NSAIDS, opiates Multi-shot radiotherapy or Radiopharmaceutical (for example, Strontium89	Steroids; bisphosphonates; chemotherapy
Epidural metastasis and cord compression	See p.341	
Plexopathies (rare, caused by direct tumour extension)	Medical: NSAIDS, opiates Radiotherapy; nerve blocks	Tricyclics; anticonvulsants
Other pain syndromes: skull/cranial nerve, liver, rectum/perineum	Radiotherapy; Medical: NSAIDS, opiates, steroids	Intrathecal chemotherapy for meningeal involvement

Anaemia, thrombocytopaenia, and coagulopathy

Some patients with extensive bone marrow replacement by tumour rapidly and regularly become symptomatic with anaemia. This tends to be normochromic and normocytic, often occurring without other symptoms and with normal renal function. They require regular blood transfusions. Platelet transfusions are rarely required for bleeding/thrombocytopaenia. Terminal patients may develop a clinical picture similar to disseminated intravascular coagulation leading to problematic haematuria.

Malignant ureteric obstruction

Locally-advanced prostate cancer, bladder, or ureteric cancer may cause unilateral or bilateral ureteric obstruction.

Unilateral obstruction is often asymptomatic, an incidental ultrasound finding that requires no specific treatment in the presence of a normal contralateral kidney. Occasionally, systemic symptoms and/or loin pain may develop. Infection of the obstructed upper urinary tract may occur: in this circumstance, drainage by nephrostomy or stenting is required.

Bilateral ureteric obstruction is a urological emergency. The patient presents either with symptoms and signs of renal failure, or anuric without a palpable bladder. A mass will probably be palpable on rectal examination. Investigations: renal ultrasound will demonstrate bilateral hydronephrosis and an empty bladder; CT urography will confirm the presence of dilated ureters down to a mass at the bladder base.

Immediate treatment of bilateral ureteric obstruction

After treating any life-threatening hyperkalaemia, options include bilateral percutaneous nephrostomies or ureteric stenting. A clotting screen is required prior to nephrostomy insertion. Insertion of retrograde ureteric stents in this setting is usually unsuccessful because tumour involving the trigone obscures the location of the ureteric orifices. More successful is antegrade ureteric stenting following nephrostomy insertion, both of which are performed under sedo-analgesia. The full-length double-J silicone or polyurethane ureteric stents require periodic (4–6 monthly) changes to prevent calcification or blockage. In the case of prostate cancer, hormone therapy should be commenced if not previously used; even in patients with androgen-independent disease, high-dose parenteral oestrogens have been used to relieve ureteric obstruction.

Long-term treatment of bilateral ureteric obstruction

Longer term treatment options include urinary diversion by formation of ileal conduit, ureteric re-implantation, insertion of short 'permanent' metallic ureteric stents, or ureteric replacement with isolated ileal segments or prosthetic graft material. Such procedures are often complicated and inappropriate in these poor-prognosis patients.

Spinal cord and cauda equina compression

Spinal cord compression

This is a uro-oncological emergency; failure to diagnose and treat promptly can lead to permanent paraplegia and autonomic dysfunction. Due to epidural compression, arising from prostate cancer vertebral body metastasis in the majority of cases, 95% of patients will complain of back pain and have a positive bone scan. 5% do not exhibit these features because their disease is paravertebral. Patients with back pain should be examined neurologically and evaluated radiologically. Pain usually precedes cord compression by about 4 months. Other clinical features include sensory changes and muscle weakness in the lower limbs, bladder, and bowel dysfunction, and these can progress rapidly to become irreversible.

If cord compression is suspected, the investigation of choice is spinal MRI. This will reveal the deposits, which are multiple in 20% of cases.

Initial treatment is with high-dose intravenous corticosteroids, for example, dexamethasone 10 mg followed by 4 mg 6-hourly for 2–3 weeks. Without delay, further treatment with radiotherapy or neurosurgical decompression is carried out. Surgery should be considered preferable if there is pathological fracture, unknown tissue diagnosis or a history of previous radiotherapy.

Cauda equina compression

The adult spinal cord tapers below L2 vertebral level into the conus medullaris. The cauda equina consists of the nerve roots of all spinal cord segments below L2, as they run in the subarachnoid space to their exit levels in the lower lumbar and sacral spines.

Pathophysiology: the cauda equina may be compressed by central intervertebral disc prolapse (1–15% of cases), spinal stenosis, or by a benign or malignant tumour within the lower lumbar or sacral vertebral canal.

Symptoms: the diagnosis should be considered in any female or young male presenting with difficulty voiding or in urinary retention. There may be back pain.

Signs: palpable bladder, loss of peri-anal (S2–4) and lateral foot sensation (S1–2), reduced anal tone; priapism.

Investigations: MRI lumbosacral spine; urodynamic studies reveal a normally-compliant, but areflexic bladder.

Treatment: intermittent self-catheterization, neurosurgery.

Urethral cancer

Primary urethral cancer is rare, occurring in elderly patients, 4 times more commonly in women.

Risk factors: urethral stricture and sexually-transmitted disease are implicated. Direct spread from tumour in the bladder or prostate is more common.

Pathology and staging

75% are squamous cell carcinomas occurring in the anterior urethra, 15% are TCC occurring in the posterior/prostatic urethra, 10% are adenocarcinomas, and the remainder include sarcoma and melanoma.

Urethral cancer metastasizes to the pelvic lymph nodes from the posterior urethra and to the inguinal nodes from the anterior urethra in 50% of patients. Staging is by the TNM system (Table 7.15).

Presentation

- Often late; many patients have metastatic disease at presentation
- Painless haematuria, initial, terminal or a bloody urethral discharge
- Voiding-type LUTS (less common)
- Perineal pain (less common)
- Peri-urethral abscess or urethro-cutaneous fistula (rare)
- Past history of sexually-transmitted or stricture disease.

Examination may reveal a hard palpable mass at the female urethral meatus, or along the course of the male anterior urethra. Inguinal lymphadenopathy, chest signs and hepatomegaly may suggest metastatic disease.

The differential diagnosis in men is:
- Urethral stricture
- Perineal abscess
- Metastatic disease involving the corpora cavernosa
- Urethro-cutaneous fistula.

The differential diagnosis in women is:
- Urethral caruncle
- Urethral cyst
- Urethral diverticulum
- Urethral wart (Condylomata acuminata)
- Urethral prolapse
- Peri-urethral abscess.

Investigations

Cysto-urethroscopy, biopsy, and bimanual examination under anaesthesia will obtain a diagnosis and local clinical staging. Chest radiography and abdomino-pelvic CT scan will enable distant staging.

Treatment

For localized anterior urethral cancer, radical surgery or radiotherapy are the options. Results are better with anterior urethral disease. Male patients would require perineal urethrostomy. Postoperative incontinence due to disruption of the external sphincter mechanism is minimal unless the bladder neck is involved, but the patient would need to sit to void. For posterior/prostatic urethral cancer, cystoprostatourethrectomy should be considered for fit men, while anterior pelvic exenteration (excision of the pelvic lymph nodes, bladder, urethra, uterus, ovaries, and part of the vagina) should be considered for women. In the absence of distant metastases, inguinal lymphadenectomy is performed if nodes are palpable, since 80% contain metastatic tumour.

For locally-advanced disease, a combination of preoperative radiotherapy and surgery is recommended.

For metastatic disease, cytotoxic chemotherapy is the only option.

5-year survival

Surgery: anterior urethra	50%
Surgery: posterior urethra:	15%
Radiotherapy:	34%
Radiotherapy and surgery:	55%

Staging is by the TNM (1997) classification following histological confirmation of the diagnosis (Table 7.16). All rely upon physical examination and imaging, the pathological classification (prefixed 'p') corresponding to the TNM categories.

Table 7.16 TNM staging of urethral carcinoma

Tx	Primary tumour cannot be assessed
T0	No evidence of primary tumour
Urethra (male and female)	
Ta	Non-invasive papillary carcinoma
Tis	Carcinoma *in situ*
T1	Tumour invades subepithelial connective tissue
T2	Tumour invades corpus spongiosum, prostate, or peri-urethral muscle
T3	Tumour invades corpus cavernosum, prostatic capsule, vagina, or bladder neck
T4	Tumour invades adjacent organs including bladder
Transitional cell carcinoma of the prostatic urethra	
Tis	Carcinoma *in situ*, prostatic urethra (pu) or prostatic ducts (pd)
T1	Tumour invades subepithelial connective tissue
T2	Tumour invades prostatic stroma, corpus spongiosum, or peri-urethral muscle
T3	Tumour invades through prostatic capsule, corpus cavernosum, or bladder neck
T4	Tumour invades adjacent organs including bladder
Nx	Regional (deep inguinal and pelvic) lymph nodes cannot be assessed
N0	No regional lymph node metastasis
N1	Metastasis in a single lymph node up to 2 cm in greatest dimension
N2	Metastasis in a single lymph node >2 cm in greatest dimension
Mx	Distant metastasis cannot be assessed
M0	No distant metastasis
M1	Distant metastasis present

Penile neoplasia: benign, viral-related and premalignant lesions

Benign tumours and lesions

Non-cutaneous

- Congenital and acquired inclusion cysts
- Retention cysts
- Syringomas (sweat gland tumours)
- Neurilemoma
- Angioma, lipoma
- Iatrogenic pseudotumour following injections
- Pyogenic granuloma following injections
- Peyronies plaque (early or atypical).

Cutaneous

- Pearly penile papules (normal in 15% of post-pubertal males)
- Zoon's balanitis (shiny, erythematous plaque on glans or prepuce)
- Lichen planus (flat-topped violacious papule).

Viral-related lesions

- **Condyloma Acuminatum:** also known as genital warts, related to human papillomavirus (HPV) infection. Soft, usually multiple benign lesions on the glans, prepuce, and shaft; may occur elsewhere on genitalia or perineum. A biopsy is worthwhile prior to topical treatment with podophyllin. 5% have urethral involvement, which may require diathermy. HPV infection (particularly types 16 and 18) is potentially carcinogenic and condylomata have been associated with penile SCC.
- **Bowenoid papulosis:** a condition resembling carcinoma *in situ*, but with a benign course. Multiple papules appear on the penile skin, or a flat glanular lesion. These should be biopsied. HPV is the suspected cause.
- **Kaposi's sarcoma:** first described in 1972, this reticulo-endothelial tumour has become the second commonest malignant penile tumour. It presents as a raised, painful, bleeding violacious papule, or as a bluish ulcer with local oedema. It is slow-growing, solitary or diffuse. It occurs in immunocompromised men, particularly in homosexuals with HIV-AIDS. Urethral obstruction may occur. Treatment is palliative; intralesional chemotherapy, laser or cryo-ablation, or radiotherapy.

Premalignant cutaneous lesions

Some histologically benign lesions are recognized to have malignant potential or occur in close association with squamous cell carcinoma (SCC) of the penis. The extent to which SCC is preceded by pre-malignant lesions is unknown.

- **Cutaneous horn:** rare solid skin overgrowth; extreme hyperkeratosis, the base may be malignant; treatment is wide local excision.
- **Pseudo-epitheliomatous micaceous and keratotic balanitis:** unusual hyperkeratotic growths on the glans; require excision, histological examination and follow-up as they may recur.

- **Balanitis Xerotica Obliterans (BXO):** also known as lichen sclerosus et atrophicus, this is a common sclerosing condition of glans and prepuce. It occurs at all ages and most commonly presents as non-retractile foreskin (phimosis). The meatus and fossa navicularis may be affected, causing obstructed and spraying voiding. The histological diagnosis is usually made after circumcision, with epithelial atrophy, loss of rete pegs and collagenization of the dermis. BXO occurs in association with penile SCC, but most pathologists would regard the lesion as benign unless epithelial dysplasia was present.
- **Leukoplakia:** solitary or multiple whiteish glanular plaques that usually involve the meatus. Treatment is excision and histology. Leukoplakia is associated with *in situ* SCC; follow-up is required.
- **Erythroplasia of Queyrat:** also known as carcinoma *in situ* or penile intraepithelial neoplasia of the glans, prepuce or penile shaft. A red velvety circumscribed painless lesion, though it may ulcerate resulting in discharge and pain. Treatment is excision biopsy if possible; radiotherapy, laser ablation or topical 5-fluorouracil may be required. Histology reveals hyperplastic mucosal cells with malignant features
- **Bowen's disease:** this is carcinoma *in situ* of the remainder of the keratinizing genital or perineal skin. Treatment is wide local excision, laser or cryo-ablation.
- **Buschke–Löwenstein tumour:** also known as verrucous carcinoma or giant condyloma acuminatum, this is an aggressive locally-invasive tumour of the glans. Metastasis is rare, but wide excision is necessary to distinguish it from SCC. Urethral erosion and fistulation may occur.

A chronic red or pale lesion on the glans or prepuce is always a cause for concern. Note should be made of its colour, size, and surface features. Early review following steroid, antibacterial, or antifungal creams is recommended; if persistent, biopsy should be recommended.

Penile cancer: epidemiology, risk factors and pathology

Squamous cell carcinoma (SCC) is the commonest primary penile cancer, accounting for 95% of penile malignancies. Others include Kaposi's sarcoma (3%); rarities include basal cell carcinoma, malignant melanoma, sarcoma, and Paget's disease. Metastases are very rarely seen from bladder, prostate, rectum and other primary sites.

Incidence and aetiology of SCC

Penile cancer is rare, representing 1% of male cancers. The incidence appears to be decreasing, most occurring in elderly men. Approximately 400 new cases and 100 deaths are reported annually in the UK.

Risk factors for SCC

Age: penile cancer incidence rises during the sixth decade and peaks in the eighth decade. It is unusual below the age of 40, but has been reported in children.

Premalignant lesions: 42% of patients with penile SCC are reported to have had a pre-existing penile lesion (see p. 346)

A prepuce (foreskin): penile cancer is rare in men circumcised neonatally. It is virtually non-existent in Israel. It is thought that chronic irritation with smegma and inflammation (balanitis) is contributory.

Geography: more common in parts of Asia, Africa and S. America, where it accounts for 10–20% of male cancers. Brazil has the highest worldwide incidence.

Human papilloma virus (HPV): wart infection, especially with types 16, 18 and 21 appear to be associated with 50–90% of cases.

Smoking and tobacco products

Pathology and staging of penile SCC

Believed to be preceded by carcinoma *in situ*, SCC starts as a slow-growing papillary, flat, or ulcerative lesion on the glans (48%), prepuce (21%), glans and prepuce (9%), coronal sulcus (6%), or shaft (2%). The remainder are indeterminate. It grows locally by superficial spread beneath the foreskin, before entering a vertical-phase growth pattern, invading the corpora cavernosa, urethra, and eventually the perineum, pelvis, and prostate. Metastasis is initially to the superficial then deep inguinal lymph nodes, and subsequently to iliac and obturator nodes. Skin necrosis, ulceration, and infection of the inguinal lymph nodes may lead to sepsis or haemorrhage from the femoral vessels. Blood-borne metastasis to lungs and liver is rare (1–10% of cases).

Histologically, SCC exhibits keratinization, epithelial pearl formation and mitoses. There are 'Classic', Baseloid, Verrucous, Sarcomatoid and Adenosquamous histological types. Grading is low (70-80%), intermediate (15%) or high (10%); grading correlates with prognosis, as does the presence of vascular invasion. Staging is by the TNM system (Fig. 7.12 and Table 7.17).

Table 7.17 1997/2002 TNM staging of penile cancer

Tx	Primary tumour cannot be assessed
T0	No evidence of primary tumour
Tis	Carcinoma *in situ*
Ta	Non-invasive verrucous carcinoma
T1	Tumour invades subepithelial connective tissue
T2	Tumour invades corpus cavernosum or spongiosum
T3	Tumour invades urethra or prostate
T4	Tumour invades other structures
Nx	Regional nodes cannot be assessed
N0	No regional lymph node metastases
N1	Single superficial inguinal lymph node metastasis
N2	Multiple or bilateral superficial inguinal lymph node metastases
N3	Metastases in deep inguinal or pelvic lymph nodes, unilateral or bilateral
Mx	Distant metastasis cannot be assessed
M0	No distant metastasis
M1	Distant metastasis

Prognostic factors for penile SCC

The presence of metastatic node disease is the best prognostic factor. Risk groups for N+ disease have been defined, based on the location, size, histological grade, depth of invasion, presence of corporal invasion, and vascular or lymphatic invasion.[1] Molecular markers under evaluation, especially p53 immunohistochemistry, may have prognostic value.

1 Stancik I and Holtl W (2003) Penile cancer: review of recent literature. *Curr Opin Urol* **13**:467–72.

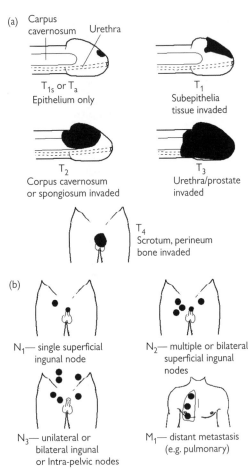

Fig. 7.12 The TNM staging of penile cancer.

Squamous cell carcinoma of the penis: management

Clinical presentation

A hard painless lump on the glans penis is the most common presentation. 15–50% of patients delay presentation for >1 year due to embarrassment, personal neglect, fear, or ignorance. A bloody discharge may be confused with haematuria. Rarely, a groin mass or urinary retention are presenting symptoms. Examination reveals a solid non-tender mass or ulcer beneath, or involving the foreskin. There is usually evidence of local infection. In more advanced disease, prepuce, glans, shaft, scrotum, and even perineum are replaced by tumour. The inguinal lymph nodes are examined.

Investigations

A biopsy is indicated. Chest and pelvic CT scan, serum calcium, and liver function tests are usually obtained. MRI may assist in assessing tumour depth of invasion.

Treatment

Following histological diagnosis, management of penile cancer should take place in supra-regional centres that can provide multidisciplinary surgical and oncological expertise for this rare disease.

The primary tumour

The first-line treatment of penile cancer, regardless of the inguinal node status, is surgery. Circumcision is appropriate for preputial lesions, but local recurrence observed in 22–50%. Penis-preserving wide excision of glanular lesions with skin graft glanular reconstruction is recommended for penile intraepithelial neoplasia (PIN), Ta-1 G1–2 and carefully selected small T1G3 or T2 tumours, giving good cosmetic and functional results. Alternatives to surgery include topical 5-fluorouracil (PIN only), laser ablation, cryo-ablation, radiotherapy or brachytherapy or photodynamic therapy.

For most T1 G3 and more advanced tumours, or for patients who may not comply with follow-up recommendations, partial or total penile amputation is required, depending on the extent of the tumour. Partial amputation is preferable, provided a 1.5 cm margin of palpably-normal shaft can be obtained. The patient must be prepared for poor cosmetic and functional results: inability to have sexual intercourse and need to sit to void urine. Local recurrence occurs in 10%, if the excision margin is positive. Total amputation involves excision of the scrotum and its contents, with formation of a perineal urethrostomy. The most common complication is urethral meatal stenosis. Radiotherapy or brachytherapy are non-surgical alternatives, though local recurrence rates of 30–50% are reported; tissue necrosis/damage leads to meatal stenosis (15–30%), urethral stricture (20–35%), fistula and pain. The use of neo-adjuvant chemotherapy is under investigation.

Lymphadenopathy

Six weeks of broad-spectrum antimicrobials (e.g. co-amoxyclav) are given after the primary tumour has been removed. In 50% of patients, nodes are reactive and become clinically insignificant.

For those with persistent inguinal lymphadenopathy, in the absence of demonstrable pelvic or metastatic disease, bilateral radical inguinal lymphadenectomy should be undertaken, since 5-year survival is 80%. The boundaries of the dissection are the inguinal ligament, the adductors and sartorius, with the femoral vessels in the floor. If lymphadenopathy is unilateral, >50% will have contralateral metastases. A modified dissection (see below) may be undertaken on the 'normal' side and extended if frozen section histology is positive. However, this major surgery has high (30-50%) morbidity (lymphoedema, thromboembolism, and skin necrosis/wound breakdown) so is not suitable for elderly or unfit men. Fine needle aspiration cytology is not recommended since a negative result will not alter treatment. Radiotherapy and chemotherapy are alternative or adjuvant treatments for metastatic nodal disease in unfit, elderly, or inoperable patients; 5-year survival 25%.

Pelvic lymphadenectomy should be considered when 2 or more positive inguinal nodes are identified at frozen section; here the likelihood of pelvic node metastasis is 23–56% and cure rates of 14–54% are reported.

There is controversy regarding the management of patients with initially non-palpable nodes. While the majority overall will not harbour metastatic disease, it is argued that delayed lymphadenectomy could reduce the chance of cure. Prophylactic modified inguinal lymphadenectomy is now recommended for high-risk G3 or pT2–4 tumours (risk of N+ disease is 70%), and should be considered for intermediate-risk pT1G2 tumours exhibiting vascular or lymphatic invasion. There is interest in dynamic sentinel node biopsy for this latter group of patients. The saphenous vein is preserved to decrease lower limb oedema, and the lateral and inferior dissections are reduced by 1–2 cm.

Fixed inguinal masses may be considered for salvage surgery following neo-adjuvant chemotherapy (response rates 20–60%), ideally within a clinical trial. Rarely, lymphadenopathy ulcerates the skin, may encase the femoral vessels and invade the deeper musculature. In these circumstances, collaboration with plastics and vascular surgeons is necessary if surgery is considered appropriate.

Distant metastatic disease is treated using single-agent systemic chemotherapy: cisplatin, bleomycin or methotrexate. Responses are partial and short-lived in 20–60% of patients. Experience with cisplatin-based combination chemotherapy is increasing, where complete responses are reported. Patients with M1 disease are offered palliative surgery for their primary tumour.

Follow-up

Careful follow-up, initially every 2–4 months, is essential after primary tumour surgery to detect and treat local recurrence (15–25%) early, since this prevents any reduction in cancer-specific survival. After removal of the primary tumour, the appearance of lymphadenopathy is almost always due to metastatic disease. Groin evaluations of patients with initially non-palpable nodes at similar intervals is necessary, since late diagnosis and treatment is a negative prognostic factor. Pelvic and chest CT imaging is justified for those patients who have undergone inguinal lymphadenectomy for metastatic disease.

5-year survival

Node-negative SCC, after surgery	65–90%
Inguinal node metastases	30%
Metastatic SCC	<10%

Carcinoma of the scrotum

Squamous cell carcinoma was originally described in Victorian chimney sweeps by Percival Pott. It was the first cancer to be associated with an occupation. A rare disease below 50 years of age, chronic exposure of the scrotal skin to soot, tar, or oil is the cause. It presents as a painless lump or ulcer, often purulent, on the anterior or posterior scrotal wall. Posterior lesions are therefore concealed if the patient is lying or sitting. Inguinal lymphadenopathy may suggest metastasis or reaction to infection. Treatment of a mass or ulcer on the scrotum is wide local excision. Antimicrobials are administered for 6 weeks if there is lymphadenopathy, after which the groins are re-evaluated. Inguinal lymphadenectomy is considered if lymphadenopathy persists, with adjuvant chemotherapy. Supraclavicular lymphadenopathy, haematogenous visceral and bony metastasis are rare and carry a poor prognosis.

Tumours of the testicular adnexa

Epithelial tumours arising from the epididymis and paratesticular tissues are rare. They are mostly of mesenchymal origin,

Adenomatoid tumours: small solid tumours arising in the epididymis or on the surface of the tunica albuginea; usually present without change for several years; benign vacuolated epithelial and stromal cells, origin unknown, treatment is local excision.

Cystadenoma of the epididymis: benign epithelial hyperplasia; young adults; often asymptomatic; one-third bilateral and associated with VHL syndrome.

Mesothelioma: presents as a firm painless scrotal mass associated with hydrocoele which gradually enlarges; any age-group; 15% metastatic to inguinal nodes; treated with orchidectomy and follow-up.

Paratesticular tumours

Rhabdomyosarcoma: scrotal mass in 1st/2nd decade; in spermatic cord; compresses testis and epididymis; lymphatic spread to para-aortic nodes; treatment is multimodal radical orchidectomy with radiotherapy and chemotherapy; 5-year survival 75%

Leiomyoma/sarcoma: scrotal mass age 40–70 years; in spermatic cord; 30% are malignant, 70% are benign; haematogenous distant spread; treatment is wide excision or radical orchidectomy.

Liposarcoma: spermatic cord tumour; 70% are malignant.

Testicular cancer

Incidence and mortality

Primary testicular cancer (TC) is the most common solid cancer in men aged 20–45, rare below 15 years and above 60 years. Constituting 1–2% of all male cancers and 5% of all urological tumours, it is considered the most curable cancer, with 1990 new cases, but only 74 deaths in the UK (2004). It's incidence is increasing in Western society, reported to affect 6 per 100,000 men. Public health campaigns encouraging testicular self-examination (TSE) for young men are ongoing.

Epidemiology and aetiology

- **Age:** the commonest affected age group is 20–45 years, with germ cell tumours. Teratomas are more common at ages 20–35, while seminoma is more common at ages 35–45 years. Rarely, infants and boys below 10 years develop yolk sac tumours and 50% men >60 years with TC have lymphoma
- **Race:** white people are three times more likely to develop TC than black people in the USA
- **Cryptorchidism:** 10% of TC's occur in undescended testes, the risk increases by 3–14 times compared with men with normally descended testes. Ultrastructural changes are present in these testes by age 3 years, although earlier orchidopexy does not completely eliminate the risk of developing TC. 5–10% of patients with a cryptorchid testis develop malignancy in the normally-descended contralateral testis
- **Intratubular germ cell neoplasia (testicular intraepithelial neoplasia, TIN):** synonymous with carcinoma *in situ*, although the disease arises from malignant change in spermatogonia. 50% of cases develop invasive germ cell TC within 5 years. The population incidence is 0.8%. Risk factors include cryptorchidism (undescended testis), extra-gonadal germ cell tumour, previous or contralateral TC (5%), atrophic contralateral testis, 45XO karyotype, Klinefelter's syndrome and infertility
- **Human immunodeficiency virus (HIV):** patients infected with the HIV virus are developing seminoma more frequently than expected
- **Genetic factors** appear to play a role, given that first-degree relatives are at higher risk, but a defined familial inheritance pattern is not apparent
- **Maternal oestrogen ingestion** during pregnancy increases the risk of cryptorchidism and TC in the male offspring.

Trauma and viral-induced atrophy have not been convincingly implicated as risk factors for TC.

Bilateral testicular cancer occurs in 1–2% of cases.

Testicular cancer (TC): pathology and staging

90% of testicular tumours are malignant germ cell tumours (GCT), split into seminomatous and non-seminomatous GCT's for clinical purposes. Seminoma, the most common germ cell tumour, appears pale and homogeneous. Teratomas are heterogeneous and sometimes contain bizarre tissues such as cartilage or hair. Metastases to the testis are rare, notably from the prostate (35%), lung (19%), colon (9%), and kidney (7%).

Table 7.18 shows the WHO histopathological classification of testicular tumours.

Table 7.18 The WHO histopathological classification of testicular tumours

Germ cell tumours (90%)	**Other tumours (7%)**
Seminoma (48%): spermatocytic, classical, and anaplastic subtypes	Epidermoid cyst (benign)
	Adenomatoid tumour
Non-seminomatous GCT (42%):	Adenocarcinoma of the rete testis
Teratoma:	
Differentiated/mature	Carcinoid
Intermediate/immature	Lymphoma (5%)
Undifferentiated/malignant	Metastatic, from another site (1%)
Yolk sac tumour	
Choriocarcinoma	
Mixed	
Mixed GCT (10%)	
Sex cord stromal tumours (3%) (10% malignant)	
Leydig cell	
Sertoli cell	
Mixed or unclassified	
Mixed germ cell/sex cord tumours (rare)	

The right testis is affected slightly more commonly than the left; synchronous bilateral TC occurs in 2.5% of cases. TC spreads by local extension into the epididymis, spermatic cord, and rarely the scrotal wall. Lymphatic spread occurs via the testicular vessels, initially to the para-aortic nodes. Involvement of the epididymis, spermatic cord or scrotum may lead to pelvic and inguinal node metastasis. Blood-borne metastasis to the lungs, liver and bones is more likely once the disease has breached the tunica albuginea.

TC is staged using various classifications, most recently the TNM (2002) system (Figs 7.13 and Table 7.19). Herein, T stage is pathological, N stage involves imaging with CT abdomen and chest; M stage involves physical examination, imaging (with CT) and biochemical investigations. An additional S category is appended for serum tumour markers (see p. 364)

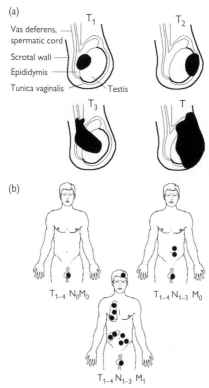

Fig. 7.13 Pathological staging of testicular cancer. (a) Primary tumours T1–4. If radical orchidectomy has not been used, T_x is used. (b) Node/metastasis: para-aortic lymphadenopathy measured in long axis on CT scan (upper figure); supraclavicular lymphadenopathy and/or pulmonary metastases—M1a, other distant metastases (e.g. liver, brain); M1b lower figure.

Table 7.19 TNM staging of testicular germ cell tumours

Tx	The primary tumour has not been assessed (no radical orchidectomy)
T0	No evidence of primary tumour
Tis	Intratubular germ cell neoplasia (carcinoma *in situ*)
T1	Tumour limited to testis and epididymis without vascular invasion; may invade tunica albuginea, but not tunica vaginalis
T2	Tumour limited to testis and epididymis with vascular/lymphatic invasion, or tumour involving tumica vaginalis
T3	Tumour invades spermatic cord with or without vascular invasion
T4	Tumour invades scrotum with or without vascular invasion
Nx	Regional lymph nodes cannot be assessed
N0	No regional lymph node metastasis
N1	Metastasis with a lymph node < or = 2 cm or multiple lymph nodes, none >2 cm
N2	Metastasis with a lymph node size 2–5 cm or multiple lymph nodes together size 2–5 cm
N3	Metastasis with a lymph node mass >5 cm
Mx	Distant metastasis cannot be assessed
M0	No distant metastasis
M1a	Non-regional lymph node or pulmonary metastasis
M1b	Distant metastasis other than to non-regional lymph node or lungs

Intratubular germ cell neoplasia (testicular intra-epithelial neoplasia, TIN)

The precursor lesion for most testicular GCTs, TIN may be observed adjacent to a tumour, and is present in the contralateral testis of up to 5% of patients with testicular GCT. Controversy exists as to whether to biopsy the contralateral testis in all cases to diagnose TIN. At particularly high risk of TIN are patients with small (<12 mL) testis, a history of cryptorchidism and age <30 years. If TIN is diagnosed, treatment is with radiotherapy. Consequently the issues of infertility and hormone replacement need to be discussed with these patients.

Testicular cancer: clinical presentation, investigation and primary treatment

Symptoms

Most patients present with a scrotal lump, usually painless. Delay in presentation is not uncommon, particularly those with metastatic disease. This may be due to patient factors (fear, self-neglect, ignorance, denial) or earlier misdiagnosis. 5% of patients develop acute scrotal pain due to intra-tumoural haemorrhage, causing diagnostic confusion. The lump may have been noted by the patient, sometimes after minor trauma, or by his partner. 10% of patients develop symptoms suggestive of advanced disease include weight loss, lumps in the neck, chest symptoms, or bone pain.

Signs

Examination of the genitalia should be carried out in a warm room with the patient relaxed. Observation may reveal asymmetry or slight scrotal skin discolouration. Using careful bimanual palpation, the normal side is first examined, followed by the abnormal side. This will reveal a hard non-tender irregular non-transilluminable mass in the testis, or replacing the testis. Care should be taken to assess the epididymis, spermatic cord, and overlying scrotal wall, which may be normal or involved in 10–15% of cases. Rarely, a secondary hydrocoele may be present if the tunica albuginea has been breached. General examination may reveal cachexia, supraclavicular lymphadenopathy, chest signs, hepatomegaly, lower limb oedema or abdominal mass, all suggestive of metastatic disease. Gynaecomastia is seen in about 5% of patients with TC, due to endocrine manifestations of some tumours.

Differential diagnoses

Hydrocoele, epididymal cyst (spermatocoele), hernia, TB, or syphilitic gumma (rare) are causes of painless scrotal swellings. Varicocoele is normally apparent only when the patient is standing. Testicular torsion and epididymo-orchitis account for most presentations of acute scrotal pain. The majority of scrotal lumps we see are harmless lesions, but no risks should be taken. Every patient who is concerned should be seen, examined and if any doubt persists, should be investigated further.

Investigations

Ultrasound (USS, 7.5 MHz) is an extension of the physical examination and will confirm that the palpable lesion is within the testis, distorting its normally regular outline and internal echo pattern. The sensitivity of USS for detecting a testicular tumour is almost 100%, including impalpable lesions of 1–2 mm and 'occult' primary tumours in patients presenting with systemic symptoms and signs. Any hypo-echoic area within the tunica albuginea should be regarded with suspicion. USS may also distinguish a primary from a secondary hydrocoele. Testicular microlithiasis is occasionally reported by USS in association with testicular tumours. There has been uncertainty regarding the significance of this anomaly in otherwise normal testes. The few prospective studies carried out have suggested no increased risk of subsequent development of testicular tumours, consequently there is no rationale for recommending serial ultrasound scans to these individuals.

Abdominal and chest CT scans are usually obtained for staging purposes if the diagnosis of TC is confirmed or considered likely. Other imaging (such as CT of brain, spine, or bone scan) is performed if clinically indicated.

Serum tumour markers (AFP and βhCG) are measured prior to any treatment of a confirmed testicular mass (□ see p. 364).

Treatment

Radical orchidectomy is both the final investigation and the definitive primary treatment for all testicular tumours, unless tissue diagnosis has been made from biopsy of a metastasis. The testis, epididymis, and spermatic cord, with their coverings, are excised through a groin incision. The cord is clamped, transfixed, and divided near the internal inguinal ring before the testis is manipulated into the wound, preventing inadvertent metastasis. A silicone prosthesis may be inserted at the time, or at a later date. Radical orchidectomy is curative in approximately 80% of patients. Fertility assessment, semen analysis, and cryo-preservation should be offered to patients without a normal contralateral testis. Contralateral testis biopsy should be considered in patients at high risk for testicular intratubular neoplasia (□ see p. 360).

Testicular cancer: serum markers

Germ cell tumours may express and secrete into the bloodstream relatively specific and readily measurable proteins. These tumour markers (with the exception of PLAP) are useful in diagnosis, staging, prognostication (📖 p. 365) and monitoring of response to treatment (📖 p. 366–9).

Onco-foetal proteins

Alpha-fetoprotein (AFP) is expressed by trophoblastic elements within 50–70% of teratomas and yolk sac tumours. With respect to seminoma, the presence of elevated serum AFP strongly suggests a non-seminomatous element. Serum half-life is 3–5 days; normal <10 ng/mL.

Human chorionic gonadotrophin (hCG) is expressed by syncytiotrophoblastic elements of choriocarcinomas (100%), teratomas (40%) and seminomas (10%). Serum half-life is 24–36 h. Laboratory assays measure the β-subunit; normal <5 mIU/mL.

When used together, 90% of patients have elevation of one or both markers; less among patients with low-stage tumours.

Cellular enzymes

Lactate dehydrogenase (LDH) is a ubiquitous enzyme, elevated in serum for various causes, therefore less specific. It is elevated in 10–20% of seminomas, correlating with tumour burden and is most useful in monitoring treatment response in advanced seminoma.

Placental alkaline phosphatase (PLAP) is a foetal iso-enzyme, elevated in up to 40% of patients with advanced germ cell tumours. It is not widely used as it is non-specific, may be elevated in smokers.

Clinical use

These markers are measured at presentation, 1–2 weeks after radical orchidectomy, and during follow-up to assess response to treatment and residual disease.

Normal markers prior to orchidectomy do not exclude metastatic disease; normalization of markers post-orchidectomy cannot be equated with absence of disease; and persistent elevations of markers post-orchidectomy may occur with liver dysfunction and hypogonadotrophism, but usually indicate metastatic disease.

S staging [part of the UICC (2002) TNM classification]

Sx	markers not available
S0	markers normal
S1	LDH <1.5 times normal upper limit; hCG <5000 mIU/mL; and AFP <1000 ng/mL
S2	LDH 1.5–10 times normal; hCG 5000–50,000 mIU/mL; and AFP 1000–10,000 ng/mL
S3	LDH >10 times normal; hCG >50,000 mIU/mL; and AFP > 10,000 ng/mL

Testicular cancer: prognostic staging system for metastatic germ cell cancer

The International Germ Cell Cancer Collaborative Group (IGCCCG) has devised a prognostic factor-based staging system for metastatic germ cell cancer that includes good and intermediate prognosis seminoma and good, intermediate, and poor prognosis non-seminomatous germ cell tumours (NSGCT) Table 7.20.

Table 7.20 IGCCCG prognostic factor-based staging system for metastatic germ cell cancer

Prognostic group	Seminoma	NSGCT
Good	90% of patients	56% of patients
5-year progression free survival (%)	86	92
All factors listed present:	Any primary site; no non-pulmonary visceral metastases; normal AFP; Any hCG or LDH	Testis or retroperitoneal primary site; no non-pulmonary visceral metastases; AFP <1000 ng/mL; HCG <5000 mIU/l; and LDH <1.5 × normal upper limit (S1)
Intermediate	10% of patients	28% of patients
5-year progression free survival (%)	73	80
All factors listed present:	Any primary site; non-pulmonary visceral metastases present; normal AFP; Any hCG or LDH	Testis or retroperitoneal primary site; no non-pulmonary visceral metastases; AFP 1000–9999 ng/mL or HCG 5000–49,999 mIU/l; LDH 1.5–10 × normal upper limit (S2)
Poor		16% of patients
5-year progression free survival (%)	No patients classified as poor prognosis	48
All factors listed present:		Mediastinal primary; non-pulmonary visceral metastases present; AFP >10,000 ng/mL or HCG >50,000 mIU/l; LDH > 10 × normal upper limit (S3).

📖 See p.364 for discussion on testicular tumour markers including S staging

Testicular cancer: management of non-seminomatous germ cell tumours (NSGCT)

Following radical orchidectomy and formal staging, the patient is normally managed by the oncologist, though the urologist may be asked to perform retroperitoneal lymph node dissection (RPLND) in selected cases. In the presence of elevated AFP, a seminoma would be managed as for teratoma. Combination chemotherapy introduced in the 1970s revolutionized the treatment of metastatic testicular teratoma, which was hitherto virtually untreatable.

Treatment and follow-up varies between the UK and USA. In the UK, it depends largely on the IGCCCG prognostic staging (📖 see p. 365), as follows:

Non-metastatic disease

T1–4N0M0S0: Surveillance or adjuvant chemotherapy (bleomycin, low-dose etoposide, cisplatin × 2 cycles) depending on risk factors for relapse (lymphatic or vascular invasion, T2–4); surveillance in presence of risk factors results in 25% relapse rate, most <1 year post-orchidectomy;

Metastatic disease

Good prognosis: chemotherapy (bleomycin, etoposide, cisplatin × 3 cycles); RPLND for residual or recurrent mass; occasionally salvage treatment with chemotherapy or radiotherapy if histology confirms tumour.

Intermediate and poor prognosis: chemotherapy (bleomycin, etoposide, cisplatin × 4 cycles); RPLND for residual or recurrent mass; occasionally salvage treatment chemotherapy or radiotherapy if histology confirms tumour.

Surveillance and follow-up after treatment

Surveillance requires the following:
- **Year 1:** monthly clinic visit, serum markers and chest X-ray, abdominal CT months 3 and 12 (MRC TE 08 study)
- **Year 2:** 2-monthly clinic visit with serum markers and chest X-ray, abdominal CT month 24
- **Years 3, 4 and 5:** 3-monthly clinic visit, serum markers and chest X-ray
- **Annual clinic visit:** serum markers and chest X-ray thereafter to 10 years
- Follow-up *after treatment* is slightly less intensive, also to 10 years
- The risk of relapse is highest in the first 2 years.

RPLND

- Retroperitoneal lymphadenopathy is usually the first and only evidence of extra-gonadal metastasis of teratoma
- In the UK, RPLND is used only to remove or de-bulk residual mass post-chemotherapy
- RPLND may remove viable tumour in 10–30% of patients, taking para-aortic nodes up to the origin of the superior mesenteric artery and down to the iliac bifurcation
- Complications: 1% mortality and 25% morbidity includes lymphocoele, pancreatitis, ileus and ejaculatory failure
- Modified techniques reduce the risk of ejaculatory disturbance, by taking nodes on the unaffected side only down to the inferior mesenteric artery
- In the USA, RPLND remains the gold standard staging investigation following radical orchidectomy.

Testicular cancer: management of seminoma, IGCN, and lymphoma

Of all seminomas, 75% are confined to the testis at presentation and are cured by radical orchidectomy; 10–15% of patients harbour regional node metastasis and 5–10% have more advanced disease.

Following radical orchidectomy and formal staging, the patient is managed by the oncologist. Treatment and follow-up depends largely on disease stage according to presence of metastases and size of nodal disease, as follows:

Non-metastatic disease

T1N0M0S0-1: Risk of subsequent para-aortic node relapse is 20%. Adjuvant treatment reduces the risk of recurrence to <1%. A randomized MRC study compared one cycle of carboplatin with radiotherapy: results suggested equivalence. Radiotherapy (RT) 20 Gy in 10 fractions includes the para-aortic nodes. Spermatocytic subtype usually warrants surveillance.

Metastatic disease

- **T1–3 N1 M0 S0–1:** RT
- **T1–3 N2 M0 S0–1:** RT; chemotherapy if nodes near kidneys
- **T1–4 N3 M0 S0–1:** chemotherapy (either bleomycin, etoposide and cisplatin or etoposide and cisplatin); if residual node mass >3 cm (rare), retroperitoneal lymph node dissection (RPLND) considered; if histology reveals tumour (30%), salvage chemotherapy
- **T1–4 N0–3 M1–2 S0–3:** chemotherapy; if residual node mass (rare), RPLND considered; if histology reveals tumour (30%), salvage chemotherapy.

Patients should also be classified into prognostic grouping classification (IGCCCG, 📖 see p. 365) as this provides an overall prognosis for patients. These patients require careful long-term follow-up, according to national guidance.

Management of intratubular germ cell neoplasia

- Observation or orchidectomy for unilateral disease
- Radiotherapy for unilateral disease in the presence of a contralateral tumour
- Radiotherapy for bilateral disease, to preserve Sertoli cells
- Systemic chemotherapy (e.g. cisplatin) controversial, not currently adopted in UK
- Sperm storage must be offered.

Management of testicular lymphoma

This may be a primary disease or a manifestation of disseminated nodal lymphoma. The median age of incidence is 60 years, but has been reported in children. 25% of patients present with systemic symptoms, 10% have bilateral testicular tumours. These patients have a poorer prognosis following radical orchidectomy and chemotherapy, while those with localized disease may enjoy long-term survival.

Miscellaneous urological disease of the kidney

Cystic renal disease: simple cysts

Simple renal cysts are single or multiple renal 'masses' ranging from a few to many centimetres in diameter that do not communicate with any part of the nephron or the renal pelvis. They are mainly confined to the renal cortex, are filled with clear fluid, and contain a membrane composed of a single layer of flattened or cuboidal epithelium. They can be unilateral or bilateral, and often affect the lower pole of the kidney. *Parapelvic cysts* describe simple parenchymal cysts located adjacent to the renal pelvis or hilum.

The prevalence of simple cysts increases with age. The precise prevalence depends on the method of diagnosis. On CT, 20% of adults have renal cysts by age 40 years and 33% by the age of 60.[1] At post-mortem, 50% of subjects aged >50 have simple cysts. Cysts do not usually increase in size with age, but may increase in number. Males and females are affected equally.

Aetiology: both congenital and acquired causes have been suggested. Chronic dialysis is associated with the formation of new simple cysts.

Presentation

Simple cysts are most commonly diagnosed as an incidental finding following a renal ultrasound or CT performed for other purposes. The great majority are asymptomatic; however, very large cysts may present as an abdominal mass or cause dull flank or back pain. Acute, severe loin pain may follow bleeding into a cyst (causing sudden distension of the wall). Rupture (spontaneous or following renal trauma) is rare. Rupture into the pelvicalyceal system can produce haematuria. Infected cysts (rare) present with flank pain and fever. Very occasionally, large cysts can cause obstruction and hydronephrosis.

Differential diagnosis

- Renal cell carcinoma
- Early autosomal dominant polycystic kidney disease (ADPKD)—diffuse, multiple, or bilateral cysts; presence of hepatic cysts
- Complex renal cysts (i.e. those which contain blood, pus, or calcification).

Investigation

Renal ultrasound

Simple cysts are round or spherical, have a smooth and distinct outline, and are 'anechoic' (no echoes within the cyst—i.e. sound waves are transmitted through the cyst). Evidence of calcification, septation, irregular margins, or clusters of cysts requires further investigation (CT ± aspiration, MRI). In the absence of these features no further investigation is required.

CT

Simple cysts are seen as round, smooth-walled lesions with homogenous fluid in the cavity (with a typical density of −10 to +20 Hounsfield units) and with no enhancement after contrast (enhancement implies that the 'mass' contains vascular tissue or communicates with the collecting system, i.e. that it is not a simple cyst). Hyperdense cysts have a density of 20–90 Hounsfield units, do not enhance with contrast media, and are <3 cm in diameter.

Treatment

A simple cyst (round or spherical, smooth wall, distinct outline, and no internal echoes) requires no further investigation, no treatment, and no follow-up. In the rare situation where the cyst is thought to be the cause of symptoms (e.g. back or flank pain) treatment options include percutaneous aspiration ± injection of sclerosing agent, or open or laparoscopic surgical excision of the cyst wall. In the rare event of cyst infection, percutaneous drainage, and antibiotics are indicated.

Cysts with features on ultrasound suggesting possible malignancy (calcification, septation, irregular margins) should be investigated by CT with contrast.

Table 8.1 Bosniak's classification of CT appearance of simple and complex cysts

Type	Description	Approx. % of such cysts which are malignant*	Treatment
I	Simple benign cyst with no smooth margins, no contrast enhancement, no septation, no calcification	None	None; no follow-up required
II	Smooth margins; thin septae; minimal calcification; no contrast enhancement. Includes high-density (hyperdense) cysts	10%	Observation—repeat ultrasound looking for increase in size or development of malignant features
III	Irregular margins; moderate calcification; thick septation (septae >1 mm thick)	40–50%	Surgical exploration ± partial nephrectomy
IV	Cystic malignant lesion; irregular margins and/or solid enhancing elements	90%	Radical nephrectomy

*From Siegel et al. (1997) Study relating CTs of cysts where pathological identification had been performed. Am J Roentgenol **169**:813–18.

1 Laucks SP Jr, McLachlan MS (1981). Aging and simple cysts of the kidney. Br J Radiol **54**:12–14.

Cystic renal disease: calyceal diverticulum

A calyceal diverticulum is an out-pocketing from the pelvicalyceal system, with which it communicates by way of a narrow neck. It is lined by a smooth layer of transitional epithelium and is covered by a thin layer of renal cortex. The aetiology of calyceal diverticula is unknown. They are usually asymptomatic and are discovered incidentally on an IVU, most commonly seen in upper pole calyces. Symptoms may result from the development of a stone or infection within the diverticulum, presumably caused by urinary stasis.

Treatment

Stones that form within the calyceal diverticulum may be treated by flexible ureteroscopy and laser lithotripsy or, if large, by percutaneous nephrolithotomy (PCNL) if percutaneous access is possible. Extracorporeal shock wave therapy (ESWL) may result in stone fragmentation, but it may be difficult for the stone fragments to get out of the diverticulum, and they may simply reform into a larger stone. Endoscopic dilatation or incision of the neck of the diverticulum may be attempted at the time of stone surgery to prevent recurrence, and this technique can also be employed if the diverticulum is thought to be the cause of recurrent urinary infection. Open surgery has also been used to remove stones and to de-roof calyceal diverticula.

Cystic renal disease: medullary sponge kidney (MSK)

Definition

A cystic condition of the kidneys characterized by dilatation of the distal collecting ducts associated with the formation of multiple cysts and diverticula within the medulla of the kidney.

Prevalence

Difficult to know as it may be asymptomatic (diagnosed on an IVU performed for other reason, or at post-mortem). Estimated to affect between 1 in 5000 to 1 in 20,000 people in the general population; 1 in 200 in those undergoing IVU (a select population). In 75% of cases both kidneys are affected.

Pathology

The renal medulla resembles a sponge in cross-section due to dilated collecting ducts in the renal papillae and the development of numerous small cysts. This is associated with urinary stasis and the formation of small calculi within the cysts. It has a reported familial inheritance and is associated with other malformations (hemihypertrophy).

Presentation

The majority of patients are asymptomatic. When symptoms do occur, they include ureteric colic, renal stone disease (calcium oxalate ± calcium phosphate), UTI, and haematuria (microscopic or macroscopic). Up to 50% have hypercalciuria due to renal calcium leak or increased gastrointestinal calcium absorption. Renal function is normal, unless obstruction occurs (secondary to renal pelvis or ureteric stones).

Differential diagnosis

Other causes of nephrocalcinosis (deposition of calcium in the renal medulla; e.g. TB, hyperparathyroidism, healed papillary necrosis, multiple myeloma).

Investigation

Intravenous urogram (IVU) (📖 See Fig. 8.1)

The characteristic radiological features of MSK, as seen on IVU, are enlarged kidneys associated with dilatation of the distal portion of the collecting ducts, along with numerous associated cysts and diverticula (the dilated ducts are said to give the appearance of 'bristles on a brush'). The collecting ducts may become filled with calcifications, giving an appearance described as a 'bouquet of flowers' or 'bunches of grapes'.

Biochemistry

24-h urinary calcium may be elevated (hypercalciuria). Detection of hypercalciuria requires further investigation to exclude other causes (i.e. raised serum parathyroid hormone levels (PTH) indicate hyperparathyroidism).

Treatment

Asymptomatic MSK disease requires no treatment. General measures to reduce urine calcium levels help reduce the chance of calcium stone formation (high fluid intake, vegetarian diet, low salt intake, consumption of fruit and citrus fruit juices). Thiazide diuretics may be required for hypercalciuria resistant to dietary measures, and are designed to lower urine calcium concentration. Intra-renal calculi are often small and, as such, may not require treatment, but if indicated this can take the form of extracorporeal shock wave therapy (ESWL), or flexible ureteroscopy and laser treatment. Ureteric stones are, again, usually small and will therefore pass spontaneously in many cases, with a period of observation. Renal function tends to remain stable in the long term. Recurrent UTI may need prophylactic antibiotics.

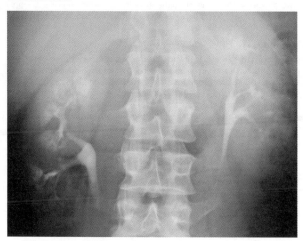

Fig. 8.1 IVU demonstrating bilateral medullary sponge kidneys.

Acquired renal cystic disease (ARCD)

A cystic degenerative disease of the kidney with ≥5 cysts visualized on CT scan. By definition this is an acquired condition, as opposed to adult polycystic kidney disease (ADPKD) which is inherited (in an autosomal dominant fashion). It is predominantly associated with chronic and end-stage renal failure, and as such is commonly found in patients undergoing haemodialysis or peritoneal dialysis. Over one third of patients develop ARCD after 3 years of dialysis. Clinically important because it may cause pain and haematuria, and is associated with the development of benign and malignant renal tumours. Male:female ratio is 3:1.

Pathology

Usually multiple, bilateral cysts found mainly within the cortex of small, contracted kidneys. Cysts vary in size (average 0.5–1 cm) and are filled with a clear fluid, which may contain oxalate crystals. They usually have cuboidal or columnar epithelial linings, and are in continuity with renal tubules (and, therefore, cannot be defined as simple cysts). Atypical cysts have a hyperplastic lining of epithelial cells, which may represent a precursor for tumour formation. Renal transplantation can cause regression of cysts in the native kidneys.

Aetiology

The exact pathogenesis is unknown, but several theories have been proposed. Obstruction or ischaemia of renal tubules may induce cyst formation. Renal failure may predispose to the accumulation of toxic endogenous substances or metabolites, alter the release of growth factors and result in changes in sex steroid production, or cause cell proliferation (secondary to immunosuppressive effects), which result in cyst formation.

Associated disorders

There is an increased risk of benign and malignant renal tumours. The chance of developing renal cell carcinoma (RCC) is ~20%; 3–6 times greater than the general population (males > females). When on dialysis, RCC usually develops within the first 10 years of treatment.

Presentation

Flank pain; UTI; macroscopic haematuria; renal colic (stone disease); hypertension.

Investigation

This depends on the presenting symptoms.
- **For suspected UTI:** culture urine
- **For haematuria:** urine cytology, flexible cystoscopy, and renal ultrasound. On ultrasound the kidneys are small and hyperechoic, with multiple cysts of varying size, many of which show calcification. If the nature of the cysts cannot be determined with certainty on ultrasound, arrange a renal CT.

Treatment

Persistent macroscopic haematuria can become problematic, exacerbated by heparinization (required for haemodialysis). Options include transferring to peritoneal dialysis, renal embolization, or nephrectomy. Infected cysts, which develop into abscesses, require percutaneous or surgical drainage. Radical nephrectomy is indicated for renal masses with features suspicious of malignancy. Smaller asymptomatic masses require surveillance. Patients with ARCD on long-term dialysis should also be considered for renal surveillance with ultrasonography or CT.

Autosomal dominant polycystic kidney disease (ADPKD)

Definition

An autosomal dominant inherited disorder involving multiple expanding renal parenchymal cysts (📖 see Fig. 8.2).

Epidemiology

Incidence is 0.1–0.5%; 95% are bilateral. ADPKD can affect children and adults, although symptoms usually occur between ages 30–50 years. ADPKD accounts for 10% of all renal failure (which usually manifests at >40 years old).

Pathology

The kidneys reach an enormous size due to multiple fluid-filled cysts and can easily be palpated on abdominal examination. Expansion of the cysts results in ischaemic atrophy of the surrounding renal parenchyma, and obstruction of normal renal tubules. End-stage renal failure occurs around age 50 years.

Associated disorders

10–30% incidence of circle of Willis berry aneurysms (associated with subarachnoid haemorrhage); cysts of the liver (33%), pancreas (10%), and spleen (<5%); mitral valve prolapse; aortic aneurysms, and diverticular disease. Of note, the incidence of renal adenoma is ~20%; however, the risk of renal cell carcinoma (RCC) is the same as the general population.

Aetiology

Two genes have been identified in ADPKD. The PKD1 gene is localized on the short arm of chromosome 16 (16p13.3) and accounts for 90% of cases. The PKD2 gene is on the long arm of chromosome 4 (4q13–23) and causes 10% of cases. A third gene, PKD3 is also implicated. Pathogenesis theories include intrinsic basement membrane abnormalities; tubular epithelial hyperplasia (causing tubular obstruction and basement membrane weakness), and alterations in the supportive extracellular matrix due to defective proteins, all of which may cause cyst formation.

Presentation

Positive family history; palpable abdominal masses; flank pain (due to mass effect, infection, stones, or following acute cystic distension due to haemorrhage or obstruction); macroscopic (and microscopic) haematuria; UTI and hypertension (75%). Renal failure may present with lethargy, nausea, vomiting, anaemia, confusion, and seizures.

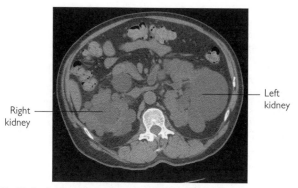

Fig. 8.2 Axial section from a CT scan demonstrating bilateral ADPKD.

Differential diagnosis

Other forms of renal cystic disease (multiple simple cysts; autosomal recessive polycystic kidney disease (ARPKD); familial juvenile nephronophthisis; medullary cystic disease; see p. 648).

Multiple renal cysts are also found in other autosomal dominant conditions. *Tuberous sclerosis* has TSC1 and 2 gene mutations on chromosomes 9 and 16. It presents with adenoma sebaceum, epilepsy, learning difficulties, polycystic kidneys and renal tumours (angiomyolipomas and more rarely RCC). *Von Hippel–Lindau (VHL) syndrome* has a VHL tumour suppressor gene mutation on the short arm of chromosome 3 (3p25), which causes hypoxia-inducible factor (HIF) to increase levels of growth factors (PDGF, TGF-α, VEGF), which can stimulate the formation of haemangioblastomas (cerebellar and retinal) and RCC. VHL syndrome also includes renal, pancreatic, and epididymal cysts, and phaeochromocytoma.

Investigation

This depends on the presenting symptoms.
- **For suspected UTI:** culture urine
- **For haematuria:** urine cytology, flexible cystoscopy, and renal ultrasound. On ultrasound the kidneys are small and hyperechoic, with multiple cysts of varying size, many of which show calcification. If the nature of the cysts cannot be determined with certainty on ultrasound, arrange a renal CT
- Renal failure will be managed by a nephrologist. Anaemia may occur, though ADPKD may cause increased erythropoietin production and polycythaemia
- Renal imaging (ultrasound, CT, and MRI are useful for initial diagnosis and investigation of complications).

Treatment

The aim is to preserve renal function as long as possible (monitor and control hypertension and UTI). Infected cysts (abscesses) should be drained. Persistent, heavy haematuria can be controlled by embolization or nephrectomy. Progressive renal failure requires dialysis, and ultimately renal transplantation.

Due to the high risk of inheritance of ADPKD, off-spring should be offered genetic testing or ultrasound screening.

Vesicoureteric reflux (VUR) in adults

VUR is the retrograde flow of urine from the bladder into the upper urinary tract with or without dilatation of the ureter, renal pelvis, and calyces (also see p. 626). It can cause symptoms and may lead to renal failure (reflux nephropathy).

Pathophysiology

Reflux is normally prevented by low bladder pressures, efficient ureteric peristalsis, and the ability of the vesicoureteric junction (VUJ) to occlude the distal ureter during bladder contraction. This is assisted by the ureters passing obliquely through the bladder wall (the 'intramural' ureter), which is 1–2 cm long. Normal intramural ureteric length to ureteric diameter ratio is 5:1. VUR of childhood tends to resolve spontaneously with increasing age because as the bladder grows, the intramural ureter lengthens.

Classification

Primary: a primary anatomical (and, therefore, functional) defect, where the intramural length of the ureter is too short (ratio <5:1).
Secondary to some other anatomical or functional problem:
- Bladder outlet obstruction (BPO, DSD, posterior urethral valves, urethral stricture), which leads to elevated bladder pressures
- Poor bladder compliance or the intermittently elevated pressures of neuropathic detrusor overactivity (due to neuropathic disorders[1]— e.g. spinal cord injury, spina bifida)
- Iatrogenic reflux following TURP or TURBT; ureteric meatotomy (incision of the ureteric orifice) for removal of ureteric stones at the VUJ; following incision of a ureterocele; ureteroneocystostomy; post pelvic radiotherapy
- Inflammatory conditions affecting function of the VUJ: TB, schistosomiasis, UTI.

Associated disorders

VUR is commonly seen in duplex ureters (the Weigert–Meyer law)[2] and associated with pelviureteric junction (PUJ) obstruction. Cystitis can cause VUR through bladder inflammation, reduced bladder compliance, increased pressures, and distortion of the VUJ. Co-existence of UTI with VUR can cause pyelonephritis. Reflux of infected urine under high pressure may lead to reflux nephropathy, resulting in renal scarring, hypertension, and renal impairment.

Presentation

- VUR may be asymptomatic, being identified during micturating cystourethrography (MCUG), IVU, or renal ultrasound performed for other reasons
- UTI symptoms
- Loin pain associated with a full bladder or immediately after micturition.

Investigation

The definitive test for the diagnosis of VUR is cystography, which may be apparent during bladder filling or during voiding (MCUG). Where clinically indicated, urodynamics establishes the presence of voiding dysfunction. If there is radiographic evidence of reflux nephropathy: check blood pressure, check the urine for proteinuria, measure serum creatinine, and arrange a ^{99m}Tc-DMSA isotope study to assess renal cortical scarring and determine split renal function.

Management

VUR is harmful to the kidney in the presence of infected urine and/or where bladder pressures are markedly elevated (due to severe BOO, poor compliance, or high-pressure overactive bladder contractions). In the absence of these factors, VUR is not harmful, at least in the short term (months). Subsequent management depends on:

- The presence and severity of symptoms
- The presence of recurrent, proven urinary infection
- The presence of already established renal damage, as indicated by radiological evidence of reflux nephropathy, hypertension, impaired renal function, or proteinuria.
- **For the patient with primary VUR**, recurrent UTIs with no symptoms between infections, no hypertension, and good renal function: treat the UTIs when they occur; consider low-dose antibiotic prophylaxis if UTIs occur frequently (>3 per year). If UTIs are regularly associated with systemic symptoms (acute pyelonephritis, rather than uncomplicated cystitis), then ureteric re-implantation is indicated
- **For the patient with primary VUR and objective evidence of deterioration** in the affected kidney: ureteric re-implantation
- **Reflux into a non-functioning kidney** (<10% function on DMSA scan) with recurrent UTIs and/or hypertension: nephro-ureterectomy
- **Primary reflux with severe recurrent loin pain:** ureteric re-implantation
- **Secondary reflux:**
  - *VUR* into a transplanted kidney: no treatment is necessary.
  - *VUR* in association with the neuropathic bladder: treat the underlying cause—relieve BOO, improve bladder compliance (options: intravesical botoxulin toxin injections, augmentation cystoplasty, sacral deafferentation)

---

1 Neuropathic disorders cause VUR because they lead to intermittently or chronically raised bladder pressure (due to bladder outlet obstruction, poor compliance, and/or detrusor overactivity).

2 The lower pole ureter inserts into the bladder in a proximal (and lateral) location to the upper pole ureter, which inserts distally, i.e. nearer the bladder neck. The lower pole ureter has a shorter intramural length and, therefore, refluxes. The upper pole ureter has a longer intramural length and tends to be obstructed. (⎕ see p. 401).

- **VUR with no symptoms, no UTI, no high bladder pressures, and no BOO:** for grades I–II reflux, monitor for infection, hypertension, and evidence of deterioration in the appearance and function of the kidneys. For grades III–V, many urologists would recommend ureteric re-implantation or an endoscopic injection of bulking agent at the ureteric orifice (📖 see Fig. 8.3 for VUR grading).

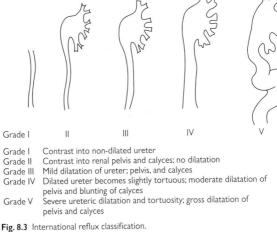

| Grade I | II | III | IV | V |

Grade I   Contrast into non-dilated ureter
Grade II   Contrast into renal pelvis and calyces; no dilatation
Grade III Mild dilatation of ureter; pelvis, and calyces
Grade IV   Dilated ureter becomes slightly tortuous; moderate dilatation of
           pelvis and blunting of calyces
Grade V   Severe ureteric dilatation and tortuosity; gross dilatation of
           pelvis and calyces

Fig. 8.3 International reflux classification.

Pelviureteric junction obstruction (PUJO) in adults

Definition An obstruction of the proximal ureter at the junction with the renal pelvis resulting in a restriction of urine flow (also 📖 see p. 634). Known as 'ureteropelvic junction obstruction'(UPJO) in North America.

Aetiology

Congenital

- **Intrinsic:** smooth muscle defect results in an aperistaltic segment of ureter at the PUJ. The ureter can insert high on the renal pelvis (which may be a primary abnormality or secondary to the pelvic dilatation)
- **Extrinsic:** compression from lower renal pole ('aberrant') vessel over which the PUJ runs. It is unlikely that these vessels are the primary cause of the obstruction. It is more probable that PUJO leads to a dilated PUJ and ballooning of the renal pelvis over the lower pole vessels, which may thus contribute to, but is not the primary cause of the obstruction.

Acquired: PUJ stricture secondary to ureteral manipulation (e.g. ureteroscopy); trauma from passage of calculi; fibro-epithelial polyps; TCC of urothelium at PUJ; external compression of ureter by retroperitoneal fibrosis or malignancy.

Presentation: flank pain precipitated by a diuresis (high fluid intake; especially precipitated by consumption of alcohol); flank mass; UTI; haematuria (after minor trauma). It may also be associated with vesicoureteric reflux (VUR).

Investigation

- **Renal ultrasound** shows renal pelvis dilatation in the absence of a dilated ureter
- **IVU** demonstrates delay of excretion of contrast and a dilated pelvicalyceal system
- **CT** to exclude a small, radiolucent stone, urothelial TCC, or retroperitoneal pathology, which may be the cause of the obstruction at the PUJ
- **MAG3 renography** (with administration of frusemide to establish a maximum diuresis) is the definitive diagnostic test for PUJO. Radioisotope accumulates in the renal pelvis, and following iv frusemide it continues to accumulate (a 'rising' curve)
- **Retrograde pyelography** to establish the exact site of the obstruction – often performed at the time of PUJ repair to avoid introducing infection into an obstructed renal pelvis.

Management

Surgery is indicated for recurrent episodes of bothersome pain, renal impairment, where a stone has developed in the obstructed kidney, and where infection (pyonephrosis) has supervened. In the absence of symptoms, consider watchful waiting with serial MAG3 renograms. If renal function remains stable and the patient remains free of symptoms, there is no need to operate.

Endopyelotomy (or pyelolysis)

A minimally invasive technique to treat PUJO. A full-thickness incision is made through the obstructing proximal ureter, from within the lumen of the ureter down into the peripelvic and peri-ureteral fat, using a sharp knife or Holmium:YAG laser. The incision is stented for 4 weeks to allow re-epithelialization of the PUJ. Generally not used for PUJO >2 cm in length. The incision may be made percutaneously or by a retrograde approach via a rigid or flexible ureteroscope, or by using a specially designed endopyelotomy balloon (the Acucise® technique).[1]

The presence of a combination of PUJO and a renal stone that is suitable for PCNL is an indication for combined PCNL and percutaneous endopyelotomy.

Success rates in terms of relieving obstruction: percutaneous endopyelotomy range from 60–100% (mean 70%); cautery wire balloon endopyelotomy 70%; ureteroscopic endopyelotomy 80%.

Pyeloplasty

- **Open:** has success rates of 95%, and may also be used after endopyelotomy failure or as a first line technique. Common techniques include dismembered pyeloplasty (also known as the Anderson–Hynes pyeloplasty: the narrowed area of PUJ is excised, the proximal ureter is spatulated and anastomosed to the renal pelvis), flap pyeloplasty (Culp), and Y–V-plasty (Foley)
- **Laparoscopic:** dismembered pyeloplasty is most commonly performed, using transperitoneal, retroperitoneal, or robotic-assisted approaches. Success rates are also ~95%.

---

1 An angioplasty-type balloon over which runs a cautery wire is inflated across the PUJ. Passage of an electrical current heats the wire and this cuts through the obstructing ring of tissue at the PUJ.

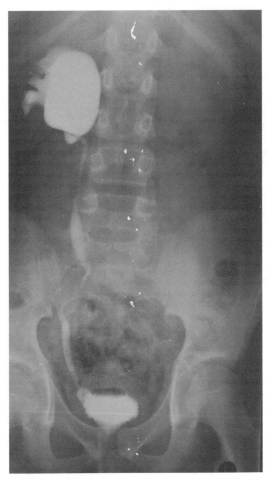

Fig. 8.4 IVU showing PUJO (with reflux and Hutch diverticulum of bladder), and absent left kidney. Image kindly provided with permission from Professor S. Reif.

Anomalies of renal fusion and ascent: horseshoe kidney, ectopic kidney

Abnormalities of renal fusion and ascent occur in weeks 6–9 of gestation, when the embryonic kidney is 'ascending' to its definitive lumbar position in the renal fossa ('ascending' as a result of rapid caudal growth of the embryo).

Horseshoe kidney

Most common example of renal fusion. Prevalence 1 in 400. Male to female ratio 2:1. The kidneys lie vertically (instead of obliquely) and are joined at their lower poles (in 95%) by midline parenchymal tissue (the isthmus). The inferior mesenteric artery obstructs ascent of the isthmus. Consequently, the horseshoe kidney lies lower in the abdomen (L3 or L4 vertebral level). Normal rotation of the kidney is also prevented and therefore the renal pelvis lies anteriorly, with the ureters also passing anteriorly over the kidneys and isthmus (but entering the bladder normally). Blood supply is variable, usually from one or more renal arteries or their branches, or from branches off the aorta or inferior mesenteric artery (📖 see Fig. 8.5).

A proportion of individuals with horseshoe kidneys have associated congenital abnormalities (Turner's syndrome, trisomy 18, genitourinary anomalies, ureteric duplication); vesicoureteric reflux; PUJ obstruction; and renal tumours (including Wilms' tumours).

Most patients with horseshoe kidneys remain asymptomatic; however, infection and calculi may develop and cause symptoms. The diagnosis is usually suggested on renal ultrasound and confirmed by IVU (calyces of the lower renal pole are seen to point medially, and lie medially in relation to the ureters) or CT. Renal function is usually normal.

Ectopic kidney

The kidney fails to achieve its normal position, and may be located in the thorax, abdomen, lumbar (in iliac fossa) or pelvis (on the contralateral side or crossed). The prevalence of renal ectopia is 1 in 900, with both sexes affected equally. The left kidney is affected more often than the right, and bilateral cases are seen in <10%. The affected kidney is smaller, with the renal pelvis positioned anteriorly (instead of medially), and the ureter is short, but enters the bladder normally. Pelvic kidneys occur in 1 in 2000–3000, and lie opposite the sacrum and below the aortic bifurcation, and are supplied by adjacent (aberrant) vessels (📖 see Fig. 8.6). Renal ectopia has an increased risk of congenital anomalies including contralateral renal agenesis and genital malformations.

Most are asymptomatic. Diagnosis is made on renal ultrasound scan, IVU, or renography. Complications include hydronephrosis (secondary to VUR, VUJO, and PUJO), stones and infection.

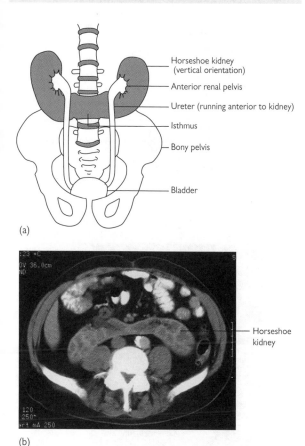

Fig. 8.5 (a) Horseshoe kidney (b) Axial section of a CT scan demonstrating a horseshoe kidney.

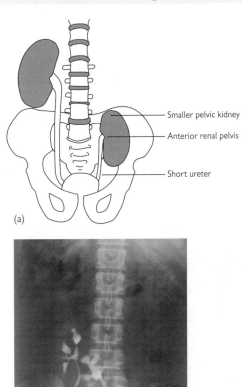

(a)

Smaller pelvic kidney

Anterior renal pelvis

Short ureter

(b)

Fig. 8.6 (a) Ectopic (pelvic) kidney (b) IVU demonstrating ectopic kidneys. Sterilization clips are also seen. Image kindly provided with permission from Prof. S. Reif.

Anomalies of renal number and rotation: renal agenesis and malrotation

Renal agenesis

Unilateral renal agenesis is the absence of one kidney due to embryological abnormality or absence of the ureteric bud. This results in failure of the ureteric bud to contact the metanephric blastema with failed induction of nephrogenesis. The incidence is 1 in 1000; left side > right; males > females. Absence of a kidney may also be caused by involution of a multicystic dysplastic kidney *in utero* or postnatally. Many patients are asymptomatic; however, it is associated with Turner's syndrome, cardiac, respiratory, gastrointestinal and musculoskeletal abnormalities. Associated genitourinary anomalies include absence of the ipsilateral ureter, abnormal trigone, VUR, PUJO, VUJO, uterine abnormalities (unicornuate-one side has failed to develop; bicornuate-partially divided uterus; didelphys—double uterus), vaginal agenesis, anomalies of seminal vesicles, and absence of vas deferens. Often discovered as an incidental finding on ultrasound performed for other reasons, or during investigation of associated abnormalities. Long-term follow-up of renal function, urinalysis and blood pressure should be considered.

Bilateral renal agenesis is rare and incompatible with life. It is associated with complete ureteric atresia, bladder hypoplasia or absence, intra-uterine growth retardation, pulmonary hypoplasia, and oligohydramnios (reduced amniotic fluid) causing characteristic 'Potter' facial features (blunted nose, low-set ears, depression on the chin) and limb abnormalities.

Malrotation

The kidney is located in a normal position, but the renal pelvis fails to rotate to the normal medial orientation. Often seen with horseshoe kidneys and renal ectopia, and associated with Turner's syndrome. The incidence is ~1 in 1000, with a male to female ratio of 2:1. The renal shape may be altered (flattened, oval, triangular or elongated) and the kidney retains its foetal lobulated outline (🕮 see Fig. 8.7). It is associated with increased deposition of fibrous tissue around the renal hilum, which can produce symptoms due to ureteric or PUJ obstruction (causing hydronephrosis, infection or stone formation). Most patients, however, remain asymptomatic. The diagnosis is made on USS, IVU or retrograde pyelography.

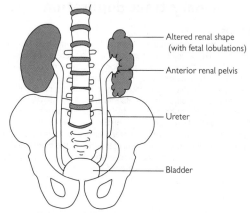

Fig. 8.7 Malrotation of the kidney.

Upper urinary tract duplication

Definitions

A duplex kidney has an upper pole and a lower pole, each with its own separate pelvicalyceal system and ureter. The two ureters may join to form a single ureter at the pelviureteric junction (bifid system; Fig. 8.8) or more distally (bifid ureter) before entering the bladder through one ureteric orifice. Alternatively, the two ureters may pass down individually to the bladder (complete duplication, Fig. 8.9). In this case, the Weigert–Meyer rule states that the upper pole ureter always opens onto the bladder medially and inferiorly to the ureter of the lower pole, thereby predisposing to ectopic placement of the ureteric orifice and obstruction (due to the longer intramural course of the ureter through the bladder wall). The lower pole ureter opens onto the bladder laterally and superiorly, reducing the intramural ureteric length, which predisposes to vesicoureteric reflux (in up to 85%; Fig. 8.10).

Epidemiology

Ureteric duplication occurs in 1 in 125 individuals. Female to male ratio is 2:1. Unilateral cases are more common than bilateral, with right and left sides affected equally. Risk of other congenital malformations is increased.

Embryology

In duplication, two ureteric buds arise from the mesonephric duct (week 4 gestation). The ureteric bud situated more distally (lower pole ureter) enters the bladder first, and so migrates a longer distance, resulting in the superior and lateral position of the ureteric orifice. The proximal bud (upper pole ureter) has less time to migrate, and consequently the ureteric orifice is inferior and medial (ectopic) (refer to p. 630). Interaction of each ureteric bud with the same metanephric tissue creates separate collecting systems within the same renal unit. With bifid ureters, a single ureteric bud splits after it has emerged from the mesonephric duct.

Complications

Ectopic ureters are associated with upper renal pole hydronephrosis (secondary to obstruction), renal hypoplasia or dysplasia (maldevelopment of the kidney correlating with the degree of ectopic displacement of ureteric orifice[1]) and ureteroceles (Fig. 8.8). Lower pole ureters are prone to reflux, resulting in hydroureter and hydronephrosis. Bifid ureters can get urine continuously passing from one collecting system to the other (yo-yo reflux), causing urinary stasis (and predisposing to infection).

Presentation

Symptoms of UTI, flank pain, or incidental finding.

---

1 Mackie GG, Stephens FD (1975). Duplex kidneys: a correlation of renal dysplasia with position of the ureteric orifice. *J Urol* **114**: 274–80.

Investigation

- **Renal ultrasound scan** demonstrates ureteric duplication ± dilatation and hydronephrosis
- **IVU** decreased contrast excretion from renal upper pole ± hydronephrosis (which may displace the lower pole downwards and outwards producing a 'drooping lily' appearance). Contrast in a ureterocele gives the appearance of a 'cobra head' (Fig. 8.8)
- **Micturating cystourethrography** (MCUG) will determine whether reflux is present
- **CT and MRI** reveals detailed anatomical information
- **Isotope renogram (^{99m}Tc-DMSA)** assesses renal function.

Management

Uncomplicated complete or incomplete ureteric duplication does not require any intervention. In symptomatic patients, the aim is to reduce obstruction and reflux, and improve function. Where renal function is reasonable, common sheath ureteric re-implantation (where a cuff of bladder tissue is taken that encompasses both duplicated ureters) can treat both conditions. A poorly functioning renal moiety (i.e. upper pole associated with ectopic ureter and/or reflux, or lower pole associated with a ureterocele) may require heminephrectomy and ureterectomy (see p. 630–2). Where both renal moieties have poor function or dysplasia, nephro-ureterectomy is indicated.

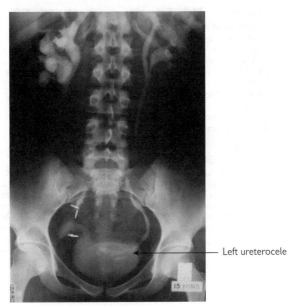

Left ureterocele

Fig. 8.8 IVU demonstrating bilateral (bifid system) renal duplication and a left ureterocele in the bladder ('cobra head' sign).

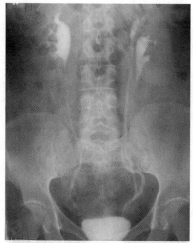

Fig. 8.9 IVU demonstrating complete left-sided renal and ureteric duplication.

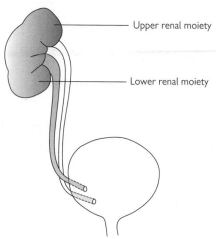

Upper renal moiety

Lower renal moiety

Fig. 8.10 Diagrammatic representation of the Weigert-Meyer rule with complete ureteric duplication.

Stone disease

Kidney stones: epidemiology

~10% of Caucasian men will develop a kidney stone by the age of 70. Within 1 year of a calcium oxalate stone, 10% of men will form another calcium oxalate stone, and 50% will have formed another stone within 10 years. The prevalence of renal tract stone disease is determined by factors *intrinsic* to the individual and by *extrinsic* (environmental) factors. A combination of factors often contribute to risk of stone formation.

Intrinsic factors

- **Age**: the peak incidence of stones occurs between the ages of 20–50 years
- **Sex**: males are affected 3 times as frequently as females. Testosterone may cause increased oxalate production in the liver (predisposing to calcium oxalate stones) and women have higher urinary citrate concentrations (citrate inhibits calcium oxalate stone formation)
- **Genetic**: kidney stones are relatively uncommon in Native Americans, Black Africans, and US Blacks, and more common in Caucasians and Asians. ~25% of patients with kidney stones report a family history of stone disease (the relative risk of stone formation remaining high after adjusting for dietary calcium intake). Familial renal tubular acidosis (predisposing to calcium phosphate stones) and cystinuria (predisposing to cystine stones) are inherited.[1]

Extrinsic (environmental) factors

- **Geographical location, climate, and season:** the relationship between these factors and stone risk is complex. While renal stone disease is more common in hot climates, some endogenous populations of hot climates have a low incidence of stones (e.g. Black Africans, Aborigines) and many temperate areas have a high incidence of stones (e.g. Northern Europe and Scandinavia). This may relate to Western lifestyle—excess food, inadequate fluid intake, limited exercise—combined with a genetic predisposition to stone formation
- **Ureteric stones become more prevalent during the summer:** the highest incidence occurs a month or so after peak summertime temperatures, presumably because of higher urinary concentration in the summer (encourages crystallization). Concentrated urine has a lower pH, encouraging cystine and uric acid stone formation. Exposure to sunlight may also increase endogenous vitamin D production, leading to hypercalciuria
- **Water intake**: low fluid intake (<1200 mL/day) predisposes to stone formation.[2] Increasing water 'hardness' (high calcium content) may reduce risk of stone formation, by decreasing urinary oxalate

- **Diet**: high animal protein intake increases risk of stone disease (high urinary oxalate, low pH, low urinary citrate).[3,4] High salt intake causes hypercalciuria. Contrary to conventional teaching, low calcium diets predispose to calcium stone disease, and high calcium intake is protective[5]
- **Occupation**: sedentary occupations predispose to stones compared with manual workers.[1]

1 Curhan GC, Willett WC, Rimm EB, Stampfer MJ (1997) Family history and risk of kidney stones. *J Am Soc Nephrol*, **8**:1568–73.

2 Borghi L, et al. (1996) Urinary volume, water and recurrences in idiopathic calcium nephrolithiasis: a 5-year randomized prospective study. *J Urol* **155**:839–43.

3 Curhan GC, et al. (1997) Comparison of dietary calcium with supplemental calcium and other nutrients as factors affecting the risk for kidney stones in women. *Ann Int Med* **126**:497–504.

4 Borghi L, et al. (2002) Comparison of 2 diets for the prevention of recurrent stones in idiopathic hypercalciuria. *N Engl J Med* **346**:77–84.

5 Curhan GC, et al. (1993) A prospective study of dietary calcium and other nutrients and the risk of symptomatic kidney stones. *N Engl J Med* **328**:833–8.

Kidney stones: types and predisposing factors

Stones may be classified according to composition, X-ray appearance, or size and shape.

Composition

Stone composition	% of all renal calculi[1]
Calcium oxalate	85%
Uric acid[2]	5–10%
Calcium phosphate + calcium oxalate	10%
Pure calcium phosphate	Rare
Struvite (infection stones)	2–20%
Cystine	1%

Other rare stone types (all of which are radiolucent): indinavir (a protease inhibitor used for treatment of HIV); triamterene (a relatively insoluble potassium sparing diuretic, most of which is excreted in urine); xanthine.

Radiodensity on X-ray

Three broad categories of stones are described, based on their X-ray appearance. This gives some indication of the likely stone composition and helps, to some extent, to determine treatment options. However, in only 40% of cases is stone composition correctly identified from visual estimation of radiodensity on plain X-ray.[3]

Radio-opaque

Opacity implies the presence of substantial amounts of calcium within the stone. Calcium phosphate stones are the most radiodense stones, being almost as dense as bone. Calcium oxalate stones are slightly less radiodense.

Relatively radiolucent

Cystine stones are relatively radiodense because they contain sulphur (Fig. 9.1). Magnesium ammonium phosphate (struvite) stones are less radiodense than calcium containing stones.

Completely radiolucent

Uric acid, triamterene, xanthine, indinavir (cannot be seen even on CTU).

Size and shape

Stones can be characterized by their size, in centimetres. Stones which grow to occupy the renal collecting system (the pelvis and one or more renal calyx) are known as staghorn calculi, since they resemble the horns of a stag (Fig. 9.2). They are most commonly composed of struvite—magnesium ammonium phosphate—(being caused by infection and forming under the alkaline conditions induced by urea-splitting bacteria), but may be composed of uric acid, cystine, or calcium oxalate monohydrate.

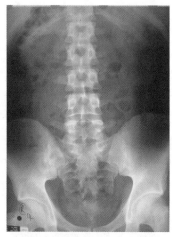

Fig. 9.1 A left cystine stone, barely visible just below the midpoint of the 12th rib.

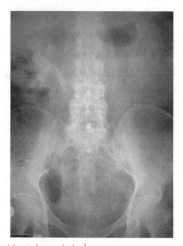

Fig. 9.2 A large, right staghorn calculus.[1]

1 The precise distribution of stone types will vary depending on the characteristics of the study population (geographical location, racial distribution, etc.). Hence, the quoted figures do not equate to 100.

2 80% of uric acid stones are pure uric acid, and 20% contain some calcium oxalate as well.

3 Ramakumar S, Patterson DE, LeRoy AJ, et al. (1999) Prediction of stone composition from plain radiographs: a prospective study. *J Endo Urol* **13**:397–401.

Kidney stones: mechanisms of formation

Urine is said to be saturated with, for example, calcium and oxalate, when the product of the concentrations of calcium and oxalate exceeds the solubility product (K_{sp}). Below the solubility product, crystals of calcium and oxalate will not form and the urine is said to be undersaturated. Above the solubility product, crystals of calcium and oxalate should form, but they do not because of the presence of *inhibitors* of crystal formation. However, above a certain concentration of calcium and oxalate, inhibitors of crystallization become ineffective, and crystals of calcium oxalate start to form. The concentration of calcium and oxalate at which this is reached (i.e. at which crystallization starts) is known as the *formation product* (K_f) and the urine is said to be *supersaturated* with the substance or substances in question at concentrations above this level. Urine is described as being *metastable* for calcium and oxalate at concentrations between the solubility product of calcium and oxalate and the formation product (📖 see Box 9.1).

The ability of urine to hold more solute in solution than can pure water is due partly to the presence of various inhibitors of crystallization (e.g. citrate forms a soluble complex with calcium, preventing it from combining with oxalate or phosphate to form calcium oxalate or calcium phosphate stones). Other inhibitors of crystallization include magnesium, glycosaminoglycans, and Tamm–Horsfall protein.

Periods of intermittent supersaturation of urine with various substances can occur as a consequence of dehydration and following meals.

The earliest phase of crystal formation is known as nucleation. Crystal nuclei usually form on the surfaces of epithelial cells or on other crystals. Crystal nuclei form into clumps—a process known as aggregation. Citrate and magnesium not only inhibit crystallization but also inhibit aggregation.

Box 9.1 Steps leading to stone formation

- Calcium and oxalate concentration < solubility product → NO STONE FORMATION
- Metastable calcium and oxalate concentrations → NO STONE FORMATION
- Calcium and oxalate concentrations > formation product → STONE FORMATION.

In the urine of subjects who do not form stones, the concentrations of most stone components are between K_{sp} and K_f.

Factors predisposing to specific stone types

Calcium oxalate (~85% of stones)

Hypercalciuria: excretion of >7 mmol of calcium per day in men and >6 mmol per day in women. A major risk factor for calcium oxalate stone formation: it increases the relative supersaturation of urine. About 50% of patients with calcium stone disease have hypercalciuria. 3 types:

- **Absorptive:** increased intestinal absorption of calcium
- **Renal:** renal leak of calcium
- **Resorptive:** increased demineralization of bone (due to hyperparathyroidism).

Hypercalcaemia: almost all patients with hypercalcaemia who form stones have primary hyperparathyroidism. Of hyperparathyroid patients, about 1% form stones (the other 99% do not because of early detection of hyperparathyroidism by screening serum calcium).

Hyperoxaluria: due to:

- Altered membrane transport of oxalate leading to increased renal leak of oxalate
- **Primary hyperoxaluria:** increased hepatic oxalate production; rare
- Increased oxalate absorption in short bowel syndrome or malabsorption (enteric hyperoxaluria)—the colon is exposed to more bile salts and this increases its permeability to oxalate.

Hypocitraturia: low urinary citrate excretion. Citrate forms a soluble complex with calcium, so preventing complexing of calcium with oxalate to form calcium oxalate stones.

Hyperuricosuria: high urinary uric acid levels lead to formation of uric acid crystals, on the surface of which calcium oxalate crystals form.

Uric acid (~5–10% of stones)

Humans are unable to convert uric acid (which is relatively insoluble) into allantoin (which is very soluble). Human urine is supersaturated with insoluble uric acid. Uric acid exists in 2 forms in urine—uric acid and sodium urate. Sodium urate is 20 times more soluble than uric acid. At a urine pH of 5, <20% of uric acid is present as soluble sodium urate. At urine pH 5.5, half the uric acid is ionized as sodium urate (soluble) and half is non-ionized as free uric acid (insoluble). At a urine pH of 6.5, >90% of uric acid is present as soluble sodium urate. Thus, uric acid is essentially insoluble in acid urine and soluble in alkaline urine. Human urine is acidic (because the end products of metabolism are acid) and this low pH, combined with supersaturation of urine with uric acid, predisposes to uric acid stone formation.

~20% of patients with gout have uric acid stones. Patients with uric acid stones may have:

- **Gout:** 50% of patients with uric acid stones have gout. The chance of forming a uric acid stone if you have gout is in the order of 1% per year from the time of the first attack of gout

- **Myeloproliferative disorders:** particularly following treatment with cytotoxic drugs, cell necrosis results in release of large quantities of nucleic acids which are converted to uric acid. A large plug of uric acid crystals may form in the collecting system of the kidney, in the absence of ureteric colic, causing oliguria or anuria
- **Idiopathic uric acid stones:** (no associated condition).

Calcium phosphate (calcium phosphate + calcium oxalate = 10% of stones)

Occur in patients with renal tubular acidosis (RTA)—a defect of renal tubular H^+ secretion resulting in impaired ability of the kidney to acidify urine. The urine is therefore of high pH, and the patient has a metabolic acidosis. The high urine pH increases supersaturation of the urine with calcium and phosphate, leading to their precipitation as stones.

Types of renal tubular acidosis
- **Type 1 or distal RTA:** the distal tubule is unable to maintain a proton gradient between the blood and the tubular fluid. 70% of such patients have stones. Urine pH is >5.5, the patient has a metabolic acidosis and hypokalaemia, urinary citrate is low, and hypercalciuria is present
- **Type 2 or proximal RTA:** due to failure of bicarbonate resorption in the proximal tubule. There is associated increased urinary citrate excretion, which protects against stone formation
- **Type 3:** a variant of type 1 RTA
- **Type 4:** seen in diabetic nephropathy and interstitial renal disease. These patients do not make stones.

If urine pH is >5.5, use the ammonium chloride loading test. Urine pH that remains above 5.5 after an oral dose of ammonium chloride = incomplete distal RTA.

Struvite (infection or triple phosphate stones) (2–20% of stones)

These stones are composed of magnesium, ammonium, and phosphate. They form as a consequence of urease-producing bacteria which produce ammonia from breakdown of urea (urease hydrolyses urea to carbon dioxide and ammonium), and in so doing alkalinize urine as in the following equation:

$$NH_2-O-NH_2 + H_2O \rightarrow 2NH_3 + CO_2$$

Under alkaline conditions, crystals of magnesium, ammonium, and phosphate precipitate.

Cystine (1% of all stones)

Occur only in patients with cystinuria—an inherited (autosomal-recessive) disorder of transmembrane cystine transport, resulting in decreased absorption of cystine from the intestine and in the proximal tubule of the kidney. Cystine is very insoluble, so reduced absorption of cystine from the proximal tubule results in supersaturation with cystine and cystine crystal formation. Cystine is poorly soluble in acid urine (300 mg/L at pH 5, 400 mg/L at pH 7).

Evaluation of the stone former

Determination of stone type and a metabolic evaluation allows identification of the factors that led to stone formation, so advice can be given to prevent future stone formation.

Metabolic evaluation depends, to an extent, on the stone type (☐ see Table 9.1). In many cases a stone is retrieved. Stone type is analysed by polarizing microscopy, X-ray diffraction, and infrared spectroscopy, rather than by chemical analysis. Where no stone is retrieved, its nature must be inferred from its radiological appearance (e.g. a completely radiolucent stone is likely to be composed of uric acid) or from more detailed metabolic evaluation.

In most patients, multiple factors are involved in the genesis of kidney stones and, as a general guide, the following evaluation is appropriate in most patients.

Risk factors for stone disease

- **Diet.:** enquire about volume of fluid intake, meat consumption (causes hypercalciuria, high uric acid levels, low urine pH, low urinary citrate), multivitamins (vitamin D increases intestinal calcium absorption), high doses of vitamin C (ascorbic acid causes hyperoxaluria)
- **Drugs:** corticosteroids (increase enteric absorption of calcium, leading to hypercalciuria); chemotherapeutic agents (breakdown products of malignant cells leads to hyperuricaemia)
- **Urinary tract infection:** urease-producing bacteria (*Proteus*, *Klebsiella*, *Serratia*, *Enterobacter*) predispose to struvite stones
- **Mobility:** low activity levels predispose to bone demineralization and hypercalciuria
- **Systemic disease:** gout, primary hyperparathyroidism, sarcoidosis
- **Family history:** cystinuria, RTA
- **Renal anatomy:** PUJO, horseshoe kidney, medullary sponge kidney (up to 2% of patients with calcium-containing stones have MSK)
- **Previous bowel resection or inflammatory bowel disease:** causes intestinal hyperoxaluria.

Metabolic evaluation of the stone former

Patients can be categorized as low risk and high risk for subsequent stone formation. High risk: previous history of a stone, family history of stones, GI disease, gout, chronic UTI, nephrocalcinosis.

Low-risk patient evaluation

Urea and electrolytes, FBC (to detect undiagnosed haematological malignancy), serum calcium (corrected for serum albumin), and uric acid, urine culture, urine dipstick for pH (☐ see p. 413).

High-risk patient evaluation

As for low-risk patients plus 24-h urine for calcium, oxalate, uric acid, cystine; evaluation for RTA.

Table 9.1 Characteristics of stone types

Stone type	Urine acidity	Mean urine pH (SEM)
Calcium oxalate	Variable	6 ($\pm$0.4)
Calcium phosphate	Tendency towards alkaline urine	>5.5
Uric acid	Acid	5.5 ($\pm$0.4)
Struvite	Alkaline*	–
Cystine	Normal (5–7)	–

* Urine pH must be above 7.2 for deposition of struvite crystals.

Urine pH

Urine pH in normal individuals shows variation, from pH 5–7. After a meal, pH is initially acid because of acid production from metabolism of purines (nucleic acids in, for example, meat). This is followed by an 'alkaline tide', pH rising to >6.5. Urine pH can help establish what type of stone the patient may have (if a stone is not available for analysis), and can help the urologist and patient in determining whether preventative measures are likely to be effective or not.

• pH <6 in a patient with radiolucent stones suggests the presence of uric acid stones
• pH consistently >5.5 suggests type 1 (distal) RTA (~70% of such patients will form calcium phosphate stones).

Evaluation for RTA

Evaluate for RTA if: calcium phosphate stones, bilateral stones, nephrocalcinosis, MSK, hypocitraturia.

• If fasting morning urine pH (i.e. first urine of the day) is >5.5, the patient has complete distal RTA
• First and second morning urine pH is a useful screening test for detection of incomplete distal RTA, over 90% of cases of RTA having a pH >6 on both specimens. The ammonium chloride loading test involves an oral dose of ammonium chloride (0.1g per kg; an acid load). If serum pH falls <7.3 or serum bicarbonate falls <16mmol/l, but urine pH remains >5.5, the patient has incomplete distal RTA.

Diagnostic tests for suspected cystinuria

Cyanide-nitroprusside colorimetric test ('cystine spot test'): if positive, a 24-h urine collection is done. A 24-h cystine >250 mg is diagnostic of cystinuria.[1]

Further reading

Millman S, Strauss AL, Parks JH, Coe FL (1982) Pathogenesis and clinical course of mixed calcium oxalate and uric acid nephrolithiasis. *Kidney Int* **22**:366–70.

Kidney stones: presentation and diagnosis

Kidney stones may present with symptoms or be found incidentally during investigation of other problems. Presenting symptoms include pain or haematuria (microscopic or occasionally macroscopic). Struvite staghorn calculi classically present with recurrent UTIs. Malaise, weakness, and loss of appetite can also occur. Less commonly, struvite stones present with infective complications (pyonephrosis, perinephric abscess, septicaemia, xanthogranulomatous pyelonephritis).

Diagnostic tests

- **Plain abdominal radiography:** calculi that contain calcium are radiodense. Sulphur-containing stones (cystine) are relatively radiolucent on plain radiography
- Radiodensity of stones in decreasing order: calcium phosphate > calcium oxalate > struvite (magnesium ammonium phosphate) >> cystine
- Completely radiolucent stones (e.g. uric acid, triamterene, indinavir) are usually suspected on the basis of the patient's history and/or urine pH (pH <6—gout; drug history—triamterene, indinavir), and the diagnosis may be confirmed by ultrasound, CTU, or MRU
- **Renal ultrasound:** its sensitivity for detecting renal calculi is ~95%[1] A combination of plain abdominal radiography and renal ultrasonography is a useful screening test for renal calculi
- **IVU:** increasingly being replaced by CTU. Useful for patients with suspected indinavir stones (which are not visible on CT)
- **CTU:** a very accurate method of diagnosing all but indinavir stones. Allows accurate determination of stone size and location and good definition of pelvicalyceal anatomy
- **MRU:** cannot visualize stones, but is able to demonstrate the presence of hydronephrosis.

1 Haddad MC, Sharif HS, Abomelha ME, *et al.* (1992) Management of renal colic: redefining the role of the urogram. *Radiology* **184**:35–6.

Kidney stone treatment options: watchful waiting

The traditional indications for intervention are pain, infection, and obstruction. Haematuria caused by a stone is only very rarely severe or frequent enough to be the only reason to warrant treatment.

Before embarking on treatment of a stone which you think is the cause of the patient's pain or infections, warn them that though you may be able to remove the stone successfully, their pain or infections may persist (i.e. the stone may be coincidental to their pain or infections, which may be due to something else). Remember, UTIs are common in women, as are stones, and it is not therefore surprising that the two may co-exist in the same patient, but be otherwise unrelated.

Options for stone treatment are watchful waiting, ESWL, flexible ureteroscopy, PCNL, open surgery, and medical 'dissolution' therapy.

When to watch and wait—and when not to

It is not necessary to treat every kidney stone. As a rule of thumb, the younger the patient, the larger the stone, and the more symptoms it is causing, the more inclined are we to recommend treatment. Thus, one would be inclined to do nothing about a 1-cm symptomless stone in the kidney of a 95-year-old patient. On the other hand, a 1-cm stone in a symptomless 20-year-old runs the risk over the remaining (many) years of the patient's life of causing problems. It could drop into the ureter causing ureteric colic, or it could increase in size and affect kidney function or cause pain.

Asymptomatic stones that are followed over a 3-year period are more likely to require intervention (surgery or ESWL) or to increase in size or cause pain if they are >4 mm in diameter and if they are located in a middle or lower pole calyx.[1] The approximate risks, over 3 years of follow-up, of requiring intervention, of developing pain, or of increase in stone size, relative to stone size, is shown in Table 9.2.

Another factor determining the need for treatment is the patient's job. Airline pilots are not allowed to fly if they have kidney stones, for fear that the stones could drop into the ureter at 30,000 ft, with disastrous consequences! They will only be deemed fit to fly when they are radiologically stone free. It is sensible to warn any one whose job entrusts them with the safety of others (pilots, train drivers, drivers of buses and lorries) that they are not fit to carry out these occupations until stone free, or at the very least that they should contact the relevant regulatory authority to seek guidance (the CAA, Civil Aviation Authority for pilots and the DVLA, Drivers Vehicle Licensing Agency for drivers).[2]

Some stones are definitely not suitable for watchful waiting. Untreated struvite (i.e. infection related) staghorn calculi will eventually destroy the kidney if untreated and are a significant risk to the patient's life. Watchful waiting is therefore NOT recommended for staghorn calculi unless patient co-morbidity is such that surgery would be a higher risk than watchful waiting. Historical series suggest that ~30% of patients with staghorn calculi who did not undergo surgical removal died of renal related causes—renal failure, urosepsis (septicaemia, pyonephrosis, perinephric abscess).[3,4] Combination of a neurogenic bladder and staghorn calculus seems to be particularly associated with a poor outcome.[5]

Table 9.2 Approximate 3-year risk of intervention, pain, or increase in stone size

	Stone size			
	<5 mm	5–10 mm	11–15 mm	>15 mm
% Requiring intervention	20%	25%	40%	30%
% Causing pain	40%	40%	40%	60%
% Increasing in size	50%	55%	60%	70%

1 Burgher A *et al.* (2004) Progression of nephrolithiasis: long-term outcomes with observation of asymptomatic calculi *J Endourol* 18:534–9.

2 Borley NC, Rainford D, Anson KM, Watkin N. (2007) What activities are safe with kidney stones? A review of occupational and travel advice in the UK. *Br J Urol Int* **99**:494–6.

3 Blandy JP, Singh M (1976) The case for a more aggressive approach to staghorn stones. *J Urol* **115**:505–6.

4 Rous SN and Turner WR (1977) Retrospective study of 95 patients with staghorn calculus disease. *J Urol* **118**:902.

5 Teichmann J (1995) Long-term renal fate and prognosis after staghorn calculus management. *J Urol* **153**:1403–7.

Stone fragmentation techniques: extracorporeal lithotripsy (ESWL)

The technique of focusing externally generated shock waves at a target (the stone). First used in humans in 1980. The first commercial lithotriptor, the Dornier HM3, became available in 1983.[1] ESWL revolutionized kidney and ureteric stone treatment.

Three methods of shock wave generation are commercially available—electrohydraulic, electromagnetic, and piezoelectric.

Electrohydraulic: application of a high voltage electrical current between 2 electrodes about 1 mm apart under water causes discharge of a spark. Water around the tip of the electrode is vaporized by the high temperature resulting in a rapidly expanding gas bubble. The rapid expansion and then the rapid collapse of this bubble generates a shock wave that is focused by a metal reflector shaped as a hemi-ellipsoid. Used in the original Dornier HM3 lithotriptor.

Electromagnetic: two electrically conducting cylindrical plates are separated by a thin membrane of insulating material. Passage of an electrical current through the plates generates a strong magnetic field between them, the subsequent movement of which generates a shock wave. An 'acoustic' lens is used to focus the shock wave.

Piezoelectric: A spherical dish is covered with about 3000 small ceramic elements, each of which expands rapidly when a high voltage is applied across them. This rapid expansion generates a shock wave.

X-ray, ultrasound, or a combination of both are used to locate the stone on which the shock waves are focused. Older machines required general or regional anaesthesia because the shock waves were powerful and caused severe pain. Newer lithotriptors generate less powerful shock waves, allowing ESWL with oral or parenteral analgesia in many cases, but they are less efficient at stone fragmentation.

Efficacy of ESWL

Likelihood of fragmentation with ESWL depends on stone size and location, anatomy of renal collecting system, degree of obesity, and stone composition. Most effective for stones <2 cm in diameter, in favourable anatomical locations. Less effective for stones >2 cm diameter, in lower pole stones in a calyceal diverticulum (poor drainage), and those composed of cystine or calcium oxalate monohydrate (very hard).

Randomized studies show that a lower shock wave rate (60 vs. 120 per min) achieves better stone fragmentation and clearance. Animal studies also demonstrate less renal injury and a smaller decrease in renal blood flow from lower shock wave rates.

Stone free rates for solitary kidney stones are 80% for stones <1 cm in diameter, 60% for those between 1–2 cm, and 50% for those >2 cm in diameter. Lower stone free rates as compared with open surgery or PCNL are accepted because of the minimal morbidity of ESWL.

There have been no randomized studies comparing stone free rates between different lithotriptors. In non-randomized studies, rather surprisingly, when it comes to efficacy of stone fragmentation, older (the original Dornier HM3 machine) is better (but higher requirement for analgesia and sedation or general anaesthesia). Less powerful (modern) lithotriptors have lower stone free rates and higher retreatment rates.

Side-effects of ESWL

ESWL causes a certain amount of structural and functional renal damage (found more frequently the harder you look). Haematuria (microscopic, macroscopic) and oedema are common, perirenal haematomas less so (0.5% detected on ultrasound with modern machines, although reported in as many as 30% with the Dornier HM3). Effective renal plasma flow (measured by renography) has been reported to fall in ~30% of treated kidneys. There is data suggesting that ESWL may increase the likelihood of development of hypertension. Acute renal injury may be more likely to occur in patients with pre-existing hypertension, prolonged coagulation time, coexisting coronary heart disease, diabetes, and in those with solitary kidneys. There is debate about whether or not ESWL causes pancreatic damage, leading to a higher risk of diabetes.

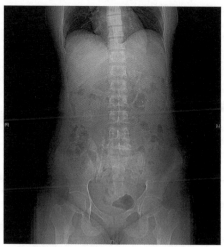

Fig. 9.3 Side-effects of ESWL: Steinstrasse (=Stone street) or 'Log-jam'.

When ESWL was first introduced, stones of all sizes were treated. It soon became apparent that multiple fragments from large stones could obstruct the ureter causing—a so-called steinstrasse. We nowadays see steinstrasse only rarely because ESWL tends to be reserved for smaller stones (<2 cm), and PCNL for larger stones.

An RCT[1] has shown that stenting prior to ESWL reduces the risk of steinstrasse (6% incidence) in stones measuring 1.5–3.5 cm diameter when compared with versus no stent (12%; incidence of steinstrasse 2.6% for stones 1.5–2 cm diameter; 56% for stones 3–3.5 cm). However, the chances of spontaneous resolution (50%) of the steinstrasse (spontaneous passage of the stones) did not differ significantly in those with or without a stent.

Steinstrasse is managed expectantly (since 50% will resolve spontaneously), with ESWL of the so-called 'lead' fragment of ureteroscopy (and only occasionally open ureterolithotomy) being required where the stones fail to pass.

Contraindications to ESWL

Absolute contraindications: pregnancy, uncorrected blood clotting disorders (including anticoagulation).

BAUS procedure-specific consent form: potential complications after ESWL

Common
- Bleeding on passing urine for short period after procedure
- Pain in the kidney as small fragments of stone pass after fragmentation
- UTI from bacteria released from the stone, needing antibiotic treatment.

Occasional
- Stone will not break as too hard, requiring an alternative treatment
- Repeated ESWL treatments may be required
- Recurrence of stones.

Rare
- Kidney damage (bruising) or infection, needing further treatment
- Stone fragments occasionally get stuck in the tube between the kidney and the bladder requiring hospital attendance, and sometimes surgery to remove the stone fragment
- Severe infection requiring intravenous antibiotics and sometimes drainage of the kidney by a small drain placed through the back into the kidney.

Alternative therapy

Telescopic surgery, open surgery, or observation to allow spontaneous passage.[1]

1 Chaussy CG, Brendel W, Schmidt E (1980) Extracorporeal induced destruction of kidney stones by shock waves. *Lancet* **2**:1265–8.

Intracorporeal techniques of stone fragmentation (fragmentation within the body)

Electrohydraulic lithotripsy (EHL)

The first technique developed for intracorporeal lithotripsy. A high voltage applied across a concentric electrode under water generates a spark. This vaporizes water, and the subsequent expansion and collapse of the gas bubble generates a shock wave. An effective form of stone fragmentation. The shock wave is not focused, so the EHL probe must be applied within 1 mm of the stone to optimize stone fragmentation.

EHL has a narrower safety margin than pneumatic, ultrasonic, or laser lithotripsy, and should be kept as far away as possible from the wall of the ureter, renal pelvis, or bladder to limit damage to these structures, and at least 2 mm away from the cystoscope, ureteroscope, or nephroscope to prevent lens fracture.

Principal uses: Bladder stones (wider safety margin than in the narrower ureter).

Pneumatic (ballistic) lithotripsy

A metal projectile contained within the handpiece is propelled backwards and forwards at great speed by bursts of compressed air (🕮 see Fig. 9.4a). It strikes a long, thin, metal probe at one end of the handpiece at 12 Hz (12 strikes/s) transmitting shock waves to the probe, which when in contact with a rigid structure such as a stone, fragments the stone. Used for stone fragmentation in the ureter (using a thin probe to allow insertion down a ureteroscope) or kidney (a thicker probe may be used, with an inbuilt suction device—'Lithovac'—to remove stone fragments).

Pneumatic lithotripsy is very safe since the excursion of the end of probe is about a millimetre and it bounces off the pliable wall of the ureter. Ureteric perforation is therefore rare. Also low cost and low maintenance. However, its ballistic effect has a tendency to cause stone migration into the proximal ureter or renal pelvis, where the stone may be inaccessible to further treatment. The metal probe cannot bend around corners, so it cannot be used for ureteroscopic treatment of stones within the kidney.

Principal uses: ureteric stones.

Ultrasonic lithotripsy

An electrical current applied across a piezoceramic plate located in the ultrasound transducer generates ultrasound waves of a specific frequency (23,000–25,000 Hz). The ultrasound energy is transmitted to a hollow metal probe, which in turn is applied to the stone (🕮 see Fig. 9.4b). The stone resonates at high frequency and this causes it to break into small fragments (the opera singer breaking a glass) which are then sucked out through the centre of the hollow probe. Soft tissues do not resonate when the probe is applied to them, and therefore are not damaged. Can only be used down straight instruments.

Principal uses: Fragmentation of renal calculi during PCNL.

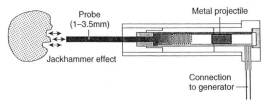

Fig. 9.4a The Lithoclast: a pneumatic lithotripsy device. (Reproduced with permission from Walsh et al. 2002).[1]

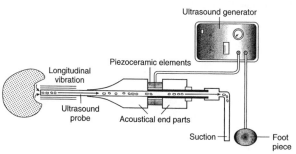

Fig. 9.4b The Calcuson: an ultrasonic lithotripsy device. (Reproduced with permission from Walsh et al. 2002).[1]

1 Walsh PC, Retik AB, Vaughan D, et al. (2002) *Campbell's Urology*, 8th edn. Amsterdam: W.B. Saunders/Elsevier, p. 3395–7.

Laser lithotripsy

The holmium: YAG laser. Principally, a photothermal mechanism of action, causing stone vaporization. Minimal shock-wave generation, and therefore less risk of causing stone migration. The laser energy is delivered down fibres which vary in diameter from 200 to 360 μ. The 200-μ fibre is very flexible and can be used to gain access to stones even within the lower pole of the kidney (□ see Figs. 9.5 and 9.6). A 275-μ fibre delivers more laser energy at the expense of a reduction in flexibility and therefore a reduced chance of lower pole access. Zone of thermal injury is limited from 0.5 to 1 mm from the laser tip. No stone can withstand the heat generated by the Ho:YAG laser. Laser lithotripsy takes time, however, since the thin laser fibre must be 'painted' over the surface of the stone to vaporize it.

Principal uses: Ureteric stones, small intrarenal stones.

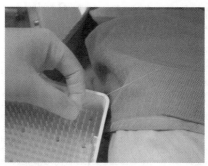

Fig. 9.5 A laser fibre.

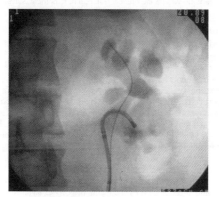

Fig. 9.6 Access to the lower pole of the kidney with a flexible ureteroscope.

Kidney stone treatment: flexible ureteroscopy and laser treatment

The development of small-calibre ureteroscopes with active deflecting mechanisms and instrument channels, in combination with the development of laser technology, small-diameter laser fibres, and stone baskets and graspers, has opened the way for intracorporeal, endoscopic treatment of kidney stones. Access to virtually the entire collecting system is possible with modern instruments. The holmium: YAG laser has a minimal effect on tissues at distances of 2–3 mm from the laser tip and so 'colateral' tissue damage is minimal with this laser type.

Flexible ureteroscopy and laser fragmentation offers a more effective treatment option compared with ESWL, with a lower morbidity than PCNL, but usually requires a general anaesthetic (some patients will tolerate it with sedation alone). It can also allow access to areas of the kidney where ESWL is less efficient or where PCNL cannot reach. It is most suited to stones <2 cm in diameter.

Indications for flexible ureteroscopic kidney stone treatment

- ESWL failure
- Lower pole stone (reduces likelihood of stone passage post ESWL—fragments have to pass 'uphill')
- Cystine stones
- Obesity such that PCNL access is technically difficult or impossible (nephroscopes may not be long enough to reach stone)
- Obesity such that ESWL is technically difficult or impossible. BMI >28 is associated with lower ESWL success rates. Treatment distance may exceed focal length of lithotriptor
- Musculoskeletal deformities such that stone access by PCNL or ESWL is difficult or impossible (e.g. kyphoscoliosis)
- Stone in a calyceal diverticulum (accessing stones in small diverticulae in upper and anterior calyces is difficult and carries significant risks)
- Stenosis of a calyceal infundibulum or 'tight' angle between renal pelvis and infundibulum. The flexible ureteroscope can negotiate acute angles and the laser can be used to divide obstructions
- Bleeding diathesis where reversal of this diathesis is potentially dangerous or difficult
- Horseshoe or pelvic kidney. ESWL fragmentation rates are only 50% in such cases[1] due to difficulties of shock-wave transmission through overlying organs (bowel). PCNL for such kidneys is difficult because of bowel proximity and variable blood supply (blood supply derived from multiple sources)
- Patient preference.

Disadvantages

Efficacy diminishes as stone burden increases—it simply takes a long time to 'paint' the surface of the stone with laser energy, so destroying it. A dust-cloud is produced as the stone fragments and this temporarily obscures the view, until it has been washed away by irrigation. Stone fragmentation rates for those expert in flexible ureteroscopy are ~70–80% for stones <2 cm in diameter and 50% for those >2 cm in diameter[2] and ~10% of patients will require 2 or more treatment sessions.[2]

1   Kupeli B, Isen K, Biri H, et al. (1999) Extracorporeal shockwave lithotripsy in anomalous kidneys. J Endourol 13:39–52.

2   Dasgupta P, et al. (2004) Flexible ureterorenoscopy: prospective analysis of the Guy's experience. Annals of the Royal College of Surgeons 86:367–70.

Kidney stone treatment: percutaneous nephrolithotomy (PCNL)

Technique

PCNL is the removal of a kidney stone via a 'track' developed between the surface of the skin and the collecting system of the kidney. The first step requires 'inflation' of the renal collecting system (pelvis and calyces) with fluid or air instilled via a ureteric catheter inserted cystoscopically (Fig. 9.7). This makes subsequent percutaneous puncture of a renal calyx with a nephrostomy needle easier (Fig. 9.8). Once the nephrostomy needle is in the calyx, a guide wire is inserted into the renal pelvis to act as a guide over which the 'track' is dilated (Fig. 9.9). An access sheath is passed down the track and into the calyx, and through this a nephroscope can be advanced into the kidney (Fig. 9.10). An ultrasonic lithotripsy probe is used to fragment the stone and remove the debris.

A posterior approach is most commonly used; below the 12th rib (to avoid the pleura and far enough away from the rib to avoid the intercostals, vessels, and nerve). The preferred approach is through a posterior calyx, rather than into the renal pelvis, because this avoids damage to posterior branches of the renal artery which are closely associated with the renal pelvis. General anaesthesia is usual, though regional or even local anaesthesia (with sedation) can be used.

Indications for PCNL

PCNL is generally recommended for stones >3 cm in diameter, those that have failed ESWL and/or an attempt at flexible ureteroscopy and laser treatment. It is the first-line option for staghorn calculi,[1] with ESWL and/or repeat PCNL being used for residual stone fragments.

For stones 2–3 cm in diameter, options include ESWL (with a JJ stent *in situ*), flexible ureteroscopy and laser treatment, and PCNL. PCNL gives the best chance of complete stone clearance with a single procedure, but this is achieved at a higher risk of morbidity. Some patients will opt for several sessions of ESWL or flexible ureteroscopy/laser treatment and the possible risk of ultimately requiring PCNL because of failure of ESWL or laser treatment, rather than proceeding with PCNL 'up front'. ~50% of stones >2 cm in diameter will be fragmented by flexible ureteroscopy and laser treatment.

Outcomes of PCNL

For small stones, the stone-free rate after PCNL is in the order of 90–95%. For staghorn stones, the stone-free rate of PCNL, when combined with post-operative ESWL for residual stone fragments, is in the order of 80–85%.

1   Segura JW, Preminger GM, Assimos DG, *et al.* (1994) Nephrolithiasis clinical guidelines panel summary report on the management of staghorn calculi. *J Urol* **151**:1648–51.

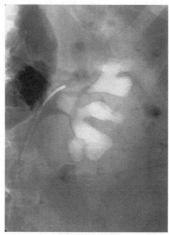

Fig. 9.7 A ureteric catheter is inserted into the renal pelvis to dilate it with air or fluid.

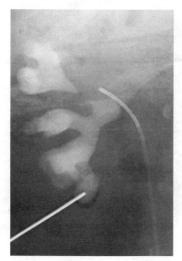

Fig. 9.8 A nephrostomy needle has been inserted into a calyx.

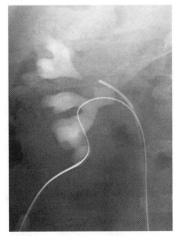

Fig. 9.9 A guide wire is inserted into the renal pelvis and down the ureter; over this guide wire the track is dilated.

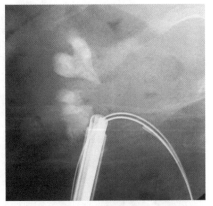

Fig. 9.10 An access sheath is passed down the track and into the calyx, and through this a nephroscope can be advanced into the kidney.

Kidney stones: open stone surgery

Indications
- Complex stone burden (projection of stone into multiple calyces, such that multiple PCNL tracks would be required to gain access to all the stone)
- Failure of endoscopic treatment (technical difficulty gaining access to the collecting system of the kidney)
- Anatomic abnormality that precludes endoscopic surgery (e.g. retrorenal colon)
- Body habitus that precludes endoscopic surgery (e.g. gross obesity, kyphoscoliosis—open stone surgery can be difficult)
- Patient request for a single procedure where multiple PCNLs might be required for stone clearance
- Non-functioning kidney.

Non-functioning kidney
Where the kidney is not working, the stone may be left *in situ* if it is not causing symptoms (e.g. pain, recurrent urinary infection, haematuria). However, staghorn calculi should be removed, unless the patient has co-morbidity that would preclude safe surgery because of the substantial risk of developing serious infective complications. If the kidney is non-functioning, the simplest way of removing the stone is to remove the kidney.

Functioning kidneys—options for stone removal
Small- to medium-sized stones
- Pyelolithotomy
- Radial nephrolithotomy.

Staghorn calculi
- Anatrophic (avascular) nephrolithotomy
- Extended pyelolithotomy with radial nephrotomies (small incisions over individual stones)
- Excision of the kidney, 'bench' surgery to remove the stones, and autotransplantation.

Specific complications of open stone surgery
Wound infection (the stones operated on are often infection stones); flank hernia; wound pain. (With PCNL these problems do not occur, blood transfusion rate is lower, analgesic requirement is less, mobilization is more rapid, and discharge earlier—all of which account for PCNL having replaced open surgery as the mainstay of treatment of large stones.) There is a significant chance of stone recurrence after open stone surgery (as for any other treatment modality) and the scar tissue that develops around the kidney will make subsequent open stone surgery technically more difficult.

Kidney stones: medical therapy (dissolution therapy)

Uric acid and cystine stones are potentially suitable for dissolution therapy. Calcium within either stone type reduces the chances of successful dissolution.

Uric acid stones

Urine is frequently supersaturated with uric acid (derived from a purine-rich diet, i.e. animal protein). 50% of patients who form uric acid stones have gout. The other 50% do so because of a high protein and low fluid intake ('Western' lifestyle). In patients with gout, the risk of developing stones is ~1% per year after the first attack of gout.

Uric acid stones form in concentrated, acid urine. Dissolution therapy is based on hydration, urine alkalinization, allopurinol, and dietary manipulation—the aim being to reduce urinary uric acid saturation. Maintain a high fluid intake (urine output 2–3 L/day), 'alkalinize' the urine to pH 6.5–7 (sodium bicarbonate 650 mg, tds or qds, or potassium citrate 30–60 mEq/day, equivalent to 15–30 mL of a potassium citrate solution tds or qds). In those with hyperuricaemia or urinary uric acid excretion >1200 mg/day, add allopurinol 300–600 mg/day (inhibits conversion of hypoxanthin and xanthine to uric acid). Dissolution of large stones (even staghorn calculi) is possible with this regimen.

Cystine stones

Cystinuria is an inherited kidney and intestinal transepithelial transport defect for the amino acids cystine, ornithine, arginine, and lysine ('COAL') leading to excessive urinary excretion of cystine. Autosomal recessive inheritance; prevalence of 1 in 700 are homozygous (i.e. both genes defective); occurs equally in both sexes. ~3% of adult stone formers are cystinuric and 6% of stone-forming children.

Most cystinuric patients excrete about 1g of cystine per day, which is well above the solubility of cystine. Cystine solubility in acid solutions is low (300 mg/l at pH 5, 400 mg/l at pH 7). Patients with cystinuria present with renal calculi, often in their teens or twenties. Cystine stones are relatively radiodense because they contain sulphur atoms. The cyanide nitroprusside test will detect most homozygote stone formers and some heterozygotes (false +ves occur in the presence of ketones).

Treatment of existing stones and prevention of further stones
The aim is to:
- Reduce cystine excretion (dietary restriction of the cystine precursor amino acid methionine and also of sodium intake to <100 mg/day)
- Increase solubility of cystine by alkalinization of the urine to >pH 7.5, maintenance of a high fluid intake, and use of drugs which convert cystine to more soluble compounds.

D-penicillamine, N-acetyl-D-penicillamine, and mercaptopropionylglycine bind to cystine—the compounds so formed are more soluble in urine than is cystine alone. D-penicillamine has potentially unpleasant and serious side-effects (allergic reactions, nephrotic syndrome, pancytopenia, proteinuria, epidermolysis, thrombocytosis, hypogeusia). Therefore, reserved for cases where alkalinization therapy and high fluid intake fail to dissolve the stones.

Treatment for failed dissolution therapy

Cystine stones are very hard and are therefore relatively resistant to ESWL. Nonetheless, for small cystine stones, a substantial proportion will still respond to ESWL. Flexible ureteroscopy (for small) and PCNL (for larger) cystine stones are used where ESWL fragmentation has failed.

Ureteric stones: presentation

Ureteric stones usually present with sudden onset of severe flank pain which is colicky (waves of increasing severity are followed by a reduction in severity, but it seldom goes away completely). It may radiate to the groin as the stone passes into the lower ureter. ~50% of patients with classic symptoms for a ureteric stone do not have a stone confirmed on subsequent imaging studies, nor do they physically ever pass a stone.

Examination

Spend a few seconds looking at the patient. Ureteric stone pain is colicky—the patient moves around, trying to find a comfortable position. They may be doubled-up with pain. Patients with conditions causing peritonitis (e.g. appendicitis, a ruptured ectopic pregnancy) lie very still: movement and abdominal palpation are very painful.

Pregnancy test

Arrange a pregnancy test in pre-menopausal women (this is mandatory in any pre-menopausal woman who is going to undergo imaging using ionizing radiation). If +ve, refer to a gynaecologist; if negative, arrange imaging to determine whether they have a ureteric stone.

Dipstick or microscopic haematuria

Many patients with ureteric stones have dipstick or microscopic haematuria (and, more rarely, macroscopic haematuria), but 10–30% have no blood in their urine.[1,2] The sensitivity of dipstick haematuria for detecting ureteric stones presenting acutely is ~95% on the first day of pain, 85% on the second day, and 65% on the third and fourth days.[2] Therefore, patients with a ureteric stone whose pain started 3–4 days ago may not have blood detectable in their urine. Dipstick testing is slightly more sensitive than urine microscopy for detecting stones (80% vs. 70%) because blood cells lyse, and therefore disappear, if the urine specimen is not examined under the microscope within a few hours. Both ways of detecting haematuria have roughly the same specificity for diagnosing ureteric stones (~60%).

Remember, blood in the urine on dipstick testing or microscopy may be a coincidental finding because of non-stone urological disease (e.g. neoplasm, infection) or a false +ve test (no abnormality is found in ~70% of patients with microscopic haematuria, despite full urological investigation).

Temperature

The most important aspect of examination in a patient with a ureteric stone confirmed on imaging is to measure their temperature. If the patient has a stone and a fever, they may have infection proximal to the stone. A fever in the presence of an obstructing stone is an indication for urine and blood culture, intravenous fluids and antibiotics, and nephrostomy drainage if the fever does not resolve within a matter of hours.[1,2]

1 Luchs JS, Katz DS, Lane DS, *et al.* (2002) Utility of hematuria testing in patients with suspected renal colic: correlation with unenhanced helical CT results. *Urology* **59**:839.

2 Kobayashi T, Nishizawa K, Mitsumori K, Ogura K (2003) Impact of date of onset on the absence of hematuria in patients with acute renal colic. *J Urol* **1770**:1093–6.

Ureteric stones: diagnostic radiological imaging

The intravenous urogram (IVU), for many years the mainstay of imaging in patients with flank pain, has been replaced by CT urography (CTU) (Fig. 9.11). Compared with IVU, CTU:

- Has greater specificity (95%) and sensitivity (97%) for diagnosing ureteric stones[1]—it can identify other, non-stone causes of flank pain (Fig. 9.12)
- Requires no contrast administration so avoiding the chance of a contrast reaction (risk of fatal anaphylaxis following the administration of low-osmolality contrast media for IVU is in the order of 1 in 100,000)[2]
- Is faster, taking just a few minutes to image the kidneys and ureters. An IVU, particularly where delayed films are required to identify a stone causing high-grade obstruction, may take hours to identify the precise location of the obstructing stone
- Is equivalent in cost to IVU, in hospitals where high volumes of CT scans are done.[3]

If you only have access to IVU, remember that it is contraindicated in patients with a history of previous contrast reactions and should be avoided in those with hay fever, a strong history of allergies, or asthma who have not been pre-treated with high-dose steroids 24 h before the IVU. Patients taking metformin for diabetes should stop this for 48 h prior to an IVU. Clearly, being able to perform an alternative test, such as CTU in such patients, is very useful.

Where 24-h CTU access is not available, admit patients with suspected ureteric colic for pain relief and arrange a CTU the following morning. When CT urography is not immediately available (between the hours of midnight and 8 a.m.) we arrange urgent abdominal ultrasonography in all patients aged >50 years who present with flank pain suggestive of a possible stone, to exclude serious pathology such as a leaking abdominal aortic aneurysm and to demonstrate any other gross abnormalities due to non-stone associated flank pain.

Plain abdominal X-ray and renal ultrasound are not sufficiently sensitive or specific for their routine use for diagnosing ureteric stones.

MR urography

This a very accurate way of determining whether a stone is present in the ureter or not.[4] However, at the present time, cost and restricted availability limit its usefulness as a routine diagnostic method of imaging in cases of acute flank pain. This may change as MR scanners become more widely available.[1,2,3,4]

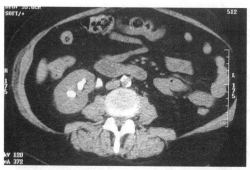

Fig. 9.11 A CT urogram.

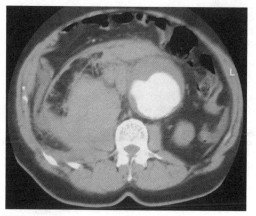

Fig. 9.12 A leaking aortic aneurysm identified on a CTU in a patient with loin pain.

1   Smith RC, Verga M, McCarthy S, Rosenfield AT (1996) Diagnosis of acute flank pain: value of unenhanced helical CT. *Am J Roentgen* **166**:97–101.

2   Caro JJ, Trindale E, McGregor M (1991) The risks of death and severe non-fatal reactions with high vs low osmolality contrast media. *Am J Roentgen* **156**:825–32.

3   Thomson JM, Glocer J, Abbott C, *et al.* (2001) Computed tomography versus intravenous urography in diagnosis of acute flank pain from urolithiasis: a randomized study comparing imaging costs and radiation dose. *Australas Radiol* **45**:291–7.

4   Louca G, Liberopoulos K, Fidas A, *et al.* (1999) MR urography in the diagnosis of urinary tract obstruction. *Eur Urol* **35**:102–8.

Ureteric stones: acute management

While appropriate imaging studies are being organized, pain relief should be given:

- A non-steroidal anti-inflammatory (e.g. diclofenac) by intramuscular or intravenous injection, by mouth or per rectum. Provides rapid and effective pain control. Analgesic effect—partly anti-inflammatory, partly by reducing ureteric peristalsis
- Where NSAIDS are inadequate, opiate analgesics such as pethidine or morphine are added.

There is no need to encourage the patient to drink copious amounts of fluids nor to give them large volumes of fluids intravenously in the hope that this will 'flush' the stone out. Renal blood flow and urine output from the affected kidney falls during an episode of acute, partial obstruction due to a stone. Excess urine output will tend to cause a greater degree of hydronephrosis in the affected kidney, which may make ureteric peristalsis* even less efficient than it already is.

The exception to this rule may be those with radiolucent uric acid stones (suspected if low urinary pH and stones not visible on plain X-ray or with lower attenuation on CT compared with calcium, cystine, and struvite stones). High fluid intake and oral potassium citrate, sodium citrate of sodium bicarbonate (to elevate urine pH to 6–7) may dissolve uric acid stones or at least reduce their size so increasing stone spontaneous passage rates.

Watchful waiting

In many instances, small ureteric stones will pass spontaneously within days or a few weeks, with analgesic supplements for exacerbations of pain.

Data on rate of spontaneous stone passage are surprisingly limited.[1] Chances of spontaneous stone passage depend principally on stone size. 68% of stones 5 mm or less will pass spontaneously (95% CI 46–85%; meta-analysis of 224 patients); 47% of stones 6–10 mm in diameter will pass spontaneously (95% CI 36–59%; meta-analysis of 104 patients).[1] Average time for spontaneous stone passage for stones 4–6mm in diameter is 3 weeks.[2] Stones that have not passed in 2 months are unlikely to do so. Of those stones that do eventually pass those 2 mm or less do so within 30 days, and those 2–6 mm in size do so within 40 days (but not all stones do pass and we cannot predict the chance of spontaneous passage in the individual patient). Therefore, accurate determination of stone size (on plain abdominal X-ray or by CTU) helps predict chances of spontaneous stone passage.

Medical expulsive therapy (MET)

There is growing evidence for the efficacy of MET, the preferred agents being the smooth muscle relaxing[1,3] alpha-1 adrenergic adrenoceptor blockers. These increase spontaneous stone passage rates, reduce stone passage time and reduce frequency of ureteric colic.[3] The EAU/AUA Nephrolithiasis Guideline Panel meta-analysis showed that 29% more patients (CI: 20–37%) taking tamsulosin passed their stones compared with controls.[1] Tamsulosin has been most studied in this setting, but terazosin and doxazosin seem to be equally effective. Whether stones in all segments of the ureter are equally responsive to alpha blockers remains to be determined.

In the same meta-analysis there was no significant difference in stone passage rates between those taking the calcium channel blocker nifedipine and control patients.

Glyceryl trinitrate patches do not aid stone passage or reduce frequency of pain episodes and corticosteroids are of minimal, if any, benefit.[3,4]

A trial of MET is a very reasonable approach for many patients, but individual circumstances may dictate 'up-front' ESWL or ureteroscopy, e.g. the possible disruption to work and daily living activities from episodes of pain occurring while a stone is progressing towards eventual spontaneous passage may prompt the patient to request ESWL or ureteroscopy (e.g. commercial airline pilots cannot fly until stone free—nor can those who fly for leisure).

MET is contraindicated where there is clinical evidence of sepsis (essentially fever) or deteriorating renal function. If you use a trial of MET, warn patients of the risks (drug side effects, possible need for intervention in the form of ESWL, ureteroscopy, or J stenting) and mention it is an 'off-label' (i.e. non-licensed) therapy. Arrange periodic follow-up imaging (usually a plain X-Ray) to monitor stone position.

---

* Peristalsis, the forward propulsion of a bolus of urine down the ureter, can only occur if the walls of the ureter above the bolus of urine can coapt i.e. close firmly together. If they cannot, as occurs in a ureter distended with urine, the bolus of urine cannot move distally).

1 Preminger GM *et al.* (2007) 2007 Guideline for the management of ureteral calculi (Joint EAU/AUA Nephrolithiasis Guideline Panel. *J Urol* **178**:2418–34.

2 Miller OF *et al.* (1999) Time to stone passage for observed ureteral calculi. *J Urol* **162**:688–91.

3 Dellabella M *et al.* (2003) Efficacy of tamsulosin in the medical management of juxtavesical ureteral stones. *J Urol* **170**:2202–5.

4 Hussain Z *et al.* (2001) Use of glyceryl trinitrate patches in patients with ureteral stones: a randomized, double-blind, placebo-controlled study. *Urology* **58**:521–5.

Ureteric stones: indications for intervention to relieve obstruction and/ or remove the stone

- **Pain** that fails to respond to analgesics or recurs and cannot be controlled with additional pain relief
- **Bacteriuria** in the presence of an obstructing stone can lead to the development of urosepsis. The EAU/AUA Nephrolithiasis Guideline Panel recommends that patients with ureteric stones and bacteriuria be treated with appropriate antibiotics (level IV evidence, i.e based on the opinions or clinical experience of respected authorities). Where intervention is planned (ESWL or ureteroscopy), appropriate antibiotics should be given in advance of the treatment
- **Fever:** have a low threshold for draining the kidney (both percutaneous nephrostomy)[1]
- **Impaired renal function** (solitary kidney obstructed by a stone, bilateral ureteric stones, or pre-existing renal impairment which gets worse as a consequence of a ureteric stone). Threshold for intervention is lower
- **Prolonged unrelieved obstruction:** this can result in long-term loss of renal function.[1] How long it takes for this loss of renal function to occur is uncertain, but generally speaking the period of watchful waiting for spontaneous stone passage tends to be limited to 4–6 weeks
- **Social reasons:** young, active patients may be very keen to opt for surgical treatment because they need to get back to work or their childcare duties, whereas some patients will be happy to sit things out. Airline pilots and some other professions are unable to work until they are stone free.

Emergency temporizing and definitive treatment of the stone

Where the pain of a ureteric stone fails to respond to analgesics or where renal function is impaired because of the stone, then temporary relief of the obstruction can be obtained by insertion of a JJ stent or percutaneous nephrostomy tube. (Percutaneous nephrostomy tube can restore efficient peristalsis by restoring the ability of the ureteric wall to coapt.)

JJ stent insertion or percutaneous nephrostomy tube can be done quickly, but the stone is still present (Fig. 9.13). It may pass down and out of the ureter with a stent or nephrostomy *in situ*, but in many instances it simply sits where it is and subsequent definitive treatment is still required. While JJ stents can relieve stone pain, they can cause bothersome irritative bladder symptoms (pain in the bladder, frequency, and urgency). JJ stents do make subsequent stone treatment in the form of ureteroscopy technically easier by causing passive dilatation of the ureter.

The patient may elect to proceed to definitive stone treatment by immediate ureteroscopy (for stones at any location in the ureter) or ESWL (if the stone is in the upper and lower ureter—ESWL cannot be used for stones in the mid-ureter because this region is surrounded by bone, which prevents penetration of the shock waves; Fig. 9.14). Local facilities and expertise will determine whether definitive treatment can be offered immediately. Not all hospitals have access to ESWL or endoscopic surgeons 365 days a year.

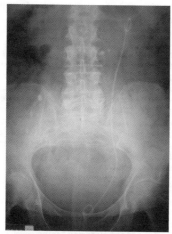

Fig. 9.13 A JJ stent.

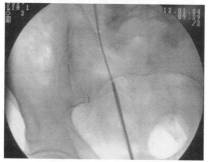

Fig. 9.14 Ureteroscopic stone fragmentation for a lower ureteric stone.

Emergency treatment of an obstructed, infected kidney

Antibiotic delivery into an obstructed collecting system is impaired and so the septic patient with an obstructing stone should undergo urgent decompression of the collecting system and definitive stone treatment (ESWL or ureteroscopy) should be delayed until the sepsis has resolved. The rationale for performing percutaneous nephrostomy, rather than JJ stent insertion for an infected, obstructed kidney is to reduce the likelihood of septicaemia occurring as a consequence of showering bacteria into the circulation. It has been theorized that this is more likely to occur with JJ stent insertion, than with percutaneous nephrostomy insertion, that J stent insertion might damage the ureter (unlikely) and that monitoring of urine output and the facility for irrigation for a viscous pyonephrosis is possible with a nephrostomy but not a J stent. Nephrostomy insertion has the advantage that it avoids the need for a general anaesthetic in fact, but J stent insertion can be done with sedation and avoids the risk of bleeding from inadvertent puncture of a branch of the renal artery.[1]

The EAU/AUA Nephrolithiasis Guideline Panel[2] recommends that the system of drainage—J stent or percutaneous nephrostomy is left to the discretion of the urologist, since both have been shown in a randomized trial of 42 patients with obstructing stones and a temperature of >38°C and/or white blood count of 17,000/mm³* to be equally effective for the management of presumed obstructive pyelonephritis or pyonephrosis[3] in terms of time to normalization of temperature and white count (which takes approximately 2-3 days) and in-hospital stay. A 6 or 7 Ch J stent was used (with a Foley bladder catheter in 70%) or 8 Ch (occasionally larger) nephrostomy (plus a urethral catheter in 33%).

---

* An arbitrary definition of leucocytosis, since patients with ureteric stones often have mildly elevated white blood count.

1 Holm–Nielsen A, Jorgensen T, Mogensen P, Fogh J (1981) The prognostic value of probe renography in ureteric stone obstruction. *Br J Urol* **53**:504–7.

2 Preminger GM *et al.* (2007) 2007 Guideline for the management of ureteral calculi Joint EAU/AUA Nephrolithiasis Guideline Panel. *J Urol* **178**:2418–34.

3 Pearle MS *et al.* (1998) Optimal method of urgent decompression of the collecting system for obstruction and infection due to ureteral calculi. *J Urol* **160**:1260.

Table 9.3 Complications and problems associated with and nephrostomy insertion and drainage ($n = 169$)[1] and J stent[2,3] (none performed for relief of obstructed, infected kidney; n=226)

Complication	J stent	Nephrostomy
Failure of insertion	16%	2%
Sepsis in previously non-septic patient		3–4%
Haemorrhage requiring transfusion		2%
Stent occlusion	1–7%	
Tube displacement (tube falling out or for J stent migrating up or down)	0.1–7%	5%
Pleural effusion		1%
Pneumonia/atelectasis		2%
Ureteric perforation	6%	
Stent symptoms	Flank pain 15–20%; suprapubic pain 20%; urinary frequency 40%; haematuria 40%	

1 Lee WJ et al. (1994) Emergency percutaneous nephrostomy: results and complications. *J Vasc Intervent Rad* **5**:135.

2 Pocock RD et al. (1986) Double J stents. A review of 100 patients. *Br J Urol* **58**:629.

3 Smedlev FH et al. (1988) J (pigtail) ureteric catheter insertions: a retrospective review. *Ann Roy Coll Surg (Engl)* **70**:377.

Ureteric stone treatment

Almost 70% of stones 5 mm or less and almost 50% of stones 6–10 mm in diameter will pass spontaneously over a period of 3–6 weeks or thereabouts.[1] Stones that have not passed in 2 months are unlikely to do so, although much to the patient's and surgeon's surprise large stones do sometimes drop out of the ureter at the last moment.

Indications for stone removal

- Pain that fails to respond to analgesics or recurs and cannot be controlled with additional pain relief
- Impaired renal function (solitary kidney obstructed by a stone, bilateral ureteric stones, or pre-existing renal impairment, which gets worse as a consequence of a ureteric stone)
- Prolonged unrelieved obstruction (generally speaking ~4–6 weeks)
- **Social reasons:** young, active patients may be very keen to opt for surgical treatment because they need to get back to work or their childcare duties, whereas some patients will be happy to sit things out. Airline pilots and some other professions are unable to work until they are stone free.

These indications need to be related to the individual patient—their stone size, their renal function, presence of a normal contralateral kidney, their tolerance of exacerbations of pain, their job and social situation, and local facilities (the availability of surgeons with appropriate skill and equipment to perform endoscopic stone treatment).

20 years ago, when the only options were watchful waiting or open surgical removal of a stone (open ureterolithotomy), surgeons, and patients were inclined to 'sit it out' for a considerable time in the hope that the stone would pass spontaneously. Nowadays, the advent of ESWL and of smaller ureteroscopes with efficient stone fragmentation devices (e.g. the holmium laser) has made stone treatment and removal a far less morbid procedure, with a far smoother and faster post-treatment recovery. It is easier for both the patient and the surgeon to opt for intervention, in the form of ESWL or surgery, as a quicker way of relieving them of their pain, and a way of avoiding unpredictable and unpleasant exacerbations of pain.

It is clearly important for the surgeon to inform the patient of the outcomes and potential complications of intervention, particularly given the fact that many of stones would pass spontaneously if left a little longer, particularly now there is evidence for MET (medical expulsive therapy).

1 Preminger et al (2007). 2007 Guideline for the management of ureteral calculi. Joint EAU/AUA Nephrolituiasis Guideline Panel. *J. Urol* **178**: 2418–34.

Treatment options for ureteric stones

- ESWL: *in situ*; or after JJ stent insertion*
- Ureteroscopy
- PCNL
- Open ureterolithotomy
- Laparoscopic ureterolithotomy
- Percutaneous antegrade ureteroscopy.

Basketing of stones (blind or under radiographic 'control') is a historical treatments (the potential for serious ureteric injury is significant).

The ureter can be divided into two halves (proximal and distal to the iliac vessels) or in thirds (upper third from the PUJ to the upper edge of the sacrum; middle third from the upper to the lower edge of the sacrum i.e. the extent of the sacroiliac joint; lower third from the lower edge of the sacrum to the VUJ).

EAU/AUA Nephrolithiasis Guideline Panel recommendations 2007[1]

These should be interpreted in the light of local facilities and expertise. Some hospitals have access to and expertise in the whole range of treatment options. Others may have limited access to a lithotriptor or may not have surgeons skilled in the use of the ureteroscope.

Smaller ureteroscopes with improved optics and larger instrument channels, and the advent of holmium laser lithotripsy have improved the efficacy of ureteroscopic stone fragmentation (to ~95% stone clearance) and reduced its morbidity. As a consequence, many surgeons and patients will opt for ureteroscopy, with its potential for a 'one-off' treatment, over ESWL where more than one treatment will be required and post-treatment imaging is required to confirm stone clearance (with ureteroscopy you can directly see that the stone has gone).

Many urology departments do not have unlimited access to ESWL and patients may, therefore, opt for ureteroscopic stone extraction.

The stone clearance rates for ESWL are stone-size dependent. ESWL is more efficient for stones <1 cm in diameter compared with those >1 cm in size. Conversely, the outcome of ureteroscopy is somewhat less dependent on stone size.

---

* (ESWL after 'push-back' of the stone into the kidney (i.e. into the renal pelvis or calyces) is a historical treatment—if the ESWL fails to fragment the stone, a relatively straightforward operation of ureteroscopy has been converted into the technically more challenging one of flexible ureterorenoscopy. So, at all costs avoid pushing the stone back into the kidney when inserting a J stent, but warn the patient of this possibility).

Efficacy outcomes (i.e. stone free rates) of EAU/AUA Nephrolithiasis Guidelines Panel 2007

Table 9.4 Median stone free rates of ESWL and ureteroscopy (figures in brackets are 95% CI)[1]

Stone position and size	ESWL	Ureteroscopy
Distal ureter <10 mm	86% (73–75)	97% (96–98)
Distal ureter >10 mm	74% (80–90)	93% (88–96)
Mid ureter <10 mm	84% (65–95)	91% (81–96)
Mid ureter >10 mm	76% (36–97)	78% (61–90)
Proximal ureter <10 mm	90% (85–93)	80% (73–85)
Proximal ureter <10 mm	68% (55–79)	79% (71–87)

RCTs comparing ESWL and ureteroscopy are generally lacking. The EAU/AUA Nephrolithiasis Guidelines Panel 2007 meta-analysis suggests that:
- **Proximal ureter <10 mm:** ESWL marginally higher stone free rate than ureteroscopy
- **Proximal ureter >10 mm:** ureteroscopy marginally higher stone free rate than ESWL
- **For all mid-ureteric stones:** ureteroscopy has a marginally higher stone free rate than ESWL, but small patient numbers make comparison difficult
- **For all distal stones ureteroscopy:** has a higher stone free rate than ESWL.

Thus, there are no great differences in stone free rates between ESWL and ureteroscopy. Precisely which technique one uses will depend to a considerable degree on local resources (e.g. ready access to ESWL) and local expertise at performing ureteroscopy, particularly for upper tract stones. Failed initial ESWL is associated with a low success rate for subsequent ESWL.[2] Therefore if no effect after 1 or 2 treatments, change tactics.

Open ureterolithotomy and laparoscopic ureterolithotomy (less invasive than open ureterolithotomy) are used in the rare cases (e.g. very impacted stones), where ESWL or ureteroscopy have been tried and failed, or were not feasible.[1] Laparoscopic ureterolithotomy for large, impacted stones has a stone-free rate averaging almost 90%.

1 Preminger GM *et al.* (2007) 2007 Guideline for the management of ureteral calculi Joint EAU/AUA Nephrolithiasis Guideline Panel. *J Urol* **178**:2418–34.

2 Pace KT *et al.* (2000) Low success rate of repeat shock wave lithotripsy for *ureteral* stones after failed initial treatment. *J Urol* **164**:1905–7.

Prevention of calcium oxalate stone formation

A series of landmark papers from Harvard Medical School[1] and other groups allow us to give rational advice on reducing the risk of future stone formation in those who have formed one or more stones. The Harvard studies stratified risk of stone formation based on intake of calcium and other nutrients (Nurses Health Study, $n = 81,000$ women; equivalent male study, $n = 45,000$).

Low fluid intake

Low fluid intake may be the single most important risk factor for recurrent stone formation. High fluid intake is protective,[1] by reducing urinary saturation of calcium, oxalate, and urate. Time to recurrent stone formation is prolonged from 2 to 3 years in previous stone formers randomized to high fluid vs. low fluid intake (averaging about 2.5 vs. 1 L/day) and over 5 years, risk of recurrent stones was 27% in low-volume controls compared with 12% in high-volume patients.[2]

Dietary calcium

Conventional teaching was that high calcium intake increases the risk of calcium oxalate stone disease. The Harvard Medical School studies have shown that low calcium intake is, paradoxically, associated with an increased risk of forming kidney stones, in both men and women (relative risk of stone formation for the highest quintile of dietary calcium intake vs. the lowest quintile = 0.65; 95% confidence intervals 0.5–0.83, i.e. high calcium intake was associated with a low risk of stone formation).

Calcium supplements

In the Harvard studies,[3] the relative risk of stone formation in women on supplemental calcium compared with those not on calcium was 1.2 (95% confidence intervals 1.02–1.4). In 67% of women on supplements, the calcium was either not consumed with a meal or was consumed with a meal with a low oxalate content. It is possible that consuming calcium supplements with a meal or with oxalate-containing foods could reduce this small risk of inducing kidney stones.

Other dietary risk factors related to stone formation

Increased risk of stone formation (relative risk of stone formation shown in brackets for highest to lowest quintiles of intake of particular dietary factor):

- Sucrose (1.5)
- Sodium (1.3): high sodium intake (leading to natriuresis) causes hypercalciuria
- Potassium (0.65).

Animal proteins

High intake of animal proteins causes increased urinary excretion of calcium, reduced pH, high urinary uric acid, and reduced urinary citrate, all of which predispose to stone formation.[4]

Alcohol

Curhan's studies from Harvard[5] suggest small quantities of wine decrease risk of stones.

Vegetarian diet

Vegetable proteins contain less of the amino acids phenylalanine, tyrosine, and tryptophan that increase the endogenous production of oxalate. A vegetarian diet may protect against the risk of stone formation.[6,7]

Dietary oxalate

A small increase in urinary oxalate concentration increases calcium oxalate supersaturation much more than does an increase in urinary calcium concentration. Mild hyperoxaluria is one of the main factors leading to calcium stone formation.[8]

1 Curhan GC, et al. (1993) A prospective study of dietary calcium and other nutrients and the risk of symptomatic kidney stones. *NEJM* **328**:833–8.

2 Borghi L, et al. (1996) Urinary volume, water and recurrences in idiopathic calcium nephrolithiasis: A 5-year randomized prospective study. *J Urol* **155**:839–43.

3 Curhan G, et al. (1997) Comparison of dietary calcium with supplemental calcium and other nutrients as factors affecting the risk for kidney stones in women. *Ann Int Med* **126**:497–504.

4 Kok DJ (1990) The effects of dietary excesses in animal protein and in sodium on the composition and crystallization kinetics of calcium oxalate monohydrate in urines of healthy men. *J Clin Endocrinol Metab* **71**:861–7.

5 Curhan G, et al. (1998) Beverage use and risk for kidney stones in women. *Ann Intern Med* **128**:534–40.

6 Robertson WG, et al. (1982) Prevalence of urinary stone disease in vegetarians. *Eur Urol* **8**:334–9.

7 Borghi, L (2002) Comparison of two diets for prevention of recurrent stones in idiopathic hypercalciuria. *NEJM* **346**:77–84.

8 Robertson WG, Peacock M, Ouimet D, et al. (1981) The main risk for calcium oxalate stone disease in man: hypercalciuria or mild hyperoxaluria? In: Smith LH, Robertson WG, Finlayson B (eds.) *Urolithiasis: Clinical and Basic Research.* New York: Plenum Press, p. 3–12.

Bladder stones

Composition

Struvite (i.e. they are infection stones) or uric acid (in non-infected urine).

Adults

Bladder calculi are predominantly a disease of men aged >50 and with bladder outlet obstruction due to BPE. They also occur in the chronically catheterized patient (e.g. spinal cord injury patients), where the chance of developing a bladder stone is 25% over 5 years (similar risk whether urethral or suprapubic location of the stone).[1]

Children

Bladder stones are still common in Thailand, Indonesia, North Africa, the Middle East, and Burma. In these endemic areas they are usually composed of a combination of ammonium urate and calcium oxalate. A low-phosphate diet in these areas (a diet of breast milk, and polished rice or millet) results in high peaks of ammonia excretion in the urine.

Symptoms

May be symptomless (incidental finding on KUB X-ray or bladder ultrasound or on cystoscopy)—the common presentation in spinal patients who have limited or no bladder sensation. In the neurologically intact patient—suprapubic or perineal pain, haematuria, urgency, and/or urge incontinence, recurrent UTI, LUTS (hesitancy, poor flow).

Diagnosis

If you suspect a bladder stone, they will be visible on KUB X-ray or renal ultrasound (Fig. 9.15).

Treatment

Most stones are small enough to be removed cystoscopically (endoscopic cystolitholapaxy), using stone-fragmenting forceps for stones that can be engaged by the jaws of the forceps and EHL or pneumatic lithotripsy for those that cannot. Large stones (☐ see Fig. 9.15) can be removed by open surgery (open cystolitholapaxy).[1]

1 Ord J (2003) Bladder management and risk of bladder stone formation in spinal cord injured patients. *J Urol.* **170**:1734–7.

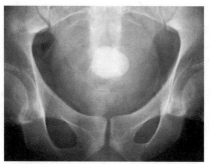

Fig. 9.15 A bladder stone.

Management of ureteric stones in pregnancy

While hypercalciuria and uric acid excretion increase in pregnancy (predisposing to stone formation), so too do urinary citrate and magnesium levels (protecting against stone formation). 'Net' effect—incidence of ureteric colic is the same as in non-pregnant women.[1] Ureteric stones occur in 1 in 1500–2500 pregnancies, mostly during the 2nd and 3rd trimesters. They are associated with a significant risk of pre-term labour[2] and the pain caused by ureteric stones can be difficult to distinguish from other causes.

Differential diagnosis of flank pain in pregnancy

Ureteric stone, placental abruption, appendicitis, pyelonephritis, and all the other (many) causes of flank pain in non-pregnant women.

Diagnostic imaging studies in pregnancy

Exposure of the foetus to ionizing radiation can cause foetal malformations, intra-uterine growth retardation, malignancies in later life (leukaemia), and mutagenic effects (damage to genes causing inherited disease in the offspring of the foetus). The foetus is most at risk during organogenesis (weeks 4–10 of gestation). Foetal radiation doses during various procedures are shown in Table 15.3. Radiation doses of <100 mGy are reported as unlikely to have an adverse effect on the foetus.[3] In the United States, the National Council on Radiation Protection has stated that 'fetal risk is considered to be negligible at <50 mGy when compared to the other risks of pregnancy, and the risk of malformations is significantly increased above control levels at doses >150 mGy'.[4] The American College of Obstetricians and Gynaecologists has stated that 'X-ray exposure to <50 mGy has not been associated with an increase in foetal anomalies or pregnancy loss'.[5] However, every effort should be made to limit exposure of the foetus to radiation.

Table 9.5 Foetal radiation dose after various radiological investigations (Note lcGy is equivalent to 10 mGy)

Procedure	Foetal dose (mGy)	Risk of inducing cancer (up to age 15 years)
KUB X-ray	1.4	1 in 24,000
IVU 6 shot	1.7	1 in 10,000
IVU 3 shot	–	–
CT: abdominal	8	1 in 4000
CT: pelvic	25	1 in 1300
Fluoroscopy for JJ stent insertion	0.4	1 in 42,000

Adapted from the Joint Guidance from the National Radiographic protection Board, College of Radiographeres Royal College of Radiologists, 1998

Plain radiography and IVU

Limited usefulness (foetal skeleton and the enlarged uterus obscure ureteric stones; delayed excretion of contrast limits opacification of ureter; theoretical risk of foetal toxicity from the contrast material). Recommendations are for a limited IVU (eg. control film followed by a 30-min film) with foetal shielding.

CTU

Very accurate method for detecting ureteric stones, but most radiologists and urologists are unhappy to recommend this form of imaging in pregnant women due to increased foetal radiation exposure. Low and ultra low dose CT protocols are being developed.

MRU

The American College of Obstetricians and Gynaecologists and the US National Council on Radiation Protection state that 'although there is no evidence to suggest that the embryo is sensitive to magnetic and radio-frequency at the intensities encountered in MRI, it might be prudent to exclude pregnant women during the first trimester'.[5,6] MRU can therefore potentially be used during the second and third trimesters, but not during the first trimester. Involves no ionizing radiation. Very accurate (100% sensitivity for detecting ureteric stones[7]), but expensive, and not readily available in most hospitals, particularly out of hours.

Management

Most (70–80%) will pass spontaneously.[3] Pain relief: opiate-based analgesics; avoid non-steroidal anti-inflammatory drugs (NSAIDs; can cause premature closure of the ductus arteriosus by blocking prostaglandin synthesis).

Indications for intervention: the same as in non-pregnant patients (pain refractory to analgesics, suspected urinary sepsis (high fever, high white count), high-grade obstruction, and obstruction in a solitary kidney).

Options for intervention

Depend on stage of pregnancy and on local facilities and expertise:

- JJ stent urinary diversion[4]. Requires regular changing (approximately 6-8 weeks to avoid encrustation)
- Nephrostomy urinary diversion
- Ureteroscopic stone removal, with laser fragmentation.

Aim to minimize radiation exposure to the foetus, and to minimize the risk of miscarriage and pre-term labour. General anaesthesia can precipitate pre-term labour and many urologists and obstetricians will err on the side of temporizing options such as nephrostomy tube drainage or JJ stent placement, rather than on operative treatment in the form of ureteroscopic stone removal.

Avoid PCNL. ESWL is contraindicated.

1   Coe FL, Parks JH, Lindhermer MD (1978) Nephrolithiasis during pregnancy. *N Engl J Med* **298**:324–6.

2   Hendricks SK (1991) An algorithm for diagnosis and therapy of urolithiasis during pregnancy *Surg Gynecol Obst* **172**:49–54.

3   Hellawell GO, Cowan NC, Holt SJ, Mutch SJ (2002) A radiation perspective for treating loin pain in pregnancy by double-pigtail stents. *Br J Urol Int* **90**:801–8.

4   National Council on Radiation Protection and Measurement (1997) *Medical radiation exposure of pregnant and potentially pregnant women*. NCRP Report no. 54. Bethesda, MD: NCRPM.

5   American College of Obstetricians and Gynaecologists Committee on Obstetric Practice (1995) *Guidelines for Diagnostic Imaging During Pregnancy*. ACOG Committee Opinion no. 158. Washington DC: ACOG.

6   Roy C (1996) Assessment of painful ureterohydronephrosis during pregnancy by MR urography. *Eur Radiol* **6**:334–8.

7   Watterson JD, Girvan AR, Beiko DT, et al. (2002) Ureteroscopy and holmium: an emerging definitive management strategy for symptomatic ureteral calculi in pregnancy. *Urology* **60**:383–7.

8   Sharp C, Shrimpton JA, Bury RF. Joint Guidance from National Radiological Protection Board, College of Radiographers and Royal College of Radiologists 1998. *Advice on Exposure to Ionizing Radiation during Pregnancy*. Produced by the National Radiological Protection Board, Chilton, Didcot, Oxon, OX11 0RQ, U.K. (www.nrpb.org)

Upper tract obstruction, loin pain, hydronephrosis

Hydronephrosis

Dilatation of the renal pelvis and calyces (Fig. 10.1). When combined with dilatation of the ureters known as hydro-ureteronephrosis.

Obstructive nephropathy is damage to the renal parenchyma resulting from an obstruction to the flow of urine anywhere along the urinary tract.

Dilatation of the renal pelvis and calyces can occur without obstruction and therefore hydronephrosis should not be taken to necessarily imply the presence of obstructive uropathy.

Ultrasound

- **False −ve (i.e. obstruction present, no hydronephrosis):** acute onset of obstruction; in the presence of an intrarenal collecting system; with dehydration; misdiagnosis of dilatation of the calyces as renal cortical cysts (in acute ureteric colic, ultrasonography fails to detect hydro-nephrosis in up to 35% of patients with proven acute obstruction on IVU)
- **False +ve (i.e. hydronephrosis, no obstruction):** capacious extrarenal pelvis; parapelvic cysts; vesicoureteric reflux; high urine flow.

Diagnostic approach to the patient with hydronephrosis

Patients with hydronephrosis may present either as an incidental finding of hydronephrosis on an ultrasound or CT done because of non-specific symptoms or it may be identified in a patient with a raised creatinine or presenting with loin pain. Symptoms, if present, will depend on the rapidity of onset of obstruction of the kidney (if that is the cause of the hydro-nephrosis), whether the obstruction is complete or partial, unilateral or bilateral, and whether the obstruction to the ureter is extrinsic to the ureter or is within its lumen.

History

- Severe flank pain suggests a more acute onset of obstruction and, if very sudden in onset, a ureteric stone may well be the cause. Pain induced by a diuresis (e.g. following consumption of alcohol) suggests a possible PUJO
- Anuria (the symptom of bilateral ureteric obstruction or complete obstruction of a solitary kidney)
- If renal function is impaired, symptoms of renal failure may be present (e.g. nausea, lethargy, anorexia)
- Extrinsic causes of obstruction (e.g. compression of the ureters by retroperitoneal malignancy) usually have a more insidious onset, whereas intrinsic obstruction (ureteric stone) is often present with severe pain of very sudden onset
- An increase in urine output may be reported by the patient due to poor renal concentrating ability
- Obstruction in the presence of bacterial urinary tract infection—signs and symptoms of pyelonephritis (flank pain and tenderness, fever) or sepsis.

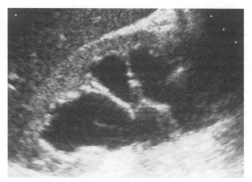

Fig. 10.1 Hydronephrosis as seen on renal ultrasonography.

Examination
- **Measure blood pressure:** elevated in high pressure chronic retention (HPCR) due to benign prostatic obstruction (caused by fluid overload)
- Bilateral oedema (due to fluid overload)
- **Abdominal examination:** percuss and palpate for an enlarged bladder.
- DRE (?prostate or rectal cancer) and in women, vaginal examination (?cervical cancer)
- Check serum creatinine to determine the functional effect of the hydronephrosis
- Renal ultrasonography (if not already done).

IVU findings in renal obstruction
- An obstructive (dense) nephrogram
- A delay in filling of the collecting system with contrast material
- Dilatation of the collecting system
- An increase in renal size
- Rupture of fornices (junction between renal papilla and its calyx) with urinary extravasation
- Ureteric dilatation and tortuosity
- A standing column of contrast material in the ureter.

Unilateral hydronephrosis
KUB X-ray (a ureteric stone may be seen); CTU (or IVU) if stone suspected.
- If no stone seen, but hydronephrosis is confirmed and ureter is non-dilated, the obstruction must be at the PUJ. In the absence of a ureteric stone visible on CTU, the diagnosis must be PUJO
- If no stone seen and ureter is dilated, as well as kidney, ureteric TCC is likely. Arrange retrograde ureterography to identify site of obstruction, and ureteroscopy/ureteric biopsy.

Bilateral hydronephrosis
- If the patient is in retention or has a substantial post-void residual urine volume, pass a catheter. If the elevated creatinine falls (and the hydronephrosis improves), the diagnosis is BOO, due, for example, to BPH, prostate cancer, urethral stricture, detrusor-sphincter dyssynergia. If the creatinine remains elevated, the obstruction affecting both ureters is higher 'up stream'
- TRUS and prostatic biopsy if prostate cancer suspected on DRE, CT scan—looking for malignant bilateral ureteric obstruction, AAA.

Causes of hydronephrosis

Unilateral
- Obstructing ureteric stone
- PUJO
- Obstructing clot in ureter
- Obstructing ureteric TCC
- (Any of the causes listed below where the pathologic process has not yet extended to involve both ureters).

Bilateral
- Bladder outlet obstruction (BOO)
  - BPH
  - Prostate cancer
  - Urethral stricture
  - Detrusor-sphincter dyssynergia
  - Posterior urethral valve
- Bilateral ureteric obstruction at their level of entry into the bladder
  - Locally advanced cervical cancer
  - Locally advanced prostate cancer
  - Locally advanced rectal cancer
  - Poor bladder compliance (often combined with detrusor-sphincter dyssynergia): neuropathic bladder (spinal cord injury, spina bifida); post-pelvic radiotherapy
- Peri-ureteric inflammation
  - From adjacent bowel involved with inflammatory bowel disease (e.g. Crohn's, ulcerative colitis) or diverticular disease
- Retroperitoneal fibrosis
  - Idiopathic (diagnosed following exclusion of other causes)
  - Peri-arteritis—aortic aneurysm, iliac artery aneurysm
  - Post-irradiation
  - Drugs—methysergide, hydralazine, haloperidol, LSD, methyldopa, beta blockers, phenacetin, amphetamines
  - Malignant—retroperitoneal malignancy (lymphoma, metastatic disease from, e.g. breast cancer), post-chemotherapy
  - Chemicals—talcum powder
  - Infection—TB, syphilis, gonorrhoea, chronic UTI
  - Sarcoidosis
- Bilateral PUJO (uncommon)
- Hydronephrosis of pregnancy (partly due to smooth muscle relaxant effect of progesterone, partly obstruction of ureters by foetus)
- Hydronephrosis in association with an ileal conduit (a substantial proportion of patients with ileal conduit urinary diversion have bilateral hydronephrosis, in the absence of obstruction)
- Bilateral ureteric stones (rare).

Management of ureteric strictures (other than PUJO)

Definition

A normal ureter undergoes peristalsis and, therefore, at any one moment at least one area of the ureter will be physiologically narrowed. A ureteric stricture is a segment of ureter that is narrowed and remains so on several images (i.e. it is a length of ureter that is constantly narrow).

Causes

Most ureteric strictures are benign and iatrogenic. Some follow impaction of ureteric stone for a prolonged period; malignant strictures—within wall of ureter (e.g. TCC ureter), extrinsic compression from outside wall of ureter (e.g. lymphoma, malignant retroperitoneal lymphadenopathy); retroperitoneal fibrosis (RPF), which may be benign (idiopathic, aortic aneurysm, post-irradiation, analgesic abuse) or malignant (retroperitoneal malignancy, post-chemotherapy).

Mechanism of iatrogenic ureteric stricture formation

Normally ischaemic:
- Usually injury at time of open or endoscopic surgery (e.g. damage to ureteric blood supply or direct damage to ureter at time of colorectal resection, AAA graft, hysterectomy); at ureteroscopy—mucosal trauma (from ureteroscope or electrohydraulic lithotripsy), perforation of ureter (urine extravasation leading to fibrosis)
- Radiotherapy in the vicinity of the ureter
- Stricture of ureteroneocystostomy of renal transplant.

Investigations

The stricture may be diagnosed following investigation for symptoms (loin pain, upper tract infection) or may be an incidental finding on an investigation done for some other reason. The stricture may be diagnosed on a renal ultrasound (hydronephrosis), an IVU or CTU. A MAG3 renogram will confirm the presence of obstruction (some minor strictures may cause no renal obstruction) and establish split renal function. Where ureteric TCC is possible proceed with ureteroscopy and biopsy.

'Treatment' options

- Nothing (symptomless stricture in an old patient with significant co-morbidity or <25% function in an otherwise healthy patient with a normally functioning contralateral kidney)
- Permanent JJ stent or nephrostomy, changed at regular intervals (symptomatic stricture in an old patient with significant co-morbidity or <25% function in affected kidney with compromised overall renal function)
- Dilatation (balloon or graduated dilator) (Figs 10.2 and 10.3)

- Incision + balloon dilatation (endo-ureterotomy by Acucise balloon; ureteroscopy or nephrostomy and incision, e.g. by laser). Leave a 12 Ch stent for 4 weeks.
- Excision of stricture and repair of ureter (open or laparoscopic approach)
- Nephrectomy.

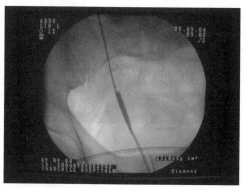

Fig. 10.2 Balloon dilatation of a lower ureteric stricture.

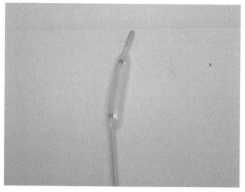

Fig. 10.3 The catheter used for balloon dilatation.

Factors associated with reduced likelihood of a good outcome after endo-ureterotomy

- <25% function in kidney
- Stricture length >1 cm
- Ischaemic stricture
- Mid-ureteric stricture (compared with upper and lower)—tenuous blood supply
- JJ stent size <12 Ch.

Ureteroenteric strictures (ileal conduits, ureteric implantation into neobladder)

These are due to ischaemia and/or peri-ureteral urine leak in the immediate post-operative period, which leads to fibrosis in the tissues around the ureter. In ileal conduits, the left ureter is affected more than right because greater mobilization is required to bring it to the right side and it may be compressed under the sigmoid mesocolon, both of which impair blood flow to the distal end of the ureter.

Pathophysiology of urinary tract obstruction

Effects of obstruction on renal blood flow and ureteric pressure

Acute unilateral obstruction of a ureter (UUO)

Leads to a triphasic relationship between renal blood flow (RBF) and ureteric pressure:

- **Phase 1** (up to 1.5 h post-obstruction): ureteric pressure rises, RBF rises (afferent arteriole dilatation)
- **Phase 2** (from 1.5–5 h post-obstruction): ureteric pressure continues to rise, RBF falls (efferent arteriole vasoconstriction)
- **Phase 3** (beyond 5 h): ureteric pressure falls, RBF continues to fall (afferent arteriole vasoconstriction).

Acute bilateral obstruction of a ureter (BUO) or obstruction of a solitary kidney

- **Phase 1** (up to 1.5 h post-obstruction): ureteric pressure rises, RBF rises (afferent arteriole dilatation).
- **Phase 2** (from 1.5–5 h post-obstruction): ureteric pressure continues to rise, RBF is significantly lower than that during unilateral ureteric obstruction.
- **Phase 3** (beyond 5 h): ureteric pressure remains elevated (in contrast to UUO). By 24 h RBF has declined to the same level for both unilateral and bilateral ureteric obstruction.

In UUO, the decrease in urine flow through the nephron results in a greater degree of Na absorption, so Na excretion falls. Water loss from the obstructed kidney increases.

Release of BUO is followed by a marked natriuresis, increased K excretion, and a diuresis (a solute diuresis). This is due to:

- An appropriate (physiological) natriuresis, to excrete excessive Na which is a consequence of BUO
- A solute diuresis from the accumulation of urea in extracellular fluid
- A diminution of the corticomedullary concentration gradient, which is normally established by the countercurrent mechanism of the loop of Henle, and is dependent on maintenance of flow through the nephron—reduction of flow, as occurs in BUO, reduces the efficiency of the countercurrent mechanism (effectively, the corticomedullary concentration gradient is 'washed out').

There may also be accumulation of natri-uretic peptides (e.g. ANP) during BUO which contributes to the natriuresis following release of the obstruction.

Likelihood of recovery of renal function after release of obstruction

In dogs with completely obstructed kidneys, full recovery of renal function after 7 days of UUO occurs within 2 weeks of relief of obstruction. 14 days of obstruction leads to a permanent reduction in renal function to 70% of control levels (recovery to this level taking 3–6 months after reversal of obstruction). There is some recovery of function after 4 weeks of obstruction, but after 6 weeks of complete obstruction there is no recovery. In humans, there is no clear relationship between the duration of BUO and the degree of recovery of renal function after relief of obstruction.

Physiology of urine flow from kidneys to bladder

Urine production by the kidneys is a continuous process. Its transport from the kidneys, down the ureter, and into the bladder occurs intermittently, by waves of peristaltic contraction of the renal pelvis and ureter (*peristalsis* = wave-like contractions and relaxations). The renal pelvis delivers urine to the proximal ureter. As the proximal ureter receives a bolus of urine it is stretched and this stimulates it to contract, while the segment of ureter just distal to the bolus of urine relaxes. Thus, the bolus of urine is projected distally.

The origin of the peristaltic wave is from collections of pacemaker cells in the proximal most regions of the renal calyces. In species with multiple calyces, such as humans, there are multiple pacemaker sites in the proximal calyces. The frequency of contraction of the calyces is independent of urine flow rate (it is the same at high and low flow rates) and it occurs at a higher rate than that of the renal pelvis. Precisely how frequency of contraction of each calyx is integrated into a single contraction of the renal pelvis is not known. All areas of the ureter are capable of acting as a pacemaker. Stimulation of the ureter at any site produces a contraction wave that propagates proximally and distally from the site of stimulation, but under normal conditions, electrical activity arises proximally and is conducted distally from one muscle cell to another (the proximal most pacemakers are dominant over these latent pacemakers).

Peristalsis persists after renal transplantation and denervation, and does not therefore appear to require innervation. The ureter does, however, receive both parasympathetic and sympathetic innervation, and stimulation of these systems can influence the frequency of peristalsis and the volume of urine bolus transmitted.

At normal urine flow, the frequency of calyceal and renal pelvic contractions is greater than that in the upper ureter, and there is a relative block of electrical activity at the PUJ. The renal pelvis fills; the ureter below it is collapsed and empty. As renal pelvic pressure rises, urine is extruded into the upper ureter. The ureteric contractile pressures that move the bolus of urine are higher than renal pelvic pressures. A closed PUJ may prevent back-pressure on the kidney. At higher urine flow rates every pacemaker-induced renal pelvic contraction is transmitted to the ureter.

To propel a bolus of urine the walls of the ureter must coapt (touch). Resting ureteric pressure is 0–5 cmH$_2$O and ureteric contraction pressures range from 20 to 80 cmH$_2$O. Ureteric peristaltic waves occur 2–6 times per min. The VUJ acts as a one-way valve under normal conditions, allowing urine transport into the bladder and preventing reflux back into the ureter.

Ureter innervation

Autonomic: the ureter has a rich autonomic innervation.
• **Sympathetic:** preganglionic fibres from spinal segments T10–L2; post-ganglionic fibres arise from the coeliac, aorticorenal, mesenteric, superior, and inferior hypogastric (pelvic) autonomic plexuses
• **Parasympathetic:** vagal fibres via coeliac to upper ureter; fibres from S2–4 to lower ureter.
Role of ureteric autonomic innervation is unclear. It is not required for ureteric peristalsis (though it may modulate this). Peristaltic waves originate from intrinsic smooth muscle pacemakers located in minor calyces of renal collecting system.

Afferent *Upper ureter*—afferents pass (alongside sympathetic nerves) to T10–L2; *lower ureter*—afferents pass (alongside sympathetic nerves and by way of pelvic plexus) to S2–4. Afferents subserve stretch sensation from renal capsule, collecting system of kidney (renal pelvis and calyces), and ureter. Stimulation of the mucosa of the renal pelvis, calyces, and ureter also stimulates nociceptors, the pain so felt being referred in a somatic distribution to T8–L2 (kidney T8–L1, ureter T10–L2), in the distribution of the subcostal, iliohypogastric, ilioinguinal, or genitofemoral nerves. Thus, ureteric pain can be felt in the flank, groin, scrotum or labia, and upper thigh depending on the precise site in the ureter from which the pain arises.

Retroperitoneal fibrosis

Retroperitoneal fibrosis (RPF) was first clearly described by the French urologist, Albarran, at the beginning of the 20th century.

Benign causes

- Idiopathic RPF comprises two-thirds of benign cases. A fibrous plaque extends laterally and downwards from the renal arteries encasing the aorta, inferior vena cava, and ureters, but rarely extends into the pelvis. The central portion of the plaque consists of woody scar tissue, while the growing margins have the histological appearance of chronic inflammation. It may be associated with mediastinal, mesenteric or bileduct fibrosis
- Drugs including methysergide, betablockers, haloperidol, amphetamines and LSD
- Chronic urinary infection including TB
- Inflammatory conditions such as Crohn's disease or sarcoidosis
- Abdominal aortic aneurysm (AAA), intra-arterial stents, and angioplasty may induce idiopathic fibrosis, due to peri-aortitis, haemorrhage or an immune response to insoluble lipoprotein.

Malignant causes

- Lymphoma is the most common cause, also sarcoma
- Metastatic or locally infiltratative carcinoma of the breast, stomach, pancreas, colon, bladder, prostate, and carcinoid tumours
- Radiotherapy may cause RPF, although rare today with precise field localization
- Chemotherapy, especially following treatment of metastatic testicular tumours, may leave fibrous masses encasing the ureters. These may or may not contain residual tumour.

Presentation

- Idiopathic retroperitoneal fibrosis classically occurs in the fifth or sixth decade of life
- Men are affected twice as commonly as women
- In the early stage, symptoms are relatively non-specific, including loss of appetite and weight, low-grade fever, sweating, and malaise. Lower limb swelling may develop. Dull, non-colicky abdominal or back pain is described in up to 90% of patients
- Later, the major complication of the disease develops: bilateral ureteric obstruction, causing anuria and renal failure
- Examination may reveal hypertension in up to 60% of patients and an underlying cause, such as an abdominal aortic aneurysm.

Investigations

- Inflammatory serum markers are elevated in idiopathic RPF (60–90% elevated ESR)
- Pyuria or bacteriuria are common
- Ultrasound will demonstrate uni- or bilateral hydronephrosis
- CT, IVU, or ureterography reveal tapering medial displacement of the ureters with proximal dilatation and will exclude calculus disease. Up to one-third of patients will have a non-functioning kidney at the time of presentation due to long standing obstruction
- CT-guided fine needle biopsy of the mass may confirm the presence of malignant disease, but a negative result does not exclude malignancy.

Management

- Emergency management of a patient presenting with established renal failure requires relief of the obstruction by percutaneous nephrostomy or ureteric stenting
- Replacement of fluid and electrolyte losses following relief of bilateral ureteric obstruction is vital due to the frequent post-obstructive diuresis
- Assess with daily weighing and measurement of blood pressure lying and standing
- Steroids may decrease the oedema often associated with retroperitoneal fibrosis and in this way help reduce the obstruction. If used, they are usually discontinued when inflammatory markers return to normal. The anti-oestrogen tamoxifen and cyclophosphamide have been used successfully in some patients
- Surgical ureterolysis with omental wrap is often necessary to free and insulate the ureters from the encasing fibrous tissue
- Biopsies are taken to exclude malignancy
- Monitor for recurrent disease with serum creatinine and ultrasound 3-6 monthly for 5 years.

Trauma to the urinary tract and other urological emergencies

Initial resuscitation of the traumatized patient

The resuscitation of the traumatized patient is usually initiated in the field by the paramedic team and is continued systematically once the patient reaches the emergency department, by a rapid, multidisciplinary, priority-based approach.

Goals of resuscitation:
- Restoration of cardiac, pulmonary and neurological function
- Diagnosis of immediate life-threatening conditions
- Prevention of complications from multisystem injuries.

The initial resuscitation process can be divided into three phases—the primary survey, the secondary survey, the definitive survey:

Primary survey

ABC: Assess the patient's Airway, Breathing, and Circulation.

Airway and Breathing
- Establish a secure airway
- Ventilate by oxygen mask, or endotracheal intubation and mechanical ventilation.
- Immobilize the cervical spine.

Circulation
Assess circulatory function by pulse rate and blood pressure.

The commonest cause of hypotension in the polytraumatized patient is hypovolaemia secondary to haemorrhage. With hypovolaemic shock an immediate bolus of intravenous isotonic crystalloid solution should be given and the patient's response (PR, BP) is assessed.

Radiological imaging

Determined by local facilities. Increasingly, in the severely traumatized patient, CT of chest, abdomen, and pelvis is used to identify significant chest, abdominal, and pelvic injuries. If not available arrange supine chest, abdomen and pelvic X-rays to identify the presence of rib and pelvic fractures, and to identify the presence of significant quantities of blood in chest, abdomen, and pelvis, and in patients with persistent hypotension from presumed bleeding, search for occult haemorrhage using a diagnostic peritoneal lavage or focused abdominal ultrasound.

Hypovolaemic shock is not always associated with hypotension. In young patients, compensatory mechanisms, e.g. rapid vasoconstriction can compensate for as much as a 35% volume loss without significant decreases in blood pressure.

Remember non-hypovolaemic causes of hypotension:
- Tension pneumothorax
- Cardiac tamponade
- Myocardial infarction
- Neurogenic (spinal cord injury).

Urinalysis

Routinely performed in every trauma patient because it provides valuable information regarding the likelihood of injuries to the upper and lower urinary tract. The absence of haematuria, however, does not exclude a urinary tract injury [e.g. haematuria may be absent in acceleration/deceleration renal injuries (see Renal Injuries below)].

As life-threatening injuries are found during the primary survey, resuscitation efforts are initiated concurrently (e.g. chest drain for pneumothorax). The decision to transfer a patient from the emergency room to either the operating room or angiography suite is made during the primary survey.

Secondary survey

Performed after completion of the primary survey. Take a complete history and perform a physical examination from head-to-toe. Arrange selective skeletal X-rays, according to physical findings.

Definitive survey

During this phase, focus attention on identifying specific organ injuries using clinical and radiographic means. Genitourinary injuries are usually recognized during the definitive survey.

During all phases of the initial resuscitation, assess vital signs (blood pressure, respiratory rate, blood gases, urinary output, and body temperature) continually. Vascular pressure monitoring, using central venous and pulmonary arterial catheters, can be performed selectively. Frequent re-evaluation should be performed to detect changes in the patient's condition and the appropriate actions taken.

Renal trauma: classification, mechanism, grading

Classification

Two categories—blunt and penetrating. Proportion of all renal injuries that are blunt—Europe 97%, USA 90%, South Africa 25–85%. Proportion depends on whether urban or non-urban community.

This classification is useful because it predicts the likely need for surgical exploration to control bleeding. Experience from large series shows that 95% of blunt injuries can be managed conservatively, whereas 50% of stab injuries and 75% of gunshot wounds require exploration.

Blunt injures
- Direct blow to the kidney
- Rapid acceleration or rapid deceleration
- A combination of the above.

Rapid deceleration frequently causes renal pedicle injuries (renal artery and vein tears or thrombosis, PUJ disruption) because renal pedicle is the site of attachment of kidney to other fixed retroperitoneal structures.

Most common cause—motor vehicle accidents (e.g. pedestrian hit by a car; direct blow combined with rapid acceleration and then deceleration). Seemingly trivial injuries (e.g. fall from a ladder), direct falls onto the flank, or sporting injuries can lead to significant renal injuries.

Penetrating injuries

Stab or gunshot injuries to the flank, lower chest, and anterior abdominal area may inflict renal damage. 50% of patients with penetrating trauma and haematuria have grade III, IV, or V renal injuries. Penetrating injuries anterior to the anterior axillary line are more likely to injure the renal vessels and renal pelvis, compared with injuries posterior to this line where less serious parenchymal injuries are more likely. Thus, renal injuries from stab wounds to the flank (i.e. posterior to anterior axillary line) can often be managed non-operatively.

Wound profile of a low-velocity gunshot wound is similar to that of a stab wound. High-velocity gunshot wounds (>350 m/s) cause greater tissue damage due to stretching of surrounding tissues ('temporary cavity').

Mechanism

The kidneys are retroperitoneal structures surrounded by peri-renal fat, the vertebral column and spinal muscles, the lower ribs, and abdominal contents. They are therefore relatively protected from injury and a considerable degree of force is usually required to injure them (only 1.5–3% of trauma patients have renal injuries). Associated injuries are therefore common (e.g. spleen, liver, mesentery of bowel). Renal injuries may not initially be obvious, hidden as they are by other structures. To confirm or exclude a renal injury, imaging studies are required. In children, there is proportionally less peri-renal fat to cushion the kidneys against injury, and thus renal injuries occur with lesser degrees of trauma.

Staging of the renal injury

Using CT, renal injuries can be staged according to the American Association for the Surgery of Trauma (AAST) Organ Injury Severity Scale. Higher injury severity scales are associated with poorer outcomes.

Grade I   Contusion (normal CT) or subcapsular haematoma with no parenchymal laceration

Grade II   <1 cm deep parenchymal laceration of cortex, no extravasation of urine (i.e. collecting system intact)

Grade III >1 cm deep parenchymal laceration of cortex, no extravasation of urine (i.e. collecting system intact)

Grade IV   Parenchymal laceration involving cortex, medulla, and collecting system OR renal artery or renal vein injury with contained haemorrhage

Grade V   Completely shattered kidney OR avulsion of renal hilum

Paediatric renal injuries

The kidneys are said to be more prone to injury in children because of the relatively greater size of the kidneys in children, the smaller protective muscle mass and cushion of peri-renal fat, and the more pliable rib cage.

Table 11.1 Summary of mechanisms, causes, grading, and treatment of renal disease

Mechanisms and cause	Blunt or penetrating
	Blunt: direct blow or acceleration/deceleration (RTAs, falls from a height, fall onto flank)
	Penetrating: knives, gunshots, iatrogenic (e.g. PCNL)
Imaging and grading	**CT:** accurate, rapid, images other intra-abdominal structures
	Staging: American Association for the Surgery of Trauma Organ Injury Severity Scale:
	I: contusion or subcapsular haematoma
	II: <1 cm laceration *without* urinary extravasation
	III: >1 cm laceration *without* urinary extravasation
	IV: laceration into collecting system, i.e urinary extravasation
	V: shattered kidney or avulsion of renal pedicle.
Treatment	**Conservative:** 95% of blunt injuries, 50% of stab injuries, 25% of gunshot wounds can be managed non-operatively (cross-match, bed rest, observation)
	Exploration if:
	• Persistent bleeding (persistent tachycardia and/or hypotension not responding to appropriate fluid and blood replacement)
	• Expanding peri-renal haematoma
	• Pulsatile peri-renal haemotoma.

See also: Santucci RA, Wessells H, Bartsch G, *et al.* (2004) Consensus on genitourinary trauma. Evaluation and management of renal injuries: consensus statement of the renal trauma subcommittee. *Br J Urol Int* **93**:937–54.

Renal trauma: clinical and radiological assessment

The haemodynamically stable patient

History: nature of trauma (blunt, penetrating)

Examination: pulse rate, systolic blood pressure, respiratory rate, location of entry and exit wounds, flank bruising, rib fractures. The *lowest recorded systolic blood pressure* is used to determine need for renal imaging.

Urinalysis: crucial for determining likelihood of renal injury and, therefore, of need for radiological tests.

Haematuria (defined as >5 erythrocytes per high-power field or dipstick positive) suggests the possibility of a renal injury; however, the amount of haematuria does not correlate consistently with the degree of renal injury.

Do a full blood count and serum chemistry profile.

Indications for renal imaging

- Macroscopic haematuria
- Penetrating chest and abdominal wounds (knives, bullets)
- Microscopic (>5 rbcs per high-powered field) or dipstick haematuria in a hypotensive patient (systolic blood pressure of <90 mmHg recorded at any time since the injury[1])
- A history of a rapid acceleration or deceleration (e.g. fall from a height, high speed motor vehicle accident). Falls from even a low height can cause serious renal injury in the absence of shock (SBP < 90mmHg) and of haematuria (PUJ disruption prevents blood reaching the bladder)
- Any child with microscopic or dipstick haematuria who has sustained trauma

Adult patients with a history of blunt trauma and microscopic or dipstick haematuria need not have their kidneys imaged as long as there is no history of acceleration/deceleration and no shock, since the chances of a significant injury being found are <0.2%.

Degree of haematuria v. severity of injury

While significant renal injury is more likely with macroscopic haematuria, in some cases of severe renal injury haematuria may be absent. Thus the relationship between the presence, absence, and degree of haematuria and the severity of trauma is not absolute. Broadly speaking, in *blunt* trauma, macroscopic haematuria predicts the likelihood of significant renal injury. Conversely, in *penetrating* trauma, haematuria may be absent in severe renal injury (renal vascular injury, PUJ, or ureter avulsion):

Blunt renal trauma in adults: chance of significant renal injury v. degree of haematuria and SBP

Degree of haematuria; systolic BP mmHg	Significant renal injury
Microhaematuria;* SBP >90	0.2%
Macroscopic haematuria; SBP >90	10%
Macroscopic haematuria; SBP <90	10%
*Dipstick or microscopic haematuria.	

The haemodynamically unstable patient

Haemodynamic instability may preclude standard imaging such as CT, the patient having to be taken to the operating theatre immediately to control the bleeding. In this situation, an on-table IVU (see box) is indicated if:
- A retroperitoneal haematoma is found and/or
- A renal injury is found which is likely to require nephrectomy.

---

1   Remember, in young adults and children, hypotension is a late manifestation of hypovolaemia: blood pressure is maintained until there has been substantial blood loss.

What imaging study?

The IVU has been replaced by contrast enhanced CT scan as the imaging study of choice in patients with suspected renal trauma. Compared with IVU, it provides clearer definition of the injury, allowing injuries to the parenchyma and collecting system to be more accurately graded, and therefore determines subsequent management. An arterial-venous phase scan is done within minutes of contrast injection, followed by a repeat scan 10–20 min after contrast administration to allow time for contrast to reach collecting system.

While ultrasound can establish the presence of two kidneys and identify blood flow in the renal vessels (power Doppler) it cannot accurately identify parenchymal tears, collecting system injuries, or extravasation of urine until a later stage when a urine collection has had time to accumulate.

Imaging is designed to:
- Grade injury
- Document presence and function of contralateral kidney
- Detect associated injuries
- Detect pre-existing renal pathology in affected kidney.

On contrast enhanced CT look for:
- Depth of parenchymal laceration
- Parenchymal enhancement (absence of enhancement suggests renal artery injury)
- Presence of urine extravasation (medial extravasation of contrast suggests disruption of PUJ or renal pelvis)
- Presence, size, and position of retroperitoneal haematoma (haematoma medial to the kidney suggests a vascular injury)
- Presence of injuries to adjacent organs (bowel, spleen, liver, pancreas, etc)
- Presence of a normal contralateral kidney.

On table IVU

When, because of shock and need for immediate laparotomy, a patient is transferred immediately to the operating theatre without having had a CT scan, and a retroperitoneal haematoma is found, a single shot abdominal X-ray, taken 10 min after contrast administration (2 mL/kg of contrast), can establish the presence/absence of a renal injury and the presence of a normally functioning contralateral kidney where the ipsilateral kidney injury is likely to necessitate a nephrectomy.

Renal trauma: treatment

Conservative (non-operative) management

Most blunt (95%) and many penetrating renal injuries (50% of stab injuries and 25% of gunshot wounds) can be managed non-operatively.

Dipstick or microscopic haematuria: if systolic BP since injury has always been >90 mmHg and no history of acceleration or deceleration, imaging and admission is not required.

Macroscopic haematuria: in a cardiovascularly stable patient, having staged the injury with CT, admit for bed rest (no hard and fast rules as to duration) and observation, until the macroscopic haematuria, if present, resolves (cross-match in case blood pressure drops); give antibiotics if urinary extravasation.

High-grade (IV and V) injuries: can be managed non-operatively if they are cardiovascularly stable. However, grade IV and, especially, grade V injuries often require nephrectomy to control bleeding (grade V injuries function poorly if repaired).

Surgical exploration

Is indicated (whether blunt or penetrating injury) if:
- The patient develops shock which does not respond to resuscitation with fluids and/or blood transfusion
- The haemoglobin decreases (there are no strict definitions of what represents a 'significant' fall in haemoglobin)
- There is urinary extravasation and associated bowel or pancreatic injury
- Expanding peri-renal haematoma (again the patient will show signs of continued bleeding)
- Pulsatile peri-renal haematoma

An expanding and/or pulsatile peri-renal haematoma suggests a renal pedicle avulsion. Haematuria is absent in 20%.

Urinary extravasation

Not in itself necessarily an indication for exploration. Almost 80–90% of these injuries will heal spontaneously. The threshold for operative repair is lower with associated bowel or pancreatic injury—bowel contents mixing with urine is a recipe for overwhelming sepsis. In these situations the renal repair should be well drained and omentum interposed between the kidney and bowel or pancreas.

If there is substantial contrast extravasation, consider placing a JJ stent. Repeat renal imaging if the patient develops a prolonged ileus or a fever, since these signs may indicate the development of a urinoma which can be drained percutaneously. Renal exploration is required for a persistent leak.

Devitalized segments

Exploration is usually not required for patients with devitalized segments of kidney and with urinary extravasation.[1]

Complications of renal injury[2-4]

Early

- **Delayed bleeding:** 1.5% of surgically treated patients, 4% of surgically treated penetrating injuries, 1–6% of paediatric blunt injuries managed non-operatively, 20% of conservatively managed stab injuries. 75% require surgery and of these 60% require nephrectomy
- **Urinary extravasation and urinoma formation:** blunt injury 2–20%; penetrating injury 10–25%. If low volume and non-infected often heal spontaneously; large volume—consider a trial of J stenting with renal repair if extravasation persists
- **Abscess formation:** flank pain; fever; ileus. CT or ultrasound is diagnostic. Treat by percutaneous drainage
- **Renal arteriovenous fistulas:** commonest cause is percutaneous renal biopsy i.e. iatrogenic. Often small and heal spontaneously, but may manifest with retroperitoneal bleeding; collecting system bleeding (heavy haematuria); microscopic haematuria; abdominal bruit; hypertension; tachycardia; high output heart failure. Diagnosis is confirmed by selective renal arteriography. Treat by arterial embolization (treatment of choice); partial nephrectomy; complete nephrectomy.

Late

- Decreased renal function
- Hypertension.

Hypertension and renal injury

Excess renin excretion occurs following renal ischaemia from renal artery injury or thrombosis or renal compression by haematoma or fibrosis (so-called 'Page' kidney). This can lead to hypertension months or years after renal injury. The exact incidence of post-traumatic hypertension is uncertain. It may occur in <1% of individuals.

1 Toutouzas KG (2002) Non-operative management of blunt renal trauma: a prospective study. *Am Surg* **68**:1097–103.

2 McAninch JW, Carroll PR, Klosterman PW *et al.* (1991) Renal reconstruction after injury. *J Urol* **145**:932.

3 Carroll PR, McAninch JW. (1985) Operative indications in penetrating renal trauma. *J Trauma* **25**:587.

4 Bernath AS, Shutte H, Fernandez RRD *et al.* (1983) Stab wounds of the kidney: conservative management in flank penetration. *J Urol* **129**:468.

Technique of renal exploration

Midline incision allows:
- Exposure of renal pedicle, so allowing early control of the renal artery and vein
- Inspection for injury to other organs.

Lift the small bowel upwards to allow access to the retroperitoneum. Incise the peritoneum over the aorta, above the inferior mesenteric artery. A large peri-renal haematoma may obscure the correct site for this incision. If this is the case, look for the inferior mesenteric vein and make your incision medial to this. Once on the aorta, the inferior vena cava may be exposed, then the renal veins and the renal arteries. Pass slings around all of these vessels. Expose the kidney by lifting the colon off of the retroperitoneum. Bleeding may be reduced by applying pressure to the vessels via the slings. Control bleeding vessels within the kidney with 4/0 vicryl or monocryl sutures. Close any defects in the collecting system with 4/0 vicryl. If your sutures cut out, place a strip of Surgicel over the site of bleeding, place your sutures through the capsule on either side of this, and tie them over the Surgicel. This will stop them from cutting through the friable renal parenchyma.

Finding a non-expanding, non-pulsatile retroperitoneal haematoma at laparotomy

The finding of an expanding and/or pulsatile retroperitoneal haematoma at laparotomy will often indicate a renal pedicle injury (avulsion or laceration), and nephrectomy may be required to stop further haemorrhage.

Controversy surrounds the correct management of the finding at laparotomy of a non-expanding, non-pulsatile retroperitoneal haematoma. Most can be left alone. Remember, exploration increases the chances of loss of the kidney (because of bleeding which can be controlled only by nephrectomy). The decision to explore is based on whether pre-operative or on-table imaging has been done and is normal or abnormal:

Pre-operative or intra-operative imaging	Action
Normal	Leave the haematoma alone
Abnormal; contralateral kidney normal	Explore and repair renal injury
Abnormal; abnormal or absent contralateral kidney	Leave the haematoma alone*
None	Explore and repair renal injury

* Exploration increases the chances of loss of the kidney (because of bleeding that can be controlled only by nephrectomy), which is a disaster if the contralateral kidney is absent or damaged.

Iatrogenic renal injury: renal haemorrhage after percutaneous nephrolithotomy (PCNL)

Significant renal injuries can occur during percutaneous nephrolithotomy (PCNL) for kidney stones. This is the surgical equivalent of a stab wound and serious haemorrhage results in 1% of cases.[1]

Bleeding during or after a PCNL can occur from vessels in the nephrostomy track itself, from an arteriovenous fistula, or from a pseudoaneurysm, which has ruptured. Track bleeding will usually tamponade around a large-bore nephrostomy tube. Traditionally persistent bleeding through the nephrostomy tube is managed by clamping the nephrostomy tube and waiting for the clot to tamponade the bleeding. While this may control bleeding in some cases, in others a rising or persistently elevated pulse rate (with later hypotension) indicates the possibility of persistent bleeding and is an indication for renal arteriography and embolization of the arteriovenous fistula or pseudoaneurysm (Figs 11.1 and 11.2). Failure to stop the bleeding by this technique is an indication for renal exploration.

Arteriovenous fistulae can sometimes occur following open renal surgery for stones or tumours, and arteriography with embolization again can be used to stop the bleeding in these cases. However, the bleeding usually occurs over a longer time course (days or even weeks), rather than as acute haemorrhage causing shock.

1   Martin X (2000) Severe bleeding after nephrolithotomy: results of hyperselective embolization. *Eur Urol* **37**:136–9.

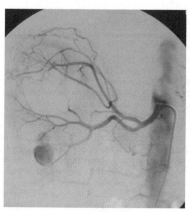

Fig. 11.1 Renal arteriography after PCNL where severe bleeding was encountered. An arteriovenous fistula was found and embolized.

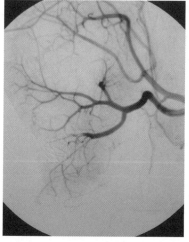

Fig. 11.2 Post-embolization of AV fistula. Note the embolization coils in the lower pole.

Ureteric injuries: mechanisms and diagnosis

Types, causes, and mechanisms
- **External:** rare—blunt (e.g. high speed road traffic accidents, fall from a height); penetrating (knife or gunshot wounds)
- **Internal trauma** (= iatrogenic): during pelvic or abdominal surgery, e.g. hysterectomy, colectomy, AAA repair; ureteroscopy. The ureter may be divided, ligated, or angulated by a suture; a segment excised or damaged by diathermy.

External injury: diagnosis
Based on a high index of suspicion for the possibility of ureteric injury in the above types of scenarios. Imaging studies: IVU or CT can be used to determine the presence of a ureteric injury. If doubt remains regarding the integrity of the ureters, retrograde ureterography should be done.

Internal (iatrogenic) injury: diagnosis
The injury may be suspected at the time of surgery, but injury may not become apparent until some days or weeks post-operatively.

Intra-operative diagnosis
For ureteric contusions and perforations seen at the time of ureteroscopy, insert a JJ stent. During abdominal or pelvic surgery firstly optimize exposure of the suspected injury site by packing bowel out of the way, controlling bleeding, and ensuring the theatre lights are appropriately positioned. Examine both ureters (bilateral injuries can occur).

Direct inspection of the ureter
A good way of inspecting the ureter for injury, but requires exposure of a considerable length of ureter to establish that it has not been injured. Lower ureteric exposure is more difficult than upper ureteric.

Extravasation after injection of methylene blue into the ureter
Look for leakage of dye from a more distant section of ureter.

On-table IVU
Technically difficult; does not always demonstrate the presence or site of injury.

On-table retrograde ureterography
Via an incision made in the bladder or via a cystoscope. A very accurate method of establishing the presence or absence of a ureteric injury (Fig. 11.3). Both ureters can easily be examined.

Post-operative diagnosis
The diagnosis is usually apparent in the first few days following surgery (see box), but it may be delayed by weeks, months, or years (presentation: flank pain; post-hysterectomy incontinence—a continuous leak of urine suggests a ureterovaginal fistula).

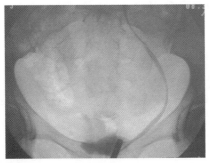

Fig. 11.3 A normal retrograde ureterogram.

Symptoms and signs of ureteric injury

May include:
- An ileus (due to urine within the peritoneal cavity)
- Prolonged post-operative fever or overt urinary sepsis
- Persistent drainage of fluid from drains, the abdominal wound, or the vagina. Send this for creatinine estimation. Creatinine level higher than that of serum = urine (creatinine level will be at least 300 µmol/L)
- Flank pain if the ureter has been ligated
- Abdominal mass, representing a urinoma (a collection of urine)
- Vague abdominal pain
- The pathology report on the organ that has been removed may note the presence of a segment of ureter!

Investigation: IVU or retrograde ureterogram. Ultrasonography may demonstrate hydronephrosis, but hydronephrosis may be absent when urine is leaking from a transected ureter into the retroperitoneum or peritoneal cavity. The IVU usually shows an obstructed ureter or occasionally a contrast leak from the site of injury.

Ureteric injuries: management

When to repair the ureteric injury

Generally, the best time to repair the ureter is as soon as the injury has been diagnosed.

Delay definitive ureteric repair when:
- The patient is unable to tolerate a prolonged procedure under general anaesthetic
- There is evidence of active infection at the site of proposed ureteric repair (infected urinoma).

A percutaneous nephrostomy should be placed, the infection drained radiologically (percutaneous drain), intravenous antibiotics given, and ureteric repair delayed until the patient is apyrexial.

Traditional teaching held that surgical repair should be delayed when the injury was diagnosed between roughly days 7 and 14 after ureteric injury, the time when maximal oedema and inflammation at the site of repair was believed to occur. However, favourable outcomes have been demonstrated after early repair and the time of the original injury is nowadays seen as a less important determinant of time of definitive repair.[1]

Definitive treatment of ureteric injuries

The options depend on:
- Whether the injury is recognized immediately
- Level of injury
- Other associated problems.

The options are:
- JJ stenting for 3–6 weeks (e.g. ligature injury recognized immediately)
- Primary closure of partial transection of the ureter
- Direct ureter to ureter anastomosis (primary uretero-ureterostomy)— if the defect between the ends of the ureter is of a length where a tension-free anastomosis is possible
- Re-implantation of the ureter into the bladder (ureteroneocystostomy) either using a psoas hitch or a Boari flap (Figs 11.4 and 11.5)
- Transuretero-ureterostomy (Fig. 11.6)
- Autotransplantation of the kidney into the pelvis—where the segment of damaged ureter is very long
- Replacement of the ureter with ileum—where the segment of damaged ureter is very long
- Permanent cutaneous ureterostomy—where the patient's life expectancy is very limited
- Nephrectomy—traditionally advocated for ureteric injury during vascular graft procedures (e.g. aortobifemoral graft for AAA), but the trend is towards ureteric repair and renal preservation, reserving nephrectomy only where a urine leak develops post-operatively (continuing drainage of urine from the drain placed at the site of ureteric anastomosis).[2]

JJ stenting

For some injuries, JJ stenting may be adequate for definitive treatment, particularly where the injury does not involve the entire circumference of the ureter and continuity is therefore maintained across the region of the ureteric injury. In situations where a ligature has been applied around the ureter, and this has been immediately recognized such that viability of the ureter has probably not been compromised, remove the ligature and place a JJ stent (cystoscopically if this is feasible or, if not, by opening the bladder). If there has been a delay in recognition of a ligature injury to the ureter, it is probably safer to remove the affected segment of ureter and perform a uretero-ureterostomy. Generally speaking the stent is maintained in position for somewhere between 3 and 6 weeks (no hard and fast rules). At the time of stent removal perform a retrograde ureterogram to confirm that there is no persistent leakage of contrast from the original site of injury, and to see if there is evidence of ureteric stricturing .

Factors other than the level of injury are important in determining the type of repair. Blast injuries characteristically cause considerable 'collateral' damage to the ureter and surrounding tissues, and this may not be apparent at the time of surgery. Delayed necrosis can occur in such apparently normal looking ureters.

1 Blandy JP et al. (1991) Early repair of iatrogenic injury to the ureter and bladder after gyneco-logical surgery. J Urol **146**:761–5.

2 McAninch JW (2002) In: Walsh PC, Retik AB, Vaughan ED, Wein AJ (eds) Campbell's Urology, 8th edn. Philadelphia: W.B. Saunders p. 3703–14.

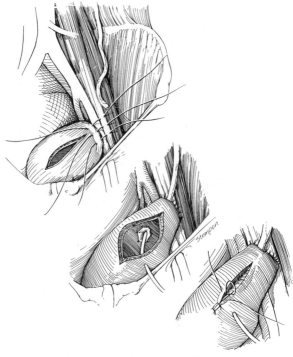

Fig. 11.4 A psoas hitch. (Reproduced with permission).[1]

General principles of ureteric repair

- The ends of the ureter should be debrided, so that the edges to be anastomosed are bleeding freely.
- The anastomosis should be tension free.
- For complete transection, the ends of the ureter should be spatulated, to allow a wide anastomosis to be done.
- A stent should be placed across the repair.
- Mucosa to mucosal anastomosis should be done, to achieve a watertight closure.
- Use 4/0 absorbable suture material.
- A drain should be placed around the site of anastomosis.

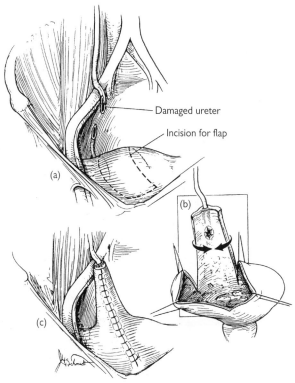

Fig. 11.5 A Boari flap (Reproduced with permission).[2]

1 Presti JC, Carroll PR. (1996) Ureteral and Renal Pelvic trauma: diagnosis and management. In Mc Aninch J.W. *Traumatic and reconstructive urology*. Philadelphia: W.B.Saunders, p. 171–79, Copyright Saunders Ltd.

2 Coburn M. (1996) Ureteral injuries from surgical trauma. McAninch J.W. *Traumatic and reconstructive urology*. Philadelphia: W.B. Saunders, p. 181–97. Copyright Saunders Ltd.

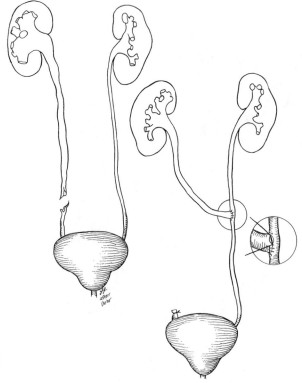

Fig. 11.6 Transuretero-ureterostomy. (Reproduced with permission).[1]

1 Presti JC, Carroll PR. (1996) Ureteral and Renal Pelvic trauma: diagnosis and management. In MeAninch J.W. Traumatic and reconstructive urology. Philadelphia: W.B.Saunders, p. 171–179. Copyright Saunders Ltd.

Pelvic fractures: bladder and ureteric injuries associated with pelvic fractures

Pelvic fractures are usually due to run-over or crush injuries, where massive force is applied to the pelvis. Associated head, chest, intra-abdominal (spleen, liver, mesentery of bowel), pelvic (bladder, urethra, vagina, rectum), and genital injuries are common and these injuries + the massive blood loss from torn pelvic veins and arteries account for the substantial (20%) mortality after pelvic fracture.

Initial assessment

Pelvic fractures are often occult. Screen run-over or crush victims with a pelvic X-ray. Assess:
- Vital signs (PR, SBP)
- Neurovascular integrity of lower limb (lumbosacral plexus, peripheral nerves, and major vessels may be damaged)
- Examine for head, chest, abdominal, and perineal injuries
- Determine stability/instability of the fracture from pelvic X-rays.

Is the fracture stable or unstable?

📖 See Box 11.1.

Abdominal and pelvic imaging in pelvic fracture

- **Abdominal/pelvic CT:** establishes presence/absence of associated pelvic (rectum, bladder) and abdominal organ injury (liver, bowel, spleen)
- **Retrograde urethrogram:** to detect urethral injury. Some hospitals perform retrograde urethrography only when blood is present at the meatus; others do this in all pelvic fracture patients where the pubic rami have been disrupted
- If the urethra is intact a retrograde cystogram is done to assess integrity of the bladder.

Box 11.1 Is the fracture stable or unstable?

Stable = the fracture can withstand normal physiologic forces.
Unstable = the fracture cannot withstand normal physiologic forces.
Instability suggests a greater degree of trauma to the pelvis and increases the likelihood of serious associated injuries. In addition, fixation of an unstable fracture reduces blood loss, mortality, hospital stay, leg length discrepancy, and long-term disability; makes nursing care easier; and reduces analgesic consumption. Stability can be defined according to the Tile classification system of pelvic ring fractures (📖 see Table 11.2)
Of unstable pelvic fractures, 70% are B2 and B3, 10–20% are open book type (B1), and 10–20% are type C.

- **Open book pelvic fracture (B1):** caused by anteroposterior compression. A dramatic rise in pelvic volume stretches vessels, nerves, and organs (e.g. bladder) (📖 see Figs. 11.7 and 11.8)
- **Closed book pelvic fracture (B2 or B3):** caused by a lateral compression force to the pelvis. The pubic rami fracture and overlap, and the ilium and sacral wings may be fractured. Nerves and vessels are not stretched, but the urethra is more likely to be damaged by scissors like action of overlapping pubic rami.
- **Vertically unstable pelvic fracture (C):** vessels and nerves can be damaged by stretching.

Radiological determination of stability

Based on inlet (for anteroposterior displacement) and outlet views (for vertical displacement) of the pelvis, the X-ray beam being angled accordingly. CT provides better definition of sacral, sacroiliac, and acetabular fractures and dislocations.

Is urethral catheterization of a pelvic fracture patient safe?

If there is no blood present at the meatus, a gentle attempt at urethral catheterization may be made. It has been suggested that this could convert a partial urethral rupture into a complete rupture. However, leading US trauma centres state 'We and others have not seen any evidence that this can convert an incomplete into a complete transection … and we usually make one gentle attempt to place a urethral catheter in suspected urethral disruption'.[1] If any resistance is encountered, stop, and obtain a retrograde urethrogram. If the retrograde urethrogram demonstrates a normal urethra, proceed with another attempt at catheterization, using plenty of lubricant. If there is a urethral rupture, insert a suprapubic catheter via a formal open approach, to allow inspection of the bladder (and repair of injuries if present).

Table 11.2 The Tile classification system of pelvic ring fractures

Type A—stable	**A1:** fracture of pelvis not involving the pelvic ring A2 Minimal displacement of pelvic ring with no instability
Type B—rotationally (horizontally) unstable	**B1:** open book B2 closed book.
	Lateral compression: ipsilateral fracture B3 closed book.
	Lateral compression: contralateral fracture (bucket handle fracture)
Type C—rotationally (horizontally) and vertically unstable	**C1:** unilateral
	C2: bilateral
	C3: with acetabular fracture

Bladder injuries associated with pelvic fractures

10% of male and 5% of female pelvic fractures are associated with a bladder injury (fracture type leading to bladder injury is usually an antero-posterior pelvic compression fracture—i.e. open book pelvic fracture; Tile classification B1). 60% of pelvic fracture bladder ruptures are extra-peritoneal, 30% intraperitoneal, and 10% combined extraperitoneal and intraperitoneal.

1 McAninch JW (2002) In: Walsh PC, Retik AB, Vaughan ED, Wein AJ (eds) *Campbell's Urology*, 8th edn. Philadelphia: W.B. Saunders p. 3703–14.

Urethral injuries associated with pelvic fractures

The posterior urethra (essentially the membranous urethra) is injured with roughly the same frequency as the bladder in subjects who sustain a pelvic fracture, occurring in 5–15% of such cases. Most posterior urethral injuries occur in association with pelvic fractures.[1] Cass found bladder ruptures in 6% of pelvic fractures, urethral rupture in 2%, and combined bladder and urethral rupture in 0.5%.[2]

Combined bladder and posterior urethral injuries following pelvic fracture

One-third of patients with a traumatic bladder rupture have injuries to other urinary structures, most commonly the urethra. 10–20% of patients with a pelvic fracture and bladder rupture also have a posterior urethral rupture.

Symptoms and signs of bladder or urethral injury in pelvic fracture

- Blood at meatus—in 40–50% of patients (no blood at meatus in 50–60%)
- Gross haematuria
- Inability to pass urine
- Perineal or scrotal bruising
- 'High riding' prostate
- Inability to pass a urethral catheter.

'High riding prostate'

The prostate and bladder become detached from the membranous urethra and are pushed upwards by the expanding pelvic haematoma. The high riding prostate is said to be a classic sign of posterior urethral rupture. Traditional teaching states that a DRE should be done in cases of pelvic trauma to determine prostatic position. However, the presence of a high riding prostate is an unreliable sign.[3] The pelvic haematoma may make it impossible to feel the prostate, so the patient may be thought to have a high riding prostate when, in fact, it is in a normal position. Conversely, what may be thought to be a normal prostate in a normal position may actually be the palpable pelvic haematoma. In pelvic fracture, a DRE is done not to identify a high riding prostate, but rather to establish the presence of an associated rectal injury (blood seen on the examining finger). However, rectal injury can still occur in the absence of rectal blood.

1 Cass AS (1984) Simultaneous bladder and prostato membranous urethral rupture from external trauma. *J Urol* **132**:907–8.

2 Cass AS (1988) *Genitourinary Trauma*. Boston: Blackwell Scientific Publications.

3 Elliott DS, Barrett DM. (1997) Long-term follow-up and evaluation of primary realignment of posterior urethral disruptions. *J Urol* **157**:814–16.

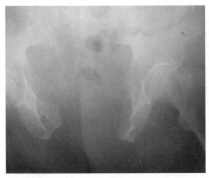

Fig. 11.7 An open book pelvic fracture before fixation.

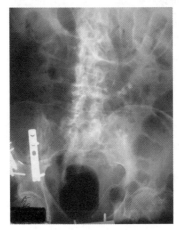

Fig. 11.8 An open book pelvic fracture after fixation.

Management of bladder injuries associated with pelvic fractures

Extraperitoneal: urethral catheter until the bladder has healed (usually 2–3 weeks)

Intraperitoneal: open surgical repair

Management of urethral injuries associated with pelvic fractures

Suprapubic catheter: placement via an open approach is generally better than a percutaneous approach, partly because it allows inspection of the bladder for associated injuries which may require repair (see below), but also because the catheter may inadvertently be placed into the large pelvic haemotoma, which always accompanies such fractures. Not only does this mean that the bladder is not being drained (so urine will leak into the pelvic haematoma and fracture site), but the suprapubic can also act as a potential source of infection of the pelvic haematoma, which can lead to life-threatening sepsis.

Management of combined urethral and bladder injuries associated with pelvic fractures

If a urethral catheter can be passed, and a cystogram shows an extra-peritoneal bladder rupture, leave a urethral catheter in place until the bladder has healed (usually 2–3 weeks).

If a urethral catheter cannot be passed (because of a complete urethral rupture), a suprapubic catheter should be placed via an open approach (rather than percutaneously), to allow inspection of the bladder (and repair if the bladder has been torn) at the same time that the suprapubic catheter is placed. The urethral rupture will prevent a cystogram from being done so *direct* inspection of the bladder is required to establish the presence/absence of a bladder injury.

Bladder injuries

Situations in which the bladder may be injured

TURBT (Figs. 11.9 and 11.10), cystoscopic bladder biopsy, TURP, cysto-litholapaxy, penetrating trauma to the lower abdomen or back, caesarean section (especially as an emergency), blunt pelvic trauma—in association with pelvic fracture or 'minor' trauma in the inebriated patient, rapid deceleration injury (e.g. seat belt injury with full bladder in the absence of a pelvic fracture), spontaneous rupture after bladder augmentation, total hip replacement (very rare).

Types of perforation

- **Intraperitoneal perforation:** the peritoneum overlying the bladder is breached allowing urine to escape into the peritoneal cavity
- **Extraperitoneal perforation:** the peritoneum is intact and urine escapes into the space around the bladder, but not into the peritoneal cavity.

Making the diagnosis

During endoscopic urological operations (e.g. TURBT, cystolitholapaxy), the diagnosis is usually obvious on visual inspection alone—a dark hole is seen in the bladder and loops of bowel may be seen on the other side. No further diagnostic tests are required.

In cases of trauma, the classic triad of symptoms and signs suggesting a bladder rupture is:

- Suprapubic pain and tenderness
- Difficulty or inability in passing urine
- Haematuria.
  Additional signs:
- Abdominal distension
- Absent bowel sounds (indicating an ileus from urine in the peritoneal cavity).

These symptoms and signs are an indication for a retrograde cystogram.

The diagnosis may be made only at operation for fixation of a pelvic fracture.

Imaging studies

Retrograde cystography or CT cystography

- Ensure the bladder is adequately distended with contrast. With inadequate distension a clot, omentum, or small bowel may 'plug' the perforation, which may not therefore be diagnosed. Use at least 400 mL of contrast in an adult and 60 mL plus 30 mL per year of age in children up to a maximum of 400 mL in children
- Obtain images after the contrast agent has been completely drained from the bladder (a post-drainage film). A whisper of contrast from a posterior perforation may be obscured by a bladder distended with contrast.

In extraperitoneal perforations, extravasation of contrast is limited to the immediate area surrounding the bladder. In intraperitoneal perforations, loops of bowel may be outlined by the contrast.

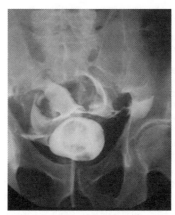

Fig. 11.9 A bladder perforation following a TURBT, as demonstrated on a cystogram (AP view).

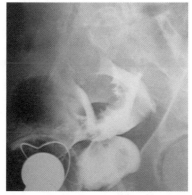

Fig. 11.10 A bladder perforation following a TURBT, as demonstrated on a cystogram (lateral view).

Treatment of bladder rupture

Extraperitoneal: bladder drainage with a urethral catheter for 2 weeks followed by a cystogram to confirm the perforation has healed.

Indications for surgical repair of extraperitoneal bladder perforation:
- If you have opened the bladder to place a suprapubic catheter for a urethral injury
- A bone spike protruding into the bladder on CT
- Associated rectal or vaginal perforation
- Where the patient is undergoing open fixation of a pelvic fracture, the bladder can be simultaneously repaired.

Intraperitoneal: usually repaired surgically to prevent complications from leakage of urine into the peritoneal cavity.

Spontaneous rupture after bladder augmentation: spontaneous bladder rupture occasionally occurs months or years after bladder augmentation, and usually with no history of trauma. If the patient has spina bifida or a spinal cord injury, they usually have limited awareness of bladder fullness and pelvic pain. Their abdominal pain may therefore be mild and vague in onset and nature. Fever or other signs of sepsis may be present. Have a high index of suspicion in patients with augmentation who present with non-specific signs of illness. A cystogram usually, although not always, confirms the diagnosis. If doubt exists, consider exploratory laparotomy.

Posterior urethral injuries in males and urethral injuries in females

Mechanisms

• External blunt	Pelvic fracture—road traffic accidents, falls from a height, crush injuries—most common cause
• External penetrating	Gunshot—rare; stab—rare
• Internal, iatrogenic	Endoscopic surgery; radical prostatectomy; TURP (more likely with vascular prostate, prostate cancer, inexperienced surgeon)
• Internal, self-inflicted	Foreign bodies inserted into urethra—rare

Male posterior urethral injuries

The great majority of posterior urethral injuries are an associated injury following pelvic fracture and their diagnosis and initial management are discussed on p. 498. Immediate (within 48 h) open repair of posterior urethral injuries is associated with a high incidence of urethral strictures (70%) and subsequent re-stenosis after stricture repair, incontinence (20%), and impotence (40%). The surrounding haematoma and tissue swelling makes it difficult to identify structures, and to mobilize the two ends of the urethra to allow tension-free anastomosis.

In the majority of male posterior urethral injuries, treatment should be deferred for 3 months to allow the oedema and haematoma to completely resolve. As this occurs, the two distracted ends of the urethra come closer together, thereby reducing the amount of mobilization that the surgeon has to do. Most such injuries can be repaired by an anastomotic urethroplasty. Optical urethrotomy (division of the stricture using an endoscopic knife or laser, via a cystoscope inserted into the urethra) is generally not recommended.

Immediate repair is indicated where there is an open wound as long as the urethral ends are close (i.e. not distracted by a large haematoma).

Urethral injuries in females

Rare, because the female urethra is short and its attachments to the pubic bone are weak, such that it is less prone to tearing during pubic bone fracture. When they do occur, such injuries are usually associated with rectal or vaginal injuries. In developing countries, prolonged labour can cause ischaemic injury to the urethra and bladder neck, leading to urethrovaginal or vesicovaginal fistula formation.

Anterior urethral injuries

These injuries are uncommon.

Mechanisms

- External blunt   Straddle injury (e.g. forceful contact of perineum with bicycle cross-bar*)—most common cause of injury; kick to perineum; penile fracture
- External penetrating   Gunshot; stab
- Internal, iatrogenic   Catheter balloon inflated in urethra; endoscopic surgery; penile surgery
- Internal, self-inflicted   Foreign bodies inserted into urethra

*Bulbar urethra being crushed against pubic bone.

History and examination

The patient usually presents with difficulty in passing urine and frank haematuria in the context of a straddle injury. Blood may be present at the end of the penis and a haematoma around the site of the rupture. If Buck's fascia has been ruptured (the deep layer of the superficial fascia of penis), urine and blood track into the scrotum causing swelling, and a 'butterfly wing' pattern of bruising, reflecting the anatomical attachments of Colles' fascia— the membranous layer of the superficial fascia of the groin and perineum (📖 see Fig. 11.11).

Confirming the diagnosis and subsequent management

Retrograde urethrography delineates the extent of urethral injury.

Extravasation of urine can create a collection of urine around the urethra (a urinoma) and generates an inflammatory reaction, with subsequent stricture formation. Super-added infection can lead to abscess formation, which may burst onto the surface of the skin leading to a urethrocutaneous fistula. More rarely, Fournier's gangrene supervenes. Urinary diversion (urethral or suprapubic catheter) prevents further extravasation of urine, and antibiotics may reduce the likelihood of superadded infection.

Anterior urethral contusion

Typical history: blood at meatus, *no* extravasation of contrast on retrograde urethrogram. Pass a small gauge urethral catheter (12 Ch in an adult), and remove a week or so later.

Partial rupture of anterior urethra

Leak of contrast from urethra with retrograde flow into bladder. Most can be managed by a period of suprapubic urinary diversion. 70% heal without stricture formation (primary closure can be difficult because of oedema and of haematoma at site of injury and can convert a short area of urethral injury into a longer one). Give a broad spectrum antibiotic to prevent infection of extravasated urine and blood. If a voiding cystogram 2 weeks later confirms urethral healing, remove suprapubic catheter. If contrast still extravasates, leave it in place a little longer.

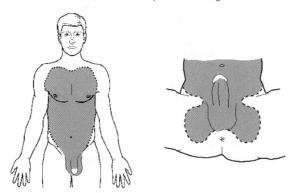

Fig. 11.11 Butterfly bruising following rupture of Buck's fascia.

Suprapubic catheterization (percutaneously) is preferred over urethral catheterization because a partial rupture can be converted to a complete rupture. If the bladder cannot be palpated, such that a suprapubic catheter cannot safely be inserted, then perform open suprapubic cystostomy (under general anaesthetic).

Complete rupture of anterior urethra

Leak of contrast from urethra on retrograde urethrogram, no filling of the posterior urethra or bladder. The urethra may either be immediately repaired (if a surgeon with sufficient experience is available) or a suprapubic catheter can be placed with delayed repair.

Penetrating partial and complete anterior urethral injuries

Knife or gunshot wound: primary (i.e. immediate) repair may be carried out, if a surgeon experienced in these techniques is available; if not, suprapubic diversion and subsequent repair by an appropriate surgeon.

Immediate surgical repair of anterior urethral injuries is only done in the context of penile fracture or where there is an open wound.

The anatomical explanation for 'butterfly wing' pattern of bruising in anterior urethral rupture

Fascial layers of penis from superficial to deep:
• Penile skin
• Superficial fascia of the penis (= dartos fascia)—continuous with the membranous layer of the superficial fascia of the groin and perineum (= Colles' fascia)
• Buck's fascia (= the deep layer of the superficial fascia)
• Deep fascia of the penis (the tunica albuginea), which covers the two dorsal rods of erectile tissue, the corpora cavernosa, and the ventrally located corpus spongiosum that surrounds the urethra (📖 see Fig. 11.12)

If Buck's fascia is intact, bruising from a urethral rupture is confined in a sleeve-like configuration, along the length of the penis. If Buck's fascia has ruptured, the extravasation of blood and thus the subsequent bruising, is limited by the attachments of Colles' fascia which forms a 'butterfly' like pattern in the perineum and is continuous in the upper abdomen and chest with Scarpa's fascia.

How to perform a retrograde urethrogram

• Aseptic technique.
• Urografin 150 ®(sodium amidotrizoate and meglumine amidotrizoate), but other contrast agents can be used
• Position the patient at an oblique angle (bottom leg flexed at the hip and knee)
• A 12 Ch catheter is placed in the fossa navicularis of the penis 1–2 cm from the external meatus, with the catheter balloon with 2 mL of water or with a penile clamp applied to prevent contrast spilling out of the urethra and to hold the catheter in place
• Continuous screening (fluoroscopy) is done as contrast is instilled until the entire length of the urethra is demonstrated. Remember, as the urethra passes through the pelvic floor (the membranous urethra) there is a normal narrowing, and similarly the prostatic urethra is narrower than the bulbar urethra.

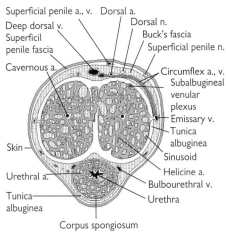

Fig. 11.12 The fascial layers of the penis.

Testicular injuries

Testicular injuries are uncommon.

Mechanisms

Blunt or penetrating. Most in civilian practice are blunt, a blow forcing the testicle against the pubis or the thigh. Bleeding occurs into the parenchyma of the testis and, if sufficient force is applied, the tunica albuginea of the testis (the tough fibrous coat surrounding the parenchyma) ruptures, allowing extrusion of seminiferous tubules.

Penetrating injuries occur as a consequence of gunshot and knife wounds and from bomb blasts; associated limb (e.g. femoral vessel), perineal (penis, urethra, rectum), pelvic, abdominal, and chest wounds may occur.

Where bleeding is confined by the tunica vaginalis, a *haematocele* is said to exist. Intraparenchymal (intratesticular) haemorrhage and bleeding beneath the parietal layer of tunica vaginalis will cause the testis to enlarge slightly. The testis may be under great pressure as a consequence of the intra-testicular haemorrhage confined by the tunica vaginalis. This can lead to ischaemia, necrosis, and atrophy of the testis.

The force is usually sufficient to rupture the tunica albuginea and the tunica vaginalis, and seminiferous tubules and blood extrude into the layers of the scrotum. This is a *haematoma*.

History and examination

Severe pain is common, as are nausea and vomiting. If the testis is surrounded by haematoma it will not be palpable. If it is possible to palpate the testis, it is usually very tender. The resulting scrotal haematoma can be very large, and the bruising and swelling so caused may spread into the inguinal region and lower abdomen.

Testicular ultrasound in cases of blunt trauma

A normal parenchymal echo pattern suggests there is no significant testicular injury (i.e. no testicular rupture). Hypo-echoic areas within the testis (indicating intraparenchymal haemorrhage) suggests testicular rupture.

Indications for exploration in scrotal trauma

- **Testicular rupture:** exploration allows evacuation of the haematoma, excision of extruded seminiferous tubules, and repair of the tear in the tunica albuginea
- **Penetrating trauma:** exploration allows repair to damaged structures (e.g. the vas deferens may have been severed and can be repaired).

Penile injuries

Amputation

Blood loss can be severe; resuscitate the shocked patient and cross-match blood. Place the penis, if found, in a wet swab inside a plastic bag, which is then placed inside another bag containing ice ('bag in a bag'). It can survive for 24 h.

Knife and gunshot wounds

Associated injuries are common (e.g. scrotum, major vessels of the lower limb). Most injuries, other than minor ones, should undergo primary repair. Remove debris from wound (e.g. particles of clothing) and debride necrotic tissue and repair as for penile fractures (see Box 11.2).

Penile fracture

Rupture of the tunica albuginea of the erect penis (i.e. rupture of one or both corpora cavernosa ± rupture of corpus spongiosum with rupture of the urethra). The tunica albuginea is 2 mm thick in the flaccid penis. It thins to 0.25 mm during erection, and is therefore vulnerable to rupture if the penis is forcibly bent (e.g. during vigorous sexual intercourse). The patient usually reports a sudden 'snapping' or 'popping' sound, and/or sensation, with sudden penile pain and detumescence of the erection.

The penis is swollen and bruised, sometimes resembling an aubergine. If Buck's fascia has ruptured, bruising extends onto the lower abdominal wall, and into the perineum and scrotum. A tender, palpable defect may be felt over the site of the tear in the tunica albuginea. If the urethra is damaged, there may be blood at the meatus or haematuria (dipstick/microscopic or macroscopic), and pain on voiding or urinary retention. Arrange a retrograde urethrogram in such cases.

Treatment

There has been a trend away from conservative management towards surgical repair (lower complication rate e.g. reduced penile deformity, less chance of penile scar tissue and prolonged penile pain).

Conservative: application of cold compresses to the penis; analgesics and anti-inflammatory drugs; abstinence from sexual activity for 6–8 weeks to allow healing.

Surgery: expose the fracture site in the tunica albuginea, evacuate the haematoma, and close the defect in the tunica.

Box 11.2 Surgical re-implantation of amputated penis

Repair the urethra first, over a catheter, to provide a stable base for subsequent neurovascular repair. Close the tunica albuginea of the corpora (4/0 absorbable suture). Cavernosal artery repair is technically very difficult and does not improve penile viability. Anastomose the dorsal artery of the penis (11/0 nylon), then the dorsal vein (9/0 nylon) to provide venous drainage, and, finally, the dorsal penile nerve (10/0 nylon).

Surgical repair of penile fracture

Expose the fracture site by degloving the penis via a circumcising incision around the subcoronal sulcus or by an incision directly over the defect if palpable. A degloving incision allows better exposure of the urethra for associated urethral injuries. Alternatively, use a midline incision extending distally from the midline raphe of the scrotum, along the shaft of the penis. This latter incision, along with a degloving incision, allows excellent exposure of both corpora cavernosa so that an unexpected bilateral injury can be repaired easily, as can a urethral injury should this have occurred.

Close the defect in the tunica with absorbable sutures or by non-absorbable sutures (bury the knots so that the patient is unable to palpate them). Non-absorbable sutures may possibly be associated with prolonged post-operative pain. Leave a urethral catheter (voiding can be difficult immediately post-operatively). Repair a urethral rupture, if present, with a spatulated single or two-layer urethral anastomosis, and splint repair with a urethral catheter for 3 weeks.

Penile bites

Clean the wound. Give broad spectrum antibiotics (e.g. cephalosporin and amoxicillin).

Zipper injuries

If the penis is still caught in the zipper, use lubricant jelly and gently attempt to open it. The zipper may have to be cut with orthopaedic cutters or prised apart with a pair of surgical clips on either side of the zipper.

Torsion of the testis and testicular appendages

Definition

A testicular torsion is a twist of the spermatic cord resulting in strangulation of the blood supply to the testis and epididymis. Testicular torsion occurs most frequently between the ages of 10–30 (peak incidence 13–15 years of age), but any age group may be affected.

History and examination

Sudden onset of severe pain in the hemiscrotum, sometimes waking the patient from sleep. It may radiate to the groin, loin, or epigastrium (reflecting its origin from the dorsal abdominal wall of the embryo and its nerve supply from T10/11). There is sometimes a history of minor trauma to the testis. Some patients report previous episodes with spontaneous resolution of the pain (suggesting previous torsion with spontaneous detorsion). The patient may have a slight fever. The testis is usually slightly swollen and very tender to touch. It may be high-riding (lying at a higher than normal position in the testis) and may be in a horizontal position due to twisting of the cord. The cremasteric reflex is usually, but not always, absent (positive Rabinowitz's sign). The cremasteric reflex may normally be elicited by stroking the finger along inside of the thigh, which results in upwards movement of the ipsilateral testis. Elevation of the involved testicle does not ameliorate the symptoms (negative Prehn's sign).

Differential diagnosis and investigations

Epididymo-orchitis, torsion of a testicular appendage, and causes of flank pain with radiation into the groin and testis (e.g. a ureteric stone). Colour Doppler ultrasound (reduced arterial blood flow in the testicular artery) and radionuclide scanning (decreased radioisotope uptake) can be used to diagnose testicular torsion, but in many hospitals these tests are not readily available and the diagnosis is based on symptoms and signs.

Surgical management

Scrotal exploration should be undertaken as a matter of urgency. Delay in relieving the twisted testis results in permanent ischaemic damage to the testis causing atrophy, loss of hormone and sperm production, and as the testis undergoes necrosis and the blood–testis barrier breaks down, an auto-immune reaction against the contralateral testis (sympathetic orchidopathia). Fix **BOTH** testes since the bell-clapper abnormality, which predisposes to torsion can occur bilaterally.

Torsion of testicular appendages

The appendix testis (hydatid of Morgagni—a remnant of the Müllerian duct) and the appendix epididymis (a remnant of a cranial mesonephric tubule of the Wolffian duct) can undergo torsion causing pain that mimicks a testicular torsion. At scrotal exploration they are easily removed with scissors or a diathermy probe.

Paraphimosis

Definition and presentation

This is where the foreskin is retracted from over the glans of the penis, becomes oedematous, and cannot then be pulled back over the glans into its normal anatomical position. It occurs most commonly in teenagers or young men and also in elderly men (who have had the foreskin retracted during catheterization, but where it has not been returned to its normal position). Paraphimosis is usually painful. The foreskin is oedematous and a small area of ulceration of the foreskin may have developed.

Treatment

The 'iced-glove' method: apply topical lignocaine gel to the glans and foreskin for 5 min. Place ice and water in a rubber glove and tie a knot in the cuff of the glove to prevent the contents from pouring out. Invaginate the penis into the thumb of the glove. This may reduce the swelling and allow reduction of the foreskin.

Granulated sugar placed in a condom or glove and applied over the end of the penis has been used to reduce the oedema by osmosis.

The Dundee technique[1]: give the patient a broad spectrum antibiotic such as 500 mg of ciprofloxacin by mouth. Apply a ring block to the base of the penis using a 26 G needle and 10–20 mL of 0.5% plain bupivicaine (children usually require general anaesthesia). Clean the skin of the foreskin and the glans with cleaning solution. Using a 25 G needle make approximately 20 punctures into the oedematous foreskin. Squeeze the oedema fluid out of the foreskin (Fig. 11.13) and return to its normal position. Approximately one-third of patients subsequently require elective circumcision for an underlying phimosis.

If this fails, the traditional surgical treatment is a dorsal slit under general anaesthetic or ring block. A longitudinal incision is made in the tight band of constricting tissue and the foreskin pulled back over the glans. Close the incision transversely to lengthen the circumference of the foreskin and prevent recurrences.

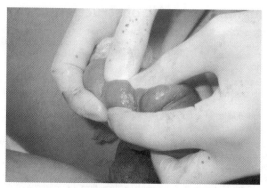

Fig. 11.13 Paraphimosis reduced by the Dundee technique. (Reproduced with kind permission of Blackwell's Publications).[1]

1 Reynard JM, Barua JM (1999) Reduction of paraphimosis the simple way—the Dundee technique. *Br J Urol Int* **83**: 859–60.

Malignant ureteric obstruction

Locally advanced prostate cancer, bladder or ureteric cancer may cause unilateral or bilateral ureteric obstruction. Locally advanced non-urological malignancies can also obstruct the ureters (e.g. cervical cancer, rectal cancer, lymphoma).

Unilateral obstruction is often asymptomatic; an incidental ultrasound finding that requires no specific treatment in the presence of a normal contralateral kidney. Occasionally, loin pain and systemic symptoms may develop due to infection of the obstructed upper urinary tract. In this circumstance, drainage by nephrostomy or stenting is required.

Bilateral ureteric obstruction is a urological emergency. The patient presents either with symptoms and signs of renal failure, or anuric without a palpable bladder. A mass will probably be palpable on rectal examination. *Investigations:* renal ultrasound will demonstrate bilateral hydronephrosis and an empty bladder; CT urography will confirm the presence of dilated ureters down to a mass at the bladder base.

Immediate treatment of bilateral ureteric obstruction

After treating any life-threatening hyperkalaemia, options include bilateral percutaneous nephrostomy or ureteric stenting. A clotting screen is required prior to nephrostomy insertion. Insertion of retrograde ureteric stents in this setting is usually unsuccessful because tumour involving the trigone obscures the location of the ureteric orifices. More successful is antegrade ureteric stenting following nephrostomy insertion, both of which are performed under sedo-analgesia. The full-length double-J silicone or polyurethane ureteric stents require periodic (4–6-monthly) changes to prevent calcification or blockage. In the case of prostate cancer, hormone therapy should be commenced if not previously used; even in patients with androgen-independent disease, high-dose parenteral oestrogens may relieve ureteric obstruction.

Long-term treatment of bilateral ureteric obstruction

Longer-term treatment options include urinary diversion by formation of ileal conduit, ureteric re-implantation, insertion of short 'permanent' metallic ureteric stents, or ureteric replacement with isolated ileal segments or prosthetic graft material. Such procedures are often complicated and inappropriate in these poor-prognosis patients.

Spinal cord and cauda equina compression

Spinal cord compression due to spinal metastases from urological cancers

This is a urological oncological emergency; failure to diagnose and treat promptly can lead to permanent paraplegia and autonomic dysfunction (failure of bladder and bowel emptying; inability to achieve an erection). Due to epidural compression arising from vertebral body metastasis in the majority of cases, 95% of patients will complain of back pain and have a positive bone scan. 10% of cases do not exhibit these features because their disease is paravertebral. Patients with back pain should be examined neurologically and evaluated radiologically. Pain usually precedes cord compression by about 4 months. Other clinical features include sensory changes and muscle weakness in the lower limbs, bladder and bowel dysfunction, and these can progress rapidly to become irreversible.

If cord compression is suspected, the investigation of choice is spinal MRI, which will reveal the deposits (multiple in 20% of cases).

Treatment

Initial treatment is with high-dose intravenous corticosteroids (e.g. dexamethasone 10 mg followed by 4 mg 6-hourly for 2–3 weeks). Without delay, further treatment with radiotherapy or neurosurgical decompression is carried out. Surgery should be considered preferable if there is pathological fracture, unknown tissue diagnosis, or previous history of radiotherapy.

Cauda equina compression

The adult spinal cord tapers below L2 vertebral level into the conus medullaris. The cauda equina consists of the nerve roots of all spinal cord segments below L2, as they run in the subarachnoid space to their exit levels in the lower lumbar and sacral spines.

Pathophysiology: the cauda equina may be compressed by central intervertebral disc prolapse (1–15% of cases), spinal stenosis, or by a benign or malignant tumour within the lower lumbar or sacral vertebral canal.

Symptoms: the diagnosis should be considered in any female or young male presenting with difficulty voiding or in urinary retention. There may be back pain.

Signs: palpable bladder, loss of peri-anal (S2–4) and lateral foot sensation (S1–2), reduced anal tone, priapism.

Investigations: MRI lumbosacral spine; urodynamic studies reveal a normally compliant but areflexic bladder.

Treatment: emergency neurosurgical decompression (laminectomy within 48 h of onset of symptoms), intermittent self-catheterization.

Infertility

Male reproductive physiology

Hypothalamic-pituitary-testicular axis

The hypothalamus secretes luteinizing hormone-releasing hormone (LHRH), also known as gonadotrophin-releasing hormone (GnRH). This causes pulsatile release of anterior pituitary gonadotrophins, called follicle stimulating hormone (FSH) and luteinizing hormone (LH), which act on the testis. FSH stimulates the seminiferous tubules to secrete inhibin and produce sperm; LH acts on Leydig cells to produce testosterone (📖 see Fig. 12.1).

Testosterone is secreted by the interstitial **Leydig cells**, which lie adjacent to the seminiferous tubules in the testis. It promotes development of the male reproductive system and secondary sexual characteristics. Steroidogenesis is stimulated by a cAMP-protein kinase C mechanism, which converts cholesterol to pregnenolone. Further steps in the biosynthesis pathway produce intermediary substances (dehydroepiandrosterone and androstenedione) prior to producing testosterone. In the blood, testosterone is attached to sex hormone binding globulin (SHBG) and albumin. At androgen-responsive target tissues, testosterone is converted into a potent androgen, dihydrotestosterone (DHT), by intracellular 5α-reductase (📖 see Fig. 16.7, p. 644).

Spermatogenesis Seminiferous tubules are lined with **Sertoli cells**, which surround developing germ cells (spermatogonium), and provide nutrients and stimulating factors, as well as secreting androgen-binding factor and inhibin (Fig. 12.2). Primordial germ cells divide to form primary spermatocytes. These undergo a first meiotic division to create secondary spermatocytes (46 chromosomes), followed by a second meiotic division to form spermatids (23 chromosomes). Finally, these differentiate into spermatozoa. This process takes 70 days. The non-motile spermatozoa leave the seminiferous tubules and pass to the epididymis, for storage and maturation (until ejaculation). Spermatozoa that are not released are reabsorbed by phagocytosis.

Mature sperm have a head, middle piece and tail (Fig. 12.3). The head is composed of a nucleus covered by an acrosome cap, containing vesicles filled with lytic enzymes. The middle piece contains mitochondria and contractile filaments, which extend into the tail to aid motility. After deposition at the cervix, sperm penetrate cervical mucus and travel through the uterus to the site of fertilization in the fallopian tube, during which time they undergo functional maturation (capacitation). Sperm start to penetrate the oocyte, and bind to the zona pellucida. The activation phase is initiated (by ZP3), triggering hyperactivated motility and the acrosomal reaction, leading to enzyme release, penetration into the cytoplasm of the oocyte, fusion, and fertilization.

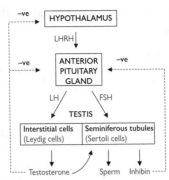

Fig. 12.1 Hypothalamic-pituitary-testicular axis.

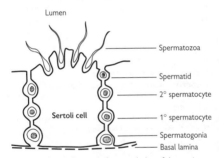

Fig. 12.2 Spermatogenesis in the seminiferous tubules of the testis.

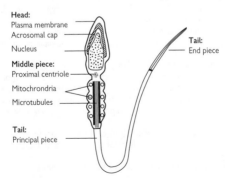

Fig. 12.3 Spermatozoon.

Aetiology and evaluation of male infertility

Definition of subfertility

Failure of conception after at least 12 months of regular unprotected intercourse. The chance of a normal couple conceiving is estimated at 20–25% per month, 75% by 6 months, and 90% at 1 year.

Epidemiology

Up to 50% of infertility is due to male factors. An estimated 14–25% of couples may be affected at some point in their reproductive years.

Pathophysiology

Failure of fertilization of the normal ovum due to defective sperm development, function, or inadequate numbers. There may be abnormalities of morphology (teratospermia), motility (asthenospermia), low sperm numbers (oligospermia), or absent sperm (azoospermia). Abnormal epididymal function may result in defective spermatozoa maturation or transport, or induce cell death.

Aetiology

- **Idiopathic** (25%)
- **Varicocele** (present in ~40%)
- **Cryptorchidism** (undescended testes)
- **Functional sperm disorders:** immunological infertility (antisperm antibodies); head or tail defects; Kartagener's syndrome (immotile cilia); dyskinetic cilia syndrome
- **Erectile or ejaculatory problems:** retrograde ejaculation causes absent or low volume ejaculate
- **Testicular injury:** orchitis (post-pubertal bilateral mumps orchitis); testicular torsion; trauma; radiotherapy
- **Endocrine disorders:** Kallmann's syndrome (isolated gonadotrophin deficiency causing hypogonadism); Prader–Willi syndrome (hypogonadism, short stature, hyperphagia, obesity); pituitary gland adenoma, radiation or infection
- **Hormone excess:** excess prolactin (pituitary tumour); excess androgen (adrenal tumour, congenital adrenal hyperplasia, anabolic steroids); excess oestrogens
- **Genetic disorders:** Kleinfelter's syndrome (47XXY) involves azoospermia, ↑FSH/LH and ↓testosterone; XX male; XYY syndrome
- **Male genital tract obstruction:** congenital absence of vas deferens; agenesis of seminal vesicles/Wolffian duct abnormalities; epididymal obstruction or infection; Müllerian prostatic cysts; groin or scrotal surgery
- **Systemic disease:** renal failure; liver cirrhosis; cystic fibrosis
- **Drugs:** chemotherapy; steroids; alcohol; marijuana; sulfasalazine; smoking
- **Environmental factors:** pesticides; heavy metals; hot baths

- **Infection:** genital tract infections are found in 10-20%. *Chlamydia trachomatis* can attach to and penetrate sperm; *Ureaplasma urealyticum* reduces sperm motility.

History

- **Sexual and reproductive:** duration of problem; frequency and timing of intercourse; use of vaginal lubricants (adversely affects sperm function); previous successful conceptions; previous birth control; erectile or ejaculatory dysfunction
- **Developmental:** age at puberty; history of cryptorchidism; gynaecomastia
- **Medical and surgical:** detailed assessment for risk factors—recent febrile illness; post-pubertal mumps orchitis; varicocele; testicular torsion, trauma or tumour; sexually transmitted infections; urinary tract infection; genitourinary and pelvic surgery; radiotherapy; respiratory diseases associated with ciliary dysfunction; diabetes
- **Drug and environmental:** previous chemotherapy; exposure to substances which impair spermatogenesis or erectile function; alcohol consumption; smoking habits; hot baths
- **Family:** hypogonadism; cryptorchidism.

Examination

Perform a full assessment of all systems, with attention to general appearance (evidence of secondary sexual development; signs of hypogonadism; gynaecomastia). *Urogenital examination* should include assessment of the penis (Peyronie's plaque, phimosis, hypospadias); measurement of testicular consistency, tenderness and volume with a Prader orchidometer (normal >20 mL—varies with race); palpate epididymis (tenderness, swelling) and spermatic cord (vas deferens present or absent; varicocele); digital rectal examination of prostate.

Investigation of male infertility

Basic investigations

Semen analysis: 2–3 specimens over several weeks, collected after 2–7 days of sexual abstinence. Deliver specimens to the laboratory within 1 hour. Ejaculate volume, liquefaction time and pH are noted (Table 12.1). Microscopy techniques measure sperm concentration, total numbers, morphology and motility (Table 12.2). The mixed antiglobulin reaction (**MAR**) test is used to detect antisperm antibodies (useful for asthenospermia, which can be associated with immunological infertility). The presence of leucocytes (>1 × 10⁶/mL of semen) suggests infection, and cultures should be requested. Low or absent ejaculate volume may suggest absence or hypoplasia of vas deferens or seminal vesicles, ejaculatory duct obstruction, hypogonadism, or retrograde ejaculation.

Hormone measurement: serum FSH, LH and testosterone (Table 12.3). In cases of isolated low testosterone level, it is recommended to test morning and free testosterone levels. Raised prolactin is associated with sexual dysfunction, and may indicate pituitary disease.

Special investigations

Chromosome analysis: indicated for clinical suspicion of an abnormality (azoospermia or oligospermia, small atrophic testes with ↑FSH).

Testicular biopsy: performed for azoospermic patients, to differentiate between obstructive and non-obstructive causes. It may also be used for simultaneous sperm retrieval.

Post-orgasmic urine analysis: the presence of >10–15 sperm per high powered field confirms the diagnosis of retrograde ejaculation.

Sperm function tests

- **Post coital test:** cervical mucus is taken just before ovulation, and within 8 h of intercourse, and microscopy performed. Normal results shows >10 sperm per high powered field, the majority demonstrating progressive motility. Abnormal results indicate inappropriate timing of the test; cervical mucus antisperm antibodies; abnormal semen; inappropriately performed coitus
- **Sperm penetration test:** a sample of semen is placed directly onto pre-ovulatory cervical mucus on a slide, and the penetrative ability of spermatozoa observed
- **Sperm-cervical mucus test:** a specimen of semen (control), and one mixed with cervical mucus are placed separately on a slide, and observed for 30 min. More than 25% exhibiting jerking movements in the mixed sample (but not the control) is a positive test for antisperm antibodies.

Imaging

Scrotal ultrasound scan is used to confirm a varicocele and assess testicular abnormalities.

Transrectal ultrasonography is indicated for low ejaculate volumes, to investigate seminal vesicle obstruction (>1.5 cm width) or absence, and ejaculatory duct obstruction (>2.3 mm).

Vasography Vas deferens is punctured at the level of the scrotum, and injected with contrast. A normal test shows the passage of contrast along the vas deferens, seminal vesicles, ejaculatory duct, and into the bladder, which rules out obstruction.

Venography Used to diagnose and guide embolization treatment of varicocele.

Table 12.1 Semen analysis: normal parameters*

Semen analysis	Normal values
Semen volume	>2.0 mL
pH	7.2–7.8
Total sperm count	$>40 \times 10^6$/ejaculate
Sperm concentration	$>20 \times 10^6$/ml
Sperm motility	>50% with progressive motility (grades >2); or >25% grade 4
Sperm morphology	>15% normal forms
Viability	>75% viable sperm
Time to liquefy	5–25 min
White blood cells (WBC)	$<1 \times 10^6$ WBC/mL
MAR-test (for anti-sperm Ab)	Negative (<10% with adherent particles)
Zinc	>2.4 mol/ejaculate
Semen fructose concentration	120–145 mg/dL

*Adapted from World Health Organization (WHO) reference values for semen analysis.

Table 12.2 Grading of sperm motility

Grade	Type of sperm motility
0	No motility
1	Sluggish; no progressive movement
2	Slow, meandering forward progression
3	Moving in a straight line with moderate speed
4	Moving in a straight line at high speed

Table 12.3 Clinical diagnosis on hormone assay

FSH*	LH**	Testosterone	Diagnosis
↑	Normal	Normal	Seminiferous tubule damage (defective spermatogenesis)
Normal	Normal	Normal	Normal or bilateral genital tract obstruction
↑	↑	Normal/↓	Testicular failure
↓	↓	↓	Hypogonadotrophism

*Follicle stimulating hormone. **Luteinizing hormone.

Oligospermia and azoospermia

Oligospermia

Defined as a sperm concentration of less than 20 million per ml of ejaculate.

Aetiology: varicoceles; idiopathic; androgen deficiency. It is identified in ~60% of patients presenting with testicular cancer or lymphoma.

Associated disorders: Often associated with abnormalities of morphology and motility. The combined disorder is called oligoasthenoteratospermia (OAT) syndrome. Common causes of OAT include varicoceles; cryptorchidism; idiopathic; drug and toxin exposure; febrile illness.

Investigations

Semen analysis: sperm counts <5-10 million/ml (severe form) require hormone investigation, including FSH and testosterone. Severe oligospermia is associated with seminiferous tubular failure, small soft testes and ↑FSH.

Hormone assays: also include prolactin levels if testosterone is low, as hyperprolactinaemia can adversely affect spermatogenesis.

Scrotal ultrasonography: to identify a varicocele.

Treatment: Correct the underlying cause (i.e. varicocele repair or embolization may improve testosterone and sperm production). Idiopathic cases may respond to empirical medical therapy (clomifene), or require assisted reproductive techniques (ART; 📖 see p. 534).

Azoospermia

Defined as an absence of sperm in the ejaculate fluid.

Aetiology

Obstructive causes

- **Vas deferens obstruction:** congenital bilateral absence of vas deferens/CBAVD;[1] post-surgery or post-vasectomy
- **Epididymal obstruction:** idiopathic, post-infective or post-surgery
- **Ejaculatory obstruction:** post-infective, post-surgery.

Non-obstructive causes

- **Hormonal abnormality:** hypogonadotrophism (Kallmann's syndrome, pituitary tumour)
- **Abnormalities of spermatogenesis:** secondary to varicocele, testicular torsion or trauma, viral orchitis or idiopathic; chromosomal anomalies (i.e. Kleinfelter's syndrome).

Investigations

- **Hormone assay:** raised FSH indicates non-obstructive cause (i.e. reduced spermatogenesis presents with ↑FSH associated with ↓inhibin). Normal FSH with normal testes indicates increased likelihood of obstruction
- **Chromosomal analysis** may be used to exclude Kleinfelter's syndrome in patients presenting with azoospermia, small soft testes, gynaecomastia, ↓FSH/LH and ↓testosterone

- **Testicular biopsy** is performed to assess if normal sperm maturation is occurring, and for sperm retrieval (for later therapeutic use)
- **Transrectal ultrasound (TRUS)** assesses absence or blockage of vas deferens, and ejaculatory duct obstruction. Exclude cystic fibrosis in patients with vas deferens defects
- **Renal tract USS** for CBAVD, as it is associated with unilateral renal agenesis
- **Vasogram** to assess for vas deferens obstruction.

Management
Treatment will depend on underlying aetiology (📖 see also p. 526).

Obstructive aetiology
- **Bilateral absence or agenesis of vas deferens:**[1] percutaneous epididymal sperm aspiration (PESA), microsurgical epididymal sperm aspiration (MESA) or testicular exploration and sperm extraction (TESE)
- **Obstructive cause with normal testis:** vasoepididymostomy or vasovasostomy if an isolated obstruction identified (i.e. epididymal obstruction or vasectomy respectively). TESE if not reconstructable.

Non-obstructive aetiology
- **Primary testicular failure with testicular atrophy:** microsurgical testicular exploration and sperm extraction (Micro-TESE) with intracytoplasmic sperm injection (ICSI) and in-vitro fertilization (IVF). Consider artificial insemination using donor (AID) if this fails
- **Primary testicular failure with normal testis:** TESE with ICSI and IVF; AID
- **Varicocele repair.**

---

1 CBAVD is associated with mutations in the cystic fibrosis transmembrane conductance regulator gene. Most of these patients are not candidates for reconstruction as they have a defect in sperm transport from mid-epididymis to seminal vesicles.

Varicocele

Definition

Dilatation of veins in the pampiniform plexus of the spermatic cord.

Prevalence

Found in 15% of men in the general population, 20–40% of males presenting with primary infertility, and 45–80% of men with secondary infertility. Rare prior to puberty; present in ~10% of adolescents. Bilateral or unilateral (left side affected in 90%).

Aetiology

Incompetent valves in the internal spermatic veins lead to retrograde blood flow, vessel dilatation, and tortuosity of the pampiniform plexus. The left internal spermatic vein enters the renal vein at right angles and is under a higher pressure than the right vein, which enters the vena cava obliquely at a lower level. As a consequence, the left side is more likely to develop a varicocele.

Pathophysiology

Testicular venous drainage is via the pampiniform plexus, a meshwork of veins encircling the testicular arteries. This arrangement normally provides a counter-current heat exchange mechanism which cools arterial blood as it reaches the testis. Varicoceles adversely affect this mechanism, resulting in elevated scrotal temperatures, and consequent deleterious effects on spermatogenesis (± loss of testicular volume over time).

Table 12.4 Varicocele grading system

Grade	Size	Definition
1	Small	Palpable only with Valsalva manoeuvre
2	Moderate	Palpable without Valsalva
3	Large	Visible through the scrotal skin

Presentation

The majority are asymptomatic, although large varicoceles may cause pain or a heavy feeling in the scrotal area. Examine both lying and standing, and ask the patient to perform the Valsalva manoeuvre (strain down). A varicocele is identified as a mass of dilated and tortuous veins above the testicle ('bag of worms'), which decompress on lying supine. Examine for testicular atrophy.

Investigation

- **Scrotal Doppler ultrasonography** is diagnostic (venous diameter >3.5 mm with patient supine)
- **Vasography** is the 'gold standard', but is reserved for patients considering embolization, or for varicocele recurring after treatment
- **Semen analysis:** varicoceles are associated with low or absent sperm counts, reduced sperm motility and abnormal morphology, either alone or in combination [oligoasthenoteratospermia (OAT) syndrome].

Management

Embolization: interventional radiological technique where the femoral vein to used to access the spermatic vein for venography and embolization (with coils or other sclerosing agents), with success rates of 83%.

Surgical ligation of spermatic veins

- **High retroperitoneal (Palomo) approach:** a muscle–splitting incision is made near the anterior superior iliac spine and the internal spermatic veins are ligated at that level
- **Inguinal (Ivanissevich) approach:** the inguinal canal is incised to access the spermatic cord, and the external spermatic veins are tied off as they exit the internal ring
- **Subinguinal approach:** external spermatic veins are accessed and ligated via a small transverse incision below the external ring. With microscopic assistance, this technique is reported to have superior outcomes to other approaches
- **Laparoscopic:** internal spermatic veins are occluded high in the retroperitoneum.

Indications for repair in adolescents are pain, bilateral large varicoceles, or varicocele in a solitary testis, persistent delayed testicular growth by >20% (as compared with non-affected side), and abnormal spermatogenesis present beyond 18 years old.

Surgical complications: varicocele recurrence; hydrocele formation; testicular atrophy, ilio-inguinal nerve damage.

Surgical outcome: 95% success rate; 70% of men have improvement of sperm parameters.

Treatment options for male factor infertility

General: Aim to identify and treat reversible causes of subfertility, and improve semen quality. Advice on modification of life style factors (i.e. reduce alcohol consumption; avoid hot baths).

Medical treatment

Antibiotics

Treat any positive semen, urine, or urethral cultures with the appropriate antibiotics.

Hormonal

- **Secondary hypogonadism** (pituitary intact) may respond to human chorionic gonadotrophin (hCG) 2000 IU subcutaneously 3 times a week, which stimulates an increase in testosterone and testicular size. If the patient remains azoospermic after 6 months of treatment, FSH is added (human recombinant FSH or human menopausal gonadotrophin). Alternatively, pulsatile LHRH can be administered subcutaneously via a minipump (used for treating Kallman's syndrome)
- **Hyperprolactinaemia** is treated with dopamine agonists
- **Anti-oestrogens** (clomiphene citrate 25 mg od) are used empirically to increase LHRH, which stimulates endogenous gonadotrophin secretion. Often used for idiopathic oligospermia.

Antioxidants

Vitamin E supplements have been shown to improve sperm function and IVF rates; zinc and folic acid may increase sperm concentrations.

Erectile and ejaculatory dysfunction

Erectile dysfunction may be treated conventionally (oral, intraurethral, intracavernosal drugs; vacuum devices or prostheses). Ejaculatory failure may respond to sympathomimetic drugs (desipramine), or electro-ejaculation (used in spinal cord injury), where an electrical stimulus is delivered via a rectal probe to the postganglionic sympathetic nerves that innervate the prostate and seminal vesicles.

Surgical treatment

Genital tract obstruction

- **Epididymal obstruction** can be overcome by microsurgical anastomosis between the epididymal tubule and vas (vasoepididymostomy)
- **Vas deferens obstruction** is treated by microsurgical reanastomosis of ends of the vas (vasovasotomy), and is used for vasectomy reversal. Highest success rates for finding viable sperm occur in the first 8 years post-vasectomy (80–90%); overall pregnancy rates are ~50%
- **Ejaculatory duct obstruction** requires transurethral resection of the ejaculatory ducts (TURED)
- **Varicocele** repaired by embolization, or open or laparoscopic surgical ligation.

Assisted reproductive techniques (ART)

Sperm extraction: sperm are removed directly from the epididymis by percutaneous epididymal sperm aspiration (**PESA**) or microsurgical epididymal sperm aspiration (**MESA**). If these methods fail, testicular exploration, and sperm extraction (**TESE**) or aspiration (**TESA**) may be tried. Sperm undergo cryopreservation until required. Later, they are separated from seminal fluid by dilution and centrifuge methods, with further selection of motile sperm and normal forms using Percoll gradient techniques.

Assisted conception

- **Intrauterine insemination (IUI):** following ovarian stimulation, sperm are placed directly into the uterus
- ***In vitro* fertilization (IVF):** controlled ovarian stimulation produces oocytes, which are then retrieved under transvaginal USS-guidance. Oocytes and sperm are placed in a Petri dish for fertilization to occur. Embryos are transferred to the uterine cavity. Pregnancy rates are 20–30% per cycle
- **Gamete intrafallopian transfer (GIFT):** oocytes and sperm are mixed and deposited into the fallopian tubes via laparoscopy. Variations include zygote intrafallopian transfer (**ZIFT**) and tubal embryo transfer (**TET**)
- **Intracytoplasmic sperm injection (ICSI)** A single spermatozoon is injected directly into the oocyte cytoplasm (through the intact zona pellucida). Pregnancy rates are 15–22% per cycle.

Sexual health

Physiology of erection and ejaculation

Innervation

Autonomic: sympathetic nerves originating from T11–L2, and parasympathetic nerves originating from S2–4, join to form the pelvic plexus. The cavernosal nerves are branches of pelvic plexus (i.e. parasympathetic) that innervate the penis. Parasympathetic stimulation causes erection; sympathetic activity causes ejaculation and detumescence (loss of erection).

Somatic: somatosensory (afferent) information travels via the dorsal penile and pudendal nerves, and enters the spinal cord at S2–4. Onuf's nucleus (segments S2–4) is the somatic centre for efferent (i.e. somatomotor) innervation of the ischiocavernosus and bulbocavernosus muscles of the penis.

Central: Medial pre-optic area (MPOA) and paraventricular nucleus (PVN) in the hypothalamus are important centres for sexual function and penile erection.

Mechanism of erection

Neuroendocrine signals from the brain, created by audiovisual or tactile stimuli, activate the autonomic nuclei of the spinal erection centre (T11–L2 and S2–4). Signals are relayed via the cavernosal nerve to the erectile tissue of the corpora cavernosa, activating the **veno-occlusive mechanism** (Table 13.1). This triggers increased arterial blood flow into sinusoidal spaces (secondary to arterial and arteriolar dilatation), relaxation of cavernosal smooth muscle, and opening of the vascular space. The result is expansion of the sinusoidal spaces against the tunica albuginea, which compresses the subtunical venous plexuses, decreasing venous outflow. Maximal stretching of the tunica albuginea, which acts to compress the emissary veins that lie within its inner circular and outer longitudinal layers, reduces venous flow even further. Rising intracavernosal pressure and contraction of the ischiocavernosus muscles produces a rigid erection. Following orgasm and ejaculation, vasoconstriction (due to increased sympathetic activity, endothelin, PGF_2 and breakdown of cGMP) produces detumescence. Noradrenaline (NA) released from sympathetic nerve terminals in the corpora acts on smooth muscle cell α_1-adrenoceptors leading to raised intracellular calcium which helps maintain penile flaccidity (Figs. 13.1 and 13.2).

Ejaculation

Tactile stimulation of the glans penis causes sensory information to travel (via the pudendal nerve) to the lumbar spinal sympathetic nuclei. Sympathetic efferent signals (travelling in the hypogastric nerve) cause contraction of smooth muscle of the epididymis, vas deferens, and secretory glands, propelling spermatozoa and glandular secretions into the prostatic urethra. There is simultaneous closure of the internal urethral sphincter and relaxation of the extrinsic sphincter, directing sperm into the bulbo-urethra (emission), but preventing sperm entering the bladder. Rhythmic contraction of the bulbocavernosus muscle (somatomotor innervation) leads to the pulsatile emission of the ejaculate from the urethra. During ejaculation, the alkaline prostatic secretion is discharged first, followed by spermatozoa and, finally, seminal vesicle secretions (ejaculate volume 2–5 mL).

Table 13.1 Phases of erectile process

Phase	Term	Description
0	Flaccid phase	Cavernosal smooth muscle contracted; sinusoids empty; minimal arterial flow
1	Latent (filling) phase	Increased pudendal artery flow; penile elongation
2	Tumescent phase	Rising intracavernosal pressure; erection forming
3	Full erection phase	Increased cavernosal pressure causes penis to become fully erect
4	Rigid erection phase	Further increases in pressure + ischiocavernosal muscle contraction
5	Detumescence phase (initial, slow and fast phases)	Following ejaculation, sympathetic discharge resumes; there is smooth muscle contraction and vasoconstriction; reduced arterial flow; blood is expelled from sinusoidal spaces

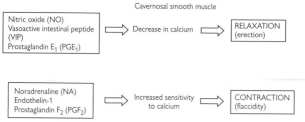

Cavernosal smooth muscle

Nitric oxide (NO)
Vasoactive intestinal peptide (VIP)
Prostaglandin E_1 (PGE_1) $\Rightarrow$ Decrease in calcium $\Rightarrow$ RELAXATION (erection)

Noradrenaline (NA)
Endothelin-1
Prostaglandin F_2 (PGF_2) $\Rightarrow$ Increased sensitivity to calcium $\Rightarrow$ CONTRACTION (flaccidity)

Fig. 13.1 Factors influencing cavernosal smooth muscle.

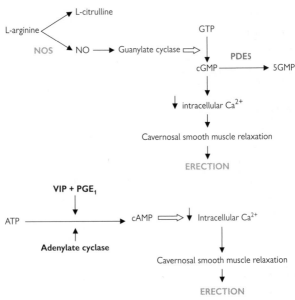

Fig. 13.2 Secondary messenger pathways involved in erection
Key: ATP adenosine triphosphate; Ca²⁺ calcium; cAMP cyclic adenosine monophosphate; cGMP cyclic guanosine monophosphate; GTP guanosine triphosphate; NA noradrenaline; NO nitric oxide; NOS nitric oxide synthase enzyme; PDE5 phosphodiesterase type 5; PGE₁ prostaglandin E₁; PGF₂ prostaglandin F₂; VIP vasoactive intestinal polypeptide.

Erectile dysfunction: evaluation

Definition

Erectile dysfunction (ED) (also called impotence) describes the 'consistent or recurrent inability to attain and/or maintain a penile erection sufficient for sexual intercourse'.[1]

Epidemiology

In men aged 40–70 years, mild ED is found in 17%; moderate ED in 25% and complete ED in 10%.[2] Incidence increases with age, affecting ~15% of men in their 70's and 30–40% in their 80's.

Aetiology

ED is generally divided into psychogenic and organic causes (Table 13.2), although it is often multifactorial.

History

Sexual: onset of ED (sudden or gradual); duration of problem; presence of erections (nocturnal, early morning, spontaneous); ability to maintain erections (early collapse, not fully rigid); loss of libido; relationship issues (frequency of intercourse and sexual desire).

Sexual function symptom questionnaires: International Index of Erectile Function (IIEF); Sexual Health Inventory for Men (SHIM); Brief Male Sexual Function Inventory (BMSFI).

Medical and surgical: enquire about risk factors including diabetes mellitus; hypertension; cardiac disease; peripheral vascular disease; endocrine or neurological disorders; pelvic surgery, radiotherapy, or trauma (damaging innervation and blood supply to the pelvis and penis).

Psychosocial: assess for social stresses, anxiety, depression, coping problems, patient expectations, and relationship details.

Drugs: enquire about current medications and ED treatments already tried (and outcome).

Social: smoking, alcohol consumption.

An **organic cause** is more likely with gradual onset (unless associated with an obvious cause such as surgery, where onset is acute); loss of spontaneous erections; intact libido and ejaculatory function; existing medical risk factors, and older age groups.

Examination

Full physical examination (CVS, abdomen, neurological); digital rectal examine to assess prostate; assess secondary sexual characteristics; external genitalia assessment to document foreskin phimosis and penile lesions (Peyronie's plaques); confirm presence, size and location of testicles. The bulbocavernosus reflex can be performed to test integrity of spinal segments S2–4 (squeezing the glans causes anal sphincter and bulbocavernosal muscle contraction).

Investigation

- **Blood tests:** U&E; fasting glucose; serum (free) testosterone (taken 8.00–11.00 a.m.); sex-hormone binding globulin; LH/FSH; prolactin; PSA; thyroid function test; fasting lipid profile (selected according to patient's history and risk factor profile)
- **Nocturnal penile tumescence and rigidity testing**: Rigiscan device contains 2 rings that are placed around base and distal penile shaft to measure tumescence, and number, duration, and rigidity of nocturnal erections. Useful for diagnosing psychogenic erectile dysfunction, and for illustrating this diagnosis to patients
- **Penile colour Doppler USS**: measures arterial peak systolic and end diastolic velocities[*], pre- and post-intracavernosal injection of PGE_1
- **Cavernosography**: imaging and measurement of blood flow of the penile after intracavernosal injection of contrast and induction of artificial erection, used to identify venous leaks
- **Penile arteriography:** reserve for trauma-related ED in younger men. Pudendal arteriography is performed before and after drug-induced erection to identify those requiring arterial by-pass surgery.

---

[*] *Normal values:* peak systolic velocity >35 cm/s; end diastolic velocity <5 cm/s.

1 Lue TF, Giuliano F, Montorsi F et al. (2004). Summary of the recommendations on sexual dysfunction in men. *J Sex Med* **1**:6–23.

2 Field HA, Goldstein I, Hatzichristou D et al. (1994) Impotence and its medical and psychological correlates: results of the Massachusetts Male Aging Study. *J Urol* **151**:54–61.

Table 13.2 Causes of erectile dysfunction 'IMPOTENCE'

Inflammatory	Prostatitis
Mechanical	Peyronie's disease
Psychological	Depression; anxiety; relationship difficulties; lack of attraction; stress
Occlusive vascular factors	*Arteriogenic:* hypertension; smoking; hyperlipidaemia; diabetes mellitus; peripheral vascular disease
	Venogenic: impairment of veno-occlusive mechanism (due to anatomical or degenerative changes)
Trauma	Pelvic fracture; spinal cord injury; penile trauma
Extra factors	*Iatrogenic:* pelvic surgery; prostatectomy
	Other: increasing age; chronic renal failure; cirrhosis, low-flow priapism (i.e. corporal fibrosis)
Neurogenic	*CNS:* Multiple sclerosis (MS); Parkinson's disease; multi-system atrophy; tumour
	Spinal cord: spina bifida; MS; syringomyelia; tumour
	PNS: Pelvic surgery or radiotherapy; peripheral neuropathy (diabetes, alcohol-related)
Chemical	Antihypertensives (β-blockers, thiazides, ACE inhibitors)
	Anti-arrhythmics (amiodarone)
	Antidepressants (tricyclics, MAOIs, SSRIs)
	Anxiolytics (benzodiazepine)
	Anti-androgens (finasteride, cyproterone acetate)
	LHRH analogues
	Anticonvulsants (phenytoin, carbamazepine)
	Anti-Parkinson drugs (levodopa)
	Statins (atorvastatin)
	Alcohol
	(Refer to BNF).
Endocrine	**Diabetes mellitus*;** hypogonadism; hyperprolactinaemia; hypo and hyperthyroidism.

*Note that this list of causes is not in the order of frequency, i.e. diabetes mellitus is one of the most important causes.
Key: MAOIs = Monoamine-oxidase inhibitors; SSRIs = Serotonin re-uptake inhibitors.
BNF = British National Formulary (bnf.org).

Erectile dysfunction: treatment

Initially correct any reversible causes (i.e. alter life-style, stop smoking, change medication etc.) 📖 see Table 13.2.

Psychosexual therapy

Aims to understand and address underlying psychological issues, and provides information and treatment in the form of sex education, psychosexual counselling, instruction on improving partner communication skills, cognitive therapy, and behavioural therapy (programmed re-learning of couple's sexual relationship).

Oral medication

Phosphodiesterase type-5 (PDE5) inhibitors: sildenafil (Viagra); tadalafil (Cialis); vardenafil (Levitra). PDE5 inhibitors enhance cavernosal smooth muscle relaxation and erection by blocking the breakdown of cGMP. Sexual stimulus is still required to initiate events. Onset of action is 15–30 min. Drug half-life is: sildenafil (100 mg) 3.82 h; vardenafil (20 mg) 4.7 h; tadalafil (20 mg) 17.5 h.

Side effects: headache; flushing; visual disturbance, backache.

Contraindications (CI): patients taking nitrates; recent myocardial infarction; recent stroke; hypotension; unstable angina; non-arteritic anterior ischaemic optic nerve neuropathy (NAOIN). *Cautions:* cardiovascular disease, Peyronie's disease and groups with predisposition to priapism.

Dopamine receptor agonist: apomorphine (Uprima). Apomorphine is administered sublingually, and acts centrally on dopaminergic receptors in the paraventricular nucleus of the hypothalamus to enhance and co-ordinate the effect of sexual stimuli. *Adverse effects:* nausea; headache; dizziness.

Intra-urethral therapy: alprostadil/caverjet (MUSE). Synthetic prostaglandin E_1 (PGE_1) pellet administered into the urethra via a specialized applicator. Once inserted, the penis is gently rolled to encourage the pellet to dissolve into the urethral mucosa, from where it enters the corpora. *Side effects:* penile pain; priapism; local reactions.

Intracavernosal injection therapy: alprostadil (synthetic PGE_1), acts to increase cAMP within corporal smooth muscle, resulting in muscle relaxation; papaverine (smooth muscle relaxant) ± phentolamine (α-adrenoceptor antagonist). Training of technique and first dose is given by health professional. Needle is inserted at right angles into the corpus cavernosum on the lateral aspects of mid-penile shaft. *CI:* sickle cell disease or high risk candidate for priapism. *Adverse effects:* pain; priapism; haematoma.

Vacuum erection device: contains 3 components: vacuum chamber, pump, and constriction band. The penis is placed in the chamber, and the vacuum created by the pump increases blood flow to the corpora cavernosa to induce an erection. The constriction band is placed onto the base of the penis to retain blood in the corpora and maintain rigidity. *Relative CI:* anticoagulation therapy. *Adverse effects:* penile coldness; bruising.

Microvascular arterial bypass and venous ligation surgery: consider in specialist centres where there is a clear-cut diagnosis of a vascular disorder. Acts to increase arterial inflow and decrease venous outflow. Success rates rarely exceed 50%.

Penile prosthesis: semi-rigid, malleable, and inflatable penile prostheses are available when other therapies have failed or are unsuitable. The device is surgically implanted into the corpora to provide penile rigidity, and generally has high satisfaction rates (Fig. 13.3). Also useful if there is co-existing penile curvature/Peyronies disease. *Side effects:* infection, erosion, mechanical failure.

Androgen replacement therapy: testosterone replacement is indicated for hypogonadism. It is available in oral, intramuscular, pellet, patch and gel forms. In older men, it is recommended that PSA is checked before and during treatment (see p. 566). It can improve the results of PDE5 inhibitors in hypogonadal men.

Treatment options for erectile dysfunction

Organic	Psychogenic
Eliminate underlying risk factors	Psychosexual counselling ± partner
Oral medication	Oral medication
Intra-urethral therapy	Intra-urethral therapy
Intracavernosal injection therapy	Intracavernosal injection therapy
Vacuum devices	
Penile prosthesis	
Androgen replacement	

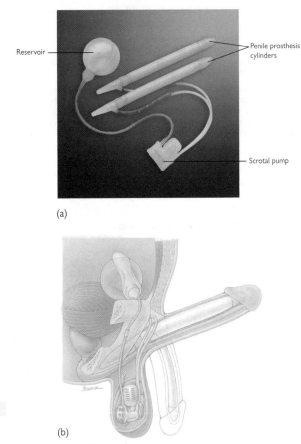

(a)

(b)

Fig. 13.3 (a) AMS 700™ Series Tactile Pump penile prosthesis. (b) Inflated prosthesis *in situ*. (Reproduced with permission, courtesy of American Medical Systems Inc., Minnesota.)

Peyronie's disease

Definition

An acquired benign penile condition characterized by curvature of the penile shaft secondary to the formation of fibrous tissue plaques within the tunica albuginea of the penis.

Epidemiology

Incidence is ~3%,[1] predominantly affecting men aged 40–60 years.

Pathophysiology

Histologically, plaques have excessive connective tissue (fibrosis) and increased cellularity with random orientation of collagen fibres. Dorsal penile plaques are most common (66%). The corpus cavernosus underlying the lesion cannot lengthen fully on erection, resulting in penile curvature. It may be associated with distal flaccidity or an unstable penis (due to waist/hourglass deformities). The disorder has 2 phases:

- **Active phase** (1–6 months): early inflammatory phase with painful erections and changing penile deformity
- **Quiescent phase** (9–12 months): disease 'burns out'. Pain disappears with resolution of inflammation, and there is stabilization of the penile deformity.

The natural history of Peyronie's plaques over 18 months is that 40% will progress, 47% will remain stable, and 13% will improve.[2]

Aetiology

The exact cause is unknown. It is likely that repeated minor trauma during intercourse causes microvascular injury and bleeding into the tunica, resulting in inflammation and fibrosis (exacerbated by transforming growth factor-β, TGF-β). There are strong associations with diabetes and vascular disease. Auto-immune disease processes have also been suggested, and there is a reported familial predisposition.

Presentation

Pain and/or curvature of the erect penis; hard area (plaque) on penis; erectile dysfunction (ED) (40%); penile shortening.

Associated disorders

Diabetes mellitus; arterial disease, Dupuytren's contractures (25%); plantar fascial contracture; tympanosclerosis; previous trauma.

Evaluation

A full medical and sexual history are taken. Either photographs or outpatient injection of intracavernosal PGE1 can be used to assess the degree of curvature. Assess the location and size of the plaque (is it tender?). *Colour Doppler USS* is used to assess the plaque, and any vascular abnormalities, whereas contrast-enhanced *MRI* is indicated for complex and extensive cavernosal fibrosis.

Management

Early disease with active inflammation (<3 months, penile pain, changing deformity) benefits most from medical therapy. Surgery is indicated for stable, mature disease, with significant deformity (preventing intercourse). Non-mechanical components of erectile dysfunction can be treated conventionally (e.g. oral or intracavernosal medications)

Conservative treatment

Medical treatment

Oral therapy: there is limited evidence for efficacy. Regimens include vitamin E (800–1000 IU daily in divided doses) for 3 months (FDA suggest <200 IU daily in long-term therapy); tamoxifen 20 mg bd for 3 months; colchicine (0.6 mg bd/tds) with checks of white blood cell counts.

Intralesional injection: verapamil (10 mg in 10 mL saline) injected into lesion every 2 weeks for 24 weeks.[3] Alternatives are collagenase and interferon alpha2-beta injection.

Iontophoresis: small amounts of electric current are used to transfer drugs (verapamil ± dexamethasone and lidocaine) transdermally to act on the plaque.[4]

- **Extracorporeal shock wave therapy (ESWL)** has little effect on penile angulation, but may help reduce pain.

Surgery

- **Nesbit procedure** The penis is de-gloved via a circumglandular incision. An artificial erection is induced by intracavernosal saline injection. On the opposite side of maximal deformity, an ellipse is excised (a width of 1 mm is taken for every 10° of penile curvature), and then closed with sutures. Success rates are 88–94%. Warn the patient that penile shortening of 2–3 cm frequently occurs.
- **Simple plication technique** sutures are placed on the opposite side of maximal deformity to straighten the penis. Success rates tend to be lower (~40%).
- **Plaque incision and grafting:** incision of plaque with insertion of venous patch, to lengthen the affected side (and minimize penile shortening). Generally reserved for patients with severe angulation (>60°) and those particularly concerned about penile shortening. Must have good erectile function. Success rates 75–96%. *Adverse effects:* erectile dysfunction 5–12%. Alternative graft materials include temporalis fascia, Surgisis (acellular biomaterial derived from porcine small intestinal submucosa) and bovine pericardium.
- **Penile prosthesis** particularly reserved for patients with moderate-severe erectile dysfunction, cavernosal fibrosis, and complex deformities,

1 Schwarzer U, Sommer F, Klotz T et al. (2001) The prevalence of Peyronie's disease: results of a large survey. *BJU Int* **88**: 727-30

2 Gelbard MK, Dorey F, James K et al. (1990) The natural history of Peyronie's disease. *J Urol* **144**: 1376-79

3 Levine LA, Goldman KE, Greenfield JM (2002) Experience with intraplaque injection of verapamil for Peyronie's disease. *J Urol* **168**: 621-5

4 Riedl CR et al. (2000) Iontophoresis for treatment of Peyronie's disease. *J Urol* **163**: 95-9

Priapism

Definition: prolonged, unwanted erection, in the absence of sexual desire or stimulus, lasting >4 h.

Epidemiology: incidence of 1.5 per 100,000,[1] with peaks at ages 5–10 and 20–50.

Classification

- **Low flow (ischaemic) priapism:** due to veno-occlusion (intracavernosal pressures of 80–120 mmHg). Most common form which manifests as a painful, rigid erection, with absent or low cavernosal blood flow. Ischaemic priapism >4 h requires emergency intervention. Blood gas analysis shows hypoxia and acidosis
- **High flow (non-ischaemic) priapism:** due to unregulated arterial blood flow, presenting with a semi-rigid, painless erection. Usually self-limiting. Blood gas analysis shows similar results to arterial blood
- **Recurrent (or stuttering) priapism:** most commonly seen in sickle cell disease. Usually high flow, but may change to low flow with anoxia.

Aetiology

Causes are primary (idiopathic) or secondary, including:

- **Intracavernosal injection therapy:** PGE_1; papaverine
- **Drugs:** α-blockers; antidepressants; antipsychotics; psychotrophics; tranquilizers; anxiolytics; anticoagulants; recreational drugs; alcohol excess; total parenteral nutrition
- **Thrombo-embolic:** sickle cell disease (may cause stuttering/recurrent priapism); leukaemia; thalassaemia; fat emboli
- **Neurogenic:** spinal cord lesion; autonomic neuropathy; anaesthesia
- **Trauma:** penile or perineal injury resulting in cavernosal artery laceration or arterio-venous fistula formation
- **Infection:** malaria; rabies; scorpion sting.

Pathophysiology

Priapism lasting for 12 h causes trabecular interstitial oedema, followed by destruction of sinusoidal endothelium and exposure of the basement membrane at 24 h, and sinusoidal thrombi, smooth muscle cell necrosis and fibrosis at 48 h.

Evaluation

- **Serum testing** to exclude sickle cell, leukaemia and thallasaemia
- **Cavernous blood samples** to determine type of priapism
- **Colour Doppler ultrasonography** of cavernosus artery and corpora cavernosa. Reduced blood flow in ischaemic priapism; ruptured artery with pooling of blood around injured area in non-ischaemic priapism.

Management in adults (Fig.13.4)

Ice packs, cold showers and exercise may be beneficial in early stages.

Low-flow priapism

Decompress urgently with aspiration of blood from corpora (5 mL portions using a 18–20 gauge butterfly needle until oxygenated red blood is obtained). If no change after 10 min, then proceed to intracavernosal injection of α_1-adrenergic agonist (phenylephrine 100–200 mcg (0.5–1 mL of a 200 mcg/mL solution to a maximum of 1 mg) every 5–10 min until detumescence occurs; see bnf.org). Monitor BP and pulse during drug administration. If this fails after 1 h, surgical intervention is needed with biopsy and shunt. If this fails, or patients present late (>72 h), consider penile prosthesis. Oral terbutaline may be effective treatment for intracavernosal injection-related cases. Sickle cell disease requires, in addition, aggressive rehydration, oxygenation, analgesia, and haematological input (consider exchange transfusion).

High flow priapism

Conservative treatment is recommended in most cases. Traumatic or delayed presentations require arteriography, and either selective or internal pudendal artery embolization with autologous blood clot. Ligation of fistula may be required.

Recurrent priapism

Optimize haematological management of sickle cell disease to reduce frequency of attacks. Androgen suppression is the most effective pharmacological therapy.

Complications: 90% of priapism >24 h develop complete erectile dysfunction.

1 Eland IA, van der Lei, Strickler BH et al. (2001) Incidence of priapism in the general population. *Urology* **57**: 970–4.

Causes of low- and high-flow priapism

Low flow priapism	High flow priapism
Intracavernosal drug injection	Arterio-venous fistula (secondary to penile or perineal trauma, or surgery)
Oral medications	
Haematological disease: Sickle cell disease, leukaemia, thalassaemia	
Fat embolus	
Spinal cord lesion	
Autonomic neuropathy	
Malignancy	

Examples of drugs which may cause priapism

Class of drug	Examples
Antihypertensives/α-blockers	Prazosin; hydralazine
Antidepressants	Sertraline; fluoxetine; lithium
Antipsychotics	Clozapine
Psychotrophics	Chlorpromazine
Tranquilizers	Mesoridazine
Anxiolytics	Hydroxyzine
Anticoagulants	Warfarin; heparin
Recreational drugs	Cocaine

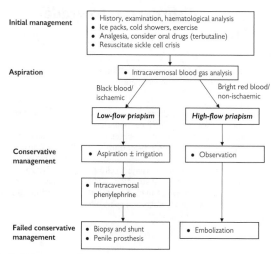

Fig. 13.4 Management of priapism.

Ejaculatory disorders: retrograde ejaculation

Definition
Failure of adequate bladder neck contraction results in the propulsion of sperm back into the bladder on ejaculation.

Aetiology
Acquired causes are due to damage or dysfunction of the bladder neck sphincter mechanism. These include **neurological** disease (spinal cord injury; neuropathy associated with diabetes mellitus; nerve damage after retroperitoneal surgery), or **anatomical disruption** following transurethral resection of ejaculatory ducts (for obstruction); bladder neck incision (BNI); transurethral resection of the prostate (TURP), or open prostatectomy. Drugs to treat bladder outflow obstruction (α-blockers) causes reversible retrograde ejaculation in 5% of men. **Congenital** causes include bladder exstrophy, ectopic ejaculatory ducts and spina bifida.

Incidence
Retrograde ejaculation following TURP or open prostatectomy occurs in 9 out of 10 men, and after BNI in 1–5 in 10.

Presentation
'Dry' ejaculation (failure to expel ejaculate fluid from the urethral meatus) or low ejaculate volume (<1 mL) and cloudy urine (containing sperm) in the first void after intercourse.

Investigation
The presence of >10–15 sperm per high powered field in post-orgasmic urine specimens confirms the diagnosis of retrograde ejaculation.

Treatment
Medical therapy is initiated in men wishing to preserve fertility, and is only effective in patients who have not had bladder neck surgery. Therapy is often given for 7–10 days prior to a planned ejaculation (co-ordinated with the partner's ovulation).

- Oral α-adrenergic receptor agonist drugs (ephedrine sulphate, pseudoephedrine) may be used to increase the sympathetic tone of the bladder neck smooth muscle sphincter mechanism.
- Imipramine, a tricyclic antidepressant drug with anticholinergic and sympathomimetic effect may also be used (25 mg bd-tds).

Sperm retrieval from urine for assisted fertility techniques

Oral sodium bicarbonate and adjustment of fluid intake is initiated to optimize urine osmolarity and pH, and enhance sperm survival. Sperm are collected by gentle urine centrifuge, and washed in insemination media in preparation for intrauterine insemination (IUI) or *in vitro* fertilization (IVF) treatments.

Ejaculatory disorders: premature ejaculation

Definition
'Persistent or recurrent ejaculation with minimal stimulation before, on, or shortly after penetration, and before the person wishes it. The disturbance causes marked distress or interpersonal difficulties'.[1] It is classified as life-long or acquired.

Aetiology
Psychological
- Early sexual experience
- Anxiety
- Reduced frequency of sexual intercourse.

Biological
- Penile hypersensitivity
- 5-Hydroxytryptamine (5-HT) receptor sensitivity (involved in the central control of ejaculation)
- Hyperexcitable ejaculatory reflex

Evaluation
Detailed medical and sexual history and physical examination. Quantitative measures of sexual intercourse include:
- Intravaginal ejaculatory latency time (IELT) - the time between vaginal penetration and ejaculation averaged over several performances. IELT <2 min suggests a diagnosis of premature ejaculation, although the DMS-IV[1] suggests IELT <15 s confirms the diagnosis
- Score of partner's sexual satisfaction
- Patient's assessment of his voluntary control over ejaculation.

Treatment
Behavioural
- Seman's stop-start manoeuvre (inhibiting the urge to ejaculate by repeatedly stopping sexual stimulation)
- Masters and Johnson's squeeze technique (inhibiting the urge to ejaculate by squeezing the glans penis)
- Sensate focus.

Pharmacological
- Selective serotonin (5-HT) reuptake inhibitors (SSRIs) (paroxetine, sertraline, fluoxetine > citalopram, fluvoxamine) taken on demand or daily. Side effects include gastrointestinal effects, anorexia, and rash
- Clomipramine (tricyclic antidepressant) given daily or as required 4–6 h before intercourse. Side effects include dry mouth, sedation, blurred vision, difficulty voiding
- Topical local anaesthetics, such as lidocaine and/or prilocaine cream, gel or spray (with condom to prevent transvaginal absorption with resultant vaginal numbness)

- Phosphodiesterase type-5 (PDE-5) inhibitors (sildenafil): limited role for acquired premature ejaculation associated with erectile dysfunction.

1 American Psychiatry Association (1994) *Diagnostic and Statistical Manual of Mental Disorders, DSM-IV*, 4th edn. Washington DC: American Psychiatric Association.

Ejaculatory disorders: inhibited ejaculation, anejaculation, and anorgasmia

Inhibited ejaculation (IE) is defined as the persistent or recurrent difficulty, delay in, or absence of attaining orgasm following sufficient stimulation, which causes personal distress.[1] It is classified as lifelong or acquired; global or situational, and the prevalence increases with age. It is caused by interference with either central control of ejaculation, afferent or efferent nerve supply to the vas, bladder neck, pelvic floor, or penis, which may be secondary to surgery, medical or psychological disease, or related to drugs. The overall result can be inhibited ejaculation, anejaculation and anorgasmia.

Anejaculation is defined as the complete absence of an antegrade or retrograde ejaculation. There is failure of emission from the seminal vesicles, prostate and ejaculatory ducts into the urethra. True anejaculation is associated with a normal orgasm sensation, and is due to drug-related causes or central or peripheral nervous system dysfunction (Table 13.3).

Table 13.3 Causes of anejaculation

Pharmacological	Neurological
Antihypertensive drugs (thiazides)	Diabetic autonomic neuropathy
Antidepressants (tricyclics, SSRIs)	Spinal cord injury
Antipsychotic drugs (phenothiazines)	Multiple sclerosis
Alcohol excess	Parkinson's disease
	Pelvic surgery (proctocolectomy)
	Para-aortic lymphadenectomy

SSRI = selective serotonin reuptake inhibitors.

Management

Detailed medical and sexual history, with full physical and neurological examination, including bulbocavernosus reflex, anal sphincter tone, and perineal sensitivity. Post-ejaculatory urinalysis can be performed to exclude retrograde ejaculation. If there is clinical suspicion of possible ejaculatory duct obstruction, consider transrectal ultrasonography, vasography or percutaneous puncture of the seminal vesicles.

Treatment

Aim to treat the specific underlying aetiology. Where the aim is to retrieve sperm for assisted reproductive techniques, methods include:

- Vibrostimulation (first-line therapy). A vibrator is applied to the penis, evoking the ejaculation reflex. It requires an intact lumbosacral spinal cord segment.
- Electro-ejaculation involves the electrical stimulation of periprostatic nerves via a rectal probe, under anaesthesia (unless the patient has a complete spinal cord injury).

Anorgasmia is defined as the inability to reach orgasm (which may give rise to anejaculation in men). The cause is usually psychological, but may also be related to drugs or decreased penile sensation (secondary to pudendal nerve dysfunction, seen in peripheral neuropathy associated with diabetes mellitus). Further neurological investigation should be considered in selected cases.

1 American Psychiatry Association (1994) *Diagnostic and Statistical Manual of Mental Disorders,* DSM-IV 4th edn. Washington DC: American Psychiatric Association.

Late-onset hypogonadism (LOH)

Late-onset hypogonadism (LOH) is defined as 'a clinical and biochemical syndrome associated with advancing age and characterized by typical symptoms and a deficiency in serum testosterone levels. It may result in significant detriment in the quality of life and adversely affect the function of multiple organ systems'.[1] It is also known as androgen decline in the ageing male (ADAM).

Pathophysiology

LOH involves components of both primary and secondary hypogonadism (p. 566), and a degree of reduced responsiveness of target organs to testosterone and its adrogenic mediators. Ageing decreases production of luteinizing hormone-releasing hormone (LHRH) and luteinizing hormone (LH) due to effects on the hypothalamus and pituitary. This causes a decline in the both the number of Leydig cells in the testes and their sensitivity to LH, so reducing testosterone levels. Sex hormone binding globulin (SHBG) binds testosterone and renders it unavailable to most tissues, and levels of SHBG increase with age. Along with age-related changes in androgen receptors and altered androgen metabolism, the result is less bioavailable testosterone.

Presentation

- Erectile dysfunction
- Reduced libido
- Reduced concentration
- Hot flushes
- Changes in mood (depression)
- Lethargy/fatigue
- Sleep disturbance
- Hair/skin changes
- Osteoporosis and muscle wasting
- Oligospermia or azoospermia

Evaluation

- History to elicit symptoms related to low testosterone levels
- Screening questionnaires:
  - The Androgen Deficiency in Aging Male (ADAM) Questionnaire
  - The Aging Male Survey (AMS)
- Examination including DRE (with PSA, to exclude prostate cancer prior to giving testosterone, and to assess prostate size)
- Flow rate and post-void residual volume to assess for bladder outflow obstruction
- Serum bloods: testosterone, PSA, full blood count (FBC), and liver function tests (LFT), fasting lipid profile.

Testosterone assessment

In a normal adult male, the serum testosterone reference range is around 10.4–34.7 nmol/L. Testosterone levels show diurnal variation, peaking in early morning, and recommendations for testing are:
• Early morning serum total testosterone (taken 8:00–11:00 a.m.)
• If low or borderline total testosterone level, perform repeat testosterone level with LH, FSH, and prolactin.

Treatment of LOH

Symptoms and biochemical evidence of testosterone deficiency indicate the need for testosterone replacement therapy (Fig. 13.5). Where testosterone levels are borderline/normal, but symptoms are present, consider an initial 3-month trial of testosterone and then review (📖 see p. 566). Residual symptoms may need specific treatment, such as phosphodiesterase type-5 (PDE5) inhibitors for erectile dysfunction.

For normal testosterone physiology, refer to p. 524; for normal androgen metabolic pathways, 📖 see p. 644.

1 Nieschlag E, Swerdloff R, Behre HM et al. (2006) Investigation, treatment and monitoring of late-onset hypogonadism in males: ISA, ISSAM, and EAU recommendations. J Androl **27**:135–7.

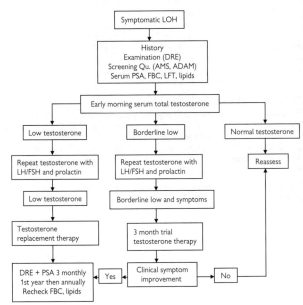

Fig. 13.5 Management pathway for symptomatic LOH.

Hypogonadism and male hormone replacement therapy

Male hypogonadism has been defined as inadequate gonadal function due to deficiencies in gametogenesis and/or the secretion of gonadal hormones. Hypogonadism may be **primary** (due to abnormal testicular function or testicular response to gonadotrophins) or **secondary** (due to failure of the hypothalamic-pituitary axis leading to inadequate gonadotrophic stimulation and reduced testicular testosterone production; Table 13.4). The result is testosterone deficiency.

Indications for testosterone treatment

Hypogonadism and related symptoms caused by low testosterone levels. Symptomatic late-onset hypogonadism (LOH) and primary hypogonadism should be treated with androgens. Patients with secondary hypogonadism may be given LH and FSH, or pulsatile LHRH if fertility is required, otherwise they should receive androgen replacement (see p. 534). The aim is to achieve normal serum testosterone levels.

Contraindications to testosterone treatment

- Male breast cancer
- Prostate cancer
- History of primary liver tumour
- Hypercalcaemia
- Clinically significant obstructive benign prostatic enlargement.

Assessment prior to testosterone treatment

- In men >45 years, DRE and serum PSA are mandatory to assess prostate health
- Fasting lipid profile
- Liver function tests (LFTs)
- Full blood count (FBC)
- Flow rate, residual volume, IPSS to assess for bladder outflow obstruction.

Assessment during testosterone treatment

- DRE and PSA every 3–6 months for the first 12 months, then yearly (for prostate cancer)
- FBC every 3–6 months for the first year and then yearly (to assess for polycythaemia)
- Fasting lipid profile (testosterone can alter total and low-density lipoprotein cholesterol).

Side effects of testosterone treatment

- Headache
- Oedema due to sodium retention
- Depression
- Gastrointestinal bleeding
- Nausea
- Cholestatic jaundice
- Liver toxicity

- Gynaecomastia
- Androgenic effects (hirsutism, male-pattern baldness)
- Polycythaemia.

Testosterone treatment

Testosterone replacement can be given by transdermal patch or gel, intramuscular injection, subdermal implant, buccal and oral administrations (Table 13.5). Transdermal preparations produce a normal testosterone level with physiological diurnal profile, although they can produce local skin reaction. Intramuscular injections are long-acting, but do not provide normal hormonal circadian rhythm. Oral preparations tend to be less used due to variable pharmacokinetics.

Metabolic syndrome is characterized by central obesity, insulin resistance, dyslipidaemia and hypertension, resulting in increased risk of cardiovascular disease and progression to diabetes mellitus. *Hypogonadism* is frequently associated with metabolic syndrome. There is evidence that testosterone treatment may help some conditions associated with the syndrome, and reduce the risk of cardiovascular complications.

Table 13.4 Causes of primary and secondary hypogonadism

Primary hypogonadism (hypergonadotrophic hypogonadism)	Secondary hypogonadism (hypogonadotrophic hypogonadism)
Congenital	*Congenital*
Chromosomal (Kleinfelter's syndrome)	Kallmann's syndrome*
Testicular maldescent	
Acquired	*Acquired*
Surgery (bilateral orchidectomy)	Hypopituitarism (pituitary lesion; surgery or radiation to the cranium)
Bilateral testicular torsion	
Radiotherapy/chemotherapy	
Infection (bilateral orchitis)	
Cirrhosis	

*Kallman's syndrome is an isolated gonadotrophin deficiency, which leads to hypogonadism.

Table 13.5 Testosterone preparations

Route of administration	Examples of preparations	Dosing regimen
Intramuscular injection	Testosterone Enantate	Initial: 250mg every 2-3 weeks Maintenance: 250mg every 3-6 weeks.
	Sustanon 250®	1ml every 3 weeks
Implant	Testosterone	100–600 mg; 600 mg maintains plasma testosterone in normal range for 4–5 months
Transdermal patch	Andropatch®	2.5–7.5 mg/24 h: dose according to plasma testosterone concentration
Transdermal gel	Testim®	5 g gel (50 mg testosterone) apply daily; adjust according to response (max 10 g gel/24 h)
	Testogel®	5 g gel (50 mg testosterone) apply daily
Buccal	Striant®	30 mg 12-hourly
Oral	Restandol® (Testosterone undecanoate)	40 mg 3–4 times per day (120–160 mg daily) for 2–3 weeks Maintenance: 40–120 mg daily

Urethritis

Urethritis is inflammation of the urethra. Infective urethritis may present with clear, mucopurulent, or purulent urethral discharge, coloured white, yellow, green, or brown. It is associated with dysuria and pain at the external urethral meatus or in the penile shaft, which persists between voiding. There may be urinary frequency and urgency.

Infective causes

- *Chlamydia trachomatis*
- *Neisseria gonorrhoeae*
- *Trichomonas vaginalis*
- *Ureaplasma urealyticum*
- *Mycoplasma genitalium*
- *Herpes simplex virus*

Evaluation

Assess symptoms, sexual history, and sexual contacts. Examine external genitalia for testicular or epididymal tenderness, discharge at the meatus, lymphadenopathy, or skin lesions. Refer to genitourinary medicine for management, and to trace and treat contacts

Investigation

Initial diagnosis of urethritis on urethral smear is defined as ≥5 polymorpho-nuclear leucocytes (PMNL) per high power field (×1000 magnification), or ≥10 PMNL per high power field (×400 magnification) in the first voiding urine specimen.

Specific tests

- Urethral swabs (with endocervical swabs in women) transported in charcoal transport medium. Used for culture and gram stain to identify *N. gonorrhoeae*. Also used for nucleic acid amplification test (NAAT) or enzyme immunoassay (EIA) to detect *N. gonorrhoeae* and *C. trachomatis*
- First 20 ml void of urine (after holding urine ≥ 1 hour). Used for EIA to identifiy *C. trachomatis*
- Midstream urine (MSU): dipstix testing ± microscopy to investigate UTI
- In selected cases, consider HIV and syphilis testing with serum rapid plasma regain (RPR) test.

Gonococcal urethritis (GU) is caused by the gram-negative dipplococcus *N. gonorrhoea*. Specific complications include haematogenous spread of infection to other sites (~1%) causing disseminated gonococcal infection (DGI) often manifest initially as tendon or joint pain.

Non-gonococcal urethritis (NGU) is mainly caused by *C. trachomatis* infection and may be asymptomatic (particularly in women). Specific complications include oculogenital syndrome (NGU and conjunctivitis). Transmission to females results in increased risk of pelvic inflammatory disease, abdominal pain, ectopic pregnancy, infertility, and perinatal infection.

General complications

- Epididymitis
- Prostatitis
- Urethral stricture.

Postgonococcal urethritis

Recurrence of symptoms and signs 4–7 days after successful single-dose therapy for gonococcal urethritis, caused by a dual urethral infection for which the NGU element was untreated. The most common cause is *C. trachomatis*.

Table 13.6 Comparison and treatment of non-gonococcal and gonococcal urethritis

	Non-gonococcal urethritis	Gonococcal urethritis
Main causative organism	*C. trachomatis*	*N. gonorrhoea*
Incubation time (days)	7–21	2–7
Onset	Gradual	Sudden
Discharge	Watery and clear	Larger volume and yellow
Dysuria	Mild	Moderate
Treatment	Azithromycin 1 g single oral dose or	Cefixime 400 mg single oral dose or
	Doxycycline 100 mg bd po 7 days	Ceftriaxone 250 mg single im dose or
		Ciprofloxacin 500 mg single oral dose

Non-specific urethritis and urethral syndrome

Non-specific urethritis (NSU) is described as the presence of polymorphonuclear leucocytes (PMNL) (≥5 per high power field at ×1000 magnification) in a male urethral smear, in the absence of any proven specific infection.

Causes of NSU

Infective causes of urethritis with false-negative laboratory results (i.e. missed STI).

Non-infective causes of urethritis

- Urethral trauma/foreign object
- Contact urethritis (spermicides, shower gel)
- Reiter's syndrome (urethritis, seronegative arthritis and conjunctivitis)
- Wegener's granulomatosis (vasculitis of unknown aetiology).

Management

Urethral swab: culture, gram stain, and nucleic acid amplification test (NAAT) to exclude sexually transmitted infection (STI). Bearing in mind that some cases of NSU may be due to STI with false-negative results, sexual contacts should be traced, and antibiotics can often alleviate symptoms. Standard *Chlamydia trachomatis* treatments are usually recommended (azithromycin 1 g single oral dose or oral doxycycline 100 mg bd 7 days) and are often effective.

Urethral syndrome is a condition of uncertain aetiology that only affects women. It manifests as dysuria, frequency, urgency, and suprapubic discomfort without any evidence of infection or urological abnormality to account for the symptoms.

Differential diagnosis

Infection, painful bladder syndrome/interstitial cystitis (PBS/IC), urethral diverticulum.

Management

It is a diagnosis of exclusion. Urethral and endocervical swabs should be taken for culture, gram stain and NAAT to exclude a STI cause, and midstream urine specimen to examine for UTI. Where indicated, consider cystoscopy to exclude PBS/IC or urethrography to investigate urethral diverticulum.

Treatment

A course of antibiotics (covering *C. trachomatis* and anaerobes) can provide symptom relief in some cases, even in the absence of positive cultures.

HIV and hepatitis in urological surgery

Human immunodeficiency virus (HIV)

Causes a spectrum of illness related to immune system deficiency (📖 see Table 13.7). HIV-1 is pandemic, and accounts for significant mortality in developing countries. HIV-2 has less pathogenicity and is predominant in West Africa. Transmission is via sexual intercourse, contaminated needles, mother-to-foetus transmission, and infected blood and blood products (blood transfusion risks are now minimal).

Pathogenesis

HIV is a retrovirus. It possesses the enzyme reverse transcriptase that enables viral RNA to be transcribed into DNA, which is then incorporated into the host cell genome. HIV binds to CD4 receptors on helper T-lymphocytes (CD4 cells), monocytes, and neural cells. After an extended latent period (8–10 years), CD4 counts decline. Acquired immunodeficiency syndrome (AIDS) is defined as HIV positivity and CD4 lymphocyte counts <200 × 10^6/L. The associated immunosuppression increases the risk of opportunistic infections and tumours (📖 see Table 13.8).

Diagnosis

ELISA[1] testing of serum detects antibodies against HIV antigens. The second confirmatory test is Western blot. Informed consent is required for the test.

Urological sequelae

- **Kidneys**: *Cytomegalovirus*, *Aspergillus*, *Toxoplasma gondii* infections, which can cause acute tubular necrosis and abscess formation; renal failure (HIV and AIDS-associated nephropathy); renal stones (secondary to indinavir treatment)
- **Ureters**: calculi
- **Bladder**: voiding dysfunction (urinary retention, bladder overactivity, outflow obstruction); UTI (opportunistic organisms); squamous cell carcinoma
- **Urethra**: Reiter's syndrome (urethritis, conjunctivitis, arthritis); bacterial urethritis
- **Prostate**: bacterial prostatitis and abscesses (opportunistic organisms)
- **External genitalia**: chronic or recurrent genital herpes; atypical syphilis; opportunistic infections of testicle and epididymis; testicular cancers (germ cell and non-germ cell, lymphoma); scrotal and penile Kaposi's sarcoma; Fournier's gangrene.

Needle stick injury: the risk of HIV transmission after percutaneous exposure to HIV-infected blood is 3 per 1000 injuries.[2] Risks are increased if patient has terminal AIDS-related complex (ARC) illness; needle is hollow bore with visible blood contamination, inserted deeply or directly into a vessel. After mucocutaneous exposure, the risk is <1 in 1000.[2] Immediately wash the area well, report to occupational health, and where appropriate, commence combination antiviral post-exposure prophylaxis (PEP) as soon as possible (zidovudine plus lamivudine plus nelfinavir[2]).

Table 13.7 Clinical syndromes of HIV infections and AIDS*

Group I	Acute seroconversion illness. Self-limiting, glandular fever-like illness ~ 6 weeks after infection.
Group II	Asymptomatic. Latent period (up to 10 years).
Group III	Persistent generalized lymphadenopathy (PGL). Nodes >1cm at >2 extra-inguinal sites.
Group IV (AIDS)	AIDS-related complex (ARC): **A:** constitutional disease (fever >1 month, weight loss >10%, diarrhoea >1 month)
	B: neurological disease (dementia, peripheral neuropathy, myelopathy)
	C: secondary infectious disease
	D: secondary cancers (Kaposi's sarcoma, non-Hodgkin's lymphoma, primary cerebral lymphoma)
	E: other conditions (lymphoid interstitial pneumonia, thrombocytopenia).

*Communicable Disease Center, USA.

Table 13.8 Examples of opportunistic infections and AIDS defining illnesses*

Bacterial infections (multiple or recurrent in children<12 years)

Candidiasis of oesophagus, trachea, bronchi

Coccidioidomycosis

Cryptococcosis

Cryptosporidiosis

Histoplasmosis

Isosporiasis

Mycobacteriosis: disseminated or extrapulmonary

Pneumocystis carinii pneumonia

Toxoplasmosis gondii

Salmonellosis: recurrent septicaemia

Cytomegalovirus

Herpes simplex virus >1 month, or bronchi, lung or oesophageal involvement

Progressive multifocal leucoencephalopathy

Oral hairy leukoplakia

Multidermatomal herpes zoster

Nocardiasis

*Valid after excluding other causes of immunodeficiency

Hepatitis B

Transmission is via sexual intercourse, infected blood, contaminated needles, and mother-to-child during parturition. The virus is carried in semen and saliva. Incubation period is 6 months. Surface antigen (HBsAg) is initially detected on blood testing from 6 to 12 weeks; persistence indicates carrier status. Antibodies to HBsAg indicates vaccination. The e-antigen (HBeAg) rises early in disease and then declines; persistence correlates with increased infectivity and severity. Antibodies to the core antigen (HBcAg) indicate past infection. Sequelae include chronic hepatitis, which may cause cirrhosis and hepatocellular carcinoma. Glomerulonephritis is a rare complication. In the investigation of testicular tumours with tumour markers, be aware that hepatitis can raise serum alpha fetoprotein (AFP) levels.

Prophylaxis: the risk of hepatitis B infection from a contaminated needle stick injury is 12%. Hospital health-care workers receive vaccination with active immunization injections at 0, 1, and 6 months. Antibodies are checked at 7–9 months, and booster doses given after 3–5 years. Passive immunization with antihepatitis B immunoglobulin may be given to non-immune contacts after high-risk exposure. Full universal theatre precautions are utilized; place patient at end of operating lists.

---

1 ELISA: enzyme-linked immunosorbant assay.

2 Chief Medical Officers' Expert Advisory Group on AIDS (2004) *HIV Post-exposure Prophylaxis Guidelines for the UK.* Available at: http://www.dh.gov.uk (accessed February 2004).

Neuropathic bladder

Innervation of the lower urinary tract (LUT)

Motor innervation of the bladder

Parasympathetic motor innervation of the bladder

Preganglionic, parasympathetic nerve cell bodies are located in the intermediolateral column of spinal segments S2–4. These preganglionic, parasympathetic fibres pass out of the spinal cord through the anterior primary rami of S2, S3, and S4 and, contained within nerves called the nervi erigentes, they head towards the pelvic plexus. In the pelvic plexus (in front of the piriformis muscle) the preganglionic, parasympathetic fibres synapse, within ganglia, with the cell bodies of the post-ganglionic parasympathetic nerves, which then run to the bladder and urethra. 50% of the ganglia of the pelvic plexus lie in the adventitia of the bladder and bladder base (the connective tissue surrounding the bladder) and 50% are within the bladder wall. The post-ganglionic axons provide cholinergic excitatory input to the smooth muscle of the bladder.

Sympathetic motor innervation of the bladder

In the male, preganglionic sympathetic nerve fibres arise from the intermediolateral column of T10–12 and L1–2. These preganglionic neurons synapse in the sympathetic chain and post-ganglionic sympathetic nerve fibres travel as the hypogastric nerves to innervate the trigone, blood vessels of the bladder, and the smooth muscle of the prostate and pre-prostatic sphincter (i.e. the bladder neck). In the female, there is sparse sympathetic innervation of the bladder neck and urethra.

In both sexes, some post-ganglionic sympathetic nerves also terminate in parasympathetic ganglia (in the adventitia surrounding the bladder and within the bladder wall) and exert an inhibitory effect on bladder smooth muscle contraction.

Afferent innervation of the bladder

Afferent nerves from receptors throughout the bladder ascend with parasympathetic neurons back to the cord and from there, up to the pontine storage and micturition centres, or to the cerebral cortex. They sense bladder filling.

Other receptors are located in the trigone and afferent neurons from these neurons ascend with sympathetic neurons up to the thoracolumbar cord, and thence to the pons and cerebral cortex.

Other receptors are located in the urethra. The afferent neurons pass through the pudendal nerve and again ascend to the pons and cerebral cortex. All these neurons have local relays in the cord.

Somatic motor innervation of the urethral sphincter: the distal urethral sphincter mechanism

Anatomically, this is located slightly distal to the apex of the prostate in the male (between the verumontanum and proximal bulbar urethra) and in the mid-urethra in the female. It has 3 components:

- **Extrinsic skeletal muscle**: this is the outermost layer, the pubo-urethral sling (part of levator ani). Composed of striated muscle and innervated by the pudendal nerve (spinal segments S2–4, somatic nerve fibres). It is activated under conditions of stress and augments urethral occlusion pressure
- **Smooth muscle within the wall of the urethra**: cholinergic innervation. Tonically active. Relaxed by nitric oxide
- **Intrinsic striated muscle** (i.e. skeletal muscle *within* the wall of the urethra, hence known as the 'intrinsic rhabdosphincter'): it forms a 'U' shape around the urethra, around the anterior and lateral aspects of the membranous urethra, and is absent posteriorly (i.e. it does not completely encircle the membranous urethra). It may produce urethral occlusion by kinking the urethra, rather than by circumferential compression.

Preganglionic **somatic** nerve fibres (i.e. neurons which innervate **striated** muscle) are, along with **parasympathetic** nerve fibres (which innervate the bladder), derived from spinal segments S2–4, specifically from Onuf's nucleus (also known as spinal nucleus X), which lies in the medial part of the anterior horn of the spinal cord. (Onuf's nucleus is the location of the cell bodies of somatic motoneurons that provide motor input to the striated muscle of the pelvic floor—the external urethral and anal sphincters.) These somatomotor nerves travel to the rhabdosphincter via the perineal branch of the pudendal nerve (documented by direct stimulation studies and horseradish peroxidase tracing—HRP accumulates in Onuf's nucleus following injection into either the pudendal or pelvic nerves). There also seems to be some innervation to the rhabdosphincter from branches of the pelvic plexus (specifically the inferior hypogastric plexus) via pelvic nerves. In dogs, complete silence of the rhabdosphincter is seen only if both the pudendal and pelvic efferents are sectioned. Thus, pudendal nerve block or pudendal neurectomy does not cause incontinence.

The nerve fibres that pass distally to the distal sphincter mechanism are located in a dorsolateral position (5 and 7 o'clock). More distally, they adopt a more lateral position.

Sensory innervation of the urethra

Afferent neurons from the urethra travel in the pudendal nerve. Their cell bodies lie in the dorsal root ganglia, and they terminate in the dorsal horn of the spinal cord at S2–4, connecting with neurons that relay sensory information to the brainstem and cerebral cortex.

The pudendal nerve—a somatic nerve derived from spinal segments S2–4—innervates striated muscle of the pelvic floor (levator ani—i.e. the pubo-urethral sling). Bilateral pudendal nerve block[1] does not lead to incontinence because of maintenance of internal (sympathetic innervation) and external sphincter function (somatic innervation, S2–4, nerve fibres travelling to the external sphincter alongside parasympathetic neurons in the nervi erigentes).

Clinical consequences of damage to the nerves innervating the LUT

Bladder neck function in the female

~75% of continent young women and 50% of perimenopausal continent women have a closed bladder neck during the bladder filling phase. 25% of continent young women and 50% of perimenopausal continent women have an open bladder neck and yet they remain continent (because of their functioning distal sphincter mechanism, the external sphincter).[2,3] Presacral neurectomy (to destroy afferent pain pathways) does not lead to incontinence because of maintenance of the somatic innervation of the external sphincter.

Sympathetic motor innervation of the bladder

Division of the hypogastric plexus of nerves during a retroperitoneal lymph node dissection for metastatic testis tumours results in paralysis of the bladder neck. This is of significance during ejaculation, where normally sympathetic activity results in closure of the bladder neck so that the ejaculate is directed distally into the posterior and then anterior urethra. If the bladder neck is incompetent, the patient develops retrograde ejaculation; they remain continent of urine because the distal urethral sphincter remains functional, being innervated by somatic neurons from S2–4.

During pelvic fracture, the external sphincter and/or its somatic motor innervation may be damaged, such that it is incompetent and unable to maintain continence of urine. Preservation of bladder neck function (the sympathetic innervation of the bladder neck usually remains intact) can preserve continence. However, if in later life the patient undergoes a TURP or bladder neck incision for symptomatic prostatic obstruction, they may well be rendered incontinent because their one remaining sphincter mechanism (the bladder neck) will be divided during these operations.

1 Brindley GS (1974) The pressure exerted by the external sphincter of the urethra when its motor nerve fibres are stimulated electrically. *Br J Urol* **46**:453–62.

2 Chapple CR, *et al.* (1989) Asymptomatic bladder neck incompetence in nulliparous females. *Br J Urol* **64**:357–9.

3 Versi E, *et al.* (1990) Distal urethral compensatory mechanisms in women with an incompetent bladder neck who remain continent and the effect of the menopause. *Neurourol Urodyn* **9**:579–90.

The physiology of urine storage and micturition

Urine storage

During bladder filling, bladder pressure remains low despite a substantial increase in volume. The bladder is thus highly compliant. Its high compliance is partly due to the elastic properties (visco-elasticity) of the connective tissues of the bladder and partly due to the ability of detrusor smooth muscle cells to increase their length without any change in tension. The detrusor is able to do this as a consequence of prevention of transmission of activity from preganglionic parasympathetic neurons to post-ganglionic efferent neurons—a so-called 'gating' mechanism within the parasympathetic ganglia. In addition, inhibitory interneuron activity in the spinal cord prevents transmission of afferent activity from sensors of bladder filling.

Micturition

A spino-bulbar-spinal reflex, co-ordinated in the pontine micturition centre in the brainstem (also known as Barrington's nucleus or the M region), results in simultaneous detrusor contraction, urethral relaxation, and subsequent micturition. Receptors located in the bladder wall sense increasing *tension* as the bladder fills (rather than stretch). This information is relayed, by afferent neurons, to the dorsal horn of the sacral cord. Neurons project from here to the peri-aqueductal gray matter (PAG) in the pons. The PAG is thus informed about the state of bladder filling. The PAG and other areas of the brain (limbic system, orbitofrontal cortex) input into the PMC and determine whether it is appropriate to start micturition.

At times when it is appropriate to void, micturition is initiated by relaxation of the external urethral sphincter and pelvic floor. Urine enters the posterior urethra and this, combined with pelvic floor relaxation, activates afferent neurons, which results in stimulation of the pontine micturition centre (located in the brainstem). Activation of the PMC switches on a detrusor contraction via a direct communication between neurons of the PMC and the cell bodies of parasympathetic, preganglionic motoneurons located in the sacral intermediolateral cell column of S2–4. At the same time that the detrusor contracts, the urethra (the external sphincter) relaxes. The PMC inhibits the somatic motoneurons located in Onuf's nucleus (the activation of which causes external sphincter contraction) by exciting GABA and glycine-containing, inhibitory neurons in the intermediolateral cell column of the sacral cord, which in turn project to the motoneurons in Onuf 's nucleus. In this way, the PMC relaxes the external sphincter.

Micturition is an example of a positive feedback loop, the aim being to maintain bladder contraction until the bladder is empty. As the detrusor contracts, tension in the bladder wall rises. The bladder wall tension receptors are stimulated and the detrusor contraction is driven harder. One of the problems of positive feedback loops is their instability. Several inhibitory pathways exist to stabilize the storage–micturition 'loop'.

- Tension receptors activate bladder afferents, which via the pudendal and hygastric nerves inhibit S2–4 parasympathetic motor nerve output. An ongoing detrusor contraction cannot be over-ridden

- Afferents in the anal and genital regions and in the distribution of the posterior tibial nerve stimulate inhibitory neurons in the sacral cord, and these neurons inhibit S2–4 parasympathetic motor nerve output. This pathway can override an ongoing detrusor contraction.
  It is hypothesized that this system prevents involuntary detrusor contraction during sexual activity, defaecation, and while walking, running, and jumping.

Excitatory neurotransmission in the normal detrusor is exclusively cholinergic, and reciprocal relaxation of the urethral sphincter and bladder neck is mediated by NO, released from post-ganglionic parasympathetic neurons.

Further reading

De Groat WC (1993) Anatomy and physiology of the lower urinary tract. *Urol Clin* NA **20**: 383–401

Bladder and sphincter behaviour in the patient with neurological disease

A variety of neurological conditions are associated with abnormal bladder and sphincter function [e.g. spinal cord injury (SCI), spina bifida (myelomeningocele), MS]. The bladder and sphincters of such patients are described as 'neuropathic'.

They may have abnormal bladder function or abnormal sphincter function or, more usually, both. The bladder may be over- or under-active, as may the sphincter, and any combination of bladder and sphincter over- or under-activity may co-exist. 'Activity' here means bladder and sphincter pressure.

In the normal lower urinary tract during bladder filling the detrusor muscle is inactive and the sphincter pressure is high. Bladder pressure is therefore low and the high sphincter pressure maintains continence. During voiding, the sphincter relaxes and the detrusor contracts. This leads to a short-lived increase in bladder pressure, sustained until the bladder is completely empty. The detrusor and sphincter thus function in synergy—when the sphincter is active, the detrusor is relaxed (storage phase), and when the detrusor contracts, the sphincter relaxes (voiding phase).

An overactive bladder is one that intermittently contracts during bladder filling, so developing high pressures when normally bladder pressure should be low. In between these waves of contraction, bladder pressure returns to normal or near normal levels. In a patient with an underlying neurological problem, bladder overactivity is called detrusor hyper-reflexia (DH). In other patients the bladder wall is stiffer than normal, a condition known as poor compliance. Bladder pressure rises progressively during filling, such bladders being unable to store urine at low pressures. Some patients have a combination of DH and poor compliance. The other end of the spectrum of bladder behaviour is the under-active bladder, which is low pressure during filling and voiding. This is called detrusor areflexia.

An overactive sphincter generates high pressure during bladder filling, but it also does so during voiding, when normally it should relax. This is known as detrusor-external sphincter dyssynergia (DESD or DSD; 📖 Fig. 14.1). During EMG recording, activity in the external sphincter increases during attempted voiding (the external sphincter should normally be 'quiet' during voiding; 📖 see Fig. 3.16). An under-active sphincter is unable to maintain enough pressure, in the face of normal bladder pressures, to prevent leakage of urine.

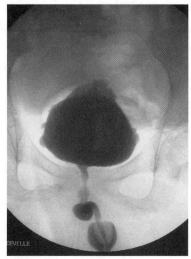

Fig. 14.1 Detrusor-external sphincter dyssynergia (DSD) seen during video-cysto-urethrography.

The neuropathic lower urinary tract: the clinical consequences of storage and emptying problems

Neuropathic patients experience two broad categories of problems—bladder filling and emptying—depending on the *balance* between bladder and sphincter pressures during filling and emptying. The effects of these bladder filling and emptying problems include incontinence, retention, recurrent UTIs, and renal failure.

High-pressure sphincter

High-pressure bladder

If the bladder is overactive (detrusor hyper-reflexia) or poorly compliant, bladder pressures during filling are high. The kidneys have to function against these chronically high pressures. Hydronephrosis develops and ultimately the kidneys fail (*renal failure*). At times the bladder pressure overcomes the sphincter pressure and the patient leaks urine (*incontinence*). If the sphincter pressure is higher than the bladder pressure during voiding (detrusor sphincter dyssynergia, DSD), bladder emptying is inefficient (*retention, recurrent UTIs*).

Low-pressure bladder

If the bladder is under-active (detrusor areflexia), pressure during filling is low. The bladder simply fills up—it is unable to generate enough pressure to empty (retention, recurrent UTIs). Urine leaks at times if the bladder pressure becomes higher than the sphincter pressure (incontinence), but this may occur only at very high bladder volumes or not at all.

Low-pressure sphincter

High-pressure bladder

If the detrusor is hyper-reflexic or poorly compliant, the bladder will only be able to hold low volumes of urine before leaking (incontinence).

Low-pressure bladder

If the detrusor is areflexic, such that it cannot develop high pressures, the patient may be dry for much of the time. They may, however, leak urine (incontinence) when abdominal pressure rises (e.g. when coughing, rising from a seated position, or when transferring to or from a wheelchair). Their low bladder pressure may compromise bladder emptying (recurrent UTIs).

Bladder management techniques for the neuropathic patient

A variety of techniques and procedures are used to treat retention, incontinence, recurrent UTIs, and hydronephrosis in the patient with a neuropathic bladder. Each of the techniques described below can be used for a variety of clinical problems. Thus, a patient with a high-pressure, hyperreflexic bladder that is causing incontinence can be managed with ISC (with intravesical botox injections if necessary), or a suprapubic catheter, or by sphincterotomy with condom sheath drainage, or by deafferentation combined with a sacral anterior root stimulator (SARS). Precisely which option to choose will depend on the individual patient's clinical problem, their hand function, their lifestyle, and other 'personal' factors, such as body image, sexual function, etc. Some patients will opt for a suprapubic catheter, as a simple, generally safe, generally very convenient and effective form of bladder drainage. Others wish to be free of external appliances and devices because of an understandable desire to look and 'feel' normal. They might opt for deafferentation with a SARS.

Intermittent self-catheterization (ISC)
📖 See p. 594.

In-dwelling catheters
📖 See p. 594.

External sphincterotomy
Deliberate division of the external sphincter to convert the high-pressure, poorly emptying bladder due to DSD to a low-pressure, efficiently emptying bladder. *Indications:* retention, recurrent UTIs, hydronephrosis.

Techniques
- Surgical (with an electrically heated 'knife' or laser). *Disadvantages:* irreversible, post-operative bleeding, septicaemia, and stricture formation[1]
- Intra-sphincteric botox (botulinum toxin). Increasingly popular because minimally invasive and reversible. *Disadvantage:* repeat injection required every 6–12 months
- A third potential option is an oral or sublingual nitric oxide (NO) donor (e.g. nifedipine, GTN). NO is a neurotransmitter which relaxes the external sphincter. Hypothesized as a treatment for DSD, and preliminary studies support this hypothesis.[2,3]

Augmentation
Technique of increasing bladder volume to lower pressure by implanting detubularized small bowel into the bivalved bladder ('clam' ileocystoplasty; Fig. 14.2) or by removing a disc of muscle from the dome of the bladder (auto-augmentation or detrusor myectomy). *Indications:* incontinence, hydronephrosis.

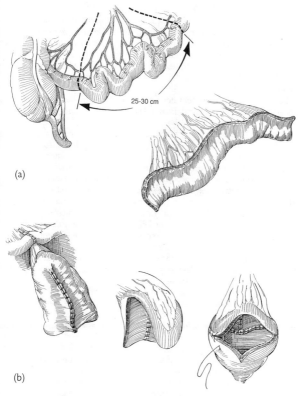

(a)

(b)

Fig. 14.2 A 'clam' ileocystoplasty. (Reproduced with permission from Elsevier).[4]

1 Reynard JM (2003) Sphincterotomy and the treatment of detrusor–sphincter dyssynergia: current status, future prospects. *Spinal Cord* **41**:1–11.

2 Keitz A, *et al.* (2004) Oral nitric oxide donors: a new pharmacological approach to detrusor-sphincter dyssynergia in spinal cord injured patients. *Eur Urol* **45**:516–20.

3 Mamas MA, Reynard JM, Brading AF (2001) Augmentation of external uretheral sphincter nitric oxide: a potential pharmacological treatment for detrusor-external sphincter dyssynergia in spinal cord injury. *Lancet* **357**:1964–7.

4 McAninch JW (1996) *Traumatic and Reconstructive Urology.* Philadelphia: W.B. Saunders© p. 301.

Intravesical injections

Recently, intravesical botulinum toxin type A injections at multiple sites in the bladder every 6–12 months have produced impressive reductions in bladder pressure and increases in volume, with minimal side-effects. As a consequence, surgical augmentation is nowadays only rarely done, being reserved for cases where botox has failed to work (where the patient is still wet between passing ISC catheters or where there is persistent hydronephrosis).

Botulinum toxin is a potent neurotoxin produced by the gram negative anaerobic bacterium Clostridium botulinum. Of the 7 serotypes only types A ('Botox®', Allergan, CA in the United States; 'Dysport®', Ipsen, Slough, UK) and B ('Myobloc®', Elan Pharmaceuticals, NJ, USA) are used clinically.

Botulinum toxin type A ('Botox®' or 'Dysport®') binds to the SV2 receptor on the presynaptic nerve terminal where it is internalized by endocytosis. It causes proteolysis of the synaptosomal associated protein, SNAP-25, which is one of a group of SNARE proteins which mediate fusion of neurotransmitter containing vesicles with neuronal cell membranes. Thus, botulinum toxin inhibits neurotransmission at motor cholinergic, noradrenergic and other (sensory) nerve terminals. It also reduces the expression of the vanilloid receptor TPRV1 and the purinoreceptor P2X3, both of which are sensory neuron receptors. Thus, while we tend to think of botulinum toxin type A as inhibit neuromuscular nerve transmission, it is likely that it also has effects on sensory nerve transmission, although its role in the management of sensory urological conditions (sensory urgency, interstitial cystitis) remains to be established.

Intravesical botox injections can be administered using a flexible cystoscope (with a flexible injection needle) or a rigid scope. Multiple techniques of injection have been described and all seem to be effective. Some surgeons dilute the botox in 5 mL of saline, whereas others use the same number of units in 20 mL of saline. Some use 'Dysport®' (Ipsen) while others use 'Botox®' (Allergan). Some inject in 20 sites, while others make 50 injections. Whether one technique or concentration or formulation of botox is superior to any other remains to be established. For intravesical injection in neuropathic patients (e.g. those with spinal cord injuries or MS) the author uses a standard dose of 1000 units of Dysport® (occasionally 1500 units), diluted in 5 mL of saline and injects 0.1–0.2 mL per site in approximately 40–50 sites (roughly 20–40 units per site), using (usually) a flexible cystoscope and injection needle. Some surgeons spare the trigone (i.e. avoid injecting the trigone), the theory (not proven) being that this avoids disrupting the valve mechanism of the vesicoureteric junction. Other surgeons (the author included) inject in the trigone.

Intravesical botox injections are indicated for hydronephrosis, which has failed to respond to increased frequency of ISC combined with oral anticholinergic medication; inter-ISC leakage, which has failed to respond to increased frequency of ISC combined with oral anticholinergic medication; urethral leakage in patients with suprapubic catheters where the leakage is thought to be due to uninhibited bladder contractions. In the author's experience intravesical botox injections are most successful for inter-ISC-leakage, they last for somewhere between 6 and 12 months, and the duration of effect of the botulinum toxin does not appear to diminish with repeat injections over, at present, 5 years of follow-up.

Side effects of botulinum toxin type A: haematuria is almost inevitable after making multiple intravescial injections sensory and is almost always self-limiting (very occasionally admission for a bladder washout of clots and irrigation via a 3-way catheter is required, but this is rare). Occasionally, systemic side effects can occur. These are rare, but can be disabling, particularly in the patient with pre-existing neurological disease. The author warns patients of the risks of generalised weakness which has occurred in 3 patients, 2 following bladder injections and one following external sphincter injections (which can impair the ability to transfer on and off a wheelchair, and affect daily living and working activities); blurring of vision (due to intraocular muscle effects—very rare, but very disabling); and difficulty breathing and/or swallowing. The latter symptoms might require a period of several weeks of in-hospital observation. All of these side effects are rare, but they can last for many months, so warn your patient that they can occur.

Deafferentation

Division of dorsal spinal nerve roots of S2–4, to convert the hyper-reflexic, high-pressure bladder into an areflexic, low-pressure one. Can be used where the hyper-reflexic bladder is the cause of incontinence or hydronephrosis. Bladder emptying can subsequently be achieved by ISC or implantation of a nerve stimulator placed on ventral roots (efferent nerves) of S2–4 to 'drive' micturition when the patient wants to void (a pager-sized externally applied radiotransmitter activates micturition (Figs 14.3 and 14.4). Also useful for DSD/incomplete bladder emptying causing recurrent UTIs and retention.

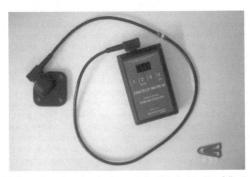

Fig. 14.3 A sacral anterior root stimulator, used to 'drive' micturition following a deafferentation (external components).

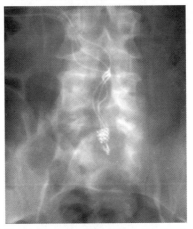

Fig. 14.4 KUB X-ray showing the sacral electrodes positioned on the ventral roots of S2, 3, and 4.

Catheters and sheaths and the neuropathic patient

Many patients manage their bladders by intermittent catheterization (IC) done by themselves (intermittent self-catheterization, ISC) or by a carer if their hand function is inadequate, as is the case with most (though remarkably not all) tetraplegics. Many others manage their bladders with an in-dwelling catheter (urethral or suprapubic). Both methods can be effective for managing incontinence, recurrent UTIs, and bladder outlet obstruction causing hydronephrosis.

Intermittent catheterization

Requires adequate hand function. The technique is a 'clean' one (simple handwashing prior to catheterization) rather than 'sterile'. Gel-coated catheters become slippery when in contact with water, so providing lubrication. Usually done 3–4-hourly.

Problems
- Recurrent UTIs
- Recurrent incontinence: check technique (adequate drainage of last few drops of urine). Suggest increasing frequency of ISC to minimize volume of urine in the bladder (reduces bacterial colonization and minimizes bladder pressure). If incontinence persists, consider intravesical botulinum toxin.

Long-term catheterization

Some patients prefer the convenience of a long-term catheter. Others regard it as a last resort when other methods of bladder drainage have failed. The suprapubic route (suprapubic catheter, SPC) is preferred over the urethral because of pressure necrosis of the ventral surface of the distal penile urethra in men (acquired hypospadias—'kippering' of the penis) and pressure necrosis of the bladder neck in women, which becomes wider and wider until urine leaks around the catheter ('patulous' urethra) or frequent expulsion of the catheter occurs with the balloon inflated.

Problems and complications of long-term catheters
- **Recurrent UTIs:** colonization with bacteria provides a potential source of recurrent infection
- **Catheter blockages are common:** due to encrustation of the lumen of the catheter with bacterial biofilms. *Proteus mirabilis*, *Morganella*, and *Providencia* species secrete a polysaccharide matrix. Within this, urease-producing bacteria generate ammonia from nitrogen in urine, raising urine pH, and precipitating magnesium and calcium phosphate crystals. The matrix-crystal complex blocks the catheter. Catheter blockage causes bypassing which soils the patient's clothes. Bladder distension can cause autonomic dysreflexia, leading to extreme rises in blood pressure, which can cause stroke and death! Regular bladder washouts and increased catheter size sometimes help. Impregnation of catheters with antibacterials (e.g. triclosan) are under investigation.[1] Intermittent filling and emptying of the bladder using a 'flip-flow' valve may reduce frequency of catheter blockages

- **Bladder stones:** develop in 1 in 4 patients over 5 years[2]
- **Bladder cancer:** chronic inflammation (from bladder stones, recurrent UTIs, long-term catheterization) may increase the risk of squamous cell carcinoma in SCI patients. Some studies report a higher incidence of bladder cancer (whether chronically catheterized or not); others do not.[3]

Condom sheaths

These are an externally worn urine collection device consisting of a tubular sheath applied over the glans and shaft of the penis (just like a contraceptive condom only without the lubrication to prevent it slipping off). Usually made of silicone rubber with a tube attached to the distal end to allow urine drainage into a leg bag. They are used as a convenient way of preventing leakage of urine, but are obviously only suitable for men. Detachment of the sheath from the penis is prevented by using adhesive gels and tapes. They are used for patients with reflex voiding (where the hyper-reflexic bladder spontaneously empties, and where bladder pressure between voids never reaches a high enough level to compromise kidney function). They are also used as a urine collection device for patients after external sphincterotomy (for combined detrusor hyper-reflexia and sphincter dysynergia where incomplete bladder emptying leads to recurrent UTIs and/or hydronephrosis).

Problems

The principal problem experienced by some patients is sheath detachment. Despite the fact that a man walked on the moon 30 years ago, we have been unable to design a condom sheath that will consistently prevent urine leakage in all men. This can be a major problem, and in some cases requires a complete change of bladder management. Skin reactions sometimes occur.

1 Stickler D, *et al.* (2003) Control of encrustation and blocked Foley catheters. *Lancet* **361:**1435–7.

2 Ord J, Lunn D, Reynard J. (2003) Bladder management and risk of bladder stone formation in spinal cord injured patients. *J Urol* **170:**1734–7.

3 Subramonian K, *et al.* (2004) Bladder cancer in patients with spinal cord injuries. *Br J Urol Int* **93:**739–43.

Management of incontinence in the neuropathic patient

Causes

High-pressure bladder (detrusor hyper-reflexia, reduced bladder compliance); sphincter weakness; UTI; bladder stones; rarely, bladder cancer (enquire for UTI symptoms and haematuria). Hyper-reflexic peripheral reflexes suggest bladder may be hyper-reflexic (increased ankle jerk reflexes, S1–2 and a +ve bulbocavernosus reflex indicating an intact sacral reflex arc—i.e. S2–4 intact). Absent peripheral reflexes suggest the bladder and sphincter may be areflexic (i.e. sphincter unable to generate pressures adequate for maintaining continence).

Initial investigations

Urine culture (for infection); KUB X-ray for bladder stones; bladder and renal ultrasound for residual urine volume and to detect hydronephrosis; cytology and cystoscopy if bladder cancer suspected.

Empirical treatment

Start with simple treatments. If the bladder residual volume is large, regular ISC may lower bladder pressure and achieve continence. Try an anticholinergic drug (e.g. oxybutynin, tolterodine). Many SCI patients are already doing ISC and simply increasing ISC frequency to 3–4 hourly may achieve continence. ISC more frequently than 3-hourly is usually impractical, particularly for paraplegic women who usually have to transfer from their wheelchair onto a toilet and then back onto their wheelchair. See Table 14.1.

Management of failed empirical treatment

Determined by VCUG, to assess bladder and sphincter behaviour.

Detrusor hyper-reflexia or poor compliance

High-pressure sphincter (i.e. DSD). Treating the high-pressure bladder is usually enough to achieve continence.

- **Bladder treatments:** intravesical *Botulinum* toxin, detrusor myectomy (auto-augmentation), bladder augmentation (ileocystoplasty). All will usually require ISC for bladder emptying
- Long-term suprapubic catheter
- Sacral deafferentation + ISC or Brindley implant (SARS—sacral anterior root stimulator).

Low-pressure sphincter. Treat the bladder first (as above). If bladder treatment alone fails, consider a urethral bulking agent, a transvaginal tape (TVT), or bladder neck closure in women or an artificial urinary sphincter in either sex (Fig. 14.5).

Detrusor areflexia + low pressure sphincter

- Urethral bulking agents
- TVT
- Bladder neck closure in women
- Artificial urinary sphincter.

The artificial urinary sphincter (AUS)

The artificial urinary sphincter essentially consists of 2 balloons connected by tubing to a control pump. One of the balloons is configured as a cuff around the bulbar urethra or bladder neck. The other balloon (placed deep to the rectus muscle) applies a constant pressure (usually 61–70 cmH$_2$O pressure) to the cuff via a control pump located in the scrotum or labia [Fig. 14.5. The AMS (American Medical Systems) 800 artificial urinary sphincter]. Pressure in the cuff is maintained until the control pump is squeezed by the patient. This forces fluid from the cuff (so it temporarily no longer occludes the urethra) into the balloon. Pressure from the balloon then refills the cuff, via delay resistors in the control pump, over a minute or so.

AUS: indications

Incontinence

- Following prostatectomy (post-TURP or radical prostatectomy)
- In the neuropathic patients (spinal cord injury, spina bifida) due to intrinsic sphincter deficiency
- Following trauma to the pelvis or perineum.

AUS: relative contraindications

- Poor bladder compliance (risk of dangerous and silent elevation of bladder pressure, with the development of hydronephrosis)
- Untreated involuntary bladder contractions (persistent incontinence common)
- Urethral stricture. Incision can expose the underlying cuff leading to AUS infection
- Poor cognitive function such that the patient is unable to appreciate the need to deflate the cuff several times a day.

Preparation prior to insertion

- Video-urodynamics (to assess bladder pressure and confirm presence of sphincter weakness incontinence). Usually not necessary in 'simple' post-radical prostatectomy patients (cause of incontinence usually obvious)
- Flexible cystoscopy to exclude urethral stricture
- Urine culture. Treat infection with an appropriate antibiotic for a week or so before insertion.

Bulbar cuff placement: for post-radical prostatectomy incontinence; previous surgery or trauma (pelvic fracture) in region of bladder neck (increased risk of rectal perforation).

Bladder neck cuff placement: women (obviously), children (bulbar urethra too small for the available cuff sizes), men who wish to maintain fertility by preserving antegrade ejaculation, neuropathic patients where ISC is or may be required.

A deactivation button prevents return of fluid from the balloon to the cuff, so allowing catheterisation or instrumentation.

Outcomes

Improved continence in 60–90%. Complications in 5–30%—infection, urethral erosion, urethral loosening under the cuff (atrophy), device ('mechanical') failure.[1]

Alternatives

- Injectable urethral bulking agents
- **Male urethral sling:** 3 types—bulbo-urethral (suprapubic to suburethral); bone anchored perineal (InVance™); transobturator (AdVance™). Said to improve continence by bulbar urethral repositioning (rather than compression). Good (short-term) outcomes for less severe incontinence—5 or fewer pads per day; poor outcome if 6 or more pads per day.[2] Long-term outcomes and those for transobturator slings remain undetermined
- **Extra-urethral retropubic adjustable compression devices:** under local or regional anaesthesia 2 small silicone balloons are introduced percutaneously via a perineal approach and positioned on each side of the urethra close to the bladder neck. Subcutaneous ports allow volume adjustment post-operatively to increase (for persistent leakage) or decrease urethral resistance (for voiding difficulty). Questions remain over its safety (e.g. 10% urethral or bladder perforation, balloon migration, fluid leakage) and continence outcomes.

1   Hussain M, Greenwell TJ, Venn SN, Mundy AR. (2005) The current role of the artificial urinary sphincter for the treatment of urinary incontinence. *J Urol* **174:**418–24.

2   Castle EP, Andrews PE, Itano N. (2005) The male sling for post-prostatectomy incontinence: mean follow-up of 18 months. *J Urol* **173:**1657.

Table 14.1 Summary of treatment for incontinence

	High bladder pressure	Low bladder pressure
High sphincter pressure	Lower bladder pressure by ISC + anticholinergics or botulinum toxin type A or augmentation	ISC*
Low sphincter pressure	Lower bladder pressure by (ISC + anticholinergics or botox or augmentation) + urethral bulking agent TVT or bladder neck closure or artificial urinary sphincter	Urethral bulking agent, TVT Bladder neck closure Artificial urinary sphincter

*High sphincter pressure is usually enough to keep patient dry.

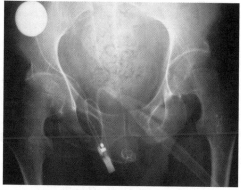

Fig. 14.5 Artificial urinary sphincter implanted around the bulbar urethra.

Management of recurrent urinary tract infections (UTIs) in the neuropathic patient

Causes of recurrent UTIs
- Incomplete bladder emptying
- Kidney stones
- Bladder stones
- Presence of an in-dwelling catheter (urethral or suprapubic).

History

What the patient interprets as a UTI may be different from your definition of UTI. The neuropathic bladder is frequently colonized with bacteria and often contains pus cells (pyuria). From time to time it becomes cloudy due to precipitation of calcium, magnesium, and phosphate salts in the absence of active infection. The presence of bacteria, pus cells, or cloudy urine in the presence of non-specific symptoms (abdominal pain, tiredness, headaches, feeling 'under the weather') is frequently interpreted as a UTI.

Indications for treatment of UTI in the neuropathic patient

It is impossible to eradicate bacteria or pus cells from the urine in the presence of a foreign body (e.g. a catheter). In the absence of fever and cloudy, smelly urine, we do not prescribe antibiotics, the indiscriminate use of which encourages growth of antibiotic-resistant organisms. We prescribe antibiotics to the chronically catheterized patient where there is a combination of fever, cloudy, smelly urine, and where the patient feels unwell. Culture urine and immediately start empirical antibiotic therapy with nitrofurantoin, ciprofoxacin, or trimethoprim (the antibiotics sensitivities of our local 'bacterial flora'), changing to a more specific antibiotic if the organism is resistant to the prescribed one.

Investigations

For recurrent UTIs (= frequent episodes of fever, cloudy, smelly urine, and feeling unwell), organize the following:
- KUB X-ray—looking for kidney and bladder stones
- Renal and bladder ultrasound to determine the presence/absence of hydronephrosis, and to measure pre-void bladder volume and post-void residual urine volume.

Treatment

In the presence of fever and cloudy, smelly urine, culture the urine and start antibiotics empirically (e.g. trimethoprim, nitrofurantoin, amoxicillin, ciprofloxacin), changing the antibiotic if the culture result suggests resistance to your empirical choice. 'Response' to treatment is suggested by the patient feeling better and their urine clearing and becoming non-offensive to smell. Persistent fever, with constitutional symptoms (malaise, rigors) despite treatment with a specific oral antibiotic in an adequate dose is an indication for admission for treatment with intravenous antibiotics.

Management of recurrent UTIs

📖 See Table 14.2.

If there is residual urine present, optimize bladder emptying by intermittent catheterization (males, females) or external sphincterotomy for DSD (males). Intermittent catheterization can be done by the patient (intermittent self-catheterization, ISC) if hand function is good (paraplegic), or by a carer if tetraplegic. An in-dwelling catheter is an option, but the presence of a foreign body in the bladder may itself cause recurrent UTIs (though in some it seems to reduce UTI frequency).

Table 14.2 Summary of treatment for recurrent UTIs

Low bladder pressure	High bladder pressure + DSD*
ISC	ISC
IDC	IDC
	External sphincterotomy—surgical, botox, stent
	Deafferentation/SARS

Remove stones if present—cystitholapxy for bladder stones, PCNL for staghorn stones.

*A new potential option for DSD is augmentation of external sphincter nitric oxide (NO), a neurotransmitter which relaxes the external sphincter, thereby encouraging antegrade flow of urine and potentially, therefore, lowering residual urine volume. NO donors such as nifedipine or GTN can be used. There is theoretical and some experimental evidence to support this.[1,2]

1   Mamas MA, Reynard JM, Brading AF (2001) Augmentation of external urethral sphincter nitric oxide: a potential pharmacological treatment for detrusor-external sphincter dyssynergia in spinal cord injury. *Lancet* **357**:1964–7.

2   Keitz A et al. (2004) Oral nitric oxide donors: a new pharmacological approach to detrusor-spincter dyssynergia in spinal cord injured patients. *Eur Urol* **45**:516–20.

Management of hydronephrosis in the neuropathic patient

An overactive bladder (detrusor hyper-reflexia) or poorly compliant bladder is frequently combined with a high-pressure sphincter (detrusor-sphincter dysynergia—DSD). Bladder pressures during both filling and voiding are high. At times the bladder pressure may overcome the sphincter pressure and the patient leaks small quantities of urine. For much of the time, however, the sphincter pressures are higher than the bladder pressures and the kidneys are chronically exposed to these high pressures. They are hydronephrotic on ultrasound and renal function slowly, but inexorably, deteriorate.

Treatment options for hydronephrosis

Bypass the external sphincter
- IDC (indwelling catheter)
- ISC (intermittent self-catheterization) + anticholinergics.

Treat the external sphincter
- Sphincterotomy: surgical incision via a cystoscope inserted down the urethra (electrically heated knife or laser), botulinum toxin type A injections into sphincter, urethral stent
- Deafferentation[1] + ISC or SARS.

Treat the bladder
- Intravesical botulinum toxin type A + ISC
- Augmentation + ISC
- Deafferentation[1] + ISC or SARS.

---

1 Deafferentation converts the high-pressure sphincter into a low-pressure sphincter and the high-pressure bladder into low-pressure bladder.

Bladder dysfunction in multiple sclerosis, in Parkinson's disease, after stroke, and in other neurological disease

Multiple sclerosis (MS)

75% of patients with MS have spinal cord involvement and, in these patients, bladder dysfunction is common. The most common symptom in patients with MS is urgency (due to DH). Bladder pressures are rarely high enough to cause upper tract problems (hydronephrosis).

Parkinson's disease (PD)

PD is a cause of parkinsonism (tremor, rigidity, bradykinesis—slow movements) and is due to degeneration of dopaminergic neurons in the substantia nigra in the basal ganglia. Frequency, urgency, and urge incontinence are common. The most common urodynamic abnormality is DH (the basal ganglia may have an inhibitory effect on the micturition reflex). L-dopa seems to have a variable effect on these symptoms and DH, improving symptoms in some and making them worse in others. LUTS in Parkinson's disease may simply be due to benign prostatic obstruction or may be due to the PD itself. Traditionally, patients with PD have had a poorer outcome after TURP than those without PD, but if the patient has urodynamically proven BOO, TURP is a treatment option.

Multiple system atrophy (MSA; formerly Shy–Drager syndrome)

A cause of parkinsonism characterized clinically by postural hypotension and detrusor areflexia. Loss of cells in the pons leads to DH (symptoms of bladder overactivity), loss of parasympathetic neurons due to cell loss in the intermediolateral cell column of the sacral cord causes poor bladder emptying, and loss of neurons in Onuf's nucleus in the sacral anterior horns leads to denervation of the striated sphincter causing incontinence. The presentation is usually with DH (i.e. symptoms of bladder overactivity), followed over the course of several years by worsening bladder emptying.

Cerebrovascular accidents

DH occurs in 70%, DSD in 15%. Detrusor areflexia can occur.[11] Frequency, nocturia, urgency, and urge incontinence are common. Retention occurs in 5% in the acute phase. Incontinence within the first 7 days after a CVA predicts poor survival.[22]

Other neurological disease

Frontal lobe lesions (e.g. tumours, AVMs)

May cause severe frequency and urgency (frontal lobe has inhibitory input to the pons).

Brainstem lesions (e.g. posterior fossa tumours)

Can cause urinary retention or bladder overactivity.

Transverse myelitis

Severe tetraparesis and bladder dysfunction, which often recovers to a substantial degree.

Peripheral neuropathies

The autonomic innervation of the bladder makes it 'vulnerable' to the effects of peripheral neuropathies such as those occurring in diabetes mellitus and amyloidosis. The picture is usually one of reduced bladder contractility (poor bladder emptying—i.e. chronic low pressure retention).

1 Sakakibara R et al. (1996) Micturitional disturbance after acute hemispheric stroke: analysis of the lesion site by CT and MRI. *J Neurol Sci* **137**:47–56.

2 Wade D et al. (1985) Outlook after an acute stroke: urinary incontinence and loss of consciousness compared in 532 patients. *Quart Med J* **56**:601–8.

Neuromodulation in lower urinary tract dysfunction

This is the electrical activation of *afferent* nerve fibres to modulate their function.

Electrical stimulation applied anywhere in the body preferentially depolarizes nerves (higher current amplitudes are required to directly depolarize muscle). In patients with LUT dysfunction, the relevant spinal segments are S2–4. *Indications:* urgency, frequency, urge incontinence, chronic urinary retention, where behavioural and drug therapy has failed.

Several sites of stimulation are available, the electrical stimulus being applied directly to nerves, or as close as possible:

- Sacral nerve stimulation (SNS)
- **Pudendal nerve:** direct pelvic floor electrical stimulation (of bladder, vagina, anus, pelvic floor muscles) or via stimulation of dorsal penile or clitoral nerve (DPN, DCN)
- Posterior tibial nerve stimulation (PTNS).[1]

PTNS

PTN (L4,5; S1–3) shares common nerve roots with those innervating the bladder. PTNS can be applied transcutaneously (stick-on surface electrodes) or percutaneously (needle electrodes). Percutaneous needle systems include the SANS (Stoller) and the UrgentPC system. Stimulation is applied via an acupuncture needle inserted just above the medial malleolus with a reference (or returns) electrode—30 min of stimulation per week, over 12 weeks. Thereafter, 30 min of treatment every 2–3 weeks can be used to maintain the treatment effect in those who respond. PTNS has not been compared with placebo ('sham' stimulation) and therefore reported efficacy may represent a placebo response.

SNS (Sacral nerve modulation—SNM)

A sacral nerve stimulator (Medtronic Interstim) delivers continuous electrical pulses to sacral nerve root 3 via an electrode inserted through the sacral foramina and connected to an electrical pulse generator which is implanted subcutaneously. Supported by NICE[2] for patients with urge incontinence who have failed lifestyle modification, behaviour, and drug therapy.

A test stimulation (the peripheral nerve evaluation, PNE) is performed, under local anaesthetic, by a percutaneous test electrode placed in S3 foramina to confirm an appropriate clinical response (a reduction in urgency, frequency, or incontinence episodes). A permanent implant is offered if there is a 50% reduction in frequency and urgency. This is placed in a subcutaneous pocket and is connected to the sacral electrode. It can be switched on and off and the amplitude varied within set limits. ~50–60% of patients have a successful PNE[3] and, of this, 50–60% who undergo subsequent permanent implantation, 50–70% report resolution of their urge incontinence and 80% report >50% reduction in incontinence episodes, persisting for at least 3–5 years.

The exact mechanism of action of SNM in patients with bladder dysfunction is not known.

1 Andrews B, Reynard J (2003) Transcutaneous posterior tibial nerve stimulation for the treatment of detrusor hyper-reflexia in spinal cord injury. *J Urol* **170**:926

2 NICE (June 2004) Interventional Procedure Guidance 64. *www.nice.org.uk/ip082systematic* review.

3 Schmidt RA, Jonas U, Oleson KA et al (1999). Sacral nerve stimulation for treatment of refractory urinary incontinence. Sacral Nerve Stimulation Study Group. *J Urol* **162**:325–7.

Urological problems in pregnancy

Physiological and anatomical changes in the urinary tract

Upper urinary tract

- **Renal size enlarges** by 1 cm, secondary to increased interstitial volume and distended renal vasculature, with renal volume increasing up to 30%
- **Dilatation of the collecting systems** producing a physiological hydronephrosis and hydro-ureters (right>left side). It is caused by mechanical obstruction by the uterus, and smooth muscle relaxation due to progesterone
- **Renal plasma flow rate (RPF)** increases early in the 1st trimester and rises by up to 80% by the beginning of the 3rd trimester, before a slight decline towards term
- **Glomerular filtration rate (GFR)** increases by 50% by the 3rd trimester, and tends to plateau at term
- **Renal function and biochemical parameters** are affected by changes in RPF and GFR. Creatinine clearance increases, and serum levels of creatinine, urea and urate fall in normal pregnancy (see Table 15.1). Raised GFR causes an increased glucose load at the renal tubules, and results in glucose excretion (physiological glycosuria of pregnancy). 24-h protein excretion is increased. Urine output also increases
- **Salt and water handling:** a reduction in serum sodium causes reduced plasma osmolality. The kidney compensates by increasing renal tubular re-absorption of sodium. Plasma renin activity is increased 10 fold, and levels of angiotensinogen and angiotensin are increased 5-fold. Osmotic thresholds for antidiuretic hormone (ADH) and thirst decrease
- **Acid-base metabolism** Serum bicarbonate is reduced. Increased progesterone stimulates the respiratory centre resulting in reduced PCO_2.

Lower urinary tract

- **Bladder displacement** occurs (superiorly and anteriorly) due to the enlarging uterus. The bladder becomes hyperaemic, and raised oestrogen levels cause hyperplasia of muscle and connective tissues. Bladder pressures can increase over pregnancy (from 9 to 20cmH$_2$O), with associated rises in absolute and functional urethral length and pressures
- **Lower urinary tract symptoms:** urinary frequency (>7 voids during the day) and nocturia (≥1 void at night) increases over the duration of gestation (incidence of 80–90% in 3rd trimester). Urgency and urge incontinence also increase, contributed to by pressure effects from the enlarging uterus. Normal bladder function returns in the majority soon after delivery
- **Acute urinary retention** is uncommon, but may occur at 12–14 weeks' gestation in association with a retroverted uterus

- **Stress urinary incontinence** occurs in 22%, and increases with parity.[1] It is partly caused by placental production of peptide hormones (relaxin), which induces collagen remodelling and consequent softening of tissues of the birth canal. Infant weight, duration of 1st and 2nd stages of labour (vaginal delivery), and instrumental delivery (ventouse extraction or forceps delivery) increase risks of post-partum[2] stress incontinence.

Table 15.1 Biochemistry reference intervals

Substance	Non-pregnant	Pregnant
Sodium mmol/L	135–145	132–141
Urea mmol/L	2.5–6.7	2–4.2
Urate µmol/L	150–390	100–270
Creatinine µmol/L	70–150	24–68
Creatinine clearance mL/min	90–110	150–200
Bicarbonate mmol/L	24–30	20–25

---

1 Parity—pregnancies that resulted in delivery beyond 28 weeks' gestation.

2 Post partum—after delivery of the child.

Urinary tract infection (UTI)

Pregnancy does not alter the incidence of lower urinary tract infection (UTI). However, physiological and anatomical changes associated with pregnancy can alter the course of infection, causing an increased risk of recurrent UTI and progression to acute pyelonephritis.

Asymptomatic bacteriuria is an asymptomatic lower UTI which affects 4% of pregnant women, with a 20–40% risk of developing pyelonephritis during pregnancy. This risk is reduced if the bacteriuria is treated, and therefore urine screening is advocated. Asymptomatic bacteriuria is defined as 2 consecutive positive urine cultures of the same bacterial organism taken 1–2 weeks apart.

Symptomatic UTI (cystitis) affects 1–2%, and presents with urinary frequency, urgency, suprapubic pain or discomfort, and dysuria.

Acute pyelonephritis is more frequently seen than in non-pregnant women, and is most common in the 3rd trimester. It presents with fever, flank pain, nausea, and vomiting, often with an elevated white cell count.

Risk factors: previous history of recurrent UTIs; pre-existing anatomical or functional urinary tract abnormality (i.e. vesicoureteric reflux); diabetes. Physiological changes in pregnancy include hydronephrosis with decreased ureteric peristalsis causing urinary stasis. Up to 75% of pyelonephritis occurs in the third trimester when these changes are most prominent.

Pathogenesis: a common causative organism is *Escherichia coli*. An increased risk of gestational pyelonephritis is associated with *E. coli* containing the virulence factor 'Dr adhesin'.

Complications: UTI increases the risk of pre-term delivery, low foetal birth weight, intra-uterine growth retardation, and maternal anaemia.

Screening tests

Midstream urine specimen (MSU) should be obtained at the first antenatal visit (week 10), and sent for urinalysis and culture to look for bacteria, protein and blood. A second MSU investigation is recommended at later visits (week 16) to examine for bacteria, protein and glucose. High risk patients with a history of urinary tract anomalies or recurrent UTI should undergo repeat urine screening throughout pregnancy. (📖 See Table 6.1 p. 167, for the recommended criteria for diagnosing UTI.)

Treatment

All proven episodes of UTI should be treated (asymptomatic or symptomatic), guided by urine culture sensitivities for 4–7 days, with follow-up cultures 1 week later, and at one other point before delivery. Antibiotics that are safe to use during pregnancy include **penicillins** (i.e. ampicillin, amoxicillin, penicillin V), and **cephalosporins** (i.e. cefaclor, cefalexin, cefotaxime, ceftriaxone, cefuroxime). Nitrofurantoin may be used in 1st and 2nd trimesters only. Acute pyelonephritis requires hospital admission for intravenous antibiotics (cephalosporin or aminopenicillin) until apyrexial, followed by oral antibiotics for 14 days, and repeated cultures for the duration of pregnancy.

Table 15.2 Antibiotics to avoid in pregnancy*

Trimester	Antibiotic	Risk in pregnancy
1,2,3	Tetracyclines	Foetal malformation; maternal hepatotoxicity; dental discolouration.
	Quinolones	Arthropathy
1	Trimethoprim	Teratogenic risk (folate antagonist).
2,3	Aminoglycosides	Auditory or vestibular nerve damage.
3	Chloramphenicol	Neonatal 'grey' syndrome.
	Sulphonamides	Neonatal haemolysis; methaemoglobinaemia.
	Nitrofurantoin	Maternal or neonatal haemolysis (if used at term), in subjects with G6PD deficiency.

*See British National Formulary (BNF), appendix 4, for full details.
Of note, antibiotics which undergo excretion by glomerular filtration may need dose adjustment in pregnancy due to increased renal clearance of these drugs.

Hydronephrosis of pregnancy

Hydronephrosis describes dilatation of the renal collecting system (pelvis and calyces). It can be associated with hydro-ureters (dilatation of the ureters), and represents a normal physiological event in pregnancy which is usually asymptomatic. Hydronephrosis develops from ~weeks 6-10 of gestation. By week 28 of gestation, 90% of pregnant women have hydronephrosis. The incidence appears to be higher in first pregnancies. It usually resolves within 2 months of delivery.

Anatomical causes

As the uterus enlarges, it rises out of the pelvis and rests upon the ureters, compressing them at the level of the pelvic brim. In addition, the ureters become elongation and mildly tortuous, with lateral displacement due to the gravid uterus. The right ureter is generally more dilated than the left, due to extrinsic compression from the overlying congested right uterine vein, and the effect of dextrorotation of the uterus. The left ureter tends to be cushioned from compression by the colon. Ureteric dilatation tends to be from above the pelvic brim.

Physiological causes

Early onset of upper urinary tract dilatation is attributed to increased levels of progesterone, which causes smooth muscle relaxation. This mechanism, coupled with mechanical obstruction, contributes to the reduced peristalsis observed in the collecting system during pregnancy.

Diagnostic dilemmas

The hydronephrosis of pregnancy poses diagnostic difficulties in women presenting with flank pain thought to be due to a renal or ureteric stone. To avoid using ionizing radiation in pregnant women, renal ultrasonography is often used as the initial imaging technique in those presenting with flank pain. In the non-pregnant patient, the presence of hydronephrosis is taken as surrogate evidence of ureteric obstruction. Because hydronephrosis is a normal finding in the majority of pregnancies, its presence *cannot* be taken as a sign of a possible ureteric stone. Ultrasound is an unreliable way of diagnosing the presence of stones in pregnant (and in non-pregnant) women. In a series of pregnant women, ultrasound had a sensitivity of 34% (i.e. it 'misses' 66% of stones) and a specificity of 86% for detecting an abnormality in the presence of a stone (i.e. false +ve rate of 14%).[1] Calculation of resistive index (RI)* (derived from measuring the velocity of intrarenal blood flow using Doppler) may prove a helpful modification. Pregnant women with obstruction secondary to stones have a higher difference in RI between affected and unaffected kidneys than women with non-obstructive hydronephrosis. Colour Doppler and transvaginal USS may also increase the diagnostic accuracy.

---

* Resistive index (RI) = peak systolic velocity (PSV) minus end-diastolic velocity (EDV) divided by peak systolic velocity (PSV) or RI = (PSV − EDV)/PSV

1 Stothers L, Lee LM (1992) Renal colic in pregnancy. *J Urol* **148**:1383–7.

Paediatric urology

Embryology: urinary tract

Following fertilization, a blastocyte (sphere of cells) is created, which implants into the uterine endometrium on day 6. The early embryonic disc of tissue develops a yolk sac and amniotic cavity, from which are derived ectoderm, endoderm, and mesoderm. Organ formation occurs between 3 and 10 weeks gestation. Most of the genito-urinary tract is derived from mesoderm.

Upper urinary tract

The **pronephros** (precursor of the kidney; *pro* = (Gk) before) is derived from an intermediate plate of mesoderm, which functions between weeks 1–4. It then regresses. The **mesonephros** [*meso* = (Gk) middle] functions from weeks 4-8, and is also associated with 2 duct systems-the mesonephric duct and, adjacent to this, the paramesonephric duct (*para* = (Gk) beside) (Fig. 16.1a). The **mesonephric (Wolffian) ducts** develop laterally, and advances downwards to fuse with the cloaca (Latin = sewer), a part of the primitive hindgut. By week 5, ureteric buds grow from the distal part of the mesonephric ducts and induces formation of the *metanephros* [permanent kidney; *meta* = (Gk) after] in the overlying mesoderm. Branching of the ureteric bud forms the renal pelvis, calyces and collecting ducts. Glomeruli and nephrons are created from metanephric mesenchyme. During weeks 6–10, the caudal end of the kidney of the foetus grows rapidly and the foetal kidney effectively moves up the posterior abdominal wall to the lumbar region. Urine production starts at week 10.

Thus, in both males and females, the mesonephric duct forms the ureters and renal collecting system. The paramesonephric duct essentially forms the female genital system (fallopian tubes, uterus, upper vagina); in males, it regresses. The mesonephric ducts also form the male genital duct system (epididymus, vas deferens, seminal vesicles), and central zone of the prostate; in females, it regresses (p. 640).

Lower urinary tract

Bladder

The mesonephric ducts and ureters drain into the cloaca. During weeks 4–6, the cloaca is subdivided into the *urogenital canal or sinus* (anteriorly) and the *anorectal canal* (posteriorly) by a process of growth, differentiation and remodelling[1] (Fig. 16.1b). The bladder is formed by the upper part of the urogenital canal. Bladder smooth muscle (detrusor) is developed from adjacent pelvic mesenchyme. The trigone develops separately, arising from a segment of the mesonephric duct. The bladder dome is initially connected to the allantois, but this later regresses to become a fibrous cord (urachus).

Urethra

The inferior portion of the urogenital canal forms the entire urethra in females, and the posterior urethra in males. Closure of the urogenital groove creates the male anterior urethra. The mesonephric ducts separate from the ureters (Fig. 16.1c), and travel caudally to join the posterior urethra in males (where they differentiate into the male genital duct system at 8–12 weeks).

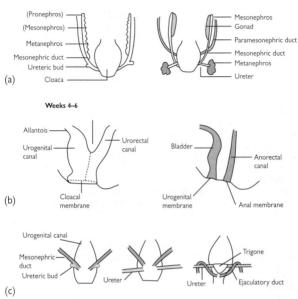

Fig. 16.1 (a) Development of the upper urinary tract (b) Development of the lower urinary tract (bladder) (c) Development of the distal ureters and mesonephric ducts.

1 Penington EC, Hutson JM (2003) The absence of lateral fusion in cloacal partition. *J Paediatr Surg* **38**:1287–95.

Undescended testes (UDT)

The testes descend into the scrotum in the third trimester (passing through the inguinal canal at 24–28 weeks). Failure of testicular descent results in cryptorchidism (or congenital undescended testes/UDT).

Incidence

4% at birth for a full-term neonate (unilateral UDT > bilateral). About 80% will spontaneously descend by 6 months. The incidence at 1 year is 1.3–1.8%.

Classification

- **Retractile:** an intermittent active cremasteric reflex causes the testis to retract up and out of the scrotum
- *Ectopic* **(<5%):** abnormal testis migration below the external ring of the inguinal canal (to perineum, base of penis or femoral areas)
- **Incomplete descent (~ 95%):** testis may be intra-abdominal, intra-inguinal or pre-scrotal
- **Atrophic/absent**
- **Acquired UDT (or testicular ascent):** testes that were down in the scrotum have ascended. Risk higher with retractile testes, and with a patent processus vaginalis. The incidence is 1–2%.[1]

Risk factors

- Pre-term infants (incidence at <30 weeks' gestation is 40%)
- Low birth weight or small for gestational age
- Twins.

Aetiology

- Abnormal testis or gubernaculum (tissue that guides the testis into the scrotum during development)
- Endocrine abnormalities: low level of androgens, human chorionic gonadotrophin (HCG), luteinizing hormone (LH), calcitonin gene-related peptide, Müllerian inhibiting substance (MIS)
- Decreased intra-abdominal pressure (prune-belly syndrome, gastroschisis).

Pathology

UDT demonstrate degeneration of Sertoli cells, loss of Leydig cells, atrophy and abnormal spermatogenesis, which usually starts in 2nd year and is irreversible by 2 years old.

Long-term complications

- Relative risk of cancer is 8-fold higher in UDT. There is a 4% lifelong risk of cancer with an intra-abdominal testis. Majority are seminomas. There is a slightly increased risk of cancer in the contra-lateral, normally descended testis
- Reduced fertility (history of unilateral UDT is associated with 12-18% risk of couple infertility)
- Increased risk of testicular torsion or trauma
- Increased risk of indirect inguinal hernias (due to a patent processus vaginalis).

Evaluation

Full examination to elucidate if testis is palpable, and to identify location. Assess for associated congenital defects. If neither testis is palpable, consider chromosome analysis (to exclude an androgenized female), and endocrine analysis (high LH and FSH with a low testosterone indicates anorchia, confirmed with serum inhibin B). For the impalpable testis, imaging with USS inguinal canal may be considered, but most recommend proceeding directly to examination under anaesthetic ± diagnostic laparoscopy.

Treatment

Orchidopexy is recommended at 6–18 months old (many operate within the first 12 months). Surgery consists of inguinal exploration, mobilization of spermatic cord, ligation of processus vaginalis, and securing the testis into a dartos pouch in the scrotal wall. Risks include testicular atrophy (5%). Intra-abdominal testes require a laparoscopic approach to mobilize the testis for orchidopexy as a single or 2-stage (Fowler–Stephens) procedure, involving division of spermatic vessels to provide extra length (the testis then relying on collateral blood flow from the vas). Alternatives include microvascular autotransplantation. Orchidectomy for small intra-abdominal testes should be considered.

1   Hack WW, Sijstermans K, van Dijk J et al. (2007). Prevalence of acquired undescended testis in 6-year, 9-year and 13-year-old Dutch schoolboys. *Arch Dis Child* **92**:17–20.

2   S. Brewster, D. Cranston, J. Noble, J. Reynard (2001) *Urology a Handbook for Students.* ©2001 BIOS Scientific Publishers Limited.

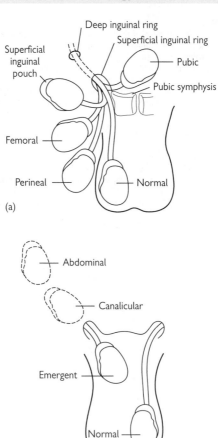

Fig. 16.2 (a) Ectopic sites for the undescended testis (b) Incomplete descent of the testis (cryptorchidism) (Reproduced with permission from Taylor & Francis Books UK).

Urinary tract infection (UTI)

Definitions UTI is a bacterial infection of the urine, which may involve the lower urinary tract/bladder (cystitis) or upper urinary tract/kidney (pyelonephritis) (📖 see p. 166).

Classification Children may be asymptomatic or symptomatic.
Simple UTI presents with mild dehydration and pyrexia.

Severe UTI presents as fever ≥38°C, unwell, vomiting with moderate to severe dehydration.

Atypical UTI includes features of serious illness/septicaemia, poor urinary flow, abnormal renal function, failure to respond to treatment <48 h; and non-*E. coli* infection.

Recurrent UTI in children describes either one episode of cystitis with one episode of pyelonephritis; ≥2 episodes of pyelonephritis or ≥3 episodes of cystitis. It may be due to bacterial persistence, unresolved infection or re-infection.

Incidence Up to age 1, the incidence in boys is higher than girls (male: female ratio is 3:1), but thereafter, the incidence in girls becomes greater (school age: males 1%; females 3%).

Pathology Common bacterial pathogens are *Escherichia coli (E. coli)*, *Enterococcus*, *Pseudomonas*, *Klebsiella*, *Proteus*, and *Staphylococcus epidermis*. Bacteria enter via the urethra to cause cystitis, and ascending infection causes pyelonephritis. Alternatively, there can be haematogenous spread from other systemic infections.

Risk factors

- **Age:** neonates and infants have increased bacterial colonization of the peri-urethral area, and an immature immune system
- **Vesicoureteric reflux (VUR):** 📖 see p. 384
- **Previous UTI**
- **Genitourinary abnormalities:** pelvi- or vesicoureteric obstruction; ureterocele; posterior urethral valves; labial adhesions
- **Voiding dysfunction:** abnormal bladder activity, compliance or emptying
- **Gender:** female>male after 1 year old
- **Foreskin:** uncircumcised boys have a 10-fold higher risk of UTI in the first year due to bacterial colonization of the glans and foreskin
- **Faecal colonization:** contributes to perineal bacterial colonization
- **Chronic constipation**.

Presentation

Neonates and infants: fever, irritability, vomiting, lethargy, diarrhoea, poor feeding.

Children: fever, nausea, suprapubic pain, dysuria, frequency, voiding difficulties, incontinence, flank pain, haematuria.

Investigation

Urine analysis and culture: advised with unexplained fever ≥38°C, or if symptomatic of UTI. Clean catch specimen where possible. In toilet trained children, a mid-stream urine (MSU) specimen is considered diagnostic with ≥10^5 cfu/mL in asymptomatic children, and ≥10^4 cfu/mL if symptomatic. In young children, a catheterized urine specimen with ≥10 colony-forming units per mL (cfu/mL) of one pathogen, or a suprapubic aspirate with ≥10^2 cfu/mL are diagnostic of UTI. Collection bag specimens are less reliable due to skin flora contamination.

Imaging Refer to NICE recommendations[1] (Tables 16.1–3).
- Ultrasound scan (USS) is the first-line investigation. It identifies bladder and kidney abnormalities (hydronephrosis, stones)
- DMSA (dimercaptosuccinic acid) renogram can demonstrate and monitor renal scarring
- Micturating cystourethrogram (MCUG) detects urethral and bladder anomalies (anatomical and functional), VUR, and ureteroceles.

Management

Infants <3months: paediatric referral and treat with intravenous (iv) 3rd generation cephalosporin antibiotic (cefotaxime or ceftriaxone).[2]

Infants and children >3 months with pyelonephritis: paediatric referral; 7–10 days of oral cephalosporin or co-amoxiclav, or iv cefotaxime or cefriaxone for 2–4 days followed by oral antibiotics for a total of 10 days.

Infants and children >3 months with cystitis: oral antibiotics for 3 days (trimethoprim, nitrofurantoin, cephalosporin, or amoxicillin), and re-assess.

Asymptomatic bacteriuria does not require antibiotics. Antibiotic prophylaxis is not recommended following a first-time simple UTI, but can be considered after recurrent UTI.

Follow-up Recurrent UTI or abnormal imaging requires paediatric assessment. Long-term follow-up is needed for bilateral renal anomalies, impaired renal function, hypertension, and/or proteinuria.

1 National Institute for Health and Excellence clinical guideline 54 (August 2007).

2 National Institute for Health and Excellence clinical guideline 47 (May 2007).

Table 16.1 Recommended imaging regimen for infants <6 months[1]

Imaging	Responds well to treatment <48 h	Atypical UTI	Recurrent UTI
USS during UTI	No	Yes	Yes
USS within 6 weeks	Yes	No	No
DMSA 4–6 months following UTI	No	Yes	Yes
MCUG	No	Yes	Yes

Table 16.2 Recommended imaging regimen for infants/children 6 months to 3 years[1]

Imaging	Responds well to treatment <48 h	Atypical UTI	Recurrent UTI
USS during UTI	No	Yes	No
USS within 6 weeks	No	No	Yes
DMSA 4–6 months following UTI	No	Yes	Yes
MCUG	No	No	No*

*MCUG may be considered for hydronephrosis, poor urinary flow, family history of VUR or non-*E. coli* UTI.

Table 16.3 Recommended imaging regimen for children >3 years[1]

Imaging	Responds well to treatment <48 h	Atypical UTI	Recurrent UTI
USS during UTI	No	Yes	No
USS within 6 weeks	No	No	Yes
DMSA 4–6 months following UTI	No	Yes	Yes
MCUG	No	No	No

Vesicoureteric reflux (VUR)

Definition VUR results from abnormal retrograde flow of urine from the bladder into the upper urinary tract.

Epidemiology Overall incidence in children is 1–2%; younger>older; girls>boys (female:male ratio 5:1); Caucasian>Afro-Caribbean. Offspring of an affected parent have up to a 70% incidence of VUR; siblings of an affected child have a 30% risk of reflux. Screening of offspring and siblings is controversial, and many would only recommend it if there is significant renal scarring in the index case.

Pathogenesis The ureter passes obliquely through the bladder wall (1–2 cm), where it is supported by muscular attachments, which prevent urine reflux during bladder filling and voiding. The normal ratio of intramural ureteric length to ureteric diameter is 5:1. Reflux occurs when the intramural length of ureter is too short (ratio < 5:1). The degree of reflux is graded I–V (□ see Fig. 8.3, p. 386). The appearance of the ureteric orifice changes with increasing severity of reflux, classically described as stadium, horseshoe, golf-hole, or patulous.

Classification

- **Primary reflux** (1%) results from a congenital abnormality of the vesicoureteric junction (VUJ). An anatomical cause is seen with duplex kidneys (and ureters): the Weigert–Meyer rule states the lower pole ureter enters the bladder proximally and laterally, resulting in a shorter intramural tunnel which predisposes to reflux (□ see Fig. 8.10, p. 401). A genetic cause is also recognized.
- **Secondary reflux** results from urinary tract dysfunction associated with elevated intravesical pressures creating damage to the VUJ. Causes include: posterior urethral valves (reflux seen in 50%); urethral stenosis; neuropathic bladder; detrusor sphincter dyssynergia. Inflammation associated with infection (acute cystitis) can also distort the VUJ causing reflux.

Complications

VUR (associated with UTI) can result in reflux nephropathy and renal scarring, causing hypertension (10–20%) and progressive renal failure (<0.1%).

Presentation

Symptoms of UTI (fever, dysuria, suprapubic, or abdominal pain), failure to thrive, vomiting, diarrhoea.

Investigation

- Urine analysis and culture to diagnose UTI
- Urinary tract USS
- DMSA renogram to detect and monitor associated renal cortical scarring
- Cystography (selected by age and sex of patient) to diagnose and grade reflux, and establish reversible causes (□ see Fig. 16.3)
- Urodynamics if suspicious of voiding dysfunction.

Management Correct problems contributing to secondary reflux. The majority of primary VUR grade I–II will resolve spontaneously (80%),[1] with 50% resolution in grade III–V.[2] A period of observation with medical treatment is therefore initially recommended. General advice includes good fluid intake, regular voiding, perineal hygiene, treatment of constipation, and use of pro-biotics.

Medical treatment Low dose antibiotic prophylaxis should be given to keep the urine sterile and lower the risk of renal damage until reflux resolves (grades III–V). Anticholinergic drugs are given to treat bladder overactivity.

Surgery

Indicated in limited cases only (NICE do not recommend routine correction of VUR). Techniques include *laparoscopic* repair and *open ureteric re-implantation* (98% success).

- **Intravesical** methods involve mobilizing the ureter, and advancing it across the trigone (Cohen repair) or reinsertion into a higher, medial position in the bladder (Politano–Leadbetter repair)
- **Extravesical** techniques involve attaching the ureter into the bladder base, and suturing muscle around it (Lich–Gregoir procedure)
- **Endoscopic injection** Deflux® is a hyaluronic acid/dextranomer bulking agent which is injected intramurally within the distal ureter, and also at the ureteric orifice ('HIT' technique), with 80–90% success rates*. It has replaced the traditional subtrigonal injection ('STING') of bulking agent (collagen) into the ureteric orifice.

---

* FDA approval for VUR.

1 Arant BS Jr. (1992) Medical management of mild and moderate vesicoureteric reflux: follow-up studies of infants and young children. A preliminary report of the Southwest Pediatric Nephrology Study Group. *J Urol* **148**:1683–7.

2 Smellie JM, Jodal U, Lax H, et al. (2001) Outcome at 10 years of severe vesicoureteric reflux managed medically: report of the International Reflux Study in Children. *J Pediatr* **139**:656–63.

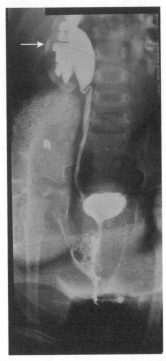

Fig. 16.3 Micturating cysto-urethrogram demonstrating grade III VUR and intrarenal reflux (shown by arrow) in a child. Image kindly provided with permission from Professor S. Reif.

Ectopic ureter

Definition The ureteric orifice is situated either below and medial, or above and lateral to the normal anatomical insertion on the trigone of the bladder.

Incidence ~1 in 1900. Female to male ratio is $\geq$ 3:1.

Pathogenesis

The ureteric bud arises from an abnormal (high or low) position on the mesonephric duct during embryological development. There is a direct correlation between the location of the ectopic ureter and the degree of ipsilateral renal hypoplasia or dysplasia.[1] 80% are associated with a duplicated collecting system (which predominantly affects females). A duplex kidney has an upper pole and a lower pole moiety, each with its own renal pelvis and ureter. The two ureters may join to form a single ureter, or they may pass down individually to the bladder (complete duplication). In this case, the upper pole ureter always opens onto the bladder below and medial to the lower pole ureter (*Weigert-Meyer rule*), predisposing to ectopic placement of the ureteric orifice (📖 see Fig. 8.10, p. 401).

Sites of ectopic ureters
- *Females:* lateral in the bladder, bladder neck, urethra, vagina, vaginal vestibule, uterus
- *Males:* lateral in the bladder, posterior urethra, seminal vesicles, ejaculatory duct, vas deferens, epididymis, bladder neck.

Presentation Most now present with an antenatal diagnosis of hydronephrosis. Later presentations include acute or recurrent UTI, which is common in both sexes. Obstruction of the ectopic ureter can lead to hydronephrosis and hydro-ureter, which may present as an abdominal mass.
- **Females:** when the ureteric opening is below the urethral sphincter, girls present with persistent vaginal discharge, or incontinence, despite successful toilet training
- **Males:** the ureter is always sited above the external urethral sphincter, so boys do not develop incontinence. UTIs may trigger epididymitis (usually recurrent).

Investigation of the urinary tract
- **USS** may demonstrate (unilateral) ureteric dilatation and hydronephrosis (often diagnosed on antenatal scan)
- **Magnetic resonance urogram (MRU)** identifies duplex systems, and gives information on renal upper and lower pole moieties
- **Micturating cystourethrography (MCUG)** assesses reflux in lower pole ureters
- **Cystourethroscopy** can directly identify a ureteric opening in the urethra
- **^{99m}Tc-DMSA renogram** assesses renal function to help plan surgery.

Treatment is mainly expectant if there are no symptoms. Where an ectopic ureter is associated with a poorly functioning renal upper pole or single-system kidney, surgery is an option. This includes open or laparoscopic upper pole nephrectomy or total nephrectomy with excision of the associated ureter. Ureteropyelostomy and uretero-ureterostomy can be considered in duplex systems where the upper renal pole has reasonable function. Where some function is retained in a single-system kidney, the distal ureter can be resected and re-implanted into the bladder.

1   Mackie GG, Stephens FD (1975) Duplex kidneys: a correlation of renal dysplasia with position of the ureteric orifice. *J Urol* **114**: 274–80.

Ureterocele

Definition A ureterocele is a cystic dilatation of the distal ureter as it drains into the bladder.

Incidence 1 in 5000–12,000 clinical paediatric admissions[1] (although 1 in 500 are found at autopsy[2]). Female to male ratio is 4:1, predominantly affecting Caucasians. 80% are associated with the upper pole of a duplex system. Single-system ureteroceles are more commonly found in males and adults. 10% are bilateral.

Classification

Intravesical or orthotopic (20%): ureterocele is completely confined within the bladder. Subtypes include:
- **Stenotic:** narrow (stenotic) orifice
- **Non-obstructed:** only visible when filled by peristalsis.

Ectopic (80%): if any part of the ureterocele extends to the bladder neck or urethra. Subtypes include:
- **Sphincteric:** wide orifice, found proximal to the bladder neck (within the internal sphincter)
- **Sphincterostenotic:** stenotic orifice, found proximal to the bladder neck
- **Ceco-ureterocele:** ectopic ureterocele that extends into the urethra, but the orifice is within the bladder.

Presentation Most present with antenatal hydronephrosis. Later presentation in infants may be with symptoms of UTI. Association with ureteric duplication increases the risk of reflux and reflux nephropathy. Ureteroceles can also cause obstruction and hydronephrosis, which may be identified on antenatal USS, or present in children with an abdominal mass or pain. A prolapsing ureterocele can present as a vaginal mass in girls.

Investigation
- **USS** shows a thin walled cyst in the bladder often associated with a duplex system
- **Micturating cystourethrogram** can identify ureterocele location, size and associated vesicoureteric reflux (reflux in the lower pole is seen in 50%)
- **Cystoscopy** may reveal a defect near the trigone
- **99mTc-DMSA** renogram assesses renal segment function.

Treatment
- **Endoscopic incision/puncture:** emergency treatment for infected or obstructed ureteroceles. Also indicated for elective management of intravesical ureteroceles. Rarely, these may require further surgery, including ureterocele excision and ureteric re-implantation to preserve renal function and prevent reflux

- **Uretero-ureterostomy or uretero-pyelostomy (from upper to lower pole moiety):** option for ectopic ureteroceles associated with a duplex system, with good function in the upper moiety, and no reflux in the lower moiety
- **Upper pole partial nephrectomy:** option for ectopic ureterocele associated with a duplex system with poor function in the upper moiety, and no reflux in the lower moiety
- **Upper pole partial nephrectomy, ureterocele excision and ureteric re-implantation:** option for ectopic ureterocele associated with a duplex system with poor function in the upper moiety, and reflux in the lower moiety
- **Nephro-ureterectomy:** indicated for significant lower pole reflux with poor function in both renal poles.

1   Malek RS, Kelalis PP, Burke EC, *et al.* (1972) Simple and ectopic ureterocele in infants and child-hood. *Surg Gynaecol Obst* **134**: 611–16.

2   Uson AC, Lattimer JK, Melicow MM (1961) Ureteroceles in infants and children: a report based on 44 cases. *Pediatrics* **27**: 971–7.

Pelviureteric junction (PUJ)* obstruction

Definition A blockage of the ureter at the junction with the renal pelvis resulting in a restriction of urine flow.

Epidemiology Childhood incidence is estimated at 1 in 1000. Boys are affected more than girls (ratio 2:1 in newborns). The left side is more often affected than the right side (ratio 2:1). They are bilateral in 10–40%.

Aetiology

In children, most PUJ obstruction is congenital, due to either an *intrinsic* narrowing (secondary to aberrant development of ureteric/renal pelvis muscle, abnormal collagen, or ureteral polyps) or *extrinsic* causes (compression of the PUJ by aberrant vessels). Co-existing vesicoureteric reflux (VUR) is found in up to 25%.

Presentation

PUJ obstruction is the most common cause of hydronephrosis found on pre-natal and early postnatal USS (differential diagnoses include 'baggy systems', VUJ obstruction, VUR, renal abnormalities, and posterior urethral valves). Infants may also present with an abdominal mass, UTI, and haematuria. Older children present with flank or abdominal pain (exacerbated by diuresis), UTI, nausea and vomiting, and haematuria following minor trauma.

Investigation

If prenatal USS has shown a large or bilateral hydronephrosis, a follow-up renal tract USS should be performed soon after birth. If there is a prenatal unilateral hydronephrosis (and the bladder is normal), the scan is deferred until day 3–7 (to allow normal physiological diuresis to occur, which may spontaneously improve or resolve the hydronephrosis).

Treatment

Conservative: Children may be observed with USS and renogram if they remain stable, with good renal function and no other complications (such as persistent infection, or stones).

Surgery: pyeloplasty is indicated if children are symptomatic, have a significant hydronephrosis (>30 mm AP renal pelvis diameter) or impaired renal function (<40%), or the obstruction has failed to resolve despite prolonged follow-up. Techniques include the Anderson–Hynes dismembered open pyeloplasty and the laparoscopic (retroperitoneal or transperitoneal approach) dismembered pyeloplasty. Post-operative follow-up is with USS (± MAG3 renogram). Where renal function is poor (<10–15%) on the side of the PUJ obstruction, options include temporary percutaneous drainage to assess the potential for recovery (i.e. suggesting a pyeloplasty could improve function), or nephrectomy where the impairment is severe or irreversible.

* PUJ also referred to as ureteropelvic junction (UPJ).

Hypospadias

Definition

Hypospadias is a congenital deformity where the opening of the urethra (the meatus) is sited on the underside (ventral) part of the penis, anywhere from the glans to the perineum. It is often associated with a 'hooded' foreskin (prepuce) and chordee (ventral curvature of the penile shaft). It occurs in 1 in 250 live male births. There is an 8% incidence in off-spring of an affected male, and a 14% risk in male siblings.

Classification

Hypospadias can be classified according to the anatomical location of the urethral meatus (see Fig. 16.4).

- **Anterior** (or distal): glandular, coronal and subcoronal (~50%)
- **Middle** distal penile, midshaft and proximal penile (~30%)
- **Posterior** (or proximal): penoscrotal, scrotal and perineal (~20%).

Aetiology

Hypospadias results from incomplete closure of urethral folds on the under-surface of the penis during embryological development. This is related to a defect in production or metabolism of foetal androgens, or the number and sensitivity of androgen receptors in the tissues. Chordee is caused by abnormal urethral plate development or an intrinsic abnormality of the corpora cavernosa, and the 'hooded' foreskin is due to failed fusion of the preputial folds (resulting in a lack of ventral foreskin).

Associated anomalies

- Undescended testes
- Inguinal hernia ± hydrocele
- Disorders of sexual development (i.e. mixed gonadal dysgenesis)
- Persistence of Müllerian structures (i.e. dilated utricle).

Diagnosis

A full clinical examination to establish the diagnosis, assess the penis and urethral plate, and detect associated abnormalities needing treatment. Patients with unilateral or bilateral absent testes and hypospadias should undergo chromosomal and endocrine investigation to exclude disorders of sex development. Posterior hypospadias can be associated with other urinary tract malformations and requires USS investigation.

Treatment

Surgery is indicated where deformity is severe, interferes with voiding or is predicted to interfere with sexual function. Repair is performed between 6–18 months of age. Local application of testosterone for 1 month pre-operatively can help increase tissue size. Surgery aims to correct penile curvature (orthoplasty), reconstruct a new urethra, and bring the new meatus to the tip of the glans using urethroplasty, glanuloplasty, and meatoplasty techniques. Some proximal defects may require a 2-stage procedure.

Distal hypospadias repairs

- Meatal advancement and glanuloplasty (MAGPI)
- Tubularization incised (urethral) plate (TIP) urethroplasty or Snodgrass procedure
- Meatal-based flaps (Mathieu procedure).

Middle hypospadias repairs

- Onlay island flap (OIF) using a preputial graft
- TIP urethroplasty
- Meatal-based flaps.

Proximal hypospadias repairs

- Transverse preputial island flap (TPIF)
- OIF repair
- Free graft (i.e. inner preputial skin used to form a neourethra as part of a 2-stage operation).

Complications

Bleeding, infection, urethral strictures, meatal stenosis, urinary dysfunction urethrocutaneous fistula, urethral diverticulum, recurrent chordee, sexual dysfunction, and failed procedures requiring re-operation.

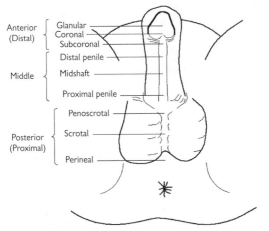

Fig. 16.4 The anatomical classification of hypospadias according to the location of the urethral meatus. (Adapted from Walsh et al. 2002)[1]

1 Walsh PC, Retik AB, Vaughan ED Jr, Wein AJ (eds) (2002) *Campbell's Urology*, 8th edn. Philadelphia: W.B. Saunders/Elsevier, p. 2287.

Normal sexual differentiation

Sexual differentiation and gonadal development is determined by the sex chromosomes (XY male, XX female). The gonads produce hormones, which influence the subsequent differentiation of internal and external genitalia.

Both sexes

Gonads develop from the **genital ridges** (formed by cells of the mesonephros and coelomic epithelium). At 5–6 weeks, primordial germ cells migrate from the yolk sac to populate the genital ridges. Primitive sex cords are formed, which support germ cell (sperm and ova) development.

From 4 weeks, the **mesonephric (Wolffian)** ducts are incorporated into the genital system, when renal function is taken over by the definitive kidney. At 6 weeks, coelomic epithelium creates the **paramesonephric (Müllerian) ducts**, which develop laterally and are fused to the urogenital sinus at their bases.

Males

The **testis-determining gene (SRY)** is located on the Y chromosome, and stimulates medullary sex cords in the primitive testis to differentiate into Sertoli cells, which produce **Müllerian inhibiting substance (MIS)** at 7–8 weeks. The sex cords also differentiate into seminiferous cords, which later form the seminiferous tubules of the testis, within which the primordial germ cells differentiate into spermatogonia. MIS also triggers regression of the paramesonephric ducts; testosterone secretion from Leydig cells of the testis, and the initial phase of testicular (abdominal) descent.

During weeks 8–12, mesonephric ducts differentiate into epididymis, vas deferens, seminal vesicles and ejaculatory ducts. The prostate capsule is formed from mesenchyme, while parenchyma (glandular acini and ducts) is derived from urethral endoderm. After week 23, the second androgen dependant phase of testicular descent occurs. The testes rapidly descend from the abdomen (via the inguinal canal during weeks 24–28), and into the scrotal sac, aided by calcitonin-related polypeptide acting on the gubernaculum. The testis is enclosed in a diverticulum of peritoneum called the processus vaginalis. The distal part persists as the tunica vaginalis around the testis, the remainder usually regresses.

Testosterone and di-hydrotestosterone (DHT) androgens are responsible for masculinization. DHT is made from testosterone by 5α-reductase enzyme in the tissues. *External genitalia* develop from week 7. Urogenital folds form around the opening of the urogenital sinus, and labioscrotal swellings develop either side. The penile shaft and glans are formed by elongation of the genital tubercle, and fusion of urogenital folds. The scrotum is created by fusion of labioscrotal folds.

Females

The genital ridge forms secondary sex cords (primitive sex cords degenerate), which surround the germ cells to create ovarian follicles (week 15). These undergo meiotic division to become primary oocytes, which are later activated to complete gametogenesis at puberty. Oestrogen is produced from week 8 under the influence of the aromatase enzyme. In the absence of MIS, the mesonephric ducts regress, and the paramesonephric ducts become the fallopian tubes, uterus and upper two-thirds of the vagina. The sinovaginal sinus is developed at the junction of the paramesonephric ducts and the urogenital sinus. This forms the lower third of the vagina.

The genital tubercle forms the clitoris; the urogenital folds become the labia minora and the labioscrotal swellings form the labia majora.

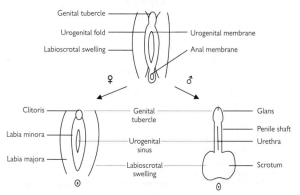

Fig. 16.5 Differentiation of external genitalia (weeks 7–16).

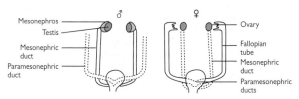

Fig. 16.6 Differentiation of the genital tract.

Abnormal sexual differentiation

Disorders of sex development (DSD) are defined as congenital conditions in which the development of chromosomal, gonadal, or anatomical sex is atypical. They are estimated to affect 1 in 4500 births, and have recently undergone changes in recommended nomenclature (Table 16.4).[1]

DSD can be divided into:

- **Sex chromosome DSD** (disorders of gonadal differentiation): these include conditions with seminiferous tubule dysgenesis (Klinefelter's syndrome 47XXY and 46XX testicular DSD); Turner's syndrome (45XO), ovotesticular DSD (46XX/46XY, 46XX, or 46XY with both ovarian and testicular tissue, and ambiguous genitalia); mixed gonadal dysgenesis 45XO/46XY mosaicism (streak gonads and a spectrum of ambiguous genitalia), and 46XX (pure) gonadal dysgenesis (females with streak gonads).
- **46XY DSD** (previously male pseudohermaphroditism): 46XY karyotype with defects of testosterone production (3β-hydroxysteroid dehydrogenase or 17α-hydroxylase enzyme deficiencies; testicular dysgenesis; Leydig cell aplasia), defects of testosterone metabolism (5α-reductase deficiency) or androgen resistance (androgen insensitivity syndrome), resulting in varying degrees of feminization. Also included are disorders of müllerian inhibiting substance (MIS) or MIS receptor defects resulting in persistent müllerian duct syndrome (male phenotype with uterus, fallopian tubes, and upper vagina).
- **46XX DSD** (previously female pseudohermaphroditism): 46XX karyotype with ovaries and internal genitalia, but a partially masculinized phenotype and ambiguous external genitalia due to intrauterine exposure to androgens. The most common type is *congenital adrenal hyperplasia (CAH)*, due to 21-hydroxylase deficiency (in 95%), an autosomal recessive disorder. Formation of hydrocortisone is impaired, resulting in a compensatory increase in adrenocorticotrophin hormone (ACTH) and testosterone production. Some forms have a 'salt wasting' aldosterone deficiency which can present in the first few weeks of life with adrenal crisis (severe vomiting and dehydration), requiring rehydration and steroid replacement therapy. Rarer causes of CAH are 11β-hydroxylase deficiency and 3β-hydroxysteroid dehydrogenase deficiency. Other causes include maternal exposure to androgens. Disorders of ovarian development (i.e. 46XX gonadal dysgenesis, 46XX testicular DSD) can also be included in this category.

Evaluation

- A detailed **history** may uncover a positive family history of DSD. Maternal ingestion of drugs such as steroids or contraceptives during pregnancy should be ascertained

- General **examination** may show associated syndrome anomalies (Klinefelter's and Turner's syndromes), or failure to thrive and dehydration (salt-wasting CAH). Assess external genitalia for phallus size and location of urethral meatus. Careful palpation may confirm the presence of testes, which excludes a diagnosis of 46 XX DSD. Patients with bilateral undescended testes, or unilateral undescended testis with hypospadias should be also suspected of having a DSD
- **Abdominal/pelvic USS** can help locate the gonads, or occasionally laparoscopy with gonadal biopsy is required for diagnosis
- **Chromosomal analysis** confirms karyotype
- **Serum tests:** serum electrolytes, testosterone and DHT analysis test for salt-wasting CAH. Serum 17-hydroxyprogesterone performed after day 3 can also diagnose 21-hydroxylase deficiency. HCG stimulation test can diagnose androgen resistance and 5α-reductase deficiency.

Management

A multidisciplinary approach is required with full parental input. Gender assignment of ambiguous genitalia is guided by the functional potential of gonadal tissue, reproductive tracts, and genitalia, with the aim of optimizing psychosocial well-being and producing a stable gender identity. Patients have a higher risk of gonadal malignancy, which requires surveillance and/or removal of gonadal tissues and hormone replacement. Patients with hypogonadism will require hormone replacement and artificial induction of puberty.

Table 16.4 Proposed revised nomenclature[1]

Previous terminology	Proposed new terminology (2007)
Intersex	Disorders of sex development (DSD)
Male pseudohermaphrodite	46,XY DSD
Female pseudohermaphrodite	46,XX DSD
True hermaphrodite	Ovotesticular DSD
Testicular feminization	Androgen insensitivity syndrome, complete (CAIS)
46XX male	46XX testicular DSD

1 Hughes IA, Houk C, Ahmed SF, et al. (2007). Consensus statement on management of intersex disorders. *Arch Dis Child* 554–63.

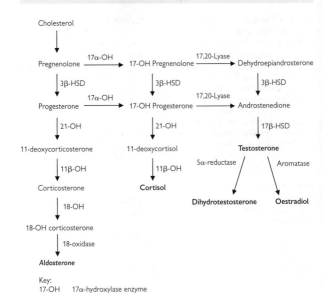

Fig. 16.7 Metabolic pathways for adrenal steroid synthesis.

Table 16.5 Disorders of sex development

Disorder	Karyotype	Gonad	Genitalia	Other features	Treatment
Disorder of gonadal differentiation					
Klinefelter's syndrome	47 XXY	Seminiferous tubule dysgenesis, small testes	Male	Tall, gynaecomastia, azoospermia, mild mental retardation, ↑FSH/LH, ↓ testosterone	Androgen replacement
46XX testicular DSD	46XX (SRY +ve)	Seminiferous tubule dysgenesis	Male	Shorter stature, gynaecomastia, infertile, hypospadias, ↑ FSH/LH, ↓ testosterone	Androgen replacement
Turner's syndrome	45XO	Streak ovaries	Female	Short stature, sexual infantilism, web neck, widespread nipples, wide carrying angle, coarctation, renal anomalies	Growth hormone; oestrogen replacement at puberty
Ovotesticular DSD	46XX, XY, 46XX/46XY	Ovary and testis	Ambiguous or male	Hypospadias (80%) in 'males.' Clitoromegaly in 'females'	Gender assignment surgery
Mixed gonadal dysgenesis	45XO/46XY	Unilateral undescended testis and streak gonad	Ambiguous	Wide phenotypic spectrum from Turner's syndrome-like female to male.	Gender assignment, gonadectomy (as ↑ cancer risk), screen for Wilms' tumour
46XX 'pure' gonadal dysgenesis	46XX	Streak ovaries	Female	Normal stature, sexual infantilism, 1° amenorrhoea	Cyclic hormone replacement
46XY DSD					
3β-hydroxysteroid dehydrogenase deficiency	46XY	Testes	Ambiguous	Salt wasting, ↓ cortisol, ↓ aldosterone	Glucocorticoid and mineralocorticoid replacement
17α-hydroxylase deficiency	46XY	Testes	Ambiguous	↓ cortisol (causing ↑ ACTH), resulting in ↓ steroids, hypokalaemia, hypertension	Glucocorticoid replacement

	Karyotype	Gonads	Phenotype	Clinical features	Management
Complete androgen insensitivity syndrome	46XY	Testes	Female	Androgen resistance, female phenotype, short blind-ending vagina, breasts at puberty	Gonadectomy after puberty, oestrogen replacement therapy
Incomplete androgen insensitivity syndrome	46XY	Testes	Ambiguous	Wide spectrum including hypospadias, infertility, gynaecomastia, pseudovagina	Gender assignment surgery +/ gonadectomy and hormone replacement.
5α-reductase deficiency	46XY	Testes	Ambiguous	Failure to convert testosterone to DHT in androgen sensitive cells, hypospadias, small phallus, short vagina, virilization at puberty	Reconstructive surgery +/- hormonal support
46XX DSD					
Congenital adrenal hyperplasia	46XX	Ovaries	Ambiguous	Simple virilization, or salt wasting aldosterone deficiency	Glucocorticoid, mineralocorticoid replacement and surgery.
Transplacental androgens	46XX	Ovaries	Ambiguous	Virilization by maternal drug use in pregnancy or maternal adrenal tumours	External genitalia reconstruction as required

Cystic kidney disease

Congenital cystic kidney disease can be is classified into genetic and non-genetic types.

Genetic

Autosomal recessive polycystic kidney disease (ARPKD)

A disease of infancy and childhood, where renal collecting tubules and ducts become cystically dilated, and numerous small cysts form in the renal cortex and medulla bilaterally. Incidence of 1 in 10,000–40,000. Severe forms present early and have a poor prognosis. Prenatal USS demonstrates oligohydramnios (amniotic fluid <200 mL), and large, 'bright' homogeneously hyperechogenic kidneys, which can cause obstructed labour and respiratory problems (secondary to pulmonary hypoplasia). Neonates have large flank masses, limb and facial anomalies. All cases are associated with congenital hepatic fibrosis. Infants may develop fatal uraemia and respiratory failure; older children present with renal failure, hypertension and portal hypertension. Most develop end-stage renal failure by adulthood requiring haemodialysis, nephrectomy (to control hypertension) and subsequent renal transplantation.

Autosomal dominant polycystic kidney disease (ADPKD)

(📖 see p. 380)

Typically presents in adulthood, although older children can present with complications of haematuria, flank pain, flank mass, UTI, proteinuria, hypertension, and intracerebral bleeds (secondary to berry aneurysm rupture). ADPKD is the most commonly inherited renal disease with an incidence of ~1 in 1000. It is characterized by multiple expanding cysts of both kidneys that ultimately destroys the intervening parenchyma, and accounts for 10% of all chronic renal failure. 90% of cases are due to a defective PKD1 gene located on chromosome 16; the remainder are due to a defective PKD2 gene on chromosome 4.

Familial juvenile nephronophthisis

An autosomal recessive disorder which develops in early childhood and accounts for up to 20% of paediatric renal failure. **Medullary cystic disease** is a similar (autosomal dominant) condition, which develops in later childhood. Histology in both conditions shows interstitial nephritis associated with corticomedullary cysts. Disease progression causes a reduction in kidney size. Features include polyuria and polydipsia (due to a salt-losing nephropathy), anaemia, growth retardation, hypertension, and chronic renal failure. Initial treatment includes salt replacement. Dialysis and renal transplantation are later options.

Others

Renal cysts are also a feature of autosomal dominant conditions including **Von-Hippel-Lindau syndrome** (cerebellar and retinal haemangioblastomas, phaeochromocytoma, pancreatic cysts, renal cell carcinoma/RCC) and **tuberous sclerosis** (adenoma sebaceum, epilepsy, learning difficulties associated with renal angiomyolipoma and RCC).

Non-genetic

Multicystic dysplastic kidney (MCDK)

The cysts of a 'multicystic' kidney are not due to dilatation of renal collecting ducts (as in polycystic disease), but instead, the entire kidney is dysplastic, with immature dysplastic stroma and cysts of various sizes. Bilateral disease is incompatible with life. The incidence of unilateral MCKD is 1 in 4000. Disease is usually detected on pre- or post-natal USS; neonates may present with an abdominal mass. Unilateral disease is often associated with vesicoureteric reflux or PUJ obstruction in the contralateral kidney. Affected kidneys may undergo renal aplasia, where they spontaneously shrink to a tiny remnant. USS and renogram (DMSA) help to distinguish this condition from hydronephrosis. Most can be treated conservatively with close surveillance and USS follow-up for the associated risks of hypertension and Wilms' tumour (both of which are very rare) which would be indications for nephrectomy.

Multilocular cystic nephroma

Presents in young children with a flank mass, loin pain, or haematuria. Diagnosis is on USS or CT, demonstrating multilocular cysts in the renal parenchyma, which may extend into the collecting system. It is included in a spectrum of disease that is closely associated with Wilms' tumour, and so the recommended treatment is partial or full nephrectomy.

Exstrophy

Exstrophy-epispadias complex describes a spectrum of congenital malformations affecting the abdominal wall, pelvis, genitourinary tract, and sometimes also the spine and anus. It includes bladder exstrophy, epispadias, and cloacal exstrophy.

Bladder exstrophy, the most common form, results from defective development of the anterior bladder and lower abdominal walls, resulting in the posterior bladder wall lying exposed on the abdomen. Virtually all cases are associated with epispadias (📖 see p. 652).

Epidemiology Incidence is ~1 in 50,000 live births. Male to female ratio is 5/6:1. Increased risk in offspring of affected patients, and with younger maternal age and increased parity.

Embryology Classically described as an embryological malformation causing abnormal over-development of the cloacal membrane, which prevents in-growth of lower abdominal (mesenchymal) tissues. The cloacal membrane normally perforates to form the urogenital and anal openings, but in exstrophy, premature rupture results in a triangular defect below the umbilicus. The timing of rupture determines the type of resulting defect (bladder exstrophy, cloacal exstrophy, or epispadias). Other theories challenge this and suggest abnormal development of the bony pelvis, or maldevelopment of the genital hillocks below their normal position, with midline fusion below, rather than above the cloacal membrane (resulting in premature cloacal rupture prior to mesenchymal in-growth).

Associated anomalies

- **Bone defects:** diastasis (widening) of the symphysis pubis due to outward rotation of the pelvic bones along the sacroiliac joints
- **Musculofascial defects:** umbilical hernias, inguinal hernias, divarication of rectus abdominis, abnormal pelvic floor, low lying umbilicus
- **Genital defects:** *Males:* short, broad penis with lateral splaying of the corporal cavernosa, short urethral plate, epispadias, deficiency of dorsal foreskin. *Females:* bifid clitoris, stenotic vaginal orifice, short anteriorly placed vaginal canal, uterine prolapse in adult life
- **Urinary tract defects:** exposed bladder plate; majority suffer vescioureteric reflux (VUR) due to lateral displacement of the ureteric orifices
- **GIT defects:** anteriorly displaced anus, rectal prolapse, abnormal anal sphincter contributes to incontinence.

Investigation

Typical features seen on prenatal USS include a lower abdominal wall mass; absent bladder filling; low-set umbilicus; small genitalia; abnormal iliac crest widening. Diagnosis can help planning of delivery in a centre with facilities to perform early surgical correction.

Management

At birth, cover the bladder with plastic film, and irrigate regularly with sterile saline. Trauma to the bladder mucosa can result in squamous metaplasia, cystitis cystica or adenocarcinoma, and squamous cell carcinoma after chronic exposure.

Surgery aims to provide a continent reservoir for urine storage, preserve renal function, and create functional and cosmetically acceptable external genitalia. Selected cases are suitable for a one-stage complete primary repair of bladder exstrophy (CPRE) involving closure of the bladder plate and epispadias repair. However, many require staged procedures:

- **Newborn:** pelvic osteotomy (cutting bone to correct deformity) with external fixation, and closure of bladder, abdominal wall and posterior urethra
- **6–18 months:** epispadias repair (see p. 652)
- **4–5 years:** bladder neck reconstruction (Young–Dees–Leadbetter procedure) and anti-reflux surgery (ureteric re-implantation) is performed when there is adequate bladder capacity and children can participate in voiding protocols. Where bladder capacity is too small, bladder augmentation or urinary diversion is required.

Surgical complications increased risk of malignancy in urinary or orthotopic bladder; fistula; hypospadias; bladder stones; infection (UTI, epididymitis); incontinence.

Primary epispadias

In epispadias, the urethra opens onto the dorsal surface of the penis, anywhere from the glans, penile shaft, or most commonly, the penopubic region. An incomplete urethral sphincter mechanism results in a high risk of incontinence. Epispadias is also associated with dorsal chordee (causing an upward curvature of the penis), and with incomplete foreskin dorsally. Epispadias is part of the exstrophy-epispadias complex (📖 see p. 650). Primary epispadias (without exstrophy) is rare.

Associated anomalies

Diastasis of the symphysis pubis results in splaying of the corpora cavernosa and shortening of the penile shaft. Females have a bifid clitoris, poorly developed labia, and demonstrate a spectrum of urethral deformities ranging from a patulous urethral orifice to a urethral cleft affecting the entire length of the urethra and sphincter. There is a 40% risk of vesicoureteric reflux (VUR).

Incidence Affects 1 in 117,000 males. Rarely seen in females (male:female ratio is 5:1).

Management

Males: urethroplasty with functional and cosmetic reconstruction of the external genitalia (penile lengthening and correction of chordee) at 6–18 months. The modified Cantwell–Ransley technique is commonly used in males. It describes mobilizing the urethra to the ventral aspect of the penis, with advancement of the urethral meatus onto the glans with a reverse MAGPI (meatal advancement-glanduloplasty). The corporal bodies are separated and rotated medially above the urethra and re-approximated. From age 4–5 years, when children can be toilet trained, bladder neck reconstruction can be performed (Youngs–Dees–Leadbetter procedure). This achieves continence, and any bladder residuals may then be emptied by urethral catheterization. If this surgery fails, insertion of artificial urinary sphincters or injection of peri-urethral bulking agents may be tried.

Females: Surgery involves urethral repair reinforced with pubic fat, along with clitoral reconstruction ± bladder neck repair.

Cloacal exstrophy

This is the most severe form of exstrophy-epispadias complex. Characterized by an exomphalos (midline abdominal defect with bowel covered in a thin sac of amnion and peritoneum), below which are two halves of an exstrophied bladder separated by an exstrophied bowel segment. It is associated with a bifid or micro-penis, and absence of one or both testes. The incidence is 1 in 300,000; male:female ratio is 6:1. There is a high risk of associated congenital anomalies. Surgical reconstruction may require terminal colostomy, pelvic osteotomy, anterior bladder reconstruction ± augmentation cystoplasty. Gender assignment may need to be considered in males.

Posterior urethral valves (PUV)

PUV are derived from an abnormal congenital membrane arising from the verumontanum and attaching obliquely to the anterior urethra (beyond the external urethral sphincter), resulting in lower urinary tract obstruction. An alternative term is COPUM or congenital obstructive post-urethral membrane. Urethral instrumentation or spontaneous partial rupture of the membrane is thought to cause the classical appearance of two valve-like folds in the prostatic urethra.

Incidence 1 in >5000 males

Pathology PUV arise through an abnormal insertion of the Wolffian ducts into the urogenital sinus during foetal development.

Presentation

Prenatal USS: the majority are diagnosed prenatally, with 60% identified on USS at 20 weeks. Features include: bilateral hydro-ureteronephrosis; dilated bladder and posterior urethra (keyhole sign); thick walled bladder; oligohydramnios (reduced amniotic fluid) and renal dysplasia. Early diagnosis is associated with poor prognosis.

Newborn and infants: respiratory distress (secondary to pulmonary hypoplasia); palpable abdominal mass (hydronephrotic kidneys or distended bladder); ascites; UTI sepsis; electrolyte abnormalities (renal impairment); failure to thrive.

Older children: milder cases may present later with recurrent UTI; poor urinary stream; incomplete bladder emptying; poor growth and incontinence. There is a risk of renal failure, vesicoureteric reflux, and voiding dysfunction (over- or under-active bladder), also described as 'valve bladder syndrome'.

Associated features: 'Pop-off valve syndrome' is seen in 20%. It describes mechanisms by which high urinary tract pressure is dissipated to allow normal renal development. It includes leaking of urine from a small bladder or renal pelvis rupture (urinary ascites), unilateral reflux into a non-functioning kidney (vesicoureteral reflux with renal dysplasia or VURD), and formation of bladder diverticuli.

Investigation

- **Bloods** to assess renal function
- **USS renal tract:** postnatal USS may show thickened bladder wall, bilateral hydronephrosis and dilated posterior urethra
- **Micturating cystourethrogram:** features of PUV include a distended posterior urethra (shield-shaped); partially filled anterior urethra; bladder neck hypertrophy; lucencies representing valve leaflets; thick walled bladder (±diverticuli); incomplete bladder emptying; vesicoureteric reflux (50%)
- **Renogram** (MAG3, DMSA): assesses renal function
- **Video-urodynamcis:** allows diagnosis of associated voiding dysfunction.

Management

Commence prophylactic antibiotics immediately, check serum electrolytes, and drain the bladder with a paediatric feeding tube. Stabilize and if necessary resuscitate patient. If there is improvement, cystoscopy and transurethral ablation of valve (cuts at 5 and 7 o'clock with either cold knife or electrocautery) is recommended (complications include urethral strictures). A temporary cutaneous vesicostomy is indicated (communicating stoma between the bladder dome and suprapubic abdominal wall, allowing free drainage of urine) when the urethra is too small for the resectoscope. Alternatives are ureterostomy drainage with valve ablation performed at a later stage. Any underlying bladder dysfunction should be diagnosed and treated.

Longer-term monitoring: Monitor children for linear growth (height, weight, and head circumference), renal function, blood pressure, urine analysis (for proteinuria, osmolality), USS, and formal glomerular flow rate (GFR) with DPTA or chromium EDTA.

Prognosis

35% have long-term poor renal function; 20% develop end-stage renal failure. Bladder dysfunction is common despite treatment of outflow obstruction. This includes bladder overactivity, incontinence and bladder underactivity associated with chronic urinary residuals and poor concentration of urine (with polyuria). From age 16 years, care should be transferred to an adult urologist or nephrologist. Problems may arise with retrograde ejaculation, impotence, and reduced libido (related to renal impairment), and abnormal prostatic or seminal vesicle secretions contributing to reduced fertility.

Non-neurogenic voiding dysfunction

Definition An abnormal voiding pattern without an underlying organic cause (neurological disease, congenital malformation or injury), which usually results in urinary incontinence (diurnal, nocturnal or both) and recurrent UTI. It is often associated with constipation and faecal retention.

Normal bladder control

- **Neonates:** sacral spinal cord reflex triggers voiding when the bladder is full
- **Infants:** primitive reflexes are suppressed, bladder capacity increases and voiding frequency is reduced
- **2–4 years:** development of conscious bladder sensation and voluntary control.

Classification

Urinary incontinence can be divided into primary types (never been dry) or secondary (re-emergence of incontinence after being dry for 6 months). Voiding dysfunction can be described as mild, moderate or major.

- **Mild:** daytime urinary frequency syndrome; post-void dribbling (urine refluxes into the vagina, then dribbles into underwear on standing); primary monosymptomatic nocturnal enuresis
- **Moderate:** 'lazy' bladder syndrome (large capacity, poor contractility, infrequent voids); overactive bladder (bladder overactivity associated with urgency and frequency). Children may demonstrate holding manoeuvres (leg crossing, squatting, Vincent's curtsey). There is increased risk of UTI, vesicoureteric reflux (VUR) and upper tract dilatation. Giggle incontinence
- **Major:** Hinman's syndrome (non-neurogenic neurogenic bladder) involves disco-ordination between the bladder muscle and external urethral sphincter activity resulting in a small, trabeculated bladder, VUR, UTI, hydronephrosis and renal damage. Caused by abnormal learned voiding patterns.

Evaluation

Aim to exclude an organic cause for the symptoms.

- **History:** enquire about UTIs; voiding habits (frequency, urgency; primary or secondary incontinence; daytime and/or night-time symptoms); family history; bowel problems; social history; behavioural problems
- **Examination:** palpate the abdomen for distended bladder or enlarged kidneys. Inspect external genitalia for congenital anomalies (i.e. epispadias). Exclude any neurological causes (hairy patch, lipoma, dimple on lower back may indicate lumbosacral spine abnormalities; examine lower limb reflexes)
- **Investigations:** urinalysis (infection, protein, glucose); voiding diary; flow rate, post-void residual volumes (PVR). In selected cases: USS renal tract (to assess for hydronephrosis, bladder size); micturating cysto-urethrogram (to assess for VUR, PVR); videourodynamics (if suspicion of neuropathic bladder or sphincter dysfunction, or difficulty in clinical diagnosis); MRI spine (if clinical suspicion of neurological cause).

Management

Behavioural (bladder retraining, timed voiding, change of voiding posture, psychological support); withdraw bladder irritants, medication (antibiotics for infection, anticholinergics for bladder overactivity and urgency, laxatives or enemas for constipation); intermittent catheterization to drain post-void residuals. Nocturnal enuresis can be treated with behavioural methods (bladder training, enuretic alarms) or with desmopressin. Surgery is rarely indicated.

Prognosis 15% spontaneously resolve per year.

Nocturnal enuresis

Enuresis is any involuntary loss of urine in the absence of any demonstrable abnormality of the urinary tract. It may occur at an inappropriate time or social setting, during the day, night or diurnally. *Nocturnal enuresis* describes loss of urine occurring during sleep. *Monosymptomatic nocturnal enuresis (MNE)* is a term used to describe bedwetting in children with no daytime urinary symptoms to suggest an underlying voiding disorder.

Prevalence

Nocturnal enuresis is estimated to affect up to 15% of 5-years olds,[1] and 10% of 7-year old children.[2] There is 15% spontaneous resolution of symptoms per year.[1] The prevalence in adults is ~0.5%.

Age (years)	Females	Males
5	10–15%	15–20%
7	7–15%	15–20%
9	5–10%	10–15%
16	1–2%	1–2%

Classification

Primary nocturnal enuresis (PNE): never been dry for more than a 6-month period.

Secondary: the re-emergence of bed wetting after a period of being dry for at least 6 months.

Pathophysiology

Three main factors that interact to produce nocturnal enuresis are:
- Altered antidiuretic hormone (ADH) secretion: an abnormal decrease in ADH levels at night causes increased urine production (nocturnal polyuria)
- Altered sleep/arousal mechanism: impaired 'arousal from sleep' response to a full bladder
- Reduced nocturnal functional bladder capacity* (± associated bladder overactivity during sleep).

Familial predisposition, psychological factors and urinary tract infection are also considered to contribute to nocturnal enuresis.

Evaluation

The aim is to establish the underlying pathophysiological factors to guide treatment.

History

Enquire about the frequency of episodes, daytime symptoms, new or recurrent problem, family history, symptoms of UTI, bowel problems, and psychosocial history.

Examination

Examine abdomen for palpable bladder; neurological exam including perineal sensation, anocutaneous reflex and lower limb sensation; examine the spine (i.e. for sacral agenesis).

Investigations

- **Voiding diary:** to assess for nocturnal polyuria and functional bladder capacity
- **Urinalysis:** to assess for infection; the presence of glucose (diabetes) or protein (UTI, renal disease).

Management

Behavioural

- **Reassurance and counselling** (including motivational techniques to improve child's self-esteem)
- **Bladder training:** regular daytime toileting, emptying the bladder before bed, avoiding bladder stimulants (i.e. blackcurrant drinks, caffeine), reduced fluid intake in the hours before sleep
- **Conditioning therapy:** an enuretic alarm is connected to the child's underwear, which is triggered with the first few drops of urine, waking the child from sleep (60–70% successful response).

Pharmacological

- Desmopressin (synthetic analogue of ADH) given intranasally or orally just before bedtime to exert an antidiuretic response
- Imipramine, a tricyclic antidepressant with anticholinergic and antispasmodic properties (used only selectively in children).

Patients with nocturnal polyuria (and normal bladder function) tend to have a good response to desmopressin. Patients with functionally reduced bladder capacity (which may be associated with occult bladder dysfunction) benefit most from a combination of enuretic alarm, bladder training and anticholinergic drugs (i.e. oxybutynin) ± desmopressin.

* Aged-based 'normal' bladder capacity in children is calculated as: Child <2 years old: bladder capacity (mL) is estimated as 7.5 mL/kg. Child >2 years old: bladder capacity in mL = 30 (age + 2).

1 Forsythe WI, Redmond A (1974) Enuresis and spontaneous cure rate: study of 1129 patients. *Arch Dis Child* **49**:259–63.

2 Hellstrom AL, Hansson E, Hansson S, *et al.* (1990) Micturition habits and incontinence in 7-year-old Swedish school entrants. *Eur J Paediatr* **149**:434–7.

Urological surgery and equipment

Preparation of the patient for urological surgery

Degree of preparation is related to the complexity of the procedure. Certain aspects of examination (pulse rate, blood pressure) and certain tests (haemoglobin, electrolytes, creatinine) are important, not only to assess fitness for surgery, but also as a baseline against which changes in the post-operative period may be measured.

- Assess cardiac status (angina, arrhythmias, previous MI, blood pressure, ECG, CXR). We assess respiratory function by pulmonary function tests (FVC, FEV_1) for all major surgery and any surgery where the patient has symptoms of respiratory problems or a history of chronic airways disease (e.g. asthma)
- Arrange an anaesthetic review where there is, for example, cardiac or respiratory co-morbidity
- Culture urine, treat active (symptomatic) infection with an appropriate antibiotic starting a week before surgery, and give prophylactic antibiotics at the induction of anaesthesia
- Consider stopping aspirin* and non-steroidal anti-inflammatory drugs 10 days prior to surgery
- Obtain consent
- Measure haemoglobin and serum creatinine, and investigate and correct anaemia, electrolyte disturbance, and abnormal renal function. If blood loss is anticipated, group and save a sample of serum or cross-match several units of blood, the precise number depending on the speed with which your blood bank can deliver blood if needed. In our own unit our policy is (other units may have a different policy):

TURBT	Group and save
TURP	Group and save
Open prostatectomy	Cross-match 2 units
Simple nephrectomy	Cross-match 2 units
Radical nephrectomy	Cross-match 4 units
(renal vein or IVC extension)	Cross match 6 units
Cystectomy	Cross-match 4 units
Radical prostatectomy	Cross-match 2 units
PCNL	Group and save

- The patient may choose to store their own blood prior to the procedure.

Should aspirin and other antiplatelet drugs be stopped prior to minor urological procedures and urological surgery?

Aspirin and TRUS biopsy

In the UK 65% of urologists routinely stop aspirin prior to TRUS biopsy; 35% do not.[1] Four of 297 urologists (1.3%) reported cerebrovascular side effects from stopping aspirin. There remains no consensus guidance on whether to stop or continue aspirin.

Aspirin and TURP

There is wide variation in management of aspirin in men undergoing TURP. In a recent audit of UK urologists, 38% said they did not stop aspirin prior to TURP, but of those that said they did stop it, a substantial number still proceeded with TURP if the aspirin had inadvertently not been stopped.[2] Overall, 75% either didn't bother stopping aspirin or proceeded with TURP if patients were inadvertently still taking it, presumably because of a perceived increased risk of serious cardiovascular events. Some studies suggest an increased risk of bleeding and need for blood transfusion in those on aspirin while others report no increased risk. There is only one RCT and this showed that aspirin did increase blood loss after TURP, but not enough to increase the requirement for blood transfusion.[3] The risks of short-term withdrawal of aspirin prior to TURP have not been established, although there are anecdotal reports of serious adverse cardiovascular events. So, should aspirin be stopped or continued prior to TURP? The short answer is that there is no substantial body of evidence to support stopping it or continuing it and as a majority continue to do TURP with patients on aspirin, but a substantial minority stop it either behaviour is reasonable. Since bleeding times return to normal within 48 h of stopping aspirin (the time taken for new platelets to reach sufficient numbers to compensate for impaired function of circulating platelets), it seems reasonable to stop it 2 days before surgery and to restart it within a few days of surgery when it is obvious that postoperative bleeding has stopped (usually when it is deemed safe to remove the catheter).

Drug eluting cardiac stents and antiplatelet agents

Be careful in patients receiving the newer antiplatelet drugs such as clopidogrel or ticlopidine (with or without aspirin), since bleeding times can increase 3 fold.[4] Severe, intractable bleeding can occur following 'minor' procedures such as prostate biopsy or bladder biopsy. Patients with coronary artery stents are treated with dual anticoagulation with aspirin and clopidogrel for several months stent insertion to reduce the risk of stent thrombosis. The precise duration of antiplatelet therapy has not been established, but 9–12 months is currently recommended by the American Heart Association. Seek advice from a cardiologist about the safety of stopping these drugs. Consider delaying invasive procedures (e.g. prostate or bladder biopsy) if the risk of bleeding is deemed to be unacceptable in the presence of the continued need for anticoagulation.

1 Masood J, Hafeez, Calleary J, Barua JM. (2007) Aspirin use and transrectal ultrasonography-guided prostate biopsy: a national survey. *Br J Urol Int* **99**:965–6.

2 Enver MK, Hoh I, Chinegwundoh FI (2006) The management of aspirin in transurethral prostatectomy: current practice in the UK. *Ann R Coll Surg Engl* **88**:280–3.

3 Nielsen JD, Holm-Nielsen A, Jespersen J, et al. (2000) The effect of low-dose acetylsalicylic acid on bleeding after transurethral prostatectomy—a prospective, randomized, double-blind, placebo-controlled study. *Scan J Urol Nephrol* **34**:194–8.

4 Stephen Jones J. (2007) Urologists: be aware of significant risks of stopping anticoagulants in patients with drug eluting coronary stents. *Br J Urol Int* **99**:1330–1.

Bowel preparation

Indicated if large bowel is to be used (bowel prep is not required if small bowel alone is to be used e.g. ileal conduit, ileal neo-bladder reconstruction). Use a simple mechanical prep (Citramag® or Picolax®—magnesium salts), 2 doses starting the morning before surgery, with clear fluid-only diet.

Antibiotic prophylaxis in urological surgery

The precise antibiotic prophylaxis policy that you use will depend on your local microbiological flora. Your local microbiology department will provide regular advice and updates on which antibiotics should be used, both for prophylaxis and treatment. The policy shown below and in Table 17.1 is our own local policy.

Since the last edition of this book there has been a move away from cefuroxime in an attempt to reduce the risk of antibiotic induced *Cl difficile* colitis. There has also been a similar move away from the use of fluoroquinolones (ciprofloxacin, norfloxacin, ofloxacin, levofloxacin) because they are a risk factor for the development of *Cl difficile* associated diarrhoea and pseudomembranous colitis (and also for MRSA since they are secreted onto the skin and many staphylococci are resistant to them).* Trimethoprim, gentamicin, penicillin and co-amoxiclav are less likely to cause *Cl difficile* associate disease.

Culture urine before any procedure, and use specific prophylaxis (based on sensitivities) if culture positive.

We avoid ciprofloxacin in inpatients because it is secreted onto the skin and causes MRSA colonization. For most purposes, nitrofurantoin provides equivalent cover without being secreted onto the skin. We do use ciprofloxacin if there is known Proteus infection (all Proteus species are resistant to nitrofurantoin).

Patients with artificial heart valves

Patients with heart murmurs and those with prosthetic heart valves: 1g of iv amoxicillin with 120 mg of gentamicin should be given at induction of anaesthesia, with an additional dose of oral amoxycillin, 500 mg 6 h later (substituting vancomycin 1 g for those who are penicillin allergic).

Patients with joint replacements

The advice is conflicting.

---

* *Cl difficile*. Gram positive, anaerobic, spore-forming bacillus. Most common cause of nosocomial diarrhoea and antibiotic associated colitis. Disease arises as a consequence of faeco-oral transmission of *Cl difficile* spores (Ribotype 027 seems to be particularly pathogenic). Once colonization has occurred, progression to diarrhoea or colitis depends on coexisting conditions and host immune response. *Cl difficile* toxins A and B are responsible for pathogenicity. They bind to intestinal epithelial receptors. Inflammatory cytokines cause fluid secretion, mucosal destruction and tissue necrosis. Other risk factors for *Cl difficile* associated disease: age >65 years. Use of proton-pump inhibitors, laxatives, nasogastric tubes, prolonged hospital stay. Treatment for diarrhoea and colitis: stop causative antibiotics, isolate and barrier nurse (wash hands with soap and water as alcohol hand rubs are ineffective against spores), oral metronidazole (oral vancomycin reserved for serious or recurrent infection).

AAOS/AUA advice

Joint advice of the American Academy of Orthopaedic Surgeons (AAOS) and the American Urological Association (AUA)—antibiotic prophylaxis is not indicated for urological patients with pins, plates, or screws, or for most patients with total joint replacements. It is recommended for all patients undergoing urological procedures, including TURP *within 2 years of a prosthetic joint replacement*, for those who are immunocompromised (e.g. rheumatoid patients, those with systemic lupus erythematosus, drug-induced immunosuppression including steroids), and for those with a history of previous joint infection, haemophilia, HIV infection, diabetes, and malignancy.

Antibiotic regime: single dose of a quinolone, such as 500 mg of ciprofloxacin, 1–2 h pre-operatively + ampicillin 2 g IV + gentamicin 1.5 mg/kg 30–60 min pre-operatively (substituting vancomycin 1 g IV for penicillin allergic patients).

UK advice

In the UK, a Working Party of the British Society for Antimicrobial Chemotherapy has stated that patients with prosthetic joint implants (including total hip replacements) do not require antibiotic prophylaxis and consider that it is unacceptable to expose patients to the adverse effects of antibiotics when there is no evidence that such prophylaxis is of any benefit. This advice is based on the rationale that joint infections are caused by skin organisms that get onto the prosthesis at the time of the operation and that the role of bacteraemia as a cause of seeding, outside the immediate post-operative period, has never been established.

We use the same antibiotic prophylaxis as for patients without joint prostheses.

Table 17.1 Oxford Urology procedure: specific antibiotic prophylaxis protocol for urological surgery

Procedure	Antibiotic prophylaxis
Catheter removal	Nitrofurantoin, 100 mg PO 30 min before catheter removal
Change of male long-term catheter	Gentamicin 1.5 mg/kg IM or IV 20 min before*
Flexible cystoscopy or GA cystoscopy	Nitrofurantoin 100 mg PO 30–60 min before procedure@
Transrectal prostatic biopsy	Ciprofloxacin 500 mg PO and metronidazole 400 mg 20 min pre-biopsy and for 48 h post-biopsy (ciprofloxacin 500 mg bds, metronidazole 400 mg tds)
ESWL	500 mg oral ciprofloxacin 30 min before treatment (nitrofurantoin does not cover *Proteus*, a common 'stone' bacterium)
PCNL	Co-amoxiclav 1.2 g IV tds starting the day before, hours before operation, and 3 doses post-operatively; gentamicin at induction
Ureteroscopy	Gentamicin 1.5 mg/kg IV at induction
Urogynaecological procedures (e.g. colposuspension)	Co-amoxiclav 1.2 g IV and metronidazole 500 mg IV at induction of anaesthesia
TURPs and TURBTs — both for non-catheterized patients (i.e. elective TURP for LUTS) and patients with catheters (undergoing TURP for retention)	Nitrofurantoin 100 mg + IV gentamicin at induction (1.5 mg/kg); nitrofurantoin 100 mg PO 30 min before catheter removal
Radical prostatectomy	Co-amoxiclav 1.2 g IV + 240 mg IV gentamicin + 500 mg IV metronidazole at induction; 240 mg of gentamicin 24 h post-op; 48 h IV Co-amoxiclav 1.2 g tds; ciprofloxacin PO 5 days

Table 17.1 Oxford Urology procedure: specific antibiotic prophylaxis protocol for urological surgery (*continued*)

Procedure	Antibiotic prophylaxis
Cystectomy or other procedures involving the use of bowel (e.g. augmentation cystoplasty)	Co-amoxiclav 1.2 g IV + 500 mg IV metronidazole at induction; further 2 doses of Co-amoxiclav 1.2 g and metronidazole (500 mg) post-operatively
Artificial urinary sphincter insertion	Vancomycin 1 g 1.5 h before leaving the ward (infuse over 100 min)** + Co-amoxiclav 1.2 g IV + 3 mg/kg IV gentamicin at induction; continue IV cefuroxime, gentamicin, and vancomycin (1 g bds) for 48 h

*Sepsis rate (necessitating admission to hospital) may be as high as 1% without antibiotic cover.

**OR teicoplanin if vancomycin allergic—400 mg at induction and bds thereafter for a total of 48 h; meropenem may be substituted for vancomycin in 'vancomycin-free' hospitals.

@ 9% of patients undergoing flexible cystoscopy develop bacteriuria (>10^5 CFU/mL of urine). A randomized, placebo controlled trial of ciprofloxacin 500 mg or trimethoprim 200 mg in 2083 patients undergoing flexible cystoscopy showed a significant reduction of bacteriuria to 3 and 5%, respectively. While both antibiotics reduce the risk of bacteriuria, ciprofloxacin is more effective—after adjustment for baseline bacteriuria (approximately 4% had bacteriuria before cystoscopy), the odds of bacteriuria for those taking trimethoprim were 4 times greater than those on ciprofloxacin. Johnson MI, Merrilees D, Robson WA *et al.* (2007) Oral ciprofloxacin or trimethoprim reduces bacteriuria after flexible cystoscopy. *Br J Urol Int* **100**:826–9.

Complications of surgery in general: DVT and PE

Venous thromboembolism (VTE) is uncommon after urological surgery, but it is considered the most important non-surgical complication of major urological procedures. Following TURP, 0.1–0.2% of patients experience a pulmonary embolus[1] and 1–5% of patients undergoing major urological surgery experience symptomatic VTE.[2] The mortality of PE is in the order of 1%.[3]

Risk factors for DVT and PE

Increased risk: open (versus endoscopic) procedures, malignancy, increasing age, duration of procedure.

Categorization of VTE risk

American College of Chest Physicians (ACCP) Guidelines on prevention of venous thromboembolism[2] and British Thromboembolic Risk Factors (THRIFT) Consensus Group[4] categorize the risk of VTE:

- **Low-risk patients**: those <40 undergoing minor surgery (surgery lasting <30 min) and no additional risk factors. No specific measures to prevent DVT are required in such patients other than early mobilization. Increasing age and duration of surgery increases risk of VTE
- **High-risk patients**: include those undergoing non-major surgery (surgery lasting >30 min) who are aged >60.

Additional risk factors (that indicate the requirement for additional prophylactic measures e.g. the addition of sc heparin and/or IPCs)

- Active heart or respiratory failure
- Active cancer or cancer treatment
- Acute medical illness
- Age over 40 years
- Antiphospholipid syndrome
- Behcet's disease
- Central venous catheter *in situ*
- Continuous travel >3 h up to 4 weeks before surgery
- Immobility (paralysis or limb in plaster)
- Inflammatory bowel disease (Crohn's disease/ulcerative colitis)
- Myeloproliferative diseases
- Nephrotic syndrome
- Obesity (body mass index >30 kg/m^2)
- Paraproteinaemia
- Paroxysmal nocturnal haemoglobinuria
- Personal or family history of VTE
- Recent myocardial infarction or stroke
- Severe infection
- Use of oral contraceptive or hormone replacement therapy
- Varicose veins with associated phlebitis
- Inherited thrombophilia

- Factor V Leiden
  - Prothrombin 2021A gene mutation
  - Antithrombin deficiency
  - Protein C or S deficiency
  - Hyperhomocyteinaemia
  - Elevated coagulation factors (e.g. Factor VIII).

Prevention of DVT and PE

See box.

Diagnosis of DVT

Signs of DVT are non-specific (i.e. cellulitis and DVT share common signs—low-grade fever, calf swelling, and tenderness). If you suspect a DVT arrange a Doppler ultrasound. If the ultrasound probe can compress the popliteal and femoral veins, there is no DVT; if it can't, there is a DVT.

Diagnosis of PE

Small PEs may be asymptomatic. **_Symptoms:_** include breathlessness, pleuritic chest pain, haemoptysis. **_Signs:_** tachycardia, tachypnoea, raised JVP, hypotension, pleural rub, pleural effusion.

Tests

- **CXR:** may be normal or show linear atelectasis, dilated pulmonary artery, oligaemia of affected segment, small pleural effusion
- **ECG:** may be normal or show tachycardia, right bundle branch block, inverted T waves in V1–V4 (evidence of right ventricular strain). The 'classic' SI, QIII, TIII pattern is rare
- **Arterial blood gases:** low PO_2 and low PCO_2
- **Imaging:** CTPA-CT pulmonary angiogram. Superior specificity and sensitivity when compared with ventilation-perfusion (VQ) radioisotope scan
- **Spiral computed tomography:** a negative CT pulmonary angiogram (CTPA) rules out a PE with similar accuracy to a normal isotope lung scan or a negative pulmonary angiogram.

Treatment of established DVT

- **Below-knee DVT:** above-knee thromboembolic stockings (AK-TEDs), if no peripheral arterial disease (enquire for claudication and check pulses) + unfractionated heparin 5000 u SC 12-hourly.
- **Above-knee DVT:** start a low molecular weight heparin and warfarin, and stop heparin when INR is between 2 and 3. Continue treatment for 6 weeks for post-surgical patient; lifelong if underlying cause (e.g. malignancy)
- Low molecular weight heparin (LMWH).

Treatment of established PE

Fixed dose, subcutaneous LMWH seems to be as effective as adjusted dose, intravenous unfractionated heparin for the treatment of PE found in conjunction with a symptomatic DVT.[3] Rates of haemorrhage are similar with both forms of heparin treatment. Start warfarin at the same time and stop heparin when INR is 2–3. Continue warfarin for 3 months.

Options for prevention of VTE

- Early mobilization
- Above-knee thromboembolic stockings (AK-TEDs) (provide graduated, static compression of the calves, thereby reducing venous stasis). More effective than below-knee TEDS for DVT prevention.[5]
- Subcutaneous heparin (low-dose unfractionated heparin—LDUH or low molecular weight heparin—LMWH). In unfractionated preparations, heparin molecules are polymerized—molecular weights from 5000–30,000 Daltons. Low molecular weight heparin is depolymerized—molecular weight 4000–5000 Daltons.
- Intermittent pneumatic calf compression (IPC) boots, which are placed around the calves, are intermittently inflated and deflated, thereby increasing the flow of blood in calf veins.[6]
- For patients undergoing major urological surgery (radical prostatectomy, cystectomy, nephrectomy), AK-TEDS with IPC intra-operatively, followed by SC heparin (LDUH or LMWH) should be used. For TURP, many urologists use a combination of AK-TEDS and IPCs; relatively few use SC heparin.[7]

Contraindications to AK-TEDS

- Any local leg conditions with which stockings would interfere, such as dermatitis, vein ligation, gangrene, recent skin grafts
- Peripheral artery occlusive disease (PAOD)
- Massive oedema of legs or pulmonary oedema from congestive cardiac failure
- Extreme deformity of the legs.

Contraindications to heparin

- Allergy to heparin
- History of haemorrhagic stroke
- Active bleeding
- Significant liver impairment—check clotting first
- Thrombocytopenia (platelet count $< 100 \times 10^9$/L).

1 Donat R, Mancey–Jones B (2002) Incidence of thromboembolism after transurethral resection of the prostate (TURP). *Scan J Urol Nephrol* **36**:119–23.

2 Geerts WH, Heit JA, Clagett PG, *et al.* (2001) Prevention of venous thromboembolism. (American College of Chest Physicians (ACCP) Guidelines on prevention of venous thrombo-embolism) *Chest* **119**:132S–175S.

3 Quinlan DJ, McQuillan A, Eikelboom JW (2004) Low molecular weight heparin compared with intravenous unfractionated heparin for treatment of pulmonary embolism. *Ann Intern Med* **140**:175–83.

4 Lowe GDO, Greer IA, Cooke TG, *et al.* (1992) Risk of and prophylaxis for venous thromboembolism in hospital patients. Thromboembolic Risk Factors (THRIFT) Consensus Group. *BMJ* **305**:567–74.

5 Howard A, *et al.* (2004) Randomized clinical trial of low molecular weight heparin with thigh-length or knee-length antiembolism stockings for patients undergoing surgery. *BJS* **91**:842–7.

6 Soderdahl DW, Henderson SR, Hansberry KL (1997) A comparison of intermittent pneumatic compression of the calf and whole leg in preventing deep venous thrombosis in urological surgery. *J Urol* **157**:1774–6.

7 Golash A, Collins PW, Kynaston HG, Jenkins BJ (2002) Venous thromboembolic prophylaxis for transurethral prostatectomy: practice among British urologists. *J Roy Soc Med* **95**:130–1.

Management of anticoagulation in the peri-operative period

Liaise with whoever is responsible for the patient's anticoagulation (e.g. anti-coagulant clinic). Warfarin should be stopped either 4 days (if the target INR is 2.5) or 5 days (if the target INR is higher) before surgery. Determine the INR the day before surgery to reduce the risk of cancellation. Administer oral vitamin K (2.5 mg) if the INR is ≥2.0. Check the INR on the day of surgery.

The main decision is whether to give bridging therapy with treatment dose heparin (UFH or LMWH) and if not whether pre-operative prophylactic LMWH is advised when the INR is <2.0. For pragmatic purposes, to save monitoring the INR as an out-patient, this could be instituted 2–3 days after warfarin is stopped, i.e. on the morning after two doses have been omitted.

	Pre-operative	Post-operative~
High Risk, e.g. VTE within 1 month. Prosthetic mitral valve AF and history of stroke	Treatment dose heparin (either IV UFH or SC LMWH)#	Treatment dose heparin (either IV UFH or SC LMWH)
Non-High Risk, e.g. AF without previous stroke	Nil/prophylactic LMWH*	Prophylactic LMWH

~ Continue until INR > 2.0 for two consecutive days.

Stop full dose iv UFH 6 h pre-operatively and check APTT, omit full dose SC LMWH on day of surgery.

* For patients with venous thromboembolism within 1–3 months or cancer we would suggest prophylactic LMWH pre-operatively.

A controversial group of patients are those with a prosthetic (non-caged) aortic valve and no other risk factor. It is acceptable not to use bridging therapy with treatment dose heparin in these patients particularly if the bleeding risk is high.[1,21,2.]

1 Dunn AS, Turpie AG (2003) Perioperative management of patients receiving oral anticoagulants: a systematic review. *Arch Intern Med* **163**:901–8.

2 Kearon, C. (2003) Managment of anticoagulation before and after elective surgery. *Am Soc Hematol Educat Program Book*, pp. 528–34.

Fluid balance and the management of shock in the surgical patient

Daily fluid requirement

Can be calculated according to patient weight:

- **For the first 10 kg:** 100 mL/kg per 24 h (=1000 mL)
- **For the next 10 kg:** (i.e. from 10–20 kg): 50 mL/kg per 24 h (=500 mL)
- **For every kg above 20 kg:** 20 mL/kg per 24 h (=1000 mL for a patient weighing 70 kg).

Thus, for every 24 h, a 70 kg adult will require 1000 mL for their first 10 kg of weight, plus 500 mL for their next 10 kg of weight, and 1000 mL for their last 50 kg of weight = total 24-h fluid requirement, 2500 mL.

Daily sodium requirement is 100 mmol, and for potassium, 70 mmol. Thus, a standard 24-h fluid regimen is 2 L of 5% dextrose + 1 L of N. saline (equivalent to about 150 mmol Na^+), with 20 mmol K^+ for every litre of infused fluid.

Fluid losses from drains or nasogastric aspirate are similar in composition to plasma and should be replaced principally with N. saline.

Shock due to blood loss

Inadequate organ perfusion and tissue oxygenation. The causes are hypovolaemia, cardiogenic, septic, anaphylactic, and neurogenic. The most common cause in the surgical patient is hypovolaemia due to blood and other fluid loss. Haemorrhage is an acute loss of circulating blood volume.

Haemorrhagic shock may be classified as:

- **Class I**: up to 750 mL of blood loss (15% of blood volume); normal pulse rate (PR), respiratory rate (RR), blood pressure, urine output, and mental status
- **Class II**: 750–1500 mL (15–30% of blood volume); PR > 100; decreased pulse pressure due to increased diastolic pressure; RR 20–30; urinary output 20–30 mL/h
- **Class III**: 1500–2000 mL (30–40% of blood volume); PR >120; decreased blood pressure and pulse pressure due to decreased systolic pressure; RR 30–40; urine output 5–15 mL/h; confusion
- **Class IV**: >2000 mL (>40% of blood volume); PR >140; decreased pulse pressure and blood pressure; RR >35; urine output <5 mL/h; cold, clammy skin.

Management

- Remember 'ABC': 100% oxygen to improve tissue oxygenation
- ECG, cardiac monitor, pulse oximetry
- Insert two short and wide intravenous cannulae in the antecubital fossa (e.g. 16 G). A central venous line may be required
- Infuse 1 L of warm Hartmann's solution or, if severe haemorrhage, then start a colloid instead (e.g. gelofusin®). Aim for a urinary output of 0.5 mL/kg/h and maintenance of blood pressure.
- Check FBC, coagulation screen, U&Es, and cardiac enzymes
- Cross-match 6 units of blood
- Arterial blood gases to assess oxygentation and pH.

Obvious and excessive blood loss may be seen from drains, but drains can block, so assume there is covert bleeding if there is a tachycardia (and low blood pressure). If this regimen fails to stabilize pulse and blood pressure, return the patient to the operating room for exploratory surgery.

Patient safety in the urology theatre

It is a fundamental part of safe surgical practice to cross-check that the following have been done prior to starting an operation or procedure. The process of cross-checking should be done with another member of staff, using several sources of information (e.g. the notes, consent form, x-ray images)) to confirm the following.

- **Patient identification:** confirm you are operating on the right patient by a process of 'active' identification (i.e. ask the patient their name, date of birth, and their address to confirm that you are talking to the correct patient)
- **Ensure you are doing the correct procedure and on the correct side by cross-checking with the notes and X-rays:** for lateralized procedures (e.g. nephrectomy, PCNL) the correct side of the operation should be confirmed by cross-checking with the X-rays and with the X-ray report, as well as referring to the notes. Where it is possible for the sides of an IVU to be incorrectly labelled, this cannot happen with a CT scan, where the location of the liver (right side) and the spleen (left side) provide confirmation of what side is what
- **Appropriate antibiotic prophylaxis has been given**
- **DVT prophylaxis has been administered** (e.g. heparin, AK-TEDS, intermittent pneumatic compression boots)
- **Blood is available, if appropriate**
- **The patient is safely and securely positioned on the operating table:** pressure points padded, not touching metal (to avoid diathermy burns), body straps securely in place.

Develop an approach to operating that involves members of your team. Listen to the opinions of staff who are junior to you. They may sometimes be able to identify errors that are not obvious to you. Cultivate the respect of the recovery room staff. They may express concern about a patient under their care—listen to their concerns, take them seriously, and, if all is well, reassure them. It does no harm for your patients or for your reputation to develop the habit of visiting every patient in the recovery room to check that all is well. You may be able to identify a problem before it has developed into a crisis and, at the very least, you will gain a reputation for being a caring surgeon.

Transurethral resection (TUR) syndrome

Arises from the infusion of a large volume of hypotonic irrigating solution into the circulation during endoscopic procedures (e.g. TURP, TURBT, PCNL). Occurs in 0.5% of TURPs.

Pathophysiology

Biochemical, haemodynamic, and neurological disturbances occur:

- Dilutional hyponatraemia is the most important—and serious—factor leading to the symptoms and signs. The serum sodium usually has to fall to <125 mmol/l before the patient becomes unwell
- Hypertension—due to fluid overload
- Visual disturbances may be due to the fact that glycine is a neurotransmitter in the retina.

Diagnosis: symptoms, signs, and tests

Confusion, nausea, vomiting, hypertension, bradycardia and visual disturbances, seizures. If the patient is awake (spinal anaesthesia) they may report visual disturbances (e.g. flashing lights).

Preventing development of TUR syndrome and definitive treatment

Use a continuous irrigating cystoscope (provides low-pressure irrigation), limit resection time, avoid aggressive resection near the capsule, and reduce the height of the irrigant solution.[1]

For prolonged procedures, where a greater degree of fluid absorption may occur, measure serum Na and give 20–40 mg of intravenous furosemide to start off-loading the excess fluid that has been absorbed. If the serum sodium comes back as being normal, you will have done little harm by giving the frusemide, but if it comes back at <125 mmol/l, you will have started treatment already and thereby may have prevented the development of severe TUR syndrome.

Techniques for measuring fluid overload

- Weighing machines can be added to the ordinary operating table[2]
- Adding a little alcohol to the irrigating fluid and constantly monitoring the expired air with a breathalyser[3] allows an estimation of the volume of excess fluid which has been absorbed.

1 Madsen PO, Naber KG (1973) The importance of the pressure in the prostatic fossa and absorption of irrigating fluid during transurethral resection of the prostate. *J Urol* **109**:446–52.

2 Coppinger SW, Lewis CA, Milroy EJG (1995) A method of measuring fluid balance during transurethral resection of the prostate. *Br J Urol* **76**:66–72.

3 Hahn RG (1993) Ethanol monitoring of extravascular absorption of irrigating fluid. *Br J Urol* **72**:766–69.

Catheters and drains in urological surgery

Catheters

Made from latex or silastic (for patients with Latex allergy or for long-term use—better tolerated by the urethral mucosa).

Types

- Self-retaining (also known as a Foley, balloon, or 2-way catheter; Fig. 17.1). An inflation channel can be used to inflate and deflate a balloon at the end of the catheter, which prevents the catheter from falling out
- 3-way catheter (also known as an irrigating catheter). Has a third channel (in addition to the balloon inflation and drainage channels) which allows fluid to be run into the bladder at the same time as it is drained from the bladder (Fig. 17.2).

Size

The size of a catheter is denoted by its circumference in mm. This is known as the 'French' or 'Charriere' (hence Ch) gauge. Thus a 12 Ch catheter has a circumference of 12 mm.

Uses

- Relief of obstruction (e.g. BOO due to BPE causing urinary retention—use the smallest catheter that you can pass; usually a 12Ch or 14Ch is sufficient in an adult)
- Irrigation of the bladder for clot retention (use a 20Ch or 22Ch 3-way catheter)
- Drainage of urine to allow the bladder to heal if it has been opened (trauma or deliberately, as part of a surgical operation)
- Prevention of ureteric reflux, maintenance of a low bladder pressure, where the ureter has been stented (post-pyeloplasty for PUJ obstruction)
- To empty the bladder before an operation on the abdomen or pelvis (deflating the bladder gets it out of harms' way)
- Monitoring of urine output post-operatively or in the unwell patient
- For delivery of bladder instillations (e.g. intravesical chemotherapy or immunotherapy)
- To allow identification of the bladder neck during surgery (e.g. radical prostatectomy, operations on or around the bladder neck).

Drains

Principally indicated for prevention of accumulation of urine, blood, lymph, or other fluids. Particularly used after the urinary tract has been opened and closed by suture repair. A suture line takes some days to become completely watertight, and during this time urine leaks from the closure site. A drain prevents accumulation of urine (a urinoma), the very presence of which can cause an ileus and, if it becomes infected, an abscess can develop.

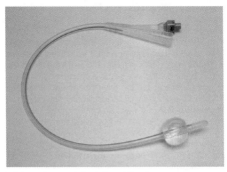

Fig. 17.1 A Foley catheter with the balloon inflated.

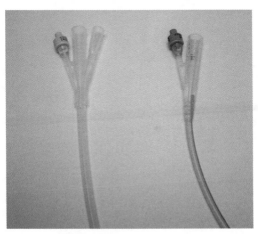

Fig. 17.2 2- and 3-way catheters.

- **Tube drains** (e.g. a Robinson's drain; Figs. 17.3 and 17.4). Provide passive drainage (i.e. no applied pressure). Used to drain suture lines at a site of repair or anastomosis of the urinary tract. Avoid placing the drain tip on the suture line, as this may prevent healing of the repair. Suture it to adjacent tissues to prevent it from being dislodged
- **Suction drains** (e.g. Hemovac®; Figs. 17.5 and 17.6). Provide active drainage (i.e. air in the drainage bottle is evacuated, producing a −ve pressure when connected to the drain tube to encourage evacuation of fluid). Used for prevention of accumulation of blood (a haematoma) in superficial wounds. Avoid in proximity to a suture line in the urinary tract—the suctioning effect may encourage continued flow of urine out of the hole, discouraging healing.

As a general principle, drains should be brought out through a separate stab wound, rather than through the main wound, since the latter may result in bacterial contamination of the main wound with subsequent risk of infection. Secure the drain with a thick suture to prevent it inadvertently 'falling out'.

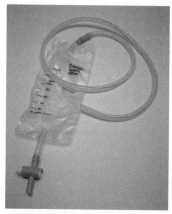

Fig. 17.3 A Robinson's (passive) drainage system.

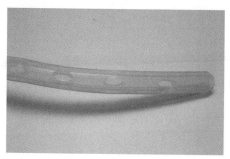

Fig. 17.4 Note the eyeholes of the Robinson's catheter.

Failure to deflate catheter balloon for removal of a urethral catheter

From time to time an inflated catheter balloon will not deflate when the time comes for removal of the catheter.

- Try inflating the balloon with air or water—this can dislodge an obstruction
- Leave a 10 mL syringe firmly inserted in the balloon channel and come back an hour or so later
- Try bursting the balloon by over-inflation
- Cut the end of the catheter off, proximal to the inflation valve—the valve may be 'stuck' and the water may drain out of the balloon
- In the female patient, introduce a needle alongside your finger into the vagina and burst the balloon by advancing the needle through the anterior vaginal and bladder wall
- In male patients, balloon deflation with a needle can also be done under ultrasound guidance. Fill the bladder with saline using a bladder syringe so that the needle can be introduced percutaneously and directed towards the balloon of the catheter under ultrasound control
- Pass a ureteroscope alongside the catheter and deflate the balloon with the rigid end of a guidewire or with a laser fibre (the end of which is sharp).

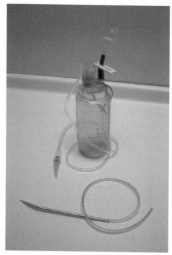

Fig. 17.5 A Redivac suction drain showing the drain tubing attached to the needle used for insertion and the suction bottle.

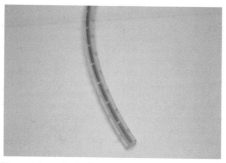

Fig. 17.6 The eye holes at the tip of the suction drain.

Guidewires

An essential tool for endourological procedures.

As a track over which catheters or instruments can be passed into the ureter, collecting system of the kidney (retrograde or antegrade), or the bladder.

Many different types of guidewire are available. They are classified according to their size, tip design, rigidity, and surface coating. These specific properties determine their use. All are radio-opaque so X-ray screening can be used to determine their position. They come prepackaged in a coiled sheath to allow ease of handling and storage (Fig. 17.7).

Size
'Size' refers to diameter measured in inches (length is usually around 150 cm). Most common size are 0.035 inches (2.7 Ch) and 0.038 inches (2.9 Ch). Also available, 0.032 inches (2.5 Ch).

Tip design
Shape of tip—straight or angle (Fig. 17.8): a straight tip is usually adequate for most uses. Occasionally, an angle tip is useful for negotiating an impacted stone or for placing the guidewire in a specific position. Similarly, a J-shaped tip can negotiate an impacted stone—the curved leading edge of this guidewire type can sometimes suddenly flick past the stone (in this situation a straight guidewire can inadvertently perforate the ureter, thereby creating a false passage).

Surface coating
Most standard guidewires are coated with polytetrafluoroethylene (PTFE), which has a low coefficient of friction, thus allowing easy passage of the guidewire through the ureter and of instruments over them. Some guidewires are coated with a polymer, which when wet is very slippery (hydrophilic coating). In some cases, the entire length of the guidewire is so coated (e.g. Terumo Glidewire) and in others, just the tip (e.g. Sensor guidewire). The virtually friction-free surface of Glidewires makes them liable to slip out of the ureter, and they therefore make unreliable safety wires (they can be exchanged for a wire with greater friction via a ureteric catheter). If allowed to become dry, these wires have a high coefficient of friction, which makes them difficult to manipulate.

Tip rigidity
The tip of all guidewires, over at least 3 cm, is soft and, therefore, flexible. This reduces—although does not completely remove—the risk of ureteric perforation.

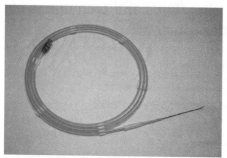

Fig. 17.7 Guidewires come prepackaged in a sheath for ease of handling.

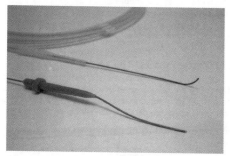

Fig. 17.8 Examples of straight-tip and angled-tip guidewires.

Shaft rigidity

Stiff guidewires are easier to manipulate than floppy ones and help to straighten a tortuous ureter (e.g. Amplatz Ultrastiff is particularly useful for this). Very malleable wires such as the Terumo Glidewire can be very useful for passing an impacted stone (for the same reason as J-tip wires).

Some guidewires provide a combination of properties—a soft, floppy, hydrophilic-coated tip with the remainder of the guidewire being stiff (e.g. Sensor guidewire).

Irrigating fluids and techniques of bladder washout

Glycine is used for endoscopic surgery requiring application of diathermy

Normal saline is used for:
- Irrigation of bladder following TURP, TURBT
- Irrigation during ureteroscopy, PCNL.

Blocked catheter post TURP and clot retention

Avoiding catheter blockage following TURP—keep the catheter bag empty; ensure a sufficient supply of irrigant solution.

The bladder will be painfully distended. Irrigant flow will have stopped. A small clot may have blocked the catheter or a chip of prostate may have stuck in the eye of the catheter. Attach a bladder syringe to the end of the catheter and pull back (Fig. 17.9). This may suck out the clot or chip of prostate and flow may restart. If it does not, draw some irrigant up into the syringe until it is about half-full and forcefully inject this fluid into the bladder. This may dislodge (and fragment) a clot that has stuck to the eye of the catheter. If the problem persists, change the catheter. You may see the obstructing chip of prostate on the end of the catheter as it is withdrawn.

Blocked catheter post TURBT

Use the same technique as for post-TURP catheter blockage, but avoid vigorous pressure on the syringe—the wall of the bladder will have been weakened at the site of tumour resection and it is possible to perforate the bladder, particularly in elderly women who have thin bladder walls.

Blocked catheters following bladder augmentation or neobladder

The suture line of the augmented bladder is weak and over-vigorous bladder washouts can rupture the bladder.

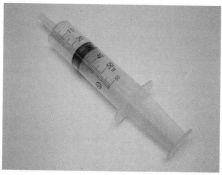

Fig. 17.9 A bladder syringe—the tip is designed to fit onto a catheter.

JJ stents

These are hollow tubes, with a coil at each end, which are inserted through the bladder (usually), into the ureter, and thence into the renal pelvis. They are designed to bypass a ureteric obstruction (e.g. due to a stone) or drain the kidney (e.g. post-renal surgery). They have a coil at each end (hence, the alternative name of 'double pigtail' stent—the coils have the configuration of a pig's tail—or the less accurate name of J stent).

These prevent migration downwards (out of the ureter) or upwards (into the ureter). They are therefore 'self-retaining'. Made of polymers of variable strength and biodurability. Some stents have a hydrophilic coating, which absorbs water and thereby makes them more slippery and easier to insert. Stents are impregnated with barium- or bismuth-containing metallic salts to make them radio-opaque, so that they can be visualized radiographically to ensure correct positioning.

Types

Classified by size and length. Common sizes are 6 or 7 Ch (Fig. 17.10). Common lengths for adults are 22–28 cm. Multi-length stents are of variable length, allowing them to accommodate to ureters of different length. A new stent design the Polaris™ loop (Boston Scientifc) is said to reduce bladder irritation and to make removal easier.

Stent materials

Polyurethane; silicone; C-flex; Silitek; Percuflex; biodegradable (experimental—obviates need for stent removal and eliminates possibility of the 'forgotten stent'). Some are coated (by chemical bonding) with a hydrogel (e.g. HydroPlus™) which provides a low friction surface so making insertion easier, encrustation less likely and in theory makes the stent more comfortable (whether this is the case in practice has not been established).

Indications and uses

- Relief of obstruction: from ureteric stones; benign (i.e. ischaemic) ureteric strictures; malignant ureteric strictures. The stent will relieve the pain caused by obstruction and reverse renal impairment if present.
- Prevention of obstruction: post ureteroscopy (routine stenting after 'uncomplicated'* ureteroscopy is not necessary)
  - Indications for J stenting post-ureteroscopy:
    - –ureteric injury
    - –solitary kidney
    - –large residual stone burden
    - –raised creatinine (implying overall impaired renal function)
    - –ureteric stricture
- Prevention of obstruction post-ESWL
  - Indications for J stenting post-ESWL:[1]
    - –stents reduce the incidence of steinstrasse with large renal calculi (1.5–3.5 cm, 6% with a stent and 13% without develop a steinstrasse post-ESWL)
    - –solitary kidney
    - –raised creatinine (implying overall impaired renal function)

(The analysis by the Joint AUA/EAU Nephrolithiasis Guideline Panel 2007[2] found no improvement in stone fragmentation with stenting i.e. stents do not enhance ESWL efficacy).
- 'Passive' dilatation of ureter prior to ureteroscopy.
- To ensure antegrade flow of urine following surgery (e.g. pyeloplasty) or injury to ureter
- Following endopyelotomy (endopyelotomy stents have a tapered end from 14 to 7 Ch, to keep the incised ureter 'open')
- Post-renal transplantation (stenting of re-implanted ureter)

An alternative to the J stent

A short term 4 or 6 Ch ureteric catheter, attached to a 12 Ch urethral catheter (to stop the ureteric catheter from falling out is an alternative form of post-ureteroscopy drainage.

In an RCT, 24 h of ureteric catheter drainage post-ureteroscopy compared with no drainage, the non-catheterized group were more likely to report renal colic (45% v 2%) and to have loin pain (76% v 20%) than the ureteric catheterized group[3]. Analgesic use was greater in the non-catheterized group (67% v 20%). 20% of non-catheterized patients and 5% of catheterized returned to hospital for analgesia (but no patient required readmission). The only disadvantage of this technique was a higher reported rate of urethral irritation (37% v 4%) in the catheterized patients. It has the obvious advantage of ease of removal of the catheter, without the need for a second procedure, and avoids the potential risk of the forgotten-stent.

---

* The definition of 'uncomplicated' ureteroscopy is not precise. 'Complicated' ureteroscopy has been variously defined as (a) ureteral perforation (i.e. mucosal injury); (b) severe ureteric oedema at the site of the stone; (c) impaction (which means difficulty getting a guidewire past the stone ('cork in a bottle' stone); (d) prolonged operation (no precise definition of what 'long' is); (e) one where ureteral dilatation was carried (to define such ureteroscopies as 'complicated' is contentious because some urologists routinely 'dilate' with a dual lumen catheter to allow double guidewire placement). Does this automatically make all their ureteroscopies 'complicated'?).

1 Al-Awadi KA et al. (1999) Steinstrasse: a comparison of incidence with and without J stenting and the effect of J stenting on subsequent management. *BJU Int* **84**:618–21.

2 Preminger GM et al. (2007) 2007 Guideline for the management of ureteral calculi, joint EAU/AUA Nephrolithiasis Guideline Panel. *J Urol* **178**:2418–34.

3 Djaladat H et al. (2007) Ureteral catheterization in uncomplicated ureterolithotripsy: a randomized, controlled trial. *Eur Urol* **52**:836–41.

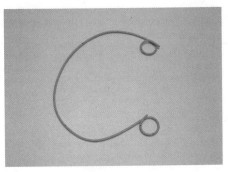

Fig. 17.10 A JJ stent.

Symptoms and complications of stents

- **Stent symptoms:** common (78%): suprapubic pain, LUTS (frequency, urgency—stent irritates trigone), haematuria, inability to work.[1] >80% of patients have stent related pain that affects daily activities, 32% report sexual dysfunction, and 58% report reduced work capacity and loss of income. Alpha blockers may help reduce pain with voiding and overall analgesic use
- **Urinary tract infection:** development of bacteriuria after stenting is common. In a small proportion sepsis can develop. In such cases consider placement of a urethral catheter to lower the pressure in the collecting system and prevent reflux of infected urine. Stents coated with the antibacterial triclosan are no better than non-coated stents in preventing stent associated UTI
- **Incorrect placement:** too high (distal end of stent in ureter; subsequent stent removal requires ureteroscopy; can be technically difficult; percutaneous removal may be required). Too low (proximal end not in renal pelvis; stent may not therefore relieve obstruction)
- **Stent migration** (up the ureter or down the ureter and into bladder)
- **Stent blockage:** catheters and stents become coated with a biofilm when in contact with urine (a protein matrix secreted by bacteria-colonizing stent). Calcium, magnesium, and phosphate salts become deposited. Biofilm build-up can lead to stent blockage or stone formation on the stent (Fig. 17.11). Stents coated with heparin are no better than non-coated stents in preventing stent biofilm formation or encrustation

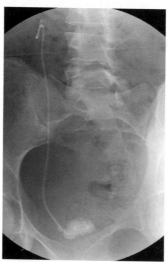

Fig. 17.11 An encrusted stent.

1 Joshi HB, Stainthorpe A, MacDonagh RP et al. Indwelling ureteral stents: evaluation of symptoms, quality of life and utility. J Urol 2003;**169**:1065-9.

- **The 'forgotten stent':** rare, but potentially very serious as biofilm may become encrusted with stone, making removal technically very difficult. If proximal end only is encrusted, PCNL may be required to remove the stone and then the stent. If the entire stent is encrusted, open removal via several incisions in the ureter may be necessary.

Commonly asked questions about stents

Does urine pass though the centre of the stent?

No, it passes around the outside of the stent. Reflux of urine occurs through the centre.

Should I place a JJ stent after ureteroscopy? (see 'Indications and uses' above)

A stent should be placed if:

- There has been ureteric injury (e.g. perforation—indicated by extravasation of contrast)
- There are residual stones that might obstruct the ureter
- The patient has had a ureteric stricture that required dilatation
- Solitary kidney
- Raised creatinine (implying overall impaired renal function).

Routine stenting after ureteroscopy for distal ureteric calculi is unnecessary.[1,2] Many urologists will place a stent after ureteroscopy for proximal ureteric stones.

Do stents cause obstruction?

In normal kidneys stents cause a significant and substantial increase in intra-renal pressure, which persists for up to 3 weeks.[3] (This can be prevented by placing a urethral catheter.)

Do stents aid stone passage?

Ureteric peristalsis requires co-aptation of the wall of the ureter proximal to the bolus of urine to be transmitted down the length of the ureter. JJ stents paralyse ureteric peristalsis. In dogs, the amplitude of each peristaltic wave (measured by an intraluminal ureteric balloon) falls (from 50 to 15 mmHg) and the frequency of ureteric peristalsis falls (from 11 to 3 waves/min). Peristalsis takes several weeks to recover. 3-mm ball bearings placed within a non-stented dog ureter take 7 days to pass, compared with 24 days in a stented ureter.

1 Srivastava A, *et al.* (2003) Routine stenting after ureteroscopy for distal ureteral calculi is unnecessary: results of a randomized controlled trial. *J Endourol* **17**:871–4.

2 Netto Jr NR *et al.* (2001) Routine ureteral stenting after ureteroscopy for ureteral lithiasis: is it really necessary? *J Urol* **166**:1252–4.

3 Ramsay JW, *et al.* (1985) The effects of double J stenting on obstructed ureters. An experimental and clinical study. *Br J Urol* **57**:630–4.

Are stents able to relieve obstruction due to extrinsic compression of a ureter?

Stents are less effective at relieving obstruction due to extrinsic obstruction by, for example, tumour or retroperitoneal obstruction.[1] They are much more effective for relieving obstruction by an intrinsic problem (e.g. a stone). Placement of two stents may provide more effective drainage (figure-of-eight configuration may produce more space around the stents for drainage).

For acute, ureteric stone obstruction with a fever, should I place a JJ stent or a nephrostomy?

In theory, one might imagine that a nephrostomy is better than a JJ stent— it can be done under local anaesthetic (JJ stent insertion may require a GA); it lowers the pressure in the renal pelvis to 0 or a negative value, whereas a JJ stent results in a persistently +ve pressure; it is less likely to be blocked by thick pus; and it allows easier subsequent imaging (contrast can be injected down the ureter—a nephrostogram—to determine if the stone has passed). A randomized trial of 42 patients with obstructing, infected stones (temperature >38°C and/or white blood count >17,000/mm^3) showed J stenting (6 or 7 Ch J stent with a Foley bladder catheter) and nephrostomy drainage (8 Ch) to be equally effective in terms of time to normalization of temperature and white count (approximately 2–3 days) and in-hospital stay. As a consequence the EAU/AUA Nephrolithiasis Guideline Panel[3] recommends that the system of drainage of the obstructed, infected kidney is left to the discretion of the urologist.

1 Docimo SG. (1989) High failure rate of indwelling ureteral stents in patients with extrinsic obstruction: experience at two institutions. *J Urol* **142**:277–9.

2 Pearle MS *et al* (1998) Optimal method of urgent decompression of the collecting system for obstruction and infection due to ureteral calculi. *J Urol* **160**:1260–4.

3 Preminger GM *et al.* (2007) 2007 Guideline for the management of ureteral calculi Joint EAU/AUA Nephrolithiasis Guideline Panel. *J Urol* **178**:2418–34.

Lasers in urological surgery

Light amplification by stimulated emission of radiation.

Photons are emitted when an atom is stimulated by an external energy source and, its electrons having been so excited, revert to their steady state. In a laser the light is coherent (all the photons are in phase with one another), collimated (the photons travel parallel to each other), and of the same wavelength (monochromatic). The light energy is thus 'concentrated', allowing delivery of high energy at a desired target.

The holmium:YAG (yttrium aluminium garnet) laser is currently the principal urological laser. It has a wavelength of 2140 nm and is highly absorbed by water and therefore by tissues which are composed mainly of water. The majority of the holmium laser energy is absorbed superficially, resulting in a superficial cutting or ablation effect. The depth of the thermal effect is no greater than 1mm. The holmium:YAG laser produces a cavitation bubble that generates only a weak shock wave as it expands and collapses. Holmium laser lithotripsy occurs primarily through a photothermal mechanism that causes stone vaporization.

Uses of the holmium:YAG laser

- Laser lithotripsy (ureteric stones, small intrarenal stones, bladder stones)
- Resection of the prostate (holmium laser prostatectomy)
- Division of urethral strictures
- Division of ureteric strictures, including PUJO
- Ablation of small bladder, ureteric, and intrarenal TCCs.

Advantages

- The holmium laser energy is delivered via a laser fibre (Fig. 17.12), which is thin enough to allow its use down a flexible instrument, without affecting the deflection of that instrument, and can therefore gain access to otherwise inaccessible parts of the kidney
- Zone of thermal injury adjacent to the tip of the laser fibre is limited to no more than 1 mm; the laser can safely be fired at a distance of 1mm from the wall of the ureter
- Can be used for all stone types
- Minimal stone migration effect because of minimal shock wave generation.

Disadvantages

- High cost
- Produces a dust cloud during stone fragmentation, which temporarily obscures the view
- Can irreparably damage endoscopes if inadvertently fired near or within the scope
- Relatively slow stone fragmentation—the laser fibre must be 'painted' over the surface of the stone to vaporize it.

Greenlight PVP for TURP

The 80 or 120 W KTP (potassium titanyl phosphate) laser is used for photoselective vaporization of the prostate. The laser is green (hence the name 'greenlight' laser) and is absorbed by haemoglobin, generating a heating effect which causes vaporization of targeted tissue.

The procedure is done under general or spinal anaesthetic.

Advantages

Saline is used for irrigation (therefore, no risk of TUR syndrome).

Disadvantages

No tissue for histological examination

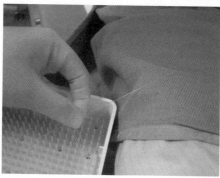

Fig. 17.12 Holmium laser fibre.

Diathermy

Diathermy is the coagulation or cutting of tissues through heat.

Monopolar diathermy

When an electric current passes between two contacts on the body there is an increase in temperature in the tissues through which the current flows. This increase in temperature depends on the volume of tissue through which the current passes, the resistance of the tissues, and the strength of the current. The stronger the current, the greater the rise in temperature. If one contact is made large, the heat is dissipated over a wide area and the rise of temperature is insignificant. This is the earth or neutral electrode and under this the rise in temperature is only 1 or 2°C. The working electrode or diathermy loop is thin so that the current density is maximal and, therefore, so is the heating effect.

When a direct current is switched on or off, nerves are stimulated and muscles will twitch. If the switching on and off is rapid enough, there is the sustained contraction familiar to the physiology class as the 'tetanic contraction'. If a high-frequency alternating current is used (300 kHz to 5 MHz), there is no time for the cell membranes of nerve or muscle to become depolarized, and nerves and muscles are not stimulated (they are stimulated at lower frequencies).

The effect of the diathermy current on the tissues depends on the heat that is generated under the diathermy loop. At relatively low temperatures, coagulation and distortion of small blood vessels occurs. If the current is increased to raise the temperature further, water within cells vaporizes and the cells explode. This explosive vaporization literally cuts the tissues apart.

Bipolar diathermy

Bipolar diathermy involves the passage of electrical current between two electrodes on the same hand piece. It is inherently safer than monopolar diathermy, since the current does not pass through the patient, and diathermy burns cannot therefore occur.

Potential problems with diathermy

The diathermy isn't working

- Do not increase the current
- Check that the irrigating fluid is glycine (sodium chloride conducts electricity causing the diathermy to short-circuit)
- Check that the diathermy plate is making good contact with the skin of the patient
- Check that the lead is undamaged
- Check that the resectoscope loop is securely fixed to the contact.

Modern diathermy machines have warning circuits which sound an alarm when there is imperfect contact between the earth plate and the patient.

Diathermy burns

If current returns to earth through a small contact rather than the broad area of the earth pad, then the tissues through which the current passes will be heated just like those under the cutting loop. If the pad is making good contact, the current will find it easier to run to earth through the pad and no harm will arise, even when there is accidental contact with some metal object. The real danger arises when the diathermy pad is not making good contact with the patient. It may not be plugged in or its wire may be broken. Under these circumstances the current must find its way to earth somehow, and any contact may then become the site of a dangerous rise in temperature.

Pacemakers and implantable cardioverter defibrillators (ICDs) and the use of diathermy

See Box 17.1 for diathermy problems and their prevention.

Box 17.1 Pacemakers, ICDs and diathermy: problems and their prevention

Diathermy can cause electrical interference of a pacemaker or ICD, leading to inhibition, triggering of electrical output from the device, reprogramming, asynchronous pacing, damage to the circuitry of the device or triggering of defibrillator discharge. An electrical current can also be induced in the pacemaker or ICD leads, which can, in turn, cause tissue heating leading to myocardial damage.

- **Pacemaker inhibition:** the high frequency of diathermy current may simulate the electrical activity of myocardial contraction so the pacemaker can be inhibited. If the patient is pacemaker-dependent, the heart may stop
- **Phantom reprogramming:** the diathermy current may also simulate the radiofrequency impulse by which the pacemaker can be reprogrammed to different settings. The pacemaker may then start to function in an entirely different mode
- **The internal mechanism of the pacemaker** may be damaged by the diathermy current if this is applied close to the pacemaker
- **Ventricular fibrillation:** if the diathermy current is channelled along the pacemaker lead, ventricular fibrillation may be induced
- **Myocardial damage:** another potential effect of channelling of the diathermy current along the pacemaker lead is burning of the myocardium at the tip of the pacemaker lead. This can subsequently result in ineffective pacing.

It was formerly recommended that a magnet was placed over the pacemaker to overcome pacemaker inhibition and to make the pacemaker function at a fixed rate. This can, however, result in phantom reprogramming. For demand pacemakers, it is better to programme the pacemaker to a fixed rate (as opposed to demand pacing) for the duration of the operation. Consult the patient's cardiologist for advice.

Other precautions

- The patient plate should be sited so that the current path does not go right through the pacemaker. Ensure that the indifferent plate is correctly applied, as an improper connection can cause grounding of the diathermy current through the ECG monitoring leads, and this can affect pacemaker function. The indifferent plate should be placed as close as possible to the pacemaker (e.g. over the thigh or buttock).
- The diathermy machine should be placed well away from the pacemaker and should certainly not be used within 15 cm of it
- The heartbeat should be continually monitored, and a defibrillator and external pacemaker should be at hand
- Try to use short bursts of diathermy at the lowest effective output
- Use bipolar diathermy in preference to monopolar (not practical for many urological procedures, where the only form of diathermy that can be used is monopolar)
- Give antibiotic prophylaxis (as for patients with artificial heart valves)
- Because the pacemaker-driven heart will not respond to fluid overload in the normal way, the resection should be as quick as possible, and fluid overload should be avoided.

Box 17.1 Pacemakers, ICDs and diathermy: problems and their prevention (continued)

Further reading

Allen M. (2006) Pacemakers and implantable cardioverter defibrillators. *Anaesthesia* **62:**852–3.

Medicines and Healthcare Products Regulatory Agency (2006) *Guidelines for the perioperative management of patients with implantable cardioverter defibrillators, where the use of diathermy is anticipated.* Available at: http://www.mhra.gov.uk

Salukhe TV, Dob D, Sutton R. (2004) Pacemakers and defibrillators: anaesthetic implications. *Br J Anaesth* **93:**95–104.

Sterilization of urological equipment

Techniques for sterilization

Autoclaving: modern cystoscopes and resectoscopes, including components such as light leads, are autoclavable. Standard autoclave regimens heat the instruments to 121°C for 15 min or 134°C for 3 min.

Chemical sterilization: this involves soaking instruments in an aqueous solution of chlorine dioxide (Tristel), an aldehyde-free chemical (there has been a move away from formaldehyde because of health and environmental concerns). Chlorine dioxide solutions kill bacteria, viruses (including HIV and hepatitis B and C), spores, and mycobacteria.

Cameras cannot be autoclaved. Use a camera sleeve or sterilize camera between cases in solutions such as Tristel.

Sterilization and prion diseases

Variant CJD (vCJD) is a neurodegenerative disease caused by a prion protein (PrP). Other examples of neurodegenerative prion diseases include classic CJD, kuru, sheep scrapie, and bovine spongiform encephalopathy (BSE). Variant CJD and BSE are caused by the same prion strain and represent a classic example of cross-species transmission of a prion disease.

There has been much recent concern about the potential for transmission of vCJD between patients via contaminated surgical instruments. Classic CJD may be transmitted by neurosurgical and other types of surgical instruments because normal hospital sterilization procedures do not completely inactivate prions.[1] It is not possible at present to quantify the risks of transmission of prion diseases by surgical instruments. To date, iatrogenic CJD remains rare, with 267 cases having been reported worldwide up to 2000.[2]

The risk of transmission of CJD may be higher with procedures performed on organs containing lymphoreticular tissue, such as tonsillectomy and adenoidectomy, because vCJD targets these tissues and is found in high concentrations there. For this reason there was a move towards the use of disposable, once-only-use instruments for procedures such as tonsillectomy. However, these instruments have been associated with a higher post-operative haemorrhage rate[3] and, as a consequence, ENT departments in the UK are no longer obliged to use disposable instruments.

In the UK, the Advisory Committee on Dangerous Pathogens and Spongiform Encephalopathy[4] provides advice on appropriate methods of cleaning and sterilization of surgical instruments. Prions are particularly resistant to conventional chemical (ethylene oxide, formaldehyde, and chlorine dioxide) and standard autoclave regimens, and dried blood or tissue remaining on an instrument could harbour prions that will not then be killed by the sterilization process. Once proteinaceous material such as blood or tissue has dried on an instrument, it is very difficult to subsequently be sure that the instrument has been sterilized. Sterilization should include:

- **Pre-sterilization cleaning**: initial low-temperature washing (<35°C) with detergents and an ultrasonic cleaning system removes and prevents coagulation of prion proteins—sonic cleaners essentially 'shake' attached material from the instrument
- **Hot wash**

- **Air drying**
- **Thermal sterilization:** longer autoclave cycles at 134–137°C for at least 18 min (or 6 successive cycles with holding times of 3 min) or 1h at conventional autoclave temperatures may result in a substantial reduction in the level of contamination with prions.

The latest models of pre-sterilization cleaning devices—automated thermal washer disinfectors—perform all of these cleaning tasks within one unit.

Enzymatic proteolytic inactivation methods are under development.

1   Collinge J (1999) Variant Creutzfeldt-Jakob disease. *Lancet* **354**:317–23.

2   Collins SJ, Lawson VA, Masters CL (2004) Transmissible spongiform encephalopathies. *Lancet* **363**:51–61.

3   Nix P (2003) Prions and disposable surgical instruments. *Int J Clin Pract* **57**:678–80.

4   The Advisory Committee on Dangerous Pathogens and Spongiform Encephalopathy (1998) *Transmissible spongiform encephalopathy agents: safe working and the prevention of infection.* London: HM Stationery Office.

Telescopes and light sources in urological endoscopy

There are 3 types of modern urological telescopes—rigid, semi-rigid, and flexible. These endoscopes may be used for inspection of the urethra and bladder (cystosco-urethroscopes—usually simply called cystoscopes), the ureter and collecting system of the kidney (ureteroscopes and ureter-orenoscopes), and, via a percutaneous access track, the kidney (nephroscopes). The light sources and image transmission systems are based on the innovative work of Professor Harold Hopkins, from the University of Reading.

The Hopkins rod-lens system

Introduced by Professor Harold Hopkins in 1959. The great advance in telescope design was the development of the rod-lens telescope, which replaced the conventional system of glass lens with rods of glass, separated by thin air spaces which, essentially, were air lenses (Fig. 17.13). By changing the majority of the light transmission medium from air to glass, the quantity of light that could be transmitted was doubled. The rods of glass were also easier to handle during manufacture, and therefore their optical quality was greater.

The angle of view of the telescope can be varied by placing a prism behind the objective lens. 0°, 12°, 30°[1] and 70° scopes are available.

Lighting

Modern endoscopes (urological and those used to image the gastrointestinal tract) use fibre optic light bundles to transmit light to the organ being inspected (developed by Karl Storz). Each glass fibre is coated with glass of a different refractive index, so that light entering at one end is totally internally reflected and emerges at the other (Fig. 17.14). These fibre optic bundles can also be used for image (as well as light) transmission, as long as the arrangement of the fibres at either end of the instrument is the same (co-ordinated fibre bundles are not required for simple light transmission). The fibre bundles are tightly bound together only at their end (for coordinated image transmission). In the middle, the bundles are not bound—this makes the instrument flexible (e.g. flexible cystoscope and flexible ureteroscope).

Digital image capture systems

Conventional analog camera systems have a 3-chip camera with separate sensors for red, green, and blue colours. They convert analog data into digital data for image storage and enhancement. Image distortion can reduce image quality (a 'spectrum' effect can occur—bands of red, green, and blue across the image). A recent innovation in scope design is chip miniaturization, which allows these sensors to be placed at the tip of the flexible cystoscope or flexible ureteroscope, so allowing a totally digital imaging system (as in a digital camera). The resolution and image quality is superior to analog systems.

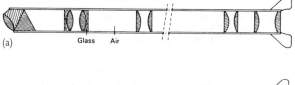

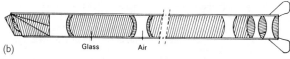

Fig. 17.13 (a) Diagram of conventional cystoscope. The glass lenses are held in place by metal spacers and separated by air spaces. (b) Rod-lens telescope with 'lenses' of air, separated by 'spaces' of glass, with no need for metal spacers. (From Blandy and Fowler 1996, reproduced with permission[2])

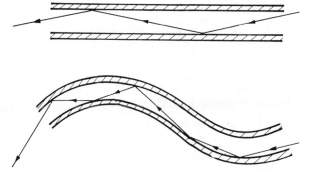

Fig. 17.14 Total internal reflection permits light to travel along a flexible glass fibre. (From Blandy and Fowler 1996, reproduced with permission from Wiley Blackwell[2])

1 In days gone by, when a tiny lamp at the end of the telescope was used for illumination, it was necessary to have a slightly angled line of vision otherwise the light bulb got in the way of the view. The 30° scope is a throw back to this historical requirement.

2 Blandy J, Fowler C (1995) *Urology*. Oxford: Blackwell Science, pp. 3–5.

Consent: general principles

Consent is required before you examine, treat, or care for a competent adult (a person aged 16 or more).

Think of obtaining consent as a *process* rather than an *event*. In order to give consent a patient must understand the nature, purpose, and likely effects (outcomes, risks) of the treatment. From the information they receive, the patient must be able to weigh up the risks against benefits, and so arrive at an informed choice. They must not be coerced into making a decision (e.g. by the doctor in a hurry). Giving the patient time to reach a decision is a good way of avoiding any accusation that they were pressured into a decision. To reiterate—think of consent as a process, rather than an event.

Giving information and level of disclosure

How much information should you give? What options and risks should you mention? The adequacy of your consent will be judged against the Bolam test: 'A doctor is not guilty of negligence if he acted in accordance with a practice accepted by a responsible body of medical men skilled in that particular art'. (That body of medical men must be a competent and reasonable body and the opinion expressed must have a logical basis—the **Bolitho** modification of the **Bolam** defence.)

You have a duty to discuss the range of treatment options available (the alternatives) regardless of their cost, in a form the patient can understand, and the side-effects and risks that are relevant to the individual patient's circumstances.

A risk is defined as a material one (one that matters, one that is important) if a reasonable person in the patient's circumstances, if warned of that risk, would attach significance to it (e.g. loss of the tip of a little finger may be of little long-term consequence to many people, but for the concert pianist it could be a disaster). In the words of Lord Scarman disclosure is necessary:

"... where the risk is such that in the court's view a prudent person in the patient's situation would have regarded it as significant."

Thus, the amount and type of information you give is different in every case. Just because there is a less than 1 in 100 chance of a particular risk materializing, does not mean you need not warn about this particular risk:

"When one refers to a 'significant risk', it is not possible to talk in precise percentages. (Lord Woolf in *Pearce v United Bristol HA* 1996)[1]"

The obvious example is the need to warn of post-vasectomy pregnancy, which occurs very infrequently (1:3000 cases). Failure to warn of such a risk would nowadays be regarded as substandard care.

Remember, it can be argued that the consent was not valid because the amount of information you gave was not enough or was in a form the patient could not understand.

---

1 Pearce and another v. United Bristol Healthcare NHS Trust, 48 *BMLR* 118. 1996.

Recording

Remember, record the consent discussion in the notes. If you do not record what you said, you might as well not bother saying it. If a patient later claims that they were not told of a particular risk or outcome, it will be difficult to refute this if your notes do not record what you said. Writing 'risks explained' is inadequate. When cases do come to court, this is usually several years after the events in question. You will have forgotten precisely what you said to the patient and it will not take much effort on the part of a barrister to suggest that you might not have said everything that you thought you said! If you give a written information sheet, record that you have done so and put a copy of the version you gave in the notes.

The consent form

The consent form is designed to record the patient's decision and, to some extent, the discussions that took place during the consent process (although the space available for recording the discussion, even on the new NHS consent form, is limited). It is not proof that the patient was properly informed—that valid consent was obtained. Avoid, if possible, technical abbreviations, such as TURBT. A patient could reasonably claim not to have understood what this was. Try to avoid standing over the patient waiting for them to sign the form. It is a good practice to leave the form with them and to return after a few minutes—they will feel less pressured and can ask further questions if they wish.

Children

Children aged less than 16 may give consent as long as they fully understand what is involved in the proposed examination or treatment (a parent cannot override the competent child's consent to treatment). However, a child cannot *refuse* consent to treatment (i.e. a parent can override a child's refusal to consent—the parent can consent on the child's behalf if the child refuses consent, although such situations are rare).

Cystoscopy

A basic skill of the urologist. Allows direct visual inspection of the urethra and bladder.

Indications

- Haematuria
- Irritative LUTS (marked frequency and urgency) where intravesical pathology is suspected (e.g. carcinoma *in situ*, bladder stone)
- For bladder biopsy
- Follow-up surveillance of patients with previously diagnosed and treated bladder cancer
- Retrograde insertion of ureteric stents and removal
- Cystoscopic removal of stones.

Technique

- **Flexible cystoscopy:** flexible cystoscope is easily passed down the urethra and into the bladder following instillation of lubricant gel (with or without local anaesthetic—a meta-analysis of 9 RCTs showed no difference in pain control between lidocaine gel and plain gel lubrication[11]). Principally diagnostic, but small biopsies can be taken with a flexible biopsy forceps, small tumours can be fulgurated (with a diathermy probe) or vaporized (with a laser fibre), and JJ stents can be inserted and removed using this type of cystoscope
- **Rigid cystoscopy:** rigid, metal instrument, which can be passed under local anaesthetic in women (short urethra), but usually requires general anaesthetic. Preferred over flexible cystoscopy where deeper biopsies will be required or as an antecedent to TURBT or cystolitholapxy where it is anticipated that other pathology will be found (tumour, stone).

The flexible cystoscope uses fibre optics for illumination and image transmission. It can be deflected through 270°.

Common post-operative complications and their management

Mild burning discomfort and haematuria are common after both flexible and rigid scopy. It usually resolves within hours. Bacteriuria after flexible cystoscopy occurs in about 8–9% of patients (4–5% have bacteriuria before cystoscopy) and this rate is reduced by prophylactic antibiotics (🕮 see Table 17.1, p. 672).

BAUS procedure specific consent form: recommended discussion of adverse events

Serious or frequently occurring complications of flexible cystoscopy

Warn the patient that if the cystoscopy is being done because of haematuria, it is possible that a bladder cancer may be found, which may require further treatment. You should specifically seek consent for biopsy (removal of tissue if an abnormality is found).

Common
- Mild burning or bleeding on passing urine for a short period after operation
- Biopsy of an abnormal area in the bladder may be required.

Occasional
Infection of bladder requiring antibiotics.

Rare
- Temporary insertion of a catheter
- Delayed bleeding requiring removal of clots or further surgery
- Injury to urethra causing delayed scar formation (a stricture).

Serious or frequently occurring complications of rigid cystoscopy
- As for flexible cystoscopy
- The use of heat (diathermy) may be required to cauterize biopsy sites
- Very rarely, perforation of the bladder can occur requiring temporary insertion of a catheter or open surgical repair.

1 Patel AR, Jones JS, Babineau D (2008). Lidocaine 2% gel versus plain lubricating gel for pain reduction during flexible cystoscopy: a meta-analysis of prospective, randomized controlled trials. *J Urol* **179**:986–90.

Transurethral resection of the prostate (TURP)

Indications

- Bothersome LUTS, which fail to respond to changes in life style or medical therapy
- Recurrent acute urinary retention
- Renal impairment due to bladder outlet obstruction (high pressure *chronic* urinary retention)
- Recurrent haematuria due to benign prostatic enlargement
- Bladder stones due to prostatic obstruction.

Post-operative care

A 3-way catheter is left *in situ* after the operation, through which irrigation fluid (normal saline) is run to dilute the blood so that a clot will not form to block the catheter. The rate of inflow of the saline is adjusted to keep the outflow a pale pink rosé colour and, as a rule, the rate of inflow can be cut down after about 20 min. The irrigation is continued for 12–24 h. The catheter is removed the day after (2nd post-operative day) if the urine has cleared to a normal colour [trial without catheter (TWOC) or trial of void (TOV)].

Common post-operative complications and their management

Blocked catheter post TURP

Common

The catheter may become blocked with clot or a prostatic 'chip', which was inadvertently left in the bladder at the end of the operation.

- Apply a bladder syringe to the end of the catheter to try to dislodge the obstruction
- If this fails, withdraw some irrigant into the syringe and flush the catheter
- If this fails, change the catheter. The obstructing chip of prostate may be found stuck in one of the eyeholes of the catheter
- Pass a new catheter, on an introducer.

If the bladder has been allowed to become so full of clot that a simple bladder washout is unable to evacuate it all, return the patient to the theatre for clot evacuation.

Haemorrhage

Minor bleeding after TURP is common and will stop spontaneously. A simple system to allow communication between staff is to describe the colour of the urine draining through the catheter as the same as a rosé wine (minor haematuria), a dark red wine (moderate haematuria), or frank blood (bright red bleeding, suggesting serious haemorrhage). The rosé urine requires no action. Dark red urine should be managed by increasing the flow of irrigant and by applying gentle traction to the catheter (with the balloon inflated to 40–50 mL), thereby pulling it onto the bladder neck or into the prostatic fossa to tamponade bleeding for 20 min or so. This will usually result in the urine clearing. An attempt at controlling heavier bleeding by these techniques may be tried, but at the same time you should make preparations to return the patient to theatre because it is unlikely that bleeding of this degree will stop. The bleeding vessel(s), if seen, is controlled with diathermy. If bleeding persists, open surgical control is required—the prostatic capsule is opened, the bleeding vessels sutured, and the prostatic bed packed. Post-operative bleeding requiring a return to theatre occurs in 0.5% of cases.[1]

BAUS procedure specific consent form—recommended discussion of adverse events

Serious or frequently occurring complications of TURP

- Temporary mild burning on passing urine, urinary frequency, haematuria
- Retrograde ejaculation in 75% of patients
- Failure of symptom resolution
- Permanent inability to achieve an erection adequate for sexual activity
- UTI requiring antibiotic therapy
- 10% of patients require re-do surgery for recurrent prostatic obstruction
- Failure to pass urine after the post-operative catheter has been removed
- In 10% of patients prostate cancer is found on subsequent pathological examination of the resected tissue
- Urethral stricture formation requiring subsequent treatment
- Incontinence (loss of urinary control)—may be temporary or permanent
- Absorption of irrigating fluid causing confusion and heart failure (TUR syndrome)
- Very rarely, perforation of the bladder requiring a temporary urinary catheter or open surgical repair.

Alternative therapy: observation, drugs, catheter, stent, laser prostatectomy, open operation.

1   Emberton M, *et al.* (1995) The National Prostatectomy Audit: the clinical management of patients during hospital admission. *Br J Urol* **75**:301–16.

Transurethral resection of bladder tumour (TURBT)

Indications
- Local control of non-muscle-invasive bladder cancer (i.e. stops bleeding tumours)
- **Staging of bladder cancer:** to determine whether the cancer is non-muscle-invasive or muscle-invasive, so that subsequent treatment and appropriate follow-up can be arranged.

Post-operative care
A 2- or 3-way catheter is left *in situ* after the operation, depending on the size of the tumour and, therefore, on the likelihood that bleeding requiring irrigation will be required. As for TURP, normal saline is run through the catheter to dilute the blood so that a clot will not form to block the catheter. It is particularly important to avoid catheter blockage post TURBT, since this could lead to distension of the bladder already weakened by resection of a tumour. The period of irrigation is usually shorter than that required after TURP and for small tumours the catheter may be removed the day after the TURBT. For larger tumours, remove it 2 days later.

Common operative and post-operative complications and their management

Bladder perforation during TURBT
Small perforations into the perivesical tissues (extraperitoneal) are not uncommon when resecting small tumours of the bladder, and so long as you have secured good haemostasis and all the irrigating fluid is being recovered, no additional steps are required except that perhaps one should leave the catheter in for 4, rather than 2 days.

Intraperitoneal perforations (through the wall of the bladder, through the peritoneum, and into the peritoneal cavity) are uncommon, but far more serious.

Is it an extraperitoneal or intraperitoneal perforation? Establishing this can be difficult. Both can cause marked distension of the lower abdomen—an intraperitoneal perforation by allowing escape of irrigating solution directly into the abdominal cavity, and an extraperitoneal perforation by expanding the retroperitoneal space, with fluid then diffusing directly into the peritoneal cavity. The fact that a suspected intraperitoneal perforation was actually extraperitoneal becomes apparent only at laparotomy when no hole can be found in the peritoneum overlying the bladder (the peritoneum over the bladder is *not* breached in an extraperitoneal perforation).

When there is no abdominal distension, the volume of extravasated fluid is likely to be low and, if the perforation is small, it is reasonable to manage the case conservatively. Achieve haemostasis and pass a catheter. Make frequent post-operative assessments of the patient's vital signs and abdomen (worsening abdominal pain, distension, and tenderness suggest the need for laparotomy).

Where there is marked abdominal distension, whether the perforation is extraperitoneal or intraperitoneal, explore the abdomen, principally to drain the large amount of fluid (which can compromise respiration in an elderly patient) by splinting the diaphragm, but also to check that loops of bowel adjacent to the site of perforation have not been injured at the same time. Failing to make the diagnosis of an intraperitoneal perforation, particularly if bowel has been injured, is a worse situation to be in than performing a laparotomy for a suspected intraperitoneal perforation but then finding that the perforation was 'only' extraperitoneal.

Open bladder repair: Pfannenstiel incision or lower midline abdominal incision, open the bladder, evacuate the clot, control bleeding, and repair the hole. Open the peritoneum, and inspect small and large bowel for perforations. Leave a urethral catheter and a drain in place.

Blocked catheter post TURBT

The catheter may become blocked with clot. Use the same technique for unblocking it as for TURP, but avoid vigorous washouts of the bladder because of the risk of bladder perforation.

Haemorrhage

Minor bleeding after TURBT is common and will stop spontaneously. The only 'technique' for controlling it is to ensure that an adequate flow of irrigant is maintained (to dilute the blood and thereby prevent clots from forming). If bleeding persists, return the patient to theatre for endoscopic control.

TUR syndrome Uncommon after TURBT, unless the tumour is large and the resection, therefore, long.

BAUS procedure specific consent form—recommended discussion of adverse events

Serious or frequently occurring complications of TURBT

Common complications

- Mild burning on passing urine
- Additional treatment (intravesical chemotherapy or immunotherapy) may be required to reduce the risk of future tumour recurrence
- UTI
- No guarantee of bladder cancer cure
- Tumour recurrence is common.

Rare complications

- Delayed bleeding requiring removal of clots or further surgery
- Damage to drainage tubes from kidney (ureters) requiring additional therapy
- Development of a urethral stricture
- Bladder perforation requiring a temporary urinary catheter or open surgical repair.

Alternative treatment: open removal of bladder; chemotherapy, radiation.

Optical urethrotomy

Indications
- Bulbar urethral stricture
- Also used for penile urethral strictures.

Anaesthesia Regional or general.

Post-operative care
- Leave a catheter for 3–5 days (longer catheterization does not reduce long-term restricturing)
- Consider ISC for 3–6 months, starting several times daily, reducing to once or twice a week towards the end of this period.

Common post-operative complications and their management
- **Septicaemia**
- **Restricturing** is the most common long-term problem occurring after optical urethrotomy.

BAUS procedure specific consent form—recommended discussion of adverse events

Common
- Mild burning on passing urine for short periods of time after operation
- Temporary insertion of a catheter
- Need for self-catheterization to keep the narrowing from closing down again.

Occasional
- Infection of bladder, requiring antibiotics
- Permission for telescopic removal/biopsy of bladder abnormality/stone if found
- Recurrence of stricture necessitating further procedures or repeat incision.

Rare
Decrease in quality of erections, requiring treatment

Alternative therapy: observation, urethral dilatation, open (non-telescopic) repair of stricture.

Circumcision

Indications
- Phimosis
- Recurrent paraphimosis
- Penile cancer confined to the foreskin
- Lesions on the foreskin of uncertain histological nature.

Contraindications
- In neonates hypospadias, chordee with hypospadias, microphallus
- In all patients – bleeding diatheses.

Circumcision in HIV prevention
Male circumcision has a significant protective effect against HIV infection.[1,2] This is thought to be due to the presence of large numbers of HIV binding target cells being present on the inner layer of the prepuce compared to the glans and outer prepuce (which is lined by squamous epithelium).

Clearly, mass circumcision programmes in Africa and other high risk areas, would be a huge task. In addition, concerns have been expressed that this beneficial effect will be negated by increased behaviour that increases HIV risk (e.g. a drop in condom use, a rise in sexual partners).

Anaesthesia Local or general.

Post-operative care
A non-adhesive dressing may be applied to the end of the penis, but this is difficult to keep on for more than an hour or two, and is unnecessary. Warn the patient that the penis may be bruised and swollen after the operation, but that this resolves spontaneously over a week or two. Sexual intercourse or masturbation should be avoided until the absorbable skin sutures have dissolved.

Common post-operative complications and their management
You might think that circumcision is about as simple an operation as you can get, but it can cause both the patient (or in the case of little boys, their parents) and you considerable concern if the cosmetic result is not what was expected, or if 'complications' occur about which the patient was not warned. As with any procedure, it should be performed with care and with the potential complications always in mind so that steps can be taken to avoid these. If complications do occur, manage them appropriately.

Haemorrhage
Most frequently occurs from the frenular artery on the ventral surface of the penis. If local pressure does not stop the bleeding (and if it is from the frenular artery, it usually won't), return the patient to theatre and, either under ring-block local anaesthesia or general anaesthetic, suture ligature the bleeding vessel. Be careful not to place the suture through the urethra!

Necrosis of the skin of the shaft of the penis

In most cases of suspected skin necrosis, there is none. Not infrequently, a crust of coagulated blood develops around the circumference of the penis after circumcision. As blood oxidizes it turns black and this appearance can be mistaken for necrosis of the end of the penis. Reassurance of the patient (and the referring doctor!) is all that is needed. If necrosis has occurred because, for example, adrenaline was used in the local anaesthetic, wait for the necrotic tissue to demarcate before assessing the extent of the problem. The penis has a superb blood supply and has remarkable healing characteristics.

Separation of the skin of the coronal sulcus from the shaft skin

If limited to a small area this will heal spontaneously. If a larger circumference of the wound has 'dehisced', resuture in theatre.

Wound infection: rare.

Urethrocutaneous fistula: due to haemostatic sutures (placed to control bleeding from the frenular) passing through the urethra; the wound later breaking down.

Urethral damage: due to a stitch placed through the urethra as the frenular artery is suture ligatured.

Excessive removal of skin

Re-epithelialization can occur if the defect between the glans and the shaft skin is not too great. If the defect is too great, the end result will be a buried penis—the glans retracts towards the skin at the base of the penis.

BAUS procedure specific consent form—recommended discussion of adverse events

Serious or frequently occurring complications of circumcision

- Bleeding of the wound occasionally needing a further procedure
- Infection of incision requiring further treatment
- Permanent altered sensation of the penis
- Persistence of absorbable stitches after 3–4 weeks, requiring removal
- Scar tenderness, rarely long-term
- You may not be completely cosmetically satisfied
- Occasional need for removal of excessive skin at a later date
- Permission for biopsy of abnormal area of glans if malignancy a concern.

Alternative therapy: drugs to relieve inflammation, leave uncircumcised.

1   Bailey RC, Moses S, Parker CB, et al. (2007) Male circumcision for HIV prevention in young men in Kisumu, Kenya: a randomized controlled trial. *Lancet* **369**:643–56.

2   Gray RH, Kigozi G, Serwadda D, et al. (2007) Male circumcision for HIV prevention in men in Rakai, Uganda: a randomised trial. *Lancet* **369**:657–66.

Hydrocele and epididymal cyst removal

Hydrocele repair (removal)

Indications: primary (idiopathic) hydrocele repair; not indicated for secondary hydrocele repair.

Anaesthesia: local or general.

Techniques
- **Lord's plication technique:** for small- to medium-sized hydroceles (minimal interference with surrounding scrotal tissues, which minimizes risk of post-operative haematoma)
- **Jaboulay procedure:** for large hydroceles. Excision of hydrocele sac.

Hydrocele aspiration
Strict attention to asepsis is vital, since introduction of infection into a closed space could lead to abscess formation. Avoid superficial blood vessels (if you hit them, a large haematoma can result).

Post-operative care: nothing specific

Post-operative complications and their management
- **Scrotal swelling:** resolves spontaneously
- **Haematoma formation:** if it is large, surgical drainage is best performed, as spontaneous resolution may take many weeks. It can be difficult to identify the bleeding vessel. Leave a small drain to prevent re-accumulation of the haematoma
- **Hydrocele recurrence.**

Epididymal cyst removal (spermatocelectomy)
- Avoid in young men who wish to maintain fertility, since epididymal obstruction can occur
- An alternative to surgical removal is aspiration, though recurrence is usual.

BAUS procedure specific consent form: recommended discussion of adverse events

Hydrocele removal
Occasional
- Recurrence of fluid collection can occur
- Collection of blood around the testes that resolves slowly or requires surgical removal
- Possible infection of incision or testis requiring further treatment.

Alternative therapy
- Observation
- Removal of fluid with a needle.

Epididymal cyst removal

Occasional

- Recurrence of fluid collection can occur
- Collection of blood around the testes that resolves slowly or requires surgical removal
- Possible infection of incision or testis requiring further treatment.

Rare

Scarring can damage the epididymis causing subfertility.

Alternative therapy: observation; removal of fluid with a needle.

Nesbit's procedure

Penile straightening procedure for correcting penile curvature. Wait for at least 6 months after the patient has experienced no more pain, and wait for the penile curvature to stabilize (there is no point in repairing the curvature if it is still progressing).

Indications Peyronie's disease

Anaesthesia Local or general

Post-operative care Avoid intercourse for 2 months. Oedema can be managed with cold compresses.

BAUS procedure specific consent form: recommended discussion of adverse events

Serious or frequently occurring complications
Common
- Some shortening of the penis
- Possible dissatisfaction with the cosmetic or functional result
- Temporary swelling and bruising of the penis and scrotum.

Occasional
- Circumcision is sometimes required as part of the procedure
- There is no guarantee of total correction of the bend
- **Bleeding or infection:** may require further treatment.

Rare
- Impotence or difficulty maintaining an erection
- Nerve injury with temporary or permanent numbness of penis.

Alternative treatment: Observation, drugs, other surgical procedures.

Vasectomy and vasovasostomy

Vasectomy

This is the removal of a section of the vas deferens from each side with the aim of achieving infertility.

Indications: a method of birth control.

Anaesthesia: local or general.

Post-operative care and common post-operative complications, and their management

Post-operative haematoma can occur. If large, evacuation may be required. Infection can occur, but is usually superficial. Two semen samples are required, usually at 10 and 12 weeks post-vasectomy, before unprotected intercourse can take place. Viable sperm can remain distal to the site of vasectomy (in the distal vas deferens or seminal vesicles) for some weeks after vasectomy, and even longer. Occasionally a persistently +ve semen analysis is an indication that the vas was not correctly identified at the time of surgery and has not been ligated (or, very rarely, that there were 2 vas deferens on one side). The potential for fertility remains in those with +ve semen analysis and re-exploration is indicated. Warn the patient that the vas deferens can later recanalize, thereby restoring fertility.

Sperm granuloma: a hard, pea-sized lump in the region of the cut ends of the vas, forming as a result of an inflammatory response to sperm leaking out of the proximal cut end of the vas. It can be a cause of persistent pain, in which case it may have to be excised or evacuated and the vas cauterized or re-ligated.

Vasovasostomy

Vasectomy reversal

Anaesthesia: this tends to be done under general or spinal anaesthesia, as it takes far longer than a vasectomy.

Post-operative care and common post-operative complications, and their management

Much the same as for vasectomy. The patient should avoid sexual intercourse for 2 weeks or so.

Vasectomy: BAUS procedure specific consent form—recommended discussion of adverse events

Serious or frequently occurring complications
Common
- Irreversible
- Small amount of scrotal bruising
- 2 semen samples are required before unprotected intercourse, both of which must show no spermatozoa.

Occasional
Bleeding requiring further surgery or bruising.

Rare

- Inflammation or infection of testis or epididymis, requiring antibiotics
- Rejoining of vas ends resulting in fertility and pregnancy (1 in 2000)
- Chronic testicular pain (5%) or sperm granuloma.

Alternative treatment: other forms of contraception (male or female).

Vasovasostomy: BAUS procedure specific consent form—
recommended discussion of adverse events

Serious or frequently occurring complications
Common

- Small amount of scrotal bruising
- No guarantee that sperm will return to semen
- Sperm may return but pregnancy not always achieved
- If storing sperm, check that appropriate forms have been filled out.

Occasional

Bleeding requiring further surgery

Rare

- Inflammation or infection of testes or epididymis, requiring antibiotics
- Chronic testicular pain (5%) or sperm granuloma.

Alternative therapy: IVF, sperm aspiration, ICSI.

Orchidectomy

Indications

Two types—radical orchidectomy and simple orchidectomy.

Radical (inguinal) orchidectomy

For excision of testicular cancer. This approach is used for 3 reasons:

- To allow ligation of the testicular lymphatics as high as possible as they pass in the spermatic cord and through the internal inguinal ring, thereby removing any cancer cells which might have started to metastasize along the cord
- To allow cross-clamping of the cord prior to manipulation of the testis which, theoretically at least, could promote dissemination of cancer cells along the lymphatics. (In reality, this probably doesn't occur)
- To prevent the potential for dissemination of tumour cells into the lymphatics that drain the scrotal skin that could occur if a scrotal approach is used. These lymphatics drain to inguinal nodes. Thus, direct spread of tumour to scrotal skin and 'violation' of another lymphatic field (the groin nodes) is avoided. Historically, this was important because the only adjuvant therapy for metastatic disease was radiotherapy. The morbidity of groin and scrotal irradiation was not inconsiderable (severe skin reactions to radiotherapy, irradiation of femoral artery and nerve).

Obtain serum markers before surgery (α-foetoprotein, βHCG, and lactic acid dehydrogenase—LDH) and get a CXR. Full staging CT scan wait till after surgery. If the contralateral testis has been removed or is small, offer sperm storage—there is usually time to do this. Warn the patient that, very occasionally, what appears clinically and on ultrasound to be a malignant testis tumour, turns out to be a benign tumour on subsequent histological examination.

Simple orchidectomy

For hormonal control of advanced prostate cancer. Done via a scrotal incision, with ligation and division of the cord and complete removal of the testis and epididymis. Alternatively, a subcapsular orchidectomy may be done, where the tunica of the testis is incised and the seminiferous tubules contained within are excised. There is the potential with this approach to leave a small number of Leydig cells which can continue to produce testosterone.

Anaesthesia Local, regional, general. Few men will require or opt for local.

Post-operative care and common post-operative complications and their management

For both simple and radical orchidectomy: scrotal haematoma. Drain it if large or enlarging or if there are signs of infection (fever, discharge of pus from the wound).

For radical orchidectomy: damage to the ilioinguinal nerve leading to an area of loss of sensation overlying the scrotum.

Orchidectomy ± testicular implant: BAUS procedure specific consent form—recommended discussion of adverse events

Serious or frequently occurring complications

Occasional

- Cancer, if found, may not be cured by orchidectomy alone
- There may be a need for additional surgery, radiotherapy, or chemotherapy
- Loss of future fertility
- Biopsy of contralateral testis may be required if an abnormality is found (small testis or history of maldescent).

Rare

- On pathological examination cancer may not be found, or the pathologic diagnosis may be uncertain
- Infection of incision may occur, requiring further treatment and possibly removal of implant if this has been inserted
- Pain requiring removal of implant
- Cosmetic expectation not always met
- Implant may lie higher in the scrotum than the normal testis did
- A palpable stitch may be felt at one end of the implant
- Long-term risks of silicone implants are not known.

Urological incisions

Midline, transperitoneal

Indications: access to peritoneal cavity and pelvis for radical nephrectomy, cystectomy, reconstructive procedures, etc.

Technique

Divide skin, subcutaneous fat. Divide fascia in midline. Find the midline between the rectus muscles. Dissect the muscles free from the underlying peritoneum. Place 2 clips on either side of the midline, pinch between the two to ensure no bowel has been trapped, elevate the clips, and divide between them with a knife. Extend the incision in the peritoneum up and down, ensuring no bowel is in the way.

Closure: use a non-absorbable (e.g. nylon) or very slowly absorbable (e.g. PDS) suture, using Jenkins rule to reduce risk of dehiscence (suture length 4× wound length).

Specific complications: dehiscence (classically around day 10 post-operatively and preceded by pink serous discharge, then sudden herniation of a bowel through incision).

Lower midline, extraperitoneal

Indications: access to pelvis (e.g. radical prostatectomy, colposuspension).

Technique: divide skin, subcutaneous fat. Divide fascia in midline. Find the midline between the rectus muscles and dissect the muscles free from the underlying peritoneum. If you make a hole in it, repair the defect with vicryl. Divide the fascia posterior to the rectus muscles in the midline, so exposing the extravesical space.

Closure: as for midline, transperitoneal.

Pfannenstiel

Indications: access to pelvis (e.g. colposuspension, open prostatectomy, open cystolithotomy).

Technique: divide the skin 2 cm above the pubis and the tissues down to the rectus sheath which is cut in an arc avoiding the inguinal canal. Apply clips to top flap (and afterwards the bottom flap) and use a combination of scissors and your fingers to separate the rectus muscle from the sheath. For maximum exposure you must elevate the anterior rectus sheath from the recti, cranially to just below the umbilicus and caudally to the pubis. Take care to diathermy a perforating branch of the inferior epigastric artery on each side. Apply 2 Babock's forceps to the inferior belly of the rectus on either side of the midline. Elevate and cut in the midline, the lower part of the fascia (transversalis fascia) between the recti. Separate the recti in the midline (do not divide them).

Closure: tack the divided transversalis fascia together and then close the transversely divided rectus sheath with vicryl.

Supra-12th rib incision

Indications: access to kidneys, renal pelvis, upper ureter.

Technique: make the incision over the tip of the 12th rib through skin and subcutaneous fascia. Palpate the tip of the 12th rib. Make a 3-cm cut with diathermy, through the muscle (latissimus dorsi) overlying the tip of the 12th rib so you come down onto the tip of the 12th rib, and then cut anterior to the tip of the 12th rib, down through external and internal oblique, transversus abdominis, to Gerota's fascia, and the perirenal fat. Sweep anteriorly with a finger to push the peritoneum and intraperitoneal organs out of harm's way. Cut the muscles overlying the rib, cutting centrally along the length of the rib, in so doing avoiding the pleura. Cut with scissors along the top edge of the rib to free the intercostal muscle from the rib—beware the pleura! Insert a Gillie's forceps between the pleura and the overlying intercostal muscle and divide the muscle fibres, so protecting the pleura. Dissect fibres of the diaphragm away from the inner surface of the 12th rib—as you do so the pleura will rise upwards with the detached diaphragmatic fibres, out of harm's way. At the posterior end of the incision feel for the sharp edge of the costovertebral ligament. Insert heavy scissors, with the blades just open, on the top of the rib (to avoid the XIth intercostal nerve) and divide the costovertebral ligament. You should now be on top of Gerota's fascia.

Specific complications
Damage to the pleura: if you make a hole in the pleura, repair it at the end of the operation. Pass a small bore catheter (e.g. Jacques) through the hole, close all the muscle layers, inflate the lung, and then, before closing the skin, remove the catheter.

Complications common to all incisions
Hernia, wound infection, chronic wound pain.

JJ stent insertion

Preparation

Can be done under sedation or general anaesthetic, using either a rigid or flexible cystoscope. The latter is particularly useful for patients who are not fit enough for a general anaesthetic. The technique described below is that used with the flexible cystoscope, but this is essentially the same if using a rigid scope.

With sedation

Oral ciprofloxacin 250 mg; lidocaine gel for urethral anaesthesia and lubrication; sedoanalgesia (diazemuls 2.5–10 mg IV, pethidine 50–100 mg IV). Monitor pulse and oxygen saturation with a pulse oximeter.

Technique

A flexible cystoscope is passed into the bladder and rotated through 180°. This allows greater deviation of the end of the cystoscope and makes identification of the ureteric orifice easier. A 0.9 mm hydrophilic guidewire (Terumo Corporation, Japan) is passed into the ureter under direct vision. The guidewire is manipulated into the renal pelvis using C-arm digital fluoroscopy. The cystoscope is placed close to the ureteric orifice and its position, relative to bony landmarks in the pelvis, is recorded by frame grabbing a fluoroscopic image. The flexible cystoscope is then removed and a 4 Ch ureteric catheter is passed over the guidewire, into the renal pelvis. A small quantity of non-ionic contrast medium is injected into the renal collecting system, to outline its position and to dilate it. The Terumo guidewire is replaced with an ultra-stiff guidewire (Cook UK Ltd, Letchworth, UK) and the 4 Ch ureteric catheter is removed. We use a variety of stent sizes depending on the patient's size (6–8 Ch, 20–26 cm; Boston Scientific Ltd, St Albans, UK). The stent is advanced to the renal pelvis under fluoroscopic control, using a 'pusher' (a hollow tube inserted over the guidewire), checking that the lower end of the stent is not inadvertently pushed up the ureter by checking the position of the ureteric orifice on the previously frame-grabbed image. The guidewire is then removed, while the pusher holds the stent in position (so that the stent is not pulled out along with the wire).

Further reading

Hellawell GO, Cowan NC, Holt SJ, Mutch SJ (2002) A radiation perspective for treating loin pain in pregnancy by double-pigtail stents. *Br J Urol Int* **90**:801–8.

McFarlane J, Cowan N, Holt S, Cowan M (2001) Outpatient ureteric procedures: a new method for retrograde ureteropyelography and ureteric stent placement. *Br J Urol Int* **87**:172–6.

Nephrectomy and nephro-ureterectomy

Indications for nephrectomy

- Renal cell cancer
- Non-functioning kidney containing a staghorn calculus
- Persistent haemorrhage following renal trauma.

Indications for nephro-ureterectomy

Transitional carcinoma of the renal pelvis and/or ureter.

Anaesthesia General

Post-operative care

Nephrectomy

Cardiovascular status and urine output should be carefully monitored in the immediate post-operative period. Haemorrhage from the renal pedicle or, for left-sided nephrectomy, the spleen, is rare, but will present with an increasing tachycardia, cool peripheries, falling urine output, and eventually a drop in blood pressure. A drain is usually not left in place, but if it is there may be excessive drainage of blood from the drain. However, do not be lulled into a false sense of security by the absence of drainage—this does not mean that haemorrhage is not occurring, as the drain may be blocked but haemorrhage may be ongoing.

For nephrectomy via a posterolateral (rib-based) incision, watch for pneumothorax. Arrange a CXR on return from the recovery room. Arrange routine chest physiotherapy to reduce the risk of chest infection. Regular chest examination is important, looking specifically for pneumothorax and pleural effusion.

Mobilize the patient as quickly as possible, to reduce the risk of DVT and PE.

Nephro-ureterectomy

Where the ureter has been excised from the bladder, a urethral catheter is left in place at the end of the procedure, to allow the hole in the bladder to heal. This is usually removed 10–14 days after surgery.

Common post-operative complications and their management

- **Haemorrhage:** see above
- **Wound infection:** rare. If superficial, treat with antibiotics. If an underlying collection of pus is suspected, open the wound to allow free drainage, and pack the wound daily
- **Pancreatic injury:** rare, but would be indicated by excessive drainage of fluid from the drain, if present, which will have a high amylase level. If no drain is present, an abdominal collection will develop, which may be manifested by a prolonged ileus.

BAUS procedure specific consent form: recommended discussion of adverse events

Serious or frequently occurring complications of nephrectomy/nephro-ureterectomy

Simple nephrectomy

Common

- Temporary insertion of a bladder catheter
- Occasional insertion of a wound drain.

Occasional

- Bleeding requiring further surgery or transfusion
- Entry into lung requiring temporary insertion of a drainage tube.

Rare

- Involvement or injury to nearby structures—blood vessels, spleen, lung, liver, pancreas, bowel, requiring further extensive surgery
- Infection, pain, or hernia of incision, requiring further treatment
- Anaesthetic or cardiovascular problems, possibly requiring intensive care admission (including chest infection, pulmonary embolus, stroke, deep vein thrombosis, heart attack).

Alternative therapy: observation, laparoscopic approach

Radical nephrectomy

As above plus:

- **Occasional:** need for further therapy for cancer
- **Rare:** may be an abnormality other than cancer on microscopic analysis
- **Alternative therapy:** observation, embolization, immunotherapy, laparoscopic approach.

Nephro-ureterectomy

As above.

Radical prostatectomy

Indications Localized prostate cancer.

Anaesthesia General or regional.

Post-operative care

Mobilize as quickly as possible and continue subcutaneous heparin and AK-TEDS until discharge, to reduce the risk of DVT and PE. Remove the drains when drainage is minimal. If there is persistent leak of fluid from the drains, send a sample for urea and creatinine, and if it is urine, get a cystogram to determine the size of the leak at the vesico-urethral junction. Urethral catheters are left *in situ* post-radical prostatectomy for a variable time depending on the surgeon who performs the operation. Some surgeons leave a catheter for 3 weeks and others for just 1 week.

Common post-operative complications and their management

Haemorrhage

Managed in the usual way (transfusion; return to theatre where bleeding persists or where there is cardiovascular compromise).

Ureteric obstruction

Usually results from oedema of the bladder, obstructing the ureteric orifices. Retrograde ureteric catheterization is rarely possible (this would require urethral catheter removal and it is difficult to see the ureteric orifices because of the oedema). Arrange placement of percutaneous nephrostomies.

Lymphocele

Drain by radiologically assisted drain placement. If the lymphocele recurs after drain removal, create a window from the lymph collection into the peritoneal cavity so the lymph drains into the peritoneum from which it is absorbed.

Displaced catheter post radical prostatectomy

If the catheter falls out a week after surgery, the patient may well void successfully, and in this situation no further action need be taken. If, however, the catheter inadvertently falls out the day after surgery, gently attempt to replace it with a 12 Ch catheter which has been well lubricated. If this fails, pass a flexible cystoscope, under local anaesthetic, into the bulbar urethra and attempt to pass a guidewire into the bladder, over which a catheter can then safely be passed. If this is not possible, another option is to hope that the patient voids spontaneously and does not leak urine at the site of the anastomosis. An ascending urethrogram may provide reassurance that there is no leak of contrast and that the anastomosis is watertight. If there is a leak or the patient is unable to void, a suprapubic catheter can be placed (percutaneously or under general anaesthetic via an open cystostomy).

Faecal fistula

Due to rectal injury, either recognized and repaired at the time of surgery, and later breaking down, or not immediately recognized. Formal closure is often required.

Contracture at the vesico-urethral anastomosis

Gentle dilatation may be tried. If the stricture recurs, instruct the patient in ISC, in an attempt to keep the stricture open. If this fails, bladder neck incision may be tried.

BAUS procedure specific consent form: recommended discussion of adverse events

Serious or frequently occurring complications of radical prostatectomy

Common

- Temporary insertion of a bladder catheter and wound drain
- High chance of impotence due to unavoidable nerve damage
- No semen is produced during orgasm causing subfertility.

Occasional

- Blood loss requiring transfusion or repeat surgery
- Urinary incontinence—temporary or permanent, requiring pads or further surgery
- Discovery that cancer cells are already outside the prostate needing observation or further treatment at a later date if required including radiotherapy or hormonal therapy.

Rare

- Anaesthetic or cardiovascular problems possibly requiring intensive care admission (including chest infection, pulmonary embolism, stroke, deep vein thrombosis, heart attack)
- Pain, infection, or hernia in area of incision
- Rectal injury, very rarely needing temporary colostomy.

Alternative therapy: watchful waiting, radiotherapy, brachytherapy, hormonal therapy, and perineal or laparoscopic removal.

Radical cystectomy

Indications

- Muscle-invasive bladder cancer
- Adenocarcinoma of bladder (radioresistant)
- Squamous carcinoma of bladder (relatively radioresistant)
- Non-muscle-invasive TCC bladder, which has failed to respond to intravesical chemotherapy or immunotherapy
- Recurrent TCC bladder post radiotherapy.

Combined with urethrectomy if:

- Multiple bladder tumours
- Involvement of bladder neck or prostatic urethra.

Anaesthesia General

Post-operative care and common post-operative complications and their management

Monitor cardiovascular status, urine output, and respiratory status carefully in the first 48 h. Routine chest physiotherapy is started early in the post-operative period to reduce the chance of chest infection. Mobilize the patient as early as possible to minimize the risk of DVT and PE. Drains are removed when they stop draining. Some surgeons prefer to leave them for a week or so, so that late leaks (urine, intestinal contents) will drain via the drain track and not cause peritonitis. Try to remove the nasogastric tube, if used, as soon as possible to assist respiration and reduce the risks of chest infection. The patient usually starts to resume their diet within a week or so. If the ileus is prolonged, start parenteral nutrition.

Haemorrhage: persistent bleeding that fails to respond to transfusion should be managed by re-exploration.

Wound dehiscence: requires resuturing under general anaesthetic.

Ileus: common. Usually resolves spontaneously within a few days.

Small bowel obstruction

From herniation of small bowel through the mesenteric defect created at the junction between the two bowel ends. Continue nasogastric aspiration. The obstruction will usually resolve spontaneously. Re-operation is occasionally required where the obstruction persists or where there are signs of bowel ischaemia.

Leakage from the intestinal anastomosis

Leading to:

- **Peritonitis:** requiring re-operation and repair or refashioning of the anastomosis
- **An enterocutaneous fistula:** bowel contents leak from the intestine and through a fistulous track onto the skin. If low-volume leak (<500 mL/24 h), will usually heal spontaneously. Normal (enteral) nutrition may be maintained until the fistula closes (which usually occurs within a

matter of days or a few weeks). If high-volume, spontaneous closure is less likely and re-operation to close the fistula may be required.

Pelvic abscess

Formal surgical (open) exploration of the pelvis is indicated with drainage of the abscess and careful inspection to see if the underlying cause is a rectal injury, in which case a defunctioning colostomy should be performed.

Partial cystectomy

Indications

Primary, solitary bladder tumours at a site that allows 2cm of normal tissue around it to be removed in a bladder that will have adequate capacity and compliance after operation. There should be:

- No prior history of bladder cancer
- No carcinoma *in situ*
- A solitary muscle-invasive tumour located well away from the ureteral orifices, which includes 2 cm of normal surrounding bladder.

High-grade tumours should not be excluded if these criteria are met. The lesions most commonly amenable to partial cystectomy are G2 or G3 TCCs or adenocarcinomas located on the posterior wall or dome.

Contraindications

Associated carcinoma *in situ*; deeply invasive tumours; tumours at the bladder base (i.e. near the ureteric orifices).

BAUS procedure specific consent form: recommended discussion of adverse events

Serious or frequently occurring complications of radical cystectomy

See also consent for ileal conduit if this is the planned form of urinary diversion.

Common

- Temporary insertion of a nasal tube, drain, and stent
- High chance of impotence (lack of erections) due to unavoidable nerve damage
- No semen is produced during orgasm (dry orgasm) causing subfertility
- Blood loss requiring transfusion or repeat surgery
- In women, pain or difficulty with sexual intercourse due to narrowing or shortening of vagina, and need for removal of uterus and ovaries (causing premature menopause in those who have not reached menopause).

Occasional

- Cancer may not be cured with surgery alone
- Need to remove penile urinary pipe as part of procedure.

Rare

- Infection or hernia of incision, requiring further treatment
- Anaesthetic or cardiovascular problems possibly requiring intensive care admission (including chest infection, pulmonary embolus, stroke, deep vein thrombosis, heart attack)
- Decreased renal function with time.

Very rarely
- Rectal injury, very rarely needing temporary colostomy
- Diarrhoea due to shortened bowel, vitamin deficiency requiring treatment
- Bowel and urine leak, requiring re-operation
- Scarring of bowel or ureters, requiring operation in the future
- Scarring, narrowing, or hernia formation around stomal opening, requiring revision.

Alternative treatment: radiotherapy, neobladder formation, rather than ileal conduit urinary diversion.

Formation of neobladder with bowel
Common: need to perform intermittent self-catheterization if bladder fails to empty.

Ileal conduit

Indications
- For urinary diversion following radical cystectomy
- Intractable incontinence for which anti-incontinence surgery has failed or is not appropriate.

Post-operative care and common post-operative complications and their management

Oliguria or anuria: try a fluid challenge.

Wound infection: treat with antibiotics and wound care. Open the superficial layers of the wound to release pus.

Wound dehiscence: rare. Requires resuturing in theatre under general anaesthetic.

Ileus: common. Usually resolves spontaneously within a few days.

Small bowel obstruction: from herniation of small bowel through the mesenteric defect created at the junction between the two bowel ends. Continue nasogastric aspiration. The obstruction will usually resolve spontaneously. Re-operation is occasionally required where the obstruction persists or where there are signs of bowel ischaemia.

Leakage from the intestinal anastomosis: Leading to:
- **Peritonitis:** requiring re-operation and repair or refashioning of the anastomosis
- **An enterocutaneous fistula:** bowel contents leak from the intestine and through a fistulous track onto the skin. If low-volume leak (<500 mL/24 h), will usually heal spontaneously. Normal (enteral) nutrition may be maintained until the fistula closes (which usually occurs within a matter of days or a few weeks. If high-volume, spontaneous closure is less likely, and re-operation to close the fistula may be required.

Leakage from the uretero-ileal junction
May be suspected because of a persistently high output of fluid from the drain. Test this for urea. Urine will have a higher urea and creatinine concentration than serum. If the fluid is lymph, the urea and creatinine concentration will be the same as that of serum. Arrange a loopgram (conduitogram). This will confirm the leak. Place a soft, small catheter (12 Ch) into the conduit to encourage antegrade flow of urine and assist healing of the uretero-ileal anastomosis. If the leakage continues, arrange bilateral nephrostomies to divert the flow of urine away from the area and encourage wound healing.

Occasionally, a uretero-ileal leak will present as a urinoma (this causes a persistent ileus). Radiologically assisted drain insertion can result in a dramatic resolution of the ileus, with subsequent healing of the uretero-ileal leak.

Hyperchloraemic acidosis
May be associated with obstruction of the stoma at its distal end or from infrequent emptying of the stoma back (leading to back pressure on the

conduit). Catheterize the stoma—this relieves the obstruction. In the long term, the conduit may have to be surgically shortened.

Acute pyelonephritis
Due to the presence of reflux combined with bacteriuria.

Stomal stenosis
The distal (cutaneous) end of the stoma may become narrowed, usually as a result of ischaemia to the distal part of the conduit. Revision surgery is required if this stenosis causes obstruction leading to recurrent UTIs or back pressure on the kidneys.

Parastomal hernia formation
Around the site through which the conduit passes, through the fascia of the anterior abdominal wall. Many hernias can be left alone. The indications for repairing a hernia are:
- Bowel obstruction
- Pain
- Difficulty with applying the stoma bag (distortion of the skin around the stoma by the hernia can lead to frequent bag detachment).

Repair the hernia defect by placing mesh over the hernia site, via an incision sited as far as possible from the stoma itself, so as to reduce the risk of wound infection.

BAUS procedure specific consent form: recommended discussion of adverse events

Serious or frequently occurring complications of ileal conduit formation
Common
- Temporary drain, stents, or nasal tube
- Urinary infections, occasionally requiring antibiotics.

Occasional
- Diarrhoea due to shortened bowel
- Blood loss requiring transfusion or repeat surgery
- Infection or hernia of incision requiring further treatment.

Rare
- Bowel and urine leakage from anastomosis requiring re-operation
- Scarring to bowel or ureters requiring operation in future
- Scarring, narrowing, or hernia formation around urine opening requiring revision
- Decreased renal function with time.

Alternative treatment: catheters, continent diversion of urine.

Percutaneous nephrolithotomy (PCNL)

Indications
- Stones >3 cm in diameter
- Stones that have failed ESWL and/or an attempt at flexible ureteroscopy and laser treatment
- Staghorn calculi.

Pre-operative preparation
- CT scan to assist planning the track position and to identify a retrorenal colon[1]
- Stop aspirin 10 days prior to surgery
- Culture urine (so appropriate antibiotic prophylaxis can be given)
- Cross-match 2 units of blood
- Start IV antibiotics the afternoon before surgery to reduce the chance of septicaemia (many of the stones treated by PCNL are infection stones). If urine is culture −ve, use 1.5 g IV cefuroxime TDS and once daily IV gentamicin (3 mg/kg). Routine antibiotic prophylaxis also reduces the incidence of post-operative UTI.[2]

Post-operative management
Once the stone has been removed, a nephrostomy tube is left *in situ* for several days (Fig. 17.15). This drains urine in the post-operative period and tamponades bleeding from the track. So-called 'tubeless' PCNL (no nephrostomy tube, although a J stent is often inserted, which has a certain morbidity) can be used in select patients (no infection—therefore, not suitable for infection staghorn stones). Less requirement for post-operative analgesia and earlier discharge has been reported.

Complications of PCNL and their management
Bleeding
Some bleeding is inevitable, but that severe enough to threaten life is uncommon. In most cases it is venous in origin and stops following placement of a nephrostomy tube (which compresses bleeding veins in the track). If bleeding persists, clamp the tube for 10 min. If bleeding continues despite this, arrange urgent angiography, looking for an arteriovenous fistula or pseudo-aneurysm, both of which will require selective renal artery embolization (required in 1% of PCNLs[3]) or open exposure of kidney to control bleeding by suture ligation, partial nephrectomy, or nephrectomy.

Septicaemia
Occurs in 1–2% of cases. Incidence is reduced by prophylactic antibiotics. Track damage. Essentially minimal. Cortical loss from track is estimated to be <0.2% of total renal cortex in animal studies.[4]

Colonic perforation
The colon is usually lateral or anterolateral to the kidney and is therefore not usually at risk of injury unless a very lateral approach is made. The colon is retrorenal in 2% of individuals (more commonly in thin females with little retroperitoneal fat[1]). The perforation usually occurs in an extraperitoneal part of the colon, and is managed by JJ stent placement

and withdrawal of the nephrostomy tube into the lumen of the colon to encourage drainage of bowel contents away from that of the urine, thereby encouraging healing without development of a fistula between bowel and kidney. A radiological contrast study a week or so later confirms that the colon has healed and that there is no leak of contrast from the bowel into the renal collecting system.

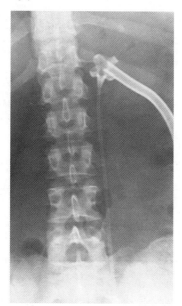

Fig. 17.15 A Malecot catheter, which has wide drainage eyeholes and an extension at the distal end which passes down the ureter to prevent fragments of stone from passing down the ureter.

1   Hopper KD, Sherman JL, Williams MD, *et al.* (1987) The variable anteroposterior position of the retroperitoneal colon to the kidneys. *Invest Radiol* **22**:298–302.

2   Inglis JA, Tolly DA (1988) Antibiotic prophylaxis at the time of percutaneous stone surgery. *J Endourol* **2**:59–62.

3   Martin X (2000) Severe bleeding after nephrolithotomy: results of hyperselective embolisation. *Eur Urol* **37**:136–9.

4   Clayman J (1987) Percutaneous nephrostomy: Assessment of renal damage associated with semi-rigid (24F) and balloon (36F) dilation. *J Urol* **138**:203–6.

Damage to the liver or spleen: very rare in the absence of splenomegaly or hepatomegaly.

Damage to the lung and pleura leading to pneumomothorax or pleural effusion: can occur with supra-12th rib puncture.

Nephrocutaneous fistula

When the nephrostomy tube is removed from the kidney, a few days after surgery, the 1cm incision usually closes within 2 or so. Occasionally, urine continues to drain percutaneously for a few days and a small 'stoma' bag must be worn. In the majority of such cases the urine leak will stop spontaneously, but if it fails to do so after a week or so, place a JJ stent to encourage antegrade drainage of urine.

Outcomes

For small stones, the stone-free rate after PCNL is in the order of 90–95%. For staghorn stones, the stone-free rate of PCNL, when combined with post-op ESWL for residual stone fragments, is in the order of 80–85%.

BAUS procedure specific consent form—recommended discussion of adverse events

Serious or frequently occurring complications of PCNL

Common

- Temporary insertion of a bladder catheter and ureteric stent/kidney tube needing later removal
- Transient haematuria
- Transient temperature.

Occasional

- More than one puncture site may be required
- No guarantee of removal of all stones and need for further operations
- Recurrence of stones.

Rare

- Severe kidney bleeding requiring transfusion, embolization, or, at last resort, surgical removal of kidney
- Damage to lung, bowel, spleen, liver requiring surgical intervention
- Kidney damage or infection needing further treatment
- Over absorption of irrigating fluids into blood system causing strain on heart function.

Alternative treatment: external shock wave treatments, open surgical removal of stones, observation.

Ureteroscopes and ureteroscopy

The instruments

Two types of ureteroscope in common use—the semi-rigid ureteroscope and the flexible ureteroscope.

Semi-rigid ureteroscopes

Have high-density fibre-optic bundles for light ('non-coherently' arranged) and image transmission ('coherently' arranged to maintain image quality). For equivalent light and image transmission using glass rod lenses, thicker lenses are required than with fibre-optic bundles. As a consequence, semi-rigid ureteroscopes can be made smaller, while maintaining the size of the instrument channel. In addition, the instrument can be bent by several degrees without the image being distorted.

The working tip of most current models is in the order of 7–8 Ch, with the proximal end of the scope being in the order of 11–12 Ch. There is usually at least one working channel of at least 3.4 Ch.

Flexible ureteroscopes

The fibre-optic bundles in flexible ureteroscopes are the same as those in semi-rigid scopes, only of smaller diameter. Thus, image quality and light transmission are not as good as with semi-rigid scopes, but are usually adequate.

The working tip of most current models is in the order of 7–8 Ch, with the proximal end of the scope being in the order of 9–10 Ch. There is usually at least one working channel of at least 3.6 Ch.

The great advantage of the flexible ureteroscope over the semi-rigid variety is the ability to perform controlled deflection of the end of the scope (active deflection). Behind the actively deflecting tip of the scope is a segment of the scope which is more flexible than the rest of the shaft. This section is able to undergo passive deflection—when the tip is fully actively deflected, by advancing the scope further, this flexible segment allows even more deflection. Flexible ureteroscopes have recently been developed which have two actively deflecting segments.

Flexible ureteroscopes are intrinsically more intricate and are therefore less durable than semi-rigid scopes.

Ureteroscopic irrigation systems

Normal saline is used (high-pressure irrigation with glycine or water would lead to fluid absorption from pyelolymphatic or venous backflow). Irrigation by gravity pressurization alone (the fluid bag suspended above the patient without any applied pressure) will produce flow that is inadequate for visualization because the long, fine-bore irrigation channels of modern ureteroscopes are inherently high-resistance. Several methods are available—hand-inflated pressure bags, foot pumps, and hand-operated syringe pumps. Whatever system is chosen, use the minimal flow required to allow a safe view so as to avoid flushing the stone out of the ureter and into the kidney, from where you may not be able to retrieve it.

Ureteric dilatation

Some surgeons do, others don't. Those who don't argue that dilatation is unnecessary in the era of modern, small-calibre ureteroscopes. Those who do cite a higher chance of being able to pass the ureteroscope all the way up to the kidney. Ureteric dilatation may be helpful where multiple passes of the ureteroscope up and down the ureter are going to be required for stone removal (alternatively, use a ureteric access sheath). Some surgeons prefer to place two guidewires into the ureter, one to pass the ureteroscope over ('railroading') and the other to act as a safety wire, so that access to the kidney is always possible if difficulties are encountered. The second guidewire is most easily placed via a dual lumen catheter which has a second channel, through which the second guidewire can be easily passed into the ureter, without requiring repeat cystoscopy. This dual lumen catheter has the added function of gently dilating the ureteric orifice to about 10 Ch. There is probably no long-term harm done to the ureter as a consequence of dilatation.[1]

Ureteric access sheaths, which have outer diameters from 10 to 14 Ch, may facilitate access to the ureter and are particularly useful if it is anticipated that the ureteroscope will have to be passed up and down the ureter on multiple occasions (to retrieve fragments of stone). In addition, they facilitate the outflow of irrigant fluid from the pelvis or the kidney, thereby maintaining the field of view and decreasing intra-renal pressures.

Patient position

The patient is positioned as flat as possible on the operating table to 'iron out' the natural curves of the ureter. A cystoscopy is performed with either a flexible or rigid instrument. A retrograde ureterogram can be done to outline pelvicalyceal anatomy. A guidewire is then passed into the renal pelvis. We use a Sensor guidewire (Microvasive, Boston Scientific) which has a 3-cm long floppy, hydrophilic tip which can usually easily be negotiated up the ureter. The remaining length of the wire is rigid and covered in a smooth PTFE. Both properties aid passage of the ureteroscope.

Technique of flexible ureteroscopy and laser treatment for intra-renal stones

Flexible ureteroscopy and laser treatment can be performed with topical urethral local anaesthesia and sedation. However, trying to fragment a moving stone with the laser can be difficult and ideally, therefore, ureteroscopy is most easily done under general anaesthesia with endotracheal intubation (rather than a laryngeal mask) to allow short periods of suspension of respiration and so stop movement of the kidney and its contained stone.

1 Garvin TJ, Clayman RV (1991) Balloon dilation of the ureter for ureteroscopy. *J Urol* **146**:742–5.

Empty the bladder to prevent 'coiling' of the scope in the bladder. Pass the scope over a guidewire. This requires two people—the surgeon holds the shaft of the scope and the assistant applies tension to the guidewire to fix the latter in position without pulling it down. This allows the scope to progress easily up the ureter. The assistant also ensures that acute angulation of the scope where the handle meets the shaft does not occur. The flexible ureteroscope should slide easily up the ureter and into the renal pelvis.

With modern active secondary deflection ureteroscopes, access to most, if not all, parts of the renal collecting system is possible.

Laser lithotripsy

The main draw back of laser lithotripsy is the dust-cloud effect that occurs as the stone is fragmented. This temporarily obscures the view and must be washed away before the laser can safely be re-applied.

The use of stone baskets to retrieve stones after ureteroscopy

The aim of ureterscopy (or flexible ureterorenoscopy) is to remove the ureteric (or renal) stone. It therefore seems intuitive to remove any large fragments—leaving them *in situ* runs the risk of ureteric colic post-ureteroscopy.

To stent or not to stent after ureteroscopy

JJ stent insertion does not increase stone-free rates and is therefore not required in 'routine' cases. A stent should be placed if:
- There has been ureteric injury (e.g. perforation—indicated by extravasation of contrast)
- There are residual stones that might obstruct the ureter
- The patient has had a ureteric stricture that required dilatation
- Solitary kidneys.

Routine stenting after ureteroscopy for distal ureteric calculi is unnecessary.[1] Many urologists will place a stent after ureteroscopy for proximal ureteric stones.

Complications of ureteroscopy

Septicaemia; ureteric perforation requiring either a JJ stent or very occasionally a nephrostomy tube where JJ stent placement is not possible; ureteric stricture (<1%).

Serious or frequently occurring complications of ureteroscopy for treatment of ureteric stones

Common

- Mild burning or bleeding on passing urine for a short period after the operation
- Temporary insertion of a bladder catheter may be required
- Insertion of a stent may be required with a further procedure to remove it
- Urinary infections occasionally requiring antibiotics.

Occasional

- Inability to get stone or movement of stone back into kidney where it is not retrievable
- Kidney damage or infection requiring further treatment
- Failure to pass scope if ureter is narrow
- Recurrence of stones.

Rare

Damage to ureter with need for open operation or placement of a nephrostomy tube into the kidney.

Alternative treatment: open surgery, shock wave therapy, or observation to allow spontaneous passage.

1 Srivastava A, et al. (2003) Routine stenting after ureteroscopy for distal ureteral calculi is unnecessary: results of a randomized controlled trial. *J Endourol* **17**:871.

Pyeloplasty

Indications PUJ obstruction.

Anaesthesia General

Post-operative care

A JJ stent, bladder catheter, and a drain are left *in situ*. The bladder catheter serves to prevent reflux of urine up the ureter, which can lead to increased leakage of urine from the anastomosis site (reflux occurs because of the presence of the JJ stent). The drain is removed when the drain output is minimal. The stent is left in position for ~6 weeks.

Common post-operative complications and their management

Haemorrhage

Usually arising from the nephrostomy track (if a nephrostomy tube has been left in place—some surgeons leave a JJ stent and a perinephric drain, with no nephrostomy). Clamp the nephrostomy tube, in an attempt to tamponade the bleeding. If the bleeding continues, consider angiography and embolization of the bleeding vessel if seen, or exploration.

Urinary leak

This can occur within the first day or so. If a urethral catheter has not been left in place, catheterize the patient, to minimize bladder pressure and therefore the chance of reflux, which might be responsible for the leak. If the drainage persists for more than a few days, shorten the drain—if it is in contact with the suture line of the anastomosis it can keep the anastomosis open, rather than letting it heal. If the leak continues, identify the site of the leak by either a nephrostogram (if a nephrostomy has been left *in situ*) or a cystogram (if a JJ stent is in place—contrast may reflux up the ureter and identify the site of leakage) or an IVU. Some form of additional drainage may help 'dry up' the leak (a JJ stent if only a nephrostomy has been left *in situ*, or a nephrostomy if one is not already in place).

Obstruction at PUJ

This is uncommon, and if it occurs it is usually detected once all the tubes have been removed and a follow-up renogram has been done. If the patient had symptomatic PUJO, but remains asymptomatic, then no further treatment may be necessary. If they develop recurrent flank pain, re-operation may be necessary.

Acute pyelonephritis

Manage with antibiotics.

BAUS procedure specific consent form: recommended discussion of adverse events

Serious or frequently occurring complications of pyeloplasty

Common
- Temporary insertion of a bladder catheter and wound drain
- Further procedure to remove ureteric stent, usually a local anaesthetic.

Occasional
Bleeding requiring further surgery or transfusion.

Rare
- Recurrent kidney or bladder infections
- Recurrence can occur, needing further surgery.

Very rarely
- Entry into lung cavity requiring insertion of temporary drainage tube
- Anaesthetic or cardiovascular problems possibly requiring intensive care admission (including chest infection, pulmonary embolus, stroke, deep vein thrombosis, heart attack)
- Need to remove kidney at a later time because of damage caused by recurrent obstruction
- Infection, pain, or hernia of incision requiring further treatment.

Alternative therapy: observation, telescopic incision, dilation of area of narrowing, temporary placement of plastic tube through narrowing, laparoscopic repair.

Laparoscopic surgery

Virtually every urological procedure can be done laparoscopically. It is particularly suited to surgery in the retroperitoneum (nephrectomy for benign and malignant disease and for kidney donation at transplantation, pyeloplasty for PUJO), but is also suited to pelvic surgery (lymph node biopsy, radical prostatectomy). Reconstructive surgery requiring laparoscopic suturing and using bowel is technically very challenging, but is possible. Laparoscopic surgery offers the advantage over open surgery of:
- Reduced post-operative pain
- Smaller scars
- Less disturbance of bowel function (less post-operative ileus)
- Reduced recovery time and reduced hospital stay.

Contraindications to laparoscopic surgery
- Severe COPD (avoid use of CO_2 for insufflation)
- Uncorrectable coagulopathy
- Intestinal obstruction
- Abdominal wall infection
- Massive haemoperitoneum
- Generalized peritonitis
- Suspected malignant ascites.

Laparoscopic surgery is difficult or potentially hazardous in the morbidly obese (inadequate instrument length, decrease range of movement of instruments, higher pneumoperitoneum pressure required to lift the heavier anterior abdominal wall, excess intra-abdominal fat limiting the view); those with extensive previous abdominal or pelvic surgery (adhesions); previous peritonitis leading to adhesion formation; in those with organomegaly; in the presence of ascites; in pregnancy; in patients with a diaphragmatic hernia; in those with aneurysms.

Potential complications unique to laparoscopic surgery

Gas embolism (potentially fatal), hypercarbia (acidosis affecting cardiac function—e.g. arrhythmias), post-operative abdominal crepitus (subcutaneous emphysema), pneumothorax, pneomomediastinum, pneumopericardium, barotraumas.

Bowel, vessel (aorta, common iliac vessels, IVC, anterior abdominal wall injury), and other viscus injury are not unique to laparoscopic surgery, but are a particular concern during port access. Perforation of small or large bowel is the most common trocar injury. Rarely, the bladder is perforated. Failure to progress with a laparoscopic approach, or vessel injury with uncontrollable haemorrhage requires conversion to an open approach. Post-operatively, bowel may become entrapped in the trocar sites, or there may be bleeding from the sheath site. An acute hydrocele can develop due to irrigation fluid accumulating in the scrotum. It resorbs spontaneously. Scrotal and abdominal wall bruising not uncommonly occurs.

BAUS procedure specific consent forms

For all laparoscopic procedures

Common
- Temporary shoulder tip pain
- Temporary abdominal bloating
- Temporary insertion of a bladder catheter and wound drain.

Occasional
Infection, pain, or hernia of incision requiring further treatment

Rare
- Bleeding requiring conversion to open surgery or transfusion
- Entry into lung cavity requiring insertion of a temporary drainage tube.

Very rarely
- Recognized (and unrecognized) injury to organs or blood vessels requiring conversion to open surgery or deferred open surgery
- Anaesthetic or cardiovascular problems possibly requiring intensive care admission (including chest infection, pulmonary embolus, stroke, deep vein thrombosis, heart attack).

Laparoscopic pyeloplasty

Common
Further procedure to remove ureteric stent, usually under local anaesthesia.

Occasional
- Recurrence can occur needing further surgery
- Short-term success rates are similar to open surgery, but long-term results unknown.

Very rarely
Need to remove kidney at a later time because of damage caused by recurrent obstruction
Alternative therapy: observation, telescopic incision, dilation of area of narrowing, temporary placement of a plastic tube through narrowing, conventional open surgical approach.

Laparoscopic simple nephrectomy

Occasional
Short-term success rates are similar to open surgery, but long-term results unknown.
Alternative therapy: observation and conventional open surgical approach.

Laparoscopic radical nephrectomy

Occasional
Short-term success rates are similar to open surgery, but long-term results unknown.

Rare
A histological abnormality other than cancer may be found.
Alternative therapy: observation, embolization, chemotherapy, immunotherapy, conventional open surgical approach.

Endoscopic cystitholapaxy and (open) cystolithotomy

Indications

- **Endoscopic cystitholapaxy:** generally indicated for small stones. The definition of 'small' is debatable. Many stones <4 cm in diameter can be removed endoscopically, but the greater the number and size of the stones, the more inclined will the surgeon be to adopt an open approach. Having said this, if you anticipate that the patient is likely to develop recurrent stones, and therefore will require multiple future procedures to remove them, then try to avoid open surgery, because each redo open cystolithotomy will be more difficult (due to the presence of scar tissue)
- **Open cystolithotomy:** for stones >4 cm in diameter and/or multiple stones (though some surgeons will be happy to 'take on' larger stones endoscopically); patients with urethral obstruction which precludes endoscopic access to bladder.

Anaesthesia Regional or general.

Post-operative care

A catheter is left in the bladder for a day or so, since haematuria is common, particularly after fragmentation of large stones. Irrigation may be required if the haematuria is heavy.

Common post-operative complications and their management

Haematuria requiring bladder washout or return to theatre is rare.

Septicaemia: uncommon

Bladder perforation: uncommon, but can occur with the use of stone 'punches' which grab the stone between powerful cutting jaws. Grasping the bladder wall in the jaws of the stone forceps or punch is easily done, and can cause perforation.

BAUS procedure specific consent form: recommended discussion of adverse events

Serious or frequently occurring complications of endoscopic cystitholapxy

Common
- Mild burning or bleeding on passing urine for short periods after operation
- Temporary insertion of a catheter.

Occasional
- Infection of bladder requiring antibiotics
- Permission for removal/biopsy of bladder abnormality if found
- Recurrence of stones or residual stone fragments.

Rare
- Delayed bleeding requiring removal of clots or further surgery
- Injury to urethra causing delayed scar formation.

Very rarely
Perforation of bladder requiring a temporary urinary catheter or return to theatre for open surgical repair.

Alternative therapy: open surgery, observation.

Scrotal exploration for torsion and orchidopexy

Indications Suspected testicular torsion

Technique

A midline incision, since this allows access to both sides so that they may both be 'fixed' within the scrotum. Untwist the testis and place in a warm, saline-soaked swab for 10 min. If it remains black, remove it, having ligated the spermatic cord with a transfixion stitch of absorbable material. If it 'pinks-up', fix it. If uncertain about its viability, make a small cut with the tip of a scalpel. If the testis bleeds actively, it should be salvaged (close the small wound with an absorbable suture). If not, it is dead and should be removed. Whatever you do, fix the other side.

Fixation technique

Some surgeons fix the testis within the scrotum with suture material, inserted at 3 points (3-point fixation). Some use absorbable sutures and others, non-absorbable. Those who use the latter argue that absorbable sutures may disappear, exposing the patient to the risk of retorsion.[1] Those who use absorbable sutures argue that the fibrous reaction around the absorbable sutures prevents retorsion and argue that the patient may be able to feel non-absorbable sutures, which can be uncomfortable. The sutures should pass through the tunica albuginea of the testis, and then through the parietal layer of the tunica vaginalis lining the inner surface of the scrotum.

Others say the testis should be fixed within a dartos pouch,[2] arguing that suture fixation breaches the blood–testis barrier, exposing both testes to the risk of sympathetic orchidopathia (an auto-immune reaction caused by development of antibodies against the testis). For dartos pouch fixation, open the tunica vaginalis, bring the testis out and untwist it. Develop a dartos pouch in the scrotum by holding the skin with forceps and dissecting with scissors between the skin and the underlying dartos muscle. Enlarge this space by inserting your two index fingers and pulling them apart. Place the testis in this pouch. Use a few absorbable sutures to attach the cord near the inside of the dartos pouch to prevent retorsion of the testes. The dartos may then be closed over the testis and the skin can be closed in a separate layer.

Post-operative care and potential complications and their management

As for all procedures involving scrotal exploration, a scrotal haematoma may result, which may have to be surgically drained.

BAUS procedure specific consent form: recommended discussion of adverse events

Serious or frequently occurring complications of scrotal exploration

Common

The testis may have to be removed if non-viable.

Occasional

- You may be able to feel the stitch used to fix the testis
- Blood collection around the testes which slowly resolves or requires surgical removal
- Possible infection of incision or testis requiring further treatment.

Rare

- Loss of testicular size or atrophy in future if testis is saved
- No guarantee of fertility.

Alternative therapy: observation—risks loss of testis and autoimmune reaction leading to subfertility and loss of hormone production in remaining testis.

1 Kuntze JR (1985) Testicular torsion after orchidopexy. *J Urol* **134**:1209–10.

2 Frank JD (2002) Fixation of the testis. *Br J Urol Int* **89**:331–3.

Electromotive drug administration (EMDA)

EMDA is a non-invasive method of enhancing drug penetration across the bladder urothelium (and prostatic urethra) resulting in greater quantities of local drug being delivered to a greater tissue depth than is achievable by passive diffusion alone. It avoids many of the side effects seen with systemic administration.

Mechanism of action

EMDA uses an electric current to accelerate and actively transport ionised molecules into tissues. Drug administration can therefore be controlled by altering the electric current intensity. The two main electrokinetic principles are: *iontophoresis* (transport of ionized molecules into tissue by applying a current across a solution containing the ions e.g. lidocaine) and *electro-osmosis* (transport of non-ionized solutes associated with the bulk transport of water e.g. mitomycin C).

Applications in urology

- Local anaesthesia (LA) of the bladder (and prostatic urethra) prior to other procedures: flexible and rigid cystoscopy with biopsy and cystodiathermy, TURBT, BNI, TUIP, intravesical capsaicin therapy and botulinum toxin-A injections
- Intravesical mitomycin C therapy for transitional cell carcinoma of the bladder
- Intravesical oxybutynin therapy for overactive bladder
- Antibiotic administration (i.e. gentamicin) for infective recalcitrant cystitis
- LA with anti-inflammatory drugs for cystodistention.

Method of EMDA LA

It can be performed as a day-case or outpatient procedure. A CE-DAS® UROGENICS® catheter-electrode* (Fig. 17.16) is inserted urethrally, and the bladder emptied and irrigated with sterile water to remove any residual urine. 150 mL of 0.5% bupivacaine and 1.5 mL (1.5 mg) of 1/1000 epinephrine is instilled into the bladder. Two dispersive electrode pads are placed on the lower abdomen (Fig. 17.17) and both the electrode pads and the catheter are connected to the PHYSIONISER® generator* (Fig. 17.18) set to +ve polarity, 25 mA current strength, a pulsed current with rise rate 50 µA/s for 23 min. The catheter is then removed, and endoscopy can proceed. EMDA LA is effective for 60 min.

Contraindications to EMDA LA

Allergy to LA: significant haematuria; patients on monoamine oxidase inhibitors.

*   Physion Srl, Medolla, Italy.

Relative contraindications

Active infection of lower genito-urinary tract, protrusion of enlarged median lobe of prostate into the bladder, urethral stricture, bladder neck stenosis.

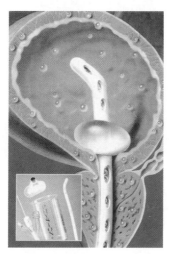

Fig. 17.16 EMDA® in bladder and prostate using catheter-electrode (Reproduced with permission from Physion S.r.l).

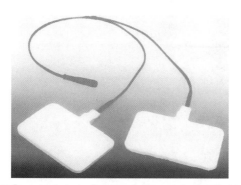

Fig. 17.17 Dispersive electrodes (Reproduced with permission from Physion S.r.l).

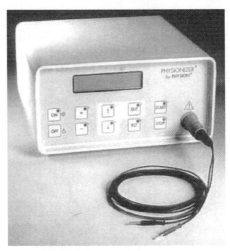

Fig. 17.18 Physionizer® 30 mini generator (Reproduced with permission from Physion S.r.l).

Basic science of relevance to urological practice

Basic physiology of bladder and urethra

Bladder

The bladder consists of an endothelial lining (urothelium) on a connective tissue base (lamina propria), surrounded by smooth muscle (the 'detrusor'), with an outer connective tissue 'adventitia'. The urothelium consists of multi-layered transitional epithelium. It has numerous tight junctions that render it impermeable to water and solutes. The detrusor muscle is a homogeneous mass of smooth muscle bundles. C-kit antigen positive 'interstitial cells' exist around detrusor bundles and in the suburothelium, and may play a role in modulating contractile behaviour of adjacent smooth muscle. The bladder base is known as the trigone—a triangular area with the two ureteric orifices and the internal urinary meatus forming the corners (Fig. 18.1). Intravesical pressure during filling is low. The main excitatory motor input to the bladder is from the autonomic nervous system, and is predominantly parasympathetic innervation (S2–4). Preganglionic nerve fibres are conveyed to the bladder in the pelvic nerves and then synapse with cholinergic postganglionic nerve cells in the pelvic plexus and on the bladder, which when activated cause muscle contraction. Sympathetic innervation (T10–L2) plays a role in urine storage (also 📖 see p. 578).

Urethra

The bladder neck (and posterior urethra) is normally closed during filling. It is composed of a circular smooth muscle (with sympathetic innervation) and is also referred to as the 'internal sphincter'. High pressure is generated at the midpoint of the urethra in women, and at the level of the membranous urethra in men, where the urethral wall is composed of a longitudinal and circular smooth muscle coat, surrounded by striated muscle (external urethral sphincter; Fig. 18.1).

The striated part of the sphincter receives motor innervation from the somatic pudendal nerve derived from (S2–4) in a region in the sacral spinal cord called 'Onuf's nucleus'. It has voluntary control, and ACh mediates contraction. The smooth muscle component of the sphincter has myogenic tone and receives excitatory and inhibitory innervation from the autonomic nervous system. Contraction is enhanced by sympathetic input (noradrenaline) and ACh. Inhibitory innervation is nitrergic (nitric oxide; also see pp. 579–80).

Micturition

As the bladder fills, sensory afferent nerves respond to stretch in bladder wall and send information about bladder filling to the central nervous system (CNS). During urine storage, the **pontine storage centre** mediates enhanced external urethral sphincter activity (so causing constriction of the sphincter). There is also somatic outflow via the pudendal nerve to the external striated sphincter muscle to cause contraction, and sympathetic outflow to constrict the (internal) smooth muscle sphincter (bladder neck) and also inhibit ganglia in the bladder wall. At a socially acceptable time, the voiding reflex is activated (Fig. 18.2). Neurones in the **peri-aqueductal grey (PAG) matter** in the pons trigger a switch to the **pontine micturition centre (PMC)** in the brainstem to activate the voiding reflex. Stimulation of detrusor smooth muscle by parasympathetic cholinergic nerves causes the bladder to contract. Simultaneous activation of nitrergic nerves reduces the intra-urethral pressure. Inhibition of somatic input relaxes the external striated sphincter muscle, and sympathetic inhibition causes coordinated bladder neck smooth muscle (internal sphincter) relaxation, resulting in bladder emptying (also 📖 see pp. 582–3).

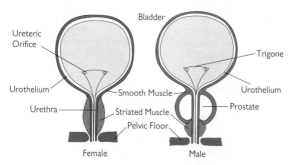

Fig. 18.1 Basic anatomy of bladder and proximal urethra.

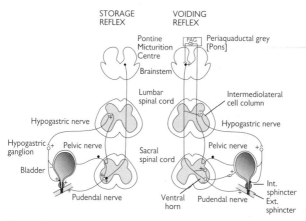

Fig. 18.2 Diagram representing the storage and voiding pathways of the micturition reflex. Micturition is stimulated by activity in the parasympathetic (pelvic) nerves, and inhibited by activity in sympathetic (hypogastric) nerves and pudendal nerves.

Basic renal anatomy

The kidneys and ureters lie within the retroperitoneum (literally behind the peritoneal cavity). The hila of the kidneys lie on the transpyloric plane (vertebral level—L1). Each kidney is composed of a cortex, surrounding the medulla, which forms projections—papillae—that drain into cup-shaped epithelial-lined pouches called calyces (the calyx draining each papilla is known as a minor calyx, and several minor calyces coalesce to form a major calyx, several of which drain into the central renal pelvis) (Fig. 18.3). The renal artery, which arises from the aorta at vertebral level L1/2, branches to form interlobar arteries, which in turn form arcuate arteries, and then cortical radial arteries from which the afferent arterioles are derived. Venous drainage occurs into the renal vein. There are two capillary networks in each kidney—a glomerular capillary network (lying within Bowman's capsule) which drains into a peritubular capillary network, surrounding the tubules (proximal tubule, loop of Henle, distal tubule, and collecting ducts).

Anatomical relations of the kidney

- Anterior relations of the right kidney are, from top to bottom, the adrenal (suprarenal) gland, the liver, and the hepatic flexure of the colon. Medially and anterior to the right renal pelvis is the second part of the duodenum. The anterior relations of the left kidney are, from top to bottom, the adrenal gland, the stomach, the spleen, and the splenic flexure of the colon. Medially lies the tail of the pancreas
- Posterior relations of both kidneys are, superiorly, the diaphragm and lower ribs, and inferiorly (from lateral to medial), transverus abdominis, quadratus lumborum, and psoas major.

The nephron

Each kidney has 1 million functional units or nephrons (Fig. 18.4). These consist of a glomerular capillary network, surrounded by podocytes (epithelial cells) that project into Bowman's capsule, which then drains into a tubular system (proximal convoluted tubule, loop of Henle, distal convoluted tubule, collecting tube, and collecting duct). Blood is delivered to the glomerular capillaries by an afferent arteriole and drained by an efferent arteriole. An ultrafiltrate of plasma is formed within the lumen of Bowman's capsule, driven by Starling forces across the glomerular capillaries. Re-absorption of salt and water occurs in the proximal tubule, loop of Henle, distal tubule, and collecting ducts.

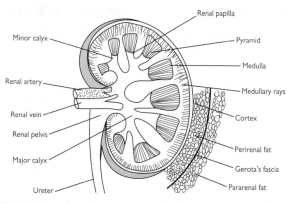

Fig. 18.3 Basic renal anatomy.

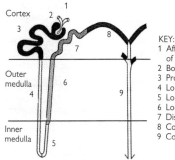

KEY:
1 Afferent and efferent arterioles of the glomerulus
2 Bowman's capsule
3 Proximal convoluted tubule
4 Loop of Henle (thin descending limb)
5 Loop of Henle (thin ascending limb)
6 Loop of Henle (thick ascending limb)
7 Distal convoluted tubule
8 Collecting tubule
9 Collecting duct

Fig. 18.4 The nephron.

Renal physiology: glomerular filtration and regulation of renal blood flow

Renal plasma clearance

Clearance is the volume of plasma that is completely cleared of solute by the kidney per minute. The clearance ratio for a substance indicates the amount of active re-absorption or excretion (i.e. ratio <1 = actively reabsorbed; >1 = actively excreted). Clearance of a substance from the plasma can be expressed mathematically as:

$$\text{Clearance} = \frac{U \times V}{P} \text{ (mL/min)}$$

$$\text{Clearance ratio} = \text{clearance/GFR}$$

where U is the concentration of a given substance in urine, P is its concentration in plasma, and V is the urine flow rate.

Glomerular filtration rate (GFR) also 📖 see p. 40–2

Glomerular filtration is driven by Starling forces: a hydrostatic pressure gradient between capillary and Bowman's capsule, which favours filtration, and colloid oncotic pressure which opposes filtration. **GFR** is the clearance for any substance which is freely filtered, and is neither re-absorbed, secreted, nor metabolized by the kidney. For a substance that is freely filtered at the glomerulus, is neither secreted nor reabsorbed by the renal tubules, and is not metabolized (catabolized), clearance is equivalent to GFR. Where a substance is both filtered at the glomerulus and secreted by the renal tubules, its clearance will be greater than GFR. Where a substance is filtered at the glomerulus, but reabsorbed by the renal tubules, its clearance will be less than GFR.

Clinically, GFR is estimated using creatinine, and is ~125 mL/min. GFR is directly related to renal plasma flow (RPF). Experimentally, GFR can be accurately calculated by measuring the clearance of inulin (a substance which is freely filtered by the glomerulus and is neither secreted nor reabsorbed by the kidneys) using the equation:

$$\text{GFR} = \frac{U \times V}{P} (= 125 \text{ mL/min})$$

Thus, the volume of plasma from which in 1 min the kidneys remove all inulin is equivalent to GFR. Factors affecting the GFR are:

- Rate of blood flow through the glomerulus
- Permeability of glomerular capillary wall (K)
- Surface area of glomerular capillary bed (S)
- Differences in hydrostatic pressure between glomerular capillary lumen (P_{gc}) and Bowmen's space (P_t)
- Differences in oncotic pressure between glomerular capillary (π_{gc}) and Bowman's space (π_t) (although autoregulation of blood flow tends to keep GFR constant despite a varying range of incoming perfusion pressures).

This can be represented by the equation:

$$\text{GFR (single nephron)} = KS([P_{gc} - P_t] - [\pi_{gc} - \pi_t])$$

Normally about one-fifth (120 mL/min) of the plasma that flows through the glomerular capillaries (600 mL/min) is filtered (filtration fraction = GFR/RPF).

Renal blood flow (RBF)

The kidneys represent <0.5% of body weight, but they receive 25% of cardiac output (~1300 mL/min through both kidneys; 650 mL/min per kidney). Combined blood flow in the two renal veins is about 1299 mL/min, and the difference in flow rates represents the urine production rate (i.e. ~1 mL/min).

Autoregulation of RBF

RBF is defined as the pressure difference between the renal artery and renal vein divided by the renal vascular resistance. The glomerular arterioles are the major determinants of vascular resistance. RBF remains essentially constant over a range of perfusion pressures (~80–180 mmHg; i.e. RBF is autoregulated). Autoregulation requires no innervation and probably occurs via:

- **A myogenic mechanism:** increased pressure in the afferent arterioles causes them to contract, thereby preventing a change in RBF
- **Tubuloglomerular feedback:** the flow rate of tubular fluid is sensed at the macula densa of the juxtaglomerular apparatus (JGA), and in some way this controls flow through the glomerulus to which the JGA is opposed

Other factors that influence RBF

Neural mechanisms

Sympathetic nerves innervate the glomerular arterioles. A reduction in circulating volume (such as blood loss) can stimulate sympathetic nerves, causing the release of noradrenaline (NA) (which acts on α1-adrenoceptors on the afferent arteriole) to cause vasoconstriction. This results in reduced RBF and GFR.

Endocrine and paracrine mechanisms:

- Angiotensin II constricts efferent arterioles and afferent arterioles and reduces RBF.
- Antidiuretic hormone (ADH), ATP, and endothelin all cause vasoconstriction and reduce RBF and GFR.
- Nitric oxide causes vasorelaxation and increases RBF.
- Atrial natriuretic peptide (ANP) causes afferent arteriole dilatation and increases RBF and GFR.

Renal physiology: regulation of water balance

Total body water (TBW) is 42 L. It is contained in 2 major compartments—the intracellular fluid (ICF or the water inside cells) which accounts for 28 L and the extracellular fluid (ECF or water outside of cells) representing 14 L. ECF is further divided into interstitial fluid (ISF, 11 L), transcellular fluid (1 L), and plasma (3 L). Hydrostatic and osmotic pressures influence movement between the compartments. Water is taken in from fluids, food and from oxidation of food. Water is lost from urine, faeces, and insensible losses. Intake and losses usually balance (~2 L/day), and TBW remains relatively constant.

Antidiuretic hormone (ADH or vasopressin)

ADH is secreted from the posterior pituitary in response to stimulus from changes in plasma osmolarity (detected by osmoreceptors in the hypothalamus), or changes in blood pressure or volume (detected by baroreceptors in the left atrium, aortic arch, and carotid sinus). These changes also stimulate the thirst centre in the brain.

The action of ADH on the kidney:

- Increases collecting duct permeability to water and urea
- Increases loop of Henle and collecting duct re-absorption of NaCl
- Vasoconstriction.

During conditions of water excess

Body fluids become hypotonic, and ADH release and thirst are suppressed. In the absence of ADH, the collecting duct is impermeable to water and a large volume of hypotonic urine is produced, so restoring normal plasma osmolarity.

During conditions of water deficit

Body fluids are hypertonic, ADH secretion, and thirst are stimulated. The collecting duct becomes permeable, water is re-absorbed into the lumen, and a small volume of hypertonic urine is excreted.

The ability to concentration or dilute urine depends on the counter-current multiplication system in the loop of Henle. Essentially, a medullary concentration gradient is generated (partly by the active transport of NaCl), which provides the osmotic driving force for the re-absorption of water from the lumen of the collecting duct when ADH is present.

Children have a circadian rhythm in ADH secretion-high at night and low during the day. Adults essentially have a constant ADH secretion over a 24-h period, with slight increases occurring around meal times. At these times, increased ADH secretion probably acts to prevent sudden increases in plasma osmolarity that would otherwise occur due to ingestion of solutes in a meal.

Renal physiology: regulation of sodium and potassium excretion

Sodium regulation

NaCl is the main determinant of ECF osmolality[1] and volume. Low-pressure receptors in the pulmonary vasculature and cardiac atria, and high-pressure baroreceptors in the aortic arch and carotid sinus, recognize changes in the circulating volume. Decreased blood volume triggers increased sympathetic nerve activity and stimulates ADH secretion, which results in reduced NaCl excretion. Conversely, when blood volumes are increased, sympathetic activity and ADH secretion are suppressed, and NaCl excretion is enhanced (natriuresis). A variety of natriuretic peptides have been isolated which cause a natriuresis. Under physiological conditions, renal natriuretic peptide (urodilatin) is the most important of these. Atrial natriuretic hormone (ANP), released after atrial distension, may influence sodium output under conditions of heart failure (acting to increase excretion of NaCl and water).

Renin-angiotensin-aldosterone system

Renin is an enzyme made and stored in the juxtaglomerular cells found in the walls of the afferent arteriole. Factors increasing renin secretion are:
- Reduced perfusion of afferent arteriole
- Sympathetic nerve activity
- Reduced Na$^+$ delivery to the macula densa.

Renin acts on angiotensin to create angiotensin I. This is converted to angiotensin II in the lungs by angiotensin converting enzyme (ACE). Angiotensin II performs several functions, which result in the retention of salt and water:
- Stimulates aldosterone secretion (resulting in NaCl re-absorption)
- Vasoconstriction of arterioles.
- Stimulates ADH secretion and thirst
- Enhances NaCl re-absorbtion by the proximal tubule.

Potassium regulation

K$^+$ is critical for many cell functions. A large concentration gradient across cell membranes is maintained by Na$^+$-K$^+$-ATPase pump. Insulin and adrenaline also promotes cellular uptake of K$^+$.

The kidney excretes up to 95% of K$^+$ ingested in the diet. The distal tubule and collecting duct are able to both reabsorb and secrete K$^+$. Factors promoting K$^+$ secretion include:
- Increased dietary K$^+$ (driven by the electrochemical gradient)
- Aldosterone
- Increased rate of flow of tubular fluid
- Metabolic alkalosis (acidosis exerts the opposite effect).

[1] Osmolality = mol/kg water. Osmolarity = mol/L of solution.

Renal physiology: acid-base balance

The normal pH of extracellular fluid (ECF) is 7.4 ($[H^+]$ = 40 nmol/L). Several mechanisms are in place to eliminate acid produced by the body, and maintain body pH within a narrow range.

Buffering systems that limit $[H^+]$ fluctuation in the blood

Buffer bases that take up H^+ ions in the body include:

Bicarbonate buffer system: $H^+ + HCO_3^- \leftrightarrows H_2CO_3 \leftrightarrows H_2O + CO_2$
Phosphate system: $H^+ + HPO_4^{2-} \leftrightarrows H_2PO_4^-$
Protein buffers: $H^+ + Protein^- \leftrightarrows HProtein$

The Henderson–Hasselbalch equation describes the relationship between pH, and the concentration of conjugate acid and base.

$$pH = 6.1 + \log \frac{[HCO_3^-]}{0.03 \, P_{CO2}}$$

From this equation, it can be seen that alterations in bicarbonate $[HCO_3^-]$ or CO_2 will affect pH. Metabolic acid-base disturbances relate to a change in bicarbonate, and respiratory acid-base disorders relate to alterations in CO_2.

Bicarbonate re-absorption along the nephron

Bicarbonate is the main buffer of ECF, and is regulated by both the kidneys and lungs. 85% is reabsorbed in the proximal convoluted tubule. Carbonic acid is first produced from CO_2 and water (accelerated by carbonic anhydrase). The carbonic acid dissociates, and an active ion pump (Na^+/H^+ antiporter) extrudes intracellular H^+ into the tubule lumen in exchange for Na^+. Secretion of H^+ ions favours a shift of the carbonic acid-bicarbonate equilibrium towards carbonic acid, which is rapidly converted into carbon dioxide and water. CO_2 diffuses into the tubular cells down its diffusion gradient and is reformed into carbonic acid by intracellular carbonic anhydrase. The bicarbonate formed by this reaction is exchanged for chloride, and passes into the circulation. Essentially, with each H^+ ion that enters the kidney a bicarbonate ion enters the blood, which bolsters the buffering capacity of the ECF.

The remaining bicarbonate is absorbed in the distal convoluted tubule, where cells actively secrete H^+ into the lumen via an ATP-dependant pump. The distal tubule is the main site that pumps H^+ into the urine to ensure the complete removal of bicarbonate. Once the bicarbonate has gone, phosphate ions and ammonia buffer any remaining H^+ ions.

Abbreviations: H_2O = water; CA = carbonic anhydrase; Cl^- = chloride ion; CO_2 = carbon dioxide; HCO_3^- = bicarbonate; H_2CO_3 = carbonic acid; H^+ = hydrogen ion; HPO_4^{2-} = phosphate ions; $H_2PO_4^-$ = phosphoric acid; Na^+ = sodium ion; P_{CO2} = partial pressure of CO_2.

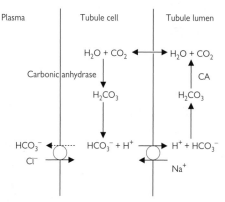

Fig. 18.5 Diagram showing bicarbonate re-absorption in the proximal convoluted tubule.

Urological eponyms

Alcock's canal: canal for the internal pudendal vessels and nerve in the ischiorectal fossa.
Benjamin Alcock (b 1801). Professor of Anatomy, Physiology, and Pathology (1837) at the Apothecaries Hall in Dublin.

Anderson–Hynes pyeloplasty: dismembered pyeloplasty for PUJO.
James Anderson and Wilfred Hynes. Surgeons, Sheffield United Hospitals.

BCG (Bacille Calmette–Guerin): attenuated TB bacillus used for immunotherapy of carcinoma *in situ* of bladder.
Leon Charles Albert Calmette (1863–1933). A pupil of Pasteur in Paris, later becoming first director of the Pasteur Institute.
Camille Guerin (b 1872). A veterinary surgeon at the Calmette Institute in Lille who, along with Calmette, developed BCG vaccine.

Bonney's test: elevation of bladder neck during vaginal examination reduces leakage of urine during coughing (used to diagnose stress incontinence).
William Bonney (1872–1953). Studied at Barts and The Middlesex Hospitals. On the staff of the Royal Masonic Hospital and The Chelsea Hospital for Women. A highly skilled surgeon with an international reputation.

Bowman's capsule: epithelial lined 'cup' surrounding the glomerulus in the kidney.
Sir William Paget Bowman (1816–1892). Surgeon to Birmingham General Hospital. Elected FRS in 1841. FRCS 1844. Won the Royal Medal of the Royal Society for his description of the Malpihgian body of the kidney. He proposed the theory of urine production by filtration of plasma. Described as the father of histology. 1846 became surgeon to Moorfields Eye Hospital. An early proponent of the opthalmoscope and the first in England to treat glaucoma by iridectomy (1862).

Camper's fascia: superficial layer of superficial fascia (fat) of abdomen and inguinal region.
Pieter Camper (1722–1789). Physician and anatomist in Leyden, The Netherlands.

Charrière system: system of measurement for 'sizing' catheters and stents.
Joseph Charrière (1803–1876). Surgical instrument maker in Paris.

Clutton's sounds: metal probes for dilating the urethra (originally used for 'sounding' for bladder stones).
Henry Clutton (1850–1909). Surgeon to St.Thomas's Hospital, London.

Colles fascia: superficial fascia of the perineum.
Abraham Colles (1773–1843). Professor of Anatomy and Surgery in Dublin.

Denonvilliers fascia: rectovesical fascia.
Charles Denonvilliers (1808–1872). Professor of Anatomy, Paris and later Professor of Surgery.

Dormia basket: basket for extracting stones from the ureter.
Enrico Dormia. Assistant Professor of Surgery, Milan.

Douglas, Pouch of: recto-uterine pouch (in females), rectovesical pouch (in males).
James Douglas (1675–1742). Anatomist; physician to the Queen.

Foley catheter: balloon catheter, designed to be self-retaining.

Foley pyeloplasty
Frederic Foley (1891–1966). Urologist, St Paul's, Minnesota.

Fournier's gangrene: fulminating gangrene of external genitalia and lower abdominal wall.
Jean Fournier (1832–1914). Professor of Dermatology, Hôpital St Louis, Paris. Also recognized the association between syphilis and tabes dorsalis.

Gerota's fascia: the renal fascia.
Dumitru Gerota (1867–1939). Professor of Surgery, University of Budapest.

(Loop of) Henle: U-shaped segment of the nephron between the proximal and distal convoluted tubules.
Friedrich Henle (1809–1885). Professor of Anatomy, Zurich and Göttingen.

von Hippel–Lindau syndrome: syndrome of multiple renal cancers
Eugen von Hippel (1867–1939). Opthalmologist in Berlin.
Arvid Lindau (b 1892). Swedish pathologist.

Hunner's ulcer: ulcer in bladder in interstitial cystitis.
Guy Hunner (1868–1957). Professor of Gynaecology, Johns Hopkins.

Jaboulay procedure: operation for hydrocele repair (excision of hydrocele sac).
Mathieu Jaboulay (1860–1913). Professor of Surgery, Lyon.

Klinefelter's syndrome: male hypogonadism with XXY chromosome complement.
Harry Klinefelter (b 1912). Associate Professor of Medicine, Johns Hopkins.

Kockerization of the duodenum: Mobilization of the 2nd part of the duodenum. Used to expose the inferior vena cava and right renal vein during radical nephrectomy.

Emil Kocker (1841–1917). Professor of Surgery, Berne University. A founder of modern surgery. Won the Nobel Prize in 1909 for work on the physiology, pathology, and surgery of the thyroid gland.

Lahey forceps: curved forceps used during surgery.
Frank Lahey (1880–1953). Head of Surgery, Lahey Clinic, Boston.

Langenbeck retractor: commonly used retractor during surgery.
Bernard von Langenbeck (1810–1887). Professor of Surgery, Kiel and Berlin. A great teacher and surgeon.

Leydig cells: interstitial cells of the testis.
Franz von Leydig (1821–1908). Professor of Histology, Würtzburg, Tübingen, Bonn.

Malécot catheter: large bore catheter, used for drainage of kidney following PCNL.
Achille Malécot (b 1852). Surgeon in Paris.

Millin's prostatectomy: retropubic open prostatectomy.
Terence Millin (d 1980). Irish Surgeon, trained in Dublin. Surgeon at the Middlesex and Guy's Hospitals and, later, the Westminster Hospital. Became President of the British Association of Urological Surgeons and then President of the Royal College of Surgeons of Ireland.

Peyronie's disease: fibrosis of shaft of penis causing a bend of the penis during erection.
Francois Peyronie (1678–1747). Surgeon to Louis XV in Paris.

Pfannenstiel incision: suprapubic incision used for surgery to the bladder and uterus.
Hermann Pfannenstiel (1862–1909). Gynaecologist from Breslau.

(Cave of) Retzius: prevesical space.
Andreas Retzius (1796–1860). Professor of Anatomy and Physiology at the Karolinska Institute, Stockholm.

Santorini's plexus: plexus of veins on the ventral surface of the prostate
Giandomenico Santorini (1681–1738). Professor of Anatomy and Medicine in Venice. Wrote a great work on anatomy, *Observationes anatomicae*, published in Venice in 1724.

Scarpa's fascia: deep layer of the superficial fascia of the abdominal wall.
Antonio Scarpa (1747–1832). Professor of Anatomy in Modena and Pavia.

Sertoli cells: supportive cells of testicular epithelium.
Entrico Sertoli (1842–1910). Professor of Experimental Physiology, Milan.

Trendelenburg position: head down operating position.
Friedrich Trendelenburg (1844–1924). Langenbeck's assistant in Berlin, and was then Professor of Surgery at Rostock, Bonn, and then Leipzig.

Weigert's law: inverse position of ectopic ureter (the ureter of the upper moiety of a duplex system) drains distally into the bladder (or below, into the urethra), whereas the lower pole ureter drains into a proximal position in the bladder.
Carl Weigert (1845–1904). German pathologist.

Wilms' tumour: nephroblastoma of kidney.
Max Wilms (1867–1918). Surgical assistant to Trandeleburg in Leipzig and subsequently Professor of Surgery in Leipzig. Later, Professor of Surgery in Basle and Heidelberg.

Young's prostatectomy: perineal prostatectomy.
Hugh Hampton Young (1870–1945). Professor of Urology, John Hopkins School of Medicine.

Index